CLINICAL IMAGING

CLINICAL IMAGING

an atlas of differential diagnosis

by

Ronald L. Eisenberg

Department of Radiology
Louisiana State University School of Medicine
Shreveport, Louisiana

AN ASPEN PUBLICATION®
Aspen Publishers, Inc.

1988

Rockville, Maryland
Royal Tunbridge Wells

Library of Congress Cataloging-in-Publication Data

Eisenberg, Ronald L.
  Clinical imaging.

  Includes index.
  1. Diagnostic imaging—Atlases. 2. Diagnostic
imaging—Handbooks, manuals, etc. 3. Diagnosis,
Differential—Atlases. 4. Diagnosis, Differential—
Handbooks, manuals, etc. I. Title. [DNLM: 1. Diagnosis,
Differential—atlases. 2. Radiography—atlases.
3. Radionuclide Imaging—atlases. 4. Tomography, X-Ray
Computed—atlases. 5. Ultrasonic Diagnosis—atlases.
                                        WN 17 E36c]
  RC78.7.D53E36   1987   616.07′57   87-14498
  ISBN: 0-87189-851-1

The authors have made every effort to ensure the accuracy of the information herein, particularly with regard to drug selection and dose. However, appropriate information sources should be consulted, especially for new or unfamiliar drugs or procedures. It is the responsibility of every practitioner to evaluate the appropriateness of a particular opinion in the context of actual clinical situations and with due consideration to new developments. Authors, editors, and the publisher cannot be held responsible for any typographical or other errors found in this book.

Editorial Services: Lisa J. McCullough

Library of Congress Catalog Card Number: 87-14498
ISBN: 0-87189-851-9

Printed in the United States of America

1   2   3   4   5

Contents

Foreword   *v*

Preface   *vii*

Acknowledgments   *ix*

1   Chest Patterns   1

2   Cardiovascular Patterns   163

3   Gastrointestinal Patterns   229

4   Genitourinary Patterns   439

5   Skeletal Patterns   559

6   Spine Patterns   723

7   Skull Patterns   775

Index   881

Foreword

Ronald Eisenberg has written six monographs in as many years, each fulfilling an important and unique need in radiology. This book is no exception.

Diagnostic radiology requires a wide variety of skills, knowledge, and experience. These include the ability to detect abnormalities on radiographs, to recognize the various diagnostic possibilities for each finding, and to select the best of these as the most likely diagnosis on the basis of the clinical findings for the patient. This book allows the reader to sharpen his or her ability in the second requirement, the differential diagnosis of radiologic findings.

Dr. Eisenberg has accomplished a Herculean task. He has outlined the characteristic radiologic features for each disease of every organ or system of the body according to radiologic patterns, provided illustrations of typical radiographic findings, and supplied succinct pathological and clinical comments. All this is presented in concise tabular fashion, so that the material is readily available for convenient use in daily practice.

More than simple lists of diagnostic possibilities for various radiologic findings are provided, and the book is not just an atlas of images. The book is unique because the major imaging findings for each disease are described and illustrated; all information is organized according to the organ or system and the disease involved and listed according to radiological pattern. It is a logical extension of the popular gamut books because it provides a verbal description of the findings, supplies illustrations, and gives information about each disease mentioned.

Dr. Eisenberg has earned the gratitude of any radiologist who, having identified a radiographic finding, has ever asked himself or herself, "What can cause this?" With this book next to the viewbox, the answers are at hand.

Robert N. Berk, MD
Editor-in-Chief
American Journal of Roentgenology

Preface

Pattern recognition leading to the development of differential diagnoses is the essence of radiology. Both the practicing radiologist faced with the reality of daily film reading and the senior resident taking the oral board examination are usually unaware of the underlying disease when they are presented with a specific finding for which they must suggest a differential diagnosis and a rational diagnostic approach. This book offers differential diagnoses for a broad spectrum of radiographic patterns, not only in conventional radiography but also in ultrasound and computed tomography. Added to these lists of differential possibilities are descriptions of the specific imaging findings to be expected for each diagnostic entity as well as differential points to aid the reader in arriving at a precise diagnosis. A wealth of illustrations is provided to point out the often subtle differences in appearance among conditions that can produce a similar overall radiographic pattern. Extensive cross referencing is provided to limit duplication and to permit the reader to find various radiographic manifestations of the same condition.

I must stress that this book in no way intends to supplant the current excellent textbooks in general radiology and imaging subspecialties. Rather, it is designed to complement these works by providing a handy reference for practicing radiologists and residents faced with the daily challenge of interpreting radiographic examinations.

Acknowledgments

I would like to express my thanks to Betty DiGrazia for the many hours she spent in the arduous task of typing and retyping the manuscript. I greatly appreciate the efforts of James Kendrick of George Washington University and the Medical Communications Department of Louisiana State University School of Medicine in Shreveport for skillfully photographing the many illustrations. Thanks also go to the many physicians who have graciously permitted me to use radiographs from their published and unpublished cases as well as to the radiology residents at LSU who continuously had eagle eyes trained to find appropriate case material. Finally, I acknowledge the unceasing encouragement and support of Anne Patterson, Editorial Director, and the entire staff at Aspen Publishers who have made the immense technical problems of preparing a book as painless as possible.

CLINICAL IMAGING

Chest Patterns

1

C1	Localized alveolar pattern	**4**
C2	Pulmonary edema pattern (symmetric bilateral alveolar pattern)	**18**
C3	Diffuse reticular or reticulonodular pattern	**26**
C4	Honeycombing	**36**
C5	Solitary pulmonary nodules	**40**
C6	Multiple pulmonary nodules	**48**
C7	Miliary nodules	**52**
C8	Cavitary lesions of the lungs	**56**
C9	Unilateral hilar enlargement	**62**
C10	Bilateral hilar enlargement	**64**
C11	Hilar and mediastinal lymph node enlargement	**66**
C12	Unilateral, lobar, or localized hyperlucency of the lung	**70**
C13	Bilateral hyperlucent lungs	**76**
C14	Lobar enlargement (bulging interlobar fissure)	**78**
C15	Lobar or segmental collapse	**80**
C16	Pulmonary parenchymal calcification	**86**
C17	Pulmonary disease with eosinophilia	**90**
C18	Skin disorder combined with widespread lung disease	**94**
C19	Meniscus (air-crescent sign)	**98**
C20	Anterior mediastinal lesions	**100**
C20A	Anterior mediastinal lesions on computed tomography	**104**
C21	Middle mediastinal lesions	**108**
C21A	Middle mediastinal lesions on computed tomography	**112**
C22	Posterior mediastinal lesions	**114**
C22A	Posterior mediastinal lesions on computed tomography	**118**
C23	Shift of the mediastinum	**122**
C24	Pneumomediastinum	**126**
C25	Pleural-based lesion	**128**
C26	Extrapleural lesion	**132**
C27	Pleural calcification	**134**
C28	Pleural effusion with otherwise normal-appearing chest	**136**
C29	Pleural effusion associated with other radiographic evidence of chest disease	**140**
C30	Chylothorax	**144**
C31	Pneumothorax	**146**
C32	Tracheal mass/narrowing	**150**
C33	Upper airway obstruction in children	**154**
C34	Elevated diaphragm	**158**
Sources		**160**

LOCALIZED ALVEOLAR PATTERN

Condition	Imaging Findings	Comments
Bacterial pneumonia *Staphylococcus* (Fig C1-1)	Rapid development of extensive alveolar infiltrates, usually involving a whole lobe or even several lobes. Air bronchograms are infrequent since the acute inflammatory exudate fills the airways, leading to segmental collapse and a loss of volume.	Most frequently occurs in children, especially during the first year of life. In adults, usually affects hospitalized patients with lowered resistance or as a complication of a viral respiratory infection. A characteristic finding in childhood disease is the development of pneumatoceles, thin-walled cystic spaces in the parenchyma that typically disappear spontaneously within several weeks. Pleural effusion (or empyema) often occurs.
Streptococcus (see Fig C14-3)	Indistinguishable from staphylococcal pneumonia. Homogeneous or patchy consolidation in a segmental distribution with a lower lobe predominance and often some loss of volume.	Uncommon condition that usually follows viral infections such as measles, pertussis, and epidemic influenza. Unlike staphylococcal infection, streptococcal pneumonia rarely causes the development of pneumatoceles. Early and rapid accumulation of empyema fluid was a characteristic feature before the advent of antibiotics.
Pneumococcus (Fig C1-2)	Homogeneous consolidation that almost invariably abuts against a visceral pleural surface and almost always contains an air bronchogram.	Most commonly occurs in alcoholics and other compromised hosts. Cavitation and pleural reaction are rare. In children, may produce the so-called round or spherical pneumonia, in which a well-circumscribed spherical consolidation on both frontal and lateral views simulates a pulmonary or mediastinal mass (Fig C1-3).
Klebsiella (Fig C1-4)	Homogeneous parenchymal consolidation containing air bronchograms (simulates pneumococcal pneumonia). Primarily involves the right upper lobe. Typically induces a large inflammatory exudate, causing increased volume of the affected lobe and characteristic bulging of an adjacent interlobar fissure (see Fig C14-1).	Most commonly develops in alcoholics and in elderly patients with chronic pulmonary disease. Unlike acute pneumococcal pneumonia, *Klebsiella* pneumonia causes frequent and rapid cavitation and there is a much greater incidence of pleural effusion and empyema.
Other enteric gram-negative bacteria (Fig C1-5)	Nonspecific, often inhomogeneous pattern of consolidation that most commonly affects the lower lobes. Cavitation is relatively common and pleural effusion may occur.	*Escherichia coli, Serratia marcescens, Enterobacteriaceae, Proteus, Pseudomonas aeruginosa, Salmonella,* and *Brucella.* Most commonly develop in debilitated or immunocompromised patients.
Hemophilus influenzae (Fig C1-6)	Nonspecific patchy pulmonary infiltrate that is often bilateral. May be unilateral lobar or segmental consolidation, simulating pneumococcal disease. Typically extensive pleural involvement that often appears out of proportion to the associated parenchymal infiltrate.	Serious infections primarily affect children under the age of 4 and older patients who have undergone antibiotic therapy or who suffer from diseases that increase their general susceptibility to infection. This organism is the leading cause of epiglottitis (see Fig C33-2), the second leading cause of childhood otitis media, and a common cause of childhood bacterial meningitis.
Hemophilus pertussis (whooping cough) (Fig C1-7)	Various combinations of atelectasis, segmental pneumonia, and hilar lymph node enlargement. Coalescence of air-space consolidation contiguous to the heart produces a typical "shaggy heart" contour.	Although often considered to have been largely eradicated by immunization, immunity is apparently not lifelong, and pertussis has become a not uncommon cause of bronchitis in adults. Acute infection most frequently affects nonimmunized children under 2 years of age.

(continued page 6)

A

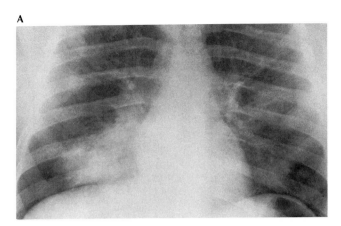

B

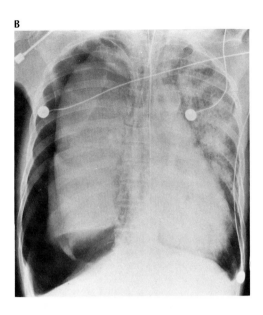

Fig C1-1. **Staphylococcal pneumonia.** (A) Ill-defined broncho-pneumonia at the right base. (B) In another patient there is consolidation in the left upper lobe and entire right lung with a moderate right pneumothorax. The extensive consolidation presents further collapse of the right lung. The pneumothorax was due to the rupture of a pneumatocele, although no pneumatocele can be identified on this film.

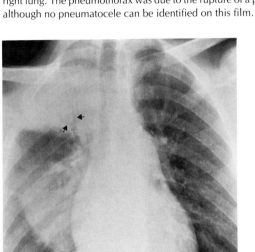

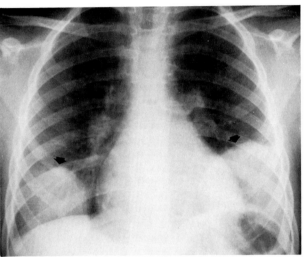

Fig C1-2. **Pneumococcal pneumonia.** Homogeneous consolidation of the right upper lobe and the medial and posterior segments of the right lower lobe. Note the associated air bronchograms (arrows).

Fig C1-3. **"Spherical" pneumonia.** Frontal view of the chest shows a rounded soft-tissue density in the posteriolateral aspects of both lower lobes (arrows) with mild bilateral hilar prominence.[1]

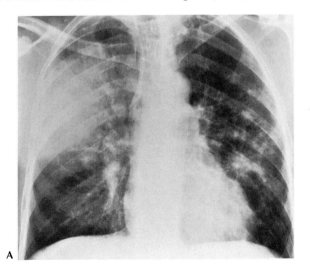

A

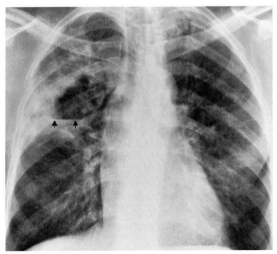

B

Fig C1-4. *Klebsiella* **pneumonia.** (A) Air-space consolidation involving much of the right upper lobe. (B) Progression of the necrotizing infection produces a large abscess cavity with an air-fluid level (arrows).

Condition	Imaging Findings	Comments
Tularemia (see Fig C11-2)	Patchy consolidations that may be bilateral, multilobar, or both. Ipsilateral hilar adenopathy and pleural effusion occur in about half the cases.	Pneumonia represents hematogenous spread or inhalation of *Francisella tularensis,* which is usually transmitted to humans from infected animals (rodents, small mammals) or insect vectors.
Yersinia pestis (see Figs C2-13 and C11-3)	Patchy segmental infiltration or dense lobar consolidation simulating pneumococcal pneumonia. Typically there is enlargement of hilar and paratracheal lymph nodes and, often, pleural effusion.	The pneumonic type of plague causes severe pulmonary consolidation, necrosis, and hemorrhage and is usually fatal. This organism is still widespread among wild rodents.
Anthrax	Patchy parenchymal infiltrates that are usually associated with pleural effusion and mediastinal widening (lymph node enlargement and hemorrhagic mediastinitis).	Bacterial disease of cattle, sheep, and goats that primarily affects humans who inhale spores from infected animals or their products (eg, wool, hides).
Legionnaires' disease (Fig C1-8)	Patchy or fluffy alveolar infiltrate that rapidly progresses to involve adjacent lobes and the contralateral side.	Acute gram-negative bacterial pneumonia that occurs in local outbreaks or as sporadic cases and may cause a fulminant, often fatal, pneumonia. Small pleural effusions are common, while cavitation and hilar adenopathy are unusual. Most patients respond well to erythromycin, though the radiographic resolution often lags behind the clinical response.
Bacteroides (Fig C1-9)	Patchy or confluent consolidation that is generally confined to the lower lobes. Cavitation and empyema are common.	Gram-negative anaerobic bacteria that are commonly found normally in the gastrointestinal and genital tracts. Pneumonia develops from aspiration of infected material or septic infarctions resulting from emboli arising in veins in the peritonsilar area or pelvis.
Fungal pneumonia **Histoplasmosis** (Fig C1-10)	In the primary form, single or multiple areas of consolidation that are most often in the lower lung and associated with hilar lymph node enlargement.	Striking hilar adenopathy, which may cause bronchial compression, may develop without radiographic evidence of parenchymal disease. Although the findings simulate primary tuberculosis, pleural effusion rarely occurs with histoplasmosis.
Blastomycosis (Fig C1-11)	Nonspecific patchy areas of air-space consolidation.	Cavitation and miliary nodules infrequently occur. Blastomycosis may appear as a solitary pulmonary mass that, when associated with unilateral lymph node enlargement, may mimic a bronchogenic carcinoma.
Coccidioidomycosis (Fig C1-12)	Pulmonary involvement usually begins as a fleeting area of patchy pneumonia that is often accompanied by ipsilateral hilar adenopathy and, less frequently, by pleural effusion.	Thin-walled cavities without surrounding reaction are suggestive of this organism (see Fig C8-5).
Cryptococcosis (**torulosis**) (Fig C1-13)	Segmental or lobar consolidation that most commonly occurs in the lower lobes.	More commonly produces a single, fairly well-circumscribed mass that is usually in the periphery of the lung and is often pleural-based. Cavitation is relatively uncommon compared with its frequency in the other mycoses.
Actinomycosis/ nocardiosis (Figs C1-14 and C1-15)	Nonsegmental air-space consolidation (may resemble pneumonia or a tumor mass). Cavitation and empyema are common if not appropriately treated.	Extension of the infection into the pleura produces an empyema, which classically leads to osteomyelitis of the ribs and the formation of a sinus tract.

(continued page 8)

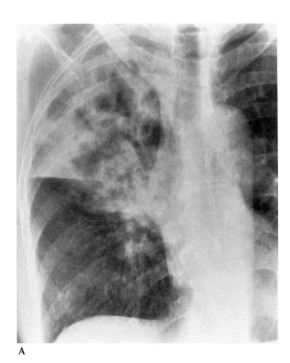

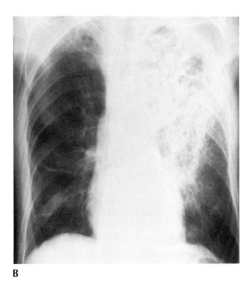

B

A

FIG C1-5. **Enteric gram-negative bacteria.** (A) *Proteus.* (B) *Pseudomonas.*[2]

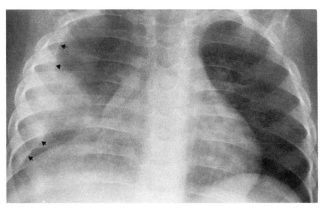

FIG C1-6. *Hemophilus influenzae* **pneumonia.** In addition to the ill-defined right lower lung consolidation, note the extensive pleural thickening or fibrinous exudate (arrows) that appears out of proportion to the associated parenchymal infiltrate.[3]

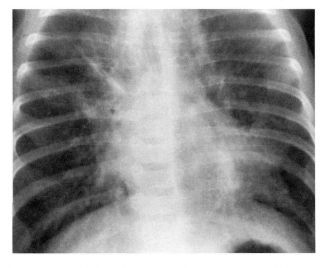

FIG C1-7. *Hemophilus pertussis.* Bilateral central parenchymal infiltrates and linear areas of atelectasis obscure the normally sharp cardiac borders to produce the shaggy heart contour.

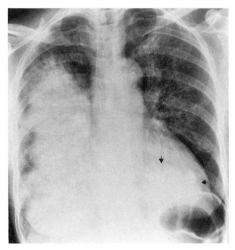

FIG C1-8. **Legionnaire's disease.** There is extensive consolidation of much of the right lung, with a smaller area of infiltrate (arrows) at the left base.

Condition	Imaging Findings	Comments
Candidiasis	Patchy, segmental, homogeneous air-space consolidation.	Reflects hematogenous dissemination. Cavitation and hilar adenopathy may occur.
Aspergillosis (see Fig C19-1)	Single or multiple areas of consolidation with poorly defined margins.	Almost always a secondary infection in which the fungus colonizes a damaged bronchial tree, pulmonary cyst, or cavity of a patient with underlying lung disease. The radiographic hallmark is a pulmonary mycetoma, a solid homogeneous rounded mass separated from the wall of the cavity by a crescent-shaped air space.
Mucormycosis (see Fig C8-7)	Progressive severe pneumonia that is widespread and confluent and often cavitates.	Occurs in patients with diabetes or an underlying malignancy (leukemia, lymphoma). Usually originates in the nose and paranasal sinuses, where the infection may destroy the walls and create an appearance that simulates a malignant neoplasm (see Fig SK17-5).
Sporotrichosis (see Fig C8-6)	Various nonspecific patterns (fibronodular infiltrates, cavitary nodular masses, chronic pneumonia). Hilar lymph node enlargement is common and may cause bronchial obstruction. Spread through the pleura into the chest wall may produce a sinus tract.	Chronic infection that is usually limited to the skin and the draining lymphatics. In rare instances, disseminated disease can involve the lungs and the skeletal system (extensive destructive arthritis with large-joint effusions).
Mycoplasma/viral infection (Figs C1-16 and C1-17)	Patchy air-space consolidation that is usually segmental and predominantly involves the lower lobes. Bilateral and multilobar involvement are common.	Initially, acute interstitial inflammation appears as a fine or coarse reticular pattern. Most infections are mild, though the radiographic signs are more extensive than might be expected from the physical examination.
Mononucleosis	Nonspecific patchy air-space consolidation.	Generalized lymphadenopathy and splenomegaly are characteristic findings. Hilar lymph node enlargement, usually bilateral, can be demonstrated in about 15% of cases (see Fig C10-1). Pneumonia is a rare complication.
Varicella	Extensive bilateral fluffy nodular infiltrate that tends to coalesce near the hilum and lung bases.	Healed varicella pneumonia classically appears as tiny miliary calcifications (see Fig C16-4), scattered widely throughout both lungs, which develop several years after the acute infection.
Cytomegalovirus	In adults, rapid development of diffuse bilateral alveolar infiltrates that are most common in the outer third of the lungs.	Primarily involves patients with underlying reticuloendothelial disease or immunologic deficiencies, or those receiving immunosuppressive therapy (especially after renal transplantation). May be radiographically indistinguishable from *Pneumocystis carinii* pneumonia.

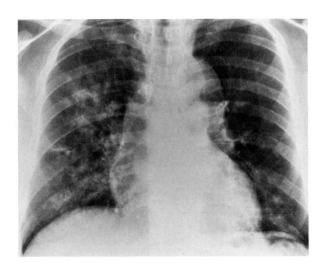

FIG C1-9. *Bacteroides* **pneumonia.** Patchy areas of consolidation primarily involve the middle and lower portions of the right lung.

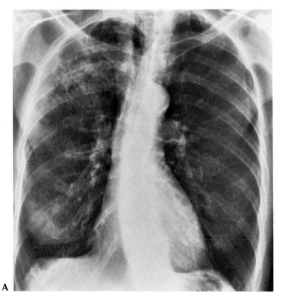

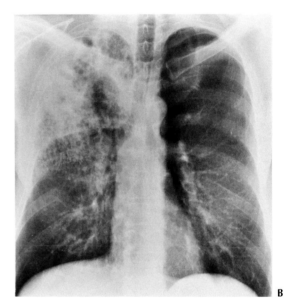

FIG C1-10. **Histoplasmosis.** (A) Initial film demonstrates an ill-defined area of parenchymal consolidation in the right upper lobe. (B) One week later there is a marked extension of the infiltrate, which now involves most of the upper half of the right lung.

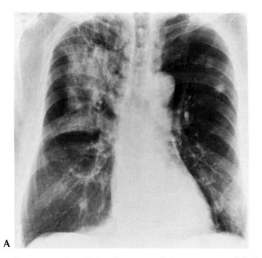

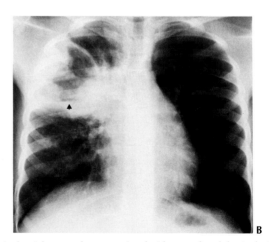

FIG C1-11. **Blastomycosis.** (A) Patchy areas of air-space consolidation in the right upper lung associated with several nodules in the left upper lung. (B) In another patient there is development of a right upper lobe cavity with thick walls and a faintly visible air-fluid level (arrow). There is an associated soft-tissue mass along the lateral wall of the cavity.[4]

Condition	Imaging Findings	Comments
Rickettsial infection (Fig C1-18)	Dense, homogeneous, segmental, or lobar consolidation simulating pneumococcal disease. Predominantly affects the lower lobes and may be bilateral.	Pneumonia develops in about half the patients with Q fever. Pleural effusion occurs in about one third of the cases, while hilar involvement and small focal lesions are rare.
Parasitic pneumonia *Pneumocystis carinii* (Fig C1-19; see Figs C2-14 and C3-19)	Initially, a hazy, perihilar granular infiltrate that spreads to the periphery and appears predominantly interstitial. In later stages, patchy areas of air-space consolidation with air bronchograms. Massive consolidation with virtually airless lungs may be a terminal appearance.	Common organism in immunosuppressed patients (especially those treated for lymphoproliferative diseases or those with renal transplants). Hilar adenopathy and significant pleural effusions are rare and should suggest an alternative diagnosis. Because the organism cannot be cultured and the disease it causes is usually fatal if untreated, an open-lung biopsy is often necessary if a sputum examination reveals no organisms in a patient suspected of having this disease.
Amebiasis	Air-space consolidation in the right lower lobe that may be obscured by an extensive pleural effusion.	Usually arises from direct extension of hepatic infection through the right hemidiaphragm (occasionally may be of hematogenous origin).
Toxoplasmosis	Combined interstitial and alveolar disease, often with hilar lymph node enlargement.	Especially virulent organism in immunocompromised patients. Central nervous system involvement is common and may lead to a brain abscess.
Ascariasis (see Fig C17-4)	Patchy or extensive areas of consolidation that are often bilateral.	Reflects an allergic response caused by larvae migrating through the lungs.
Cutaneous larva migrans (creeping eruption) (see Fig C17-7)	Transient, migratory pulmonary infiltrates associated with lung and blood eosinophilia.	Pulmonary involvement develops in about half the patients about 1 week after the skin eruption caused by penetration and migration of the larvae of the dog and cat hookworm (*Ancylostoma braziliense*).
Strongyloidiasis (see Fig C17-5)	Ill-defined patchy areas of air-space consolidation or fine miliary nodules.	Pulmonary manifestations occur during the stage of larval migration (in most patients the chest radiograph remains normal).
Paragonamiasis (see Figs C6-3 and C8-9)	Patchy air-space consolidation that primarily involves the bases of the lungs. Characteristic finding is the "ring shadow," composed of a thin-walled cyst with a prominent crescent-shaped opacity along one side of its border.	Chronic infection of the lung caused by a trematode that is acquired by eating raw, or poorly cooked, infected crabs or crayfish. Although many patients with a heavy infestation are asymptomatic, others present with cough, pain, hemoptysis, and brownish sputum.
Tuberculosis **Primary** (Fig C1-20)	In primary disease, a lobar or segmental air-space consolidation that is usually homogeneous, dense, and well defined. Associated enlargement of the hilar or mediastinal lymph nodes is very common (see Figs C9-1 and C9-2). Pleural effusion often occurs, especially in adults (see Fig C28-1).	Primary tuberculosis may affect any lobe. The diagnosis cannot be excluded because the infection is not in the upper lobe. Although traditionally considered a disease of children and young adults, with the dramatic decrease in the prevalence of tuberculosis (especially in children and young adults), primary pulmonary disease can develop at any age.

(continued page 12)

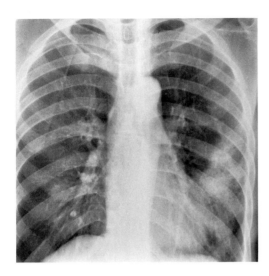

FIG C1-12. Coccidioidomycosis pneumonia. Ill-defined area of patchy infiltrate in the left lower lung.

A

B

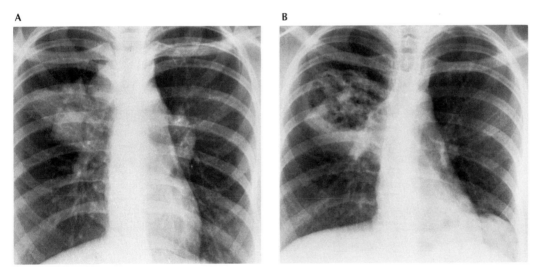

FIG C1-13. Cryptococcosis. (A) Initial film demonstrates an air-space consolidation in the right upper lung. (B) With progression of the infection, the right upper lung pneumonia has cavitated (arrows) and a left lower lobe air-space consolidation (arrows) has developed.

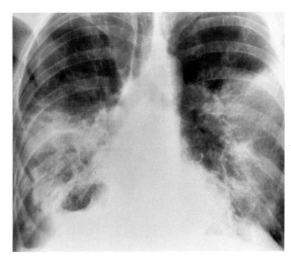

FIG C1-14. Actinomycosis. Bilateral, nonsegmental air-space consolidation.

Condition	Imaging Findings	Comments
Secondary (reactivation)	Initially a nonspecific hazy, poorly margined alveolar infiltrate that most commonly affects the upper lobes, especially the apical and posterior segments. Cavitation is common (see Fig C8-3) and may result in bronchogenic spread characterized by multiple patchy infiltrates.	Bilateral (though often asymmetric) upper lobe disease is common and is almost diagnostic of reactivation tuberculosis. Because an apical lesion may be obscured by overlying clavicle or ribs, an apical lordotic view is often of value. Pleural effusion and lymph node enlargement are rare in secondary disease.
Atypical mycobacteria (see Fig C8-4)	Often radiographically indistinguishable from primary tuberculosis, though pleural effusion and hilar adenopathy are much less common.	Often produces thin-walled cavities with minimal surrounding parenchymal disease. Patients with an atypical mycobacterial infection have a negative tuberculin test and do not respond to antituberculous therapy.
Postobstructive pneumonitis (Fig C1-21)	Homogeneous increase in density corresponding exactly to a lobe or one or more segments, usually with a substantial loss of volume.	With slowly progressive, obstructive endobronchial processes such as bronchogenic carcinoma and bronchial adenoma, infection is frequent so that there may be only slight or moderate loss of volume. Pneumonitis, bronchiectasis, and abscesses that develop behind the obstruction are usually sufficient to counteract, at least partly, collapse induced by air absorption. The characteristic radiographic picture of "obstructive pneumonitis" should immediately suggest the presence of an obstructing endobronchial lesion. Non-neoplastic causes include mucoid impaction (hypersensitivity aspergillosis), aspirated foreign bodies, and the tracheobronchial form of amyloidosis.
Pulmonary infarct (Fig C1-22)	Area of consolidation that most commonly involves the lower lobes and is often associated with pleural effusion and elevation of the ipsilateral hemidiaphragm. A highly characteristic, though uncommon, appearance is a pleural-based, wedge-shaped density that has a rounded apex (Hampton hump) and often occurs in the costophrenic sulcus. In many instances, an infarction produces a nonspecific parenchymal density that simulates an acute pneumonia.	Although it is often said that infarction invariably extends to a visceral pleural surface, this is of little diagnostic value since most pneumonias have a similar appearance. The pattern of resolution of the consolidation is of value in distinguishing among acute inflammatory processes, pulmonary hemorrhage, edema, and frank necrosis. Pulmonary infarctions tend to shrink gradually while retaining the same general configuration seen on initial views (resorption of the perimeter of the infarct with preservation of the pleural base). In contrast, the resolution of pneumonia tends to be patchy and is characterized by a fading of the radiographic density throughout the entire involved area. Parenchymal hemorrhage and edema generally clear within 4 to 7 days; the resolution of necrotic lung tissue usually requires 3 weeks or more.
Pulmonary contusion (see Figs C5-14 and C26-2)	Varies from irregular patchy areas of air-space consolidation to an extensive homogeneous density involving almost an entire lung.	Most common pulmonary complication of blunt chest trauma in which there is exudation of edema and blood into both the air spaces and the interstitium of the lung. In the absence of an appropriate clinical history of trauma or evidence of rib fractures, pulmonary contusion may be indistinguishable from pneumonia. Resolution typically occurs rapidly, with complete clearing within 2 weeks.

A

B

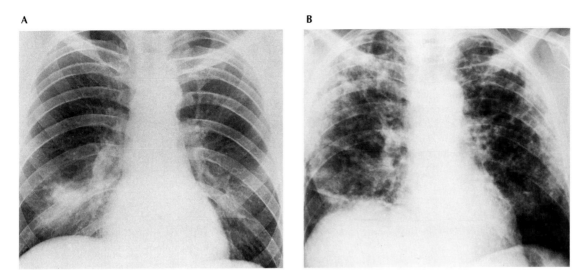

Fig C1-15. Nocardiosis. (A) Initial chest radiograph demonstrates an area of nonspecific alveolar infiltrate in the right lower lobe. (B) Without appropriate therapy, infection spreads to involve both lungs diffusely with a patchy infiltrate and multiple small cavities.

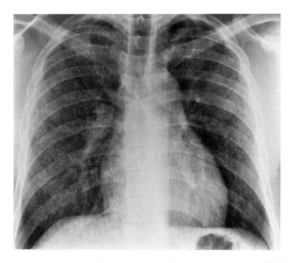

Fig C1-16. Mycoplasma pneumonia. Initial acute interstitial inflammation produces a diffuse fine reticular pattern.

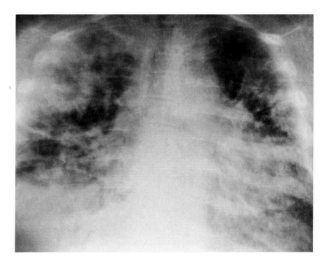

Fig C1-17. Viral pneumonia. Diffuse peribronchial infiltrate with associated air-space consolidation obscures the heart border (shaggy heart sign). A patchy alveolar infiltrate is present in the right upper lung.

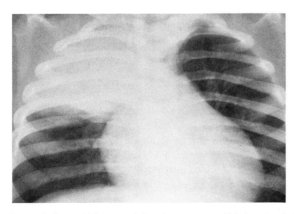

Fig C1-18. Q fever. Right upper lobe air-space consolidation simulating pneumococcal pneumonia.

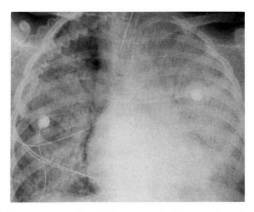

Fig C1-19. *Pneumocystis carinii* pneumonia. Severe, bilateral air-space consolidation with air bronchograms. The patient was undergoing immunosuppressive therapy for lymphoma and died shortly after this radiograph was made.

Condition	Imaging Findings	Comments
Lipoid pneumonia (**Fig C1-23**)	Granular pattern of small, scattered alveolar densities that predominantly occur in the perihilar and lower lobe areas.	Caused by the aspiration of various vegetable, animal, or mineral oils into the lungs. As the oil is taken from the alveolar spaces by macrophages that pass into the interstitial space, a fine reticular pattern is produced. Infrequently appears as a granulomatous-lipoid mass that may be huge and may simulate bronchogenic carcinoma (see Fig C5-15).
Lung torsion	Opacification of the affected lung develops if the torsion is not relieved and the vascular supply is compromised.	Rare complication of trauma that occurs almost invariably in children, presumably because of the easy compressibility of their thoracic cage. Torsion occurs through 180°, so that the base of the lung comes to lie at the apex of the hemithorax and the apex at the base. The pulmonary opacification is due to exudation of blood into the air spaces and interstitial tissues.
Localized pulmonary edema (**Fig C1-24**)	Nonsymmetric, atypical alveolar consolidation.	Most commonly occurs in patients with pre-existing lung disease such as chronic emphysema. Unilateral pulmonary edema is most frequently related to dependency.
Bronchioloalveolar (alveolar cell) carcinoma (**Fig C1-25**)	In the less common diffuse form, a pattern varying from poorly defined nodules scattered throughout both lungs to irregular pulmonary infiltrates, often with air bronchograms.	More frequently appears as a well-circumscribed, peripheral solitary nodule that often contains an air bronchogram (see Fig C5-13) (never associated with solitary nodule caused by bronchogenic carcinoma or a granuloma). Although the margins of the tumor are usually well circumscribed, the mass may be poorly defined and simulate an area of focal pneumonia.
Lymphoma	Patchy areas of parenchymal infiltrate that may coalesce to form a large homogeneous nonsegmental mass. Cavitation and pleural effusion may occur.	Pleuropulmonary involvement usually occurs by direct extension from mediastinal nodes along the lymphatics of the bronchovascular sheaths. At times, it may be difficult to distinguish a superimposed infection following radiation therapy or chemotherapy from the continued spread of lymphomatous tissue. However, any alveolar lung infiltrate in a patient with known lymphoma is more likely to represent an infectious than a lymphomatous process. Primary pulmonary lymphoma is rare and presents as a homogeneous mass that rarely obstructs the bronchial tree and thus almost invariably contains an air bronchogram. When most or all of a segment or lobe is involved, the appearance may simulate acute pneumonia.
Pseudolymphoma	Segmental consolidation extending outward from a hilum and containing an air bronchogram.	Rare benign condition that histologically closely resembles malignant lymphoma. Although apparently segmental, in most cases the consolidation stops short of the visceral pleura at the periphery of the lung.

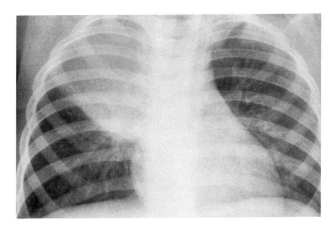

Fɪɢ C1-20. Primary tuberculosis. Consolidation of the right upper lobe.

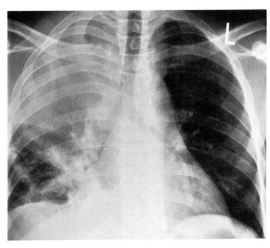

Fɪɢ C1-21. Postobstructive pneumonitis. Homogeneous increased density involving the right upper lobe secondary to carcinoma of the lung. Patchy increased opacification at the right base is due to a combination of atelectasis and infiltrate secondary to extension of the tumor into neighboring bronchi.

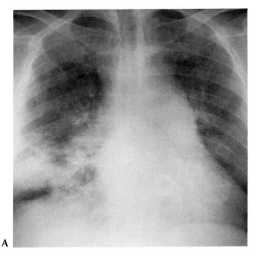

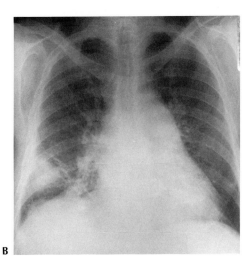

A   B

Fɪɢ C1-22. Pulmonary infarction. (A) Chest film made 3 days after open-heart surgery demonstrates a very irregular opacity at the right base (pneumonia versus pulmonary embolization with infarction). (B) On a film made 5 days later, the consolidation is seen to have reduced in size yet to have retained the same general configuration as on the initial view. The diagnosis of pulmonary embolism was confirmed by a radionuclide lung scan.[5]

A   B

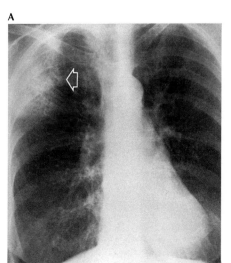

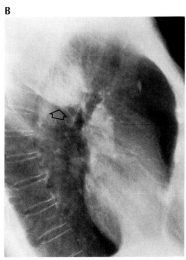

Fɪɢ C1-23. Lipoid pneumonia. (A) Frontal and (B) lateral views demonstrate an air space consolidation in the posterior segment of the right upper lobe (arrows). Note the prominence of interstitial reticular markings leading from the right hilum to the infiltrate.

Condition	Imaging Findings	Comments
Loeffler's syndrome (idiopathic eosinophilic pneumonia) (see Fig C17-1)	Transient, rapidly changing, nonsegmental areas of parenchymal consolidation associated with blood eosinophilia. The infiltrates are often located in the periphery of the lung, running more or less parallel to the lateral chest wall and simulating a pleural process.	A similar appearance can develop secondary to parasites (filariasis, ascariasis, cutaneous larva migrans), drug therapy (nitrofurantoin), and fungal infections (hypersensitivity bronchopulmonary aspergillosis). When caused by an identifiable extrinsic agent, the disease usually is acute and responds promptly to the removal of the offending organism or drug. When no obvious cause is detectable, the pulmonary consolidation and eosinophilia tend to be more prolonged and persistent, though there is usually a dramatic response to steroids.
Radiation pneumonitis (Fig C1-26)	Patchy areas of irregular consolidation that are localized to the radiation port and are often associated with a considerable loss of volume.	Acute radiation pneumonitis is rarely detectable less than 1 month after the end of treatment and must be differentiated from bacterial pneumonia. The late or chronic stage of radiation damage is characterized by extensive fibrosis and loss of volume that may be difficult to distinguish from the lymphangitic spread of a malignant tumor.
Sarcoidosis (see Fig C2-17)	Ill-defined densities that may be discrete or may coalesce into large areas of segmental consolidation. This pattern resembles an acute inflammatory process and may contain an air bronchogram.	Infrequent manifestation. More characteristic radiographic changes are a diffuse reticulonodular pattern and typical bilateral enlargement of hilar and paratracheal lymph nodes (see Figs C10-6 and C11-8).
Progressive massive fibrosis (pneumoconiosis) (see Figs C6-9 and C6-10)	Nonsegmental conglomerate masses that are usually bilateral and relatively symmetric and almost always restricted to the upper half of the lungs. They commonly develop in the mid-zone or periphery of the lung and tend to migrate later toward the hilum, leaving overinflated and emphysematous lung tissue between the consolidation and the pleural surface.	Caused by the confluence of numerous individual nodules in patients with advanced silicosis or coal-miner's pneumoconiosis. The conglomerate fibrotic lesions may cavitate as a result of central ischemic necrosis or tuberculous caseation.
Asbestosis/talcosis	In patients with extensive interstitial fibrosis, large conglomerate opacities may develop that are well or ill defined, are often multiple and nonsegmental, and predominantly involve the lower lung (in contrast to the upper lobe predominance of the conglomerate opacities in silicosis).	Pleural plaque formation, which may be massive and bizarre in shape, is characteristic of both conditions (see Figs C27-4 and C27-5). In asbestosis there is often thin, curvilinear calcification of the diaphragmatic pleura, obscuration of the heart border (shaggy heart sign), and a high incidence of associated malignancy (bronchogenic carcinoma, mesothelioma).
Systemic lupus erythematosus	Nonspecific patchy infiltrate that is more commonly situated peripherally in the lung bases.	Often associated with bilateral pleural effusions and cardiac enlargement due to pericardial effusion (see Fig C28-4).

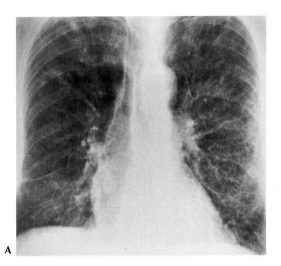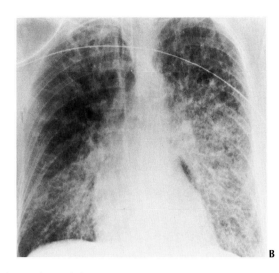

FIG C1-24. Congestive heart failure in pulmonary emphysema. (A) Initial chest radiograph demonstrates a paucity of vascular markings in the right middle and upper zones along with increased interstitial markings elsewhere. (B) With the onset of congestive heart failure, there is patchy interstitial and alveolar edema that does not affect the segments in which the vascularity had been severely diminished.

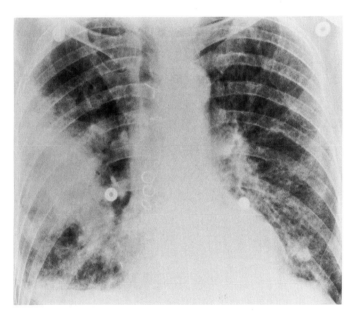

FIG C1-25. Alveolar cell carcinoma. Patchy, ill-defined right-sided mass simulates an area of focal pneumonia.

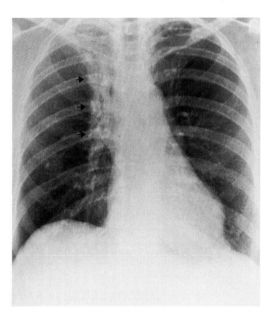

FIG C1-26. Radiation pneumonitis. After postmastectomy radiation, a mass of fibrous tissue (arrows) extends from the right hilum to parallel the right border of the mediastinum.

PULMONARY EDEMA PATTERN
(SYMMETRIC BILATERAL ALVEOLAR PATTERN)

Condition	Comments
Cardiovascular disease causing pulmonary venous hypertension **(Figs C2-1 and C2-2)**	Most common cause of the pulmonary edema pattern. Usually associated with cardiomegaly (especially if the result of left ventricular failure); other cardiogenic causes include mitral valvular disease, left atrial myxoma, and the hypoplastic left heart syndromes. Noncardiogenic causes include disorders of the pulmonary veins (primary or secondary to mediastinal fibrosis or tumor), veno-occlusive disease, and anomalous pulmonary venous return. Unilateral pulmonary edema is probably most frequently related to dependency (Fig C2-2). A patchy, asymmetric pattern may develop in patients with emphysema.
Renal failure/uremia **(Fig C2-3)**	Causes include acute glomerulonephritis and chronic renal disease. Complex mechanism (left ventricular failure, decreased oncotic pressure, hypervolemia, increased capillary permeability). May produce a dense ''butterfly'' pattern.
Fluid overload/ overtransfusion (hypervolemia, hypoproteinemia) **(Fig C2-4)**	A common cause of the pattern, particularly during the postoperative period and in elderly patients. Rapid clearing with appropriate treatment. The pulmonary edema pattern may also be the result of an incompatible blood transfusion.
Neurogenic/postictal	An often asymmetric pattern of pulmonary edema may develop after head trauma, seizures, or stroke. Related to increased intracranial pressure (typically disappears within several days following surgical relief). Normal heart size (if no underlying cardiac disease).
Inhalation of noxious gases **(Fig C2-5)**	Transient pulmonary edema pattern that develops within a few hours of exposure and clears within a few days (if not fatal). Causes include the inhalation of nitrogen dioxide (silo-filler's disease), sulfur dioxide, phosgene, chlorine, carbon monoxide, and hydrocarbon compounds.
Aspiration of gastric contents (Mendelson's syndrome)	Often an asymmetric pattern of pulmonary edema (depends on the position of the patient when aspiration occurred). Caused by vomiting related to anesthesia, seizure, or coma (alcohol or barbiturate poisoning, cerebrovascular accident). Grave prognosis unless immediate steroid and antibiotic therapy (then resolves in 7 to 10 days).

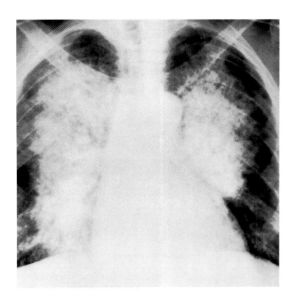

FIG C2-1. Congestive heart failure. Diffuse bilateral symmetric infiltration of the central portion of the lungs along with relative sparing of the periphery produces the butterfly, or bat's wing, pattern. The margins of the edematous lung are sharply defined. The consolidation is fairly homogeneous and is associated with a well-defined air bronchogram on both sides.[6]

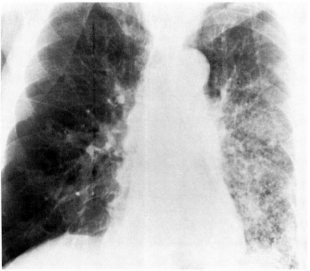

FIG C2-2. Unilateral pulmonary edema due to dependency. Diffuse alveolar pattern is limited to the left lung.

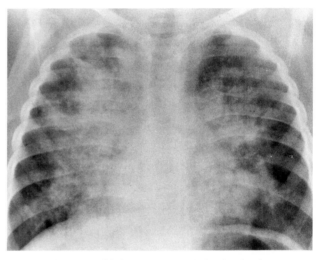

FIG C2-3. Chronic renal failure. Typical perihilar alveolar densities producing the butterfly pattern of uremic lung. Unlike pulmonary edema due to congestive heart failure, in chronic renal failure the cardiac silhouette is normal in size.

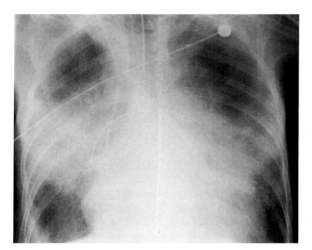

FIG C2-4. Fluid overload. Pulmonary edema pattern developing in the postoperative period in an elderly patient. Note the endotracheal tube and pulmonary artery catheter.

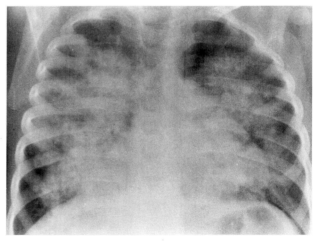

FIG C2-5. Hydrocarbon poisoning. Diffuse pulmonary edema pattern, with the alveolar consolidation most prominent in the central portions of the lung.

Condition	Comments
Near-drowning (Fig C2-6)	No radiographic difference between fresh and salt water aspiration. Complete resolution, usually in 7 to 10 days.
Aspiration of hypertonic contrast material	High osmotic force causes massive influx of fluid into the alveolar air spaces.
High altitude	Pulmonary edema pattern (often irregular and patchy) is a manifestation of mountain or altitude sickness. Rapid clearing after oxygen administration or return to sea level.
Transient tachypnea of newborn	Loss of definition of prominent vascular markings due to retained fetal lung fluid that clears rapidly in 1 to 4 days. Normal heart size. Predisposing factors include cesarean section, prematurity, breech delivery, and maternal diabetes.
Rapid re-expansion of lungs (post-thoracentesis)	Unilateral pulmonary edema pattern (unless both lungs re-expanded) that follows the rapid removal of large amounts of air or fluid from the pleural space.
Fat embolism (Fig C2-7)	Develops 1 to 2 days after trauma (usually leg fractures). The radiographic resolution requires 7 days or longer. Absence of cardiomegaly, pulmonary venous hypertension, and interstitial edema differentiates this condition from cardiogenic edema.
Amniotic fluid embolism (Fig C2-8)	Diffuse air-space consolidation that is virtually indistinguishable from the appearance caused by other forms of acute pulmonary edema. The entrance of amniotic fluid containing particulate matter into the maternal circulation during spontaneous delivery or cesarean section can cause sudden and massive obstruction of the pulmonary vascular bed, leading to shock and often death. Because the condition is often rapidly fatal, radiographs are infrequently obtained; most of the rare nonfatal cases are incorrectly diagnosed.
Thoracic trauma (contused lung) (Fig C2-9)	Alveolar edema pattern due to contusion or hemorrhage is the most common pulmonary complication of blunt chest trauma. The appearance is seldom symmetric (involvement is greater on the side of maximum impact). Unlike traumatic fat embolism, the radiographic changes of pulmonary contusion and hemorrhage are apparent soon after trauma and resolve rapidly (usually in 1 to 7 days).

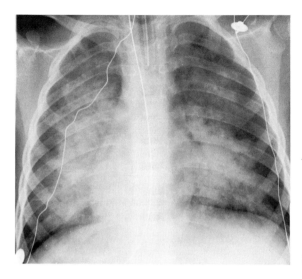

Fɪɢ C2-6. **Near-drowning.** Diffuse pulmonary edema pattern.

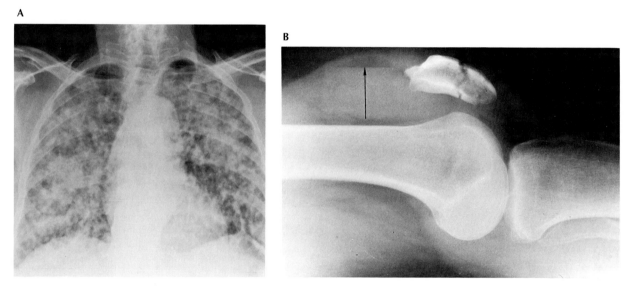

Fɪɢ C2-7. **Fat embolism.** (A) Frontal chest radiograph made 3 days after a leg fracture demonstrates diffuse bilateral air-space consolidation due to alveolar hemorrhage and edema. Unlike cardiogenic pulmonary edema, the distribution in this patient is predominantly peripheral rather than central and the heart is not enlarged. (B) Recumbent radiograph of the knee obtained with a horizontal beam demonstrates the characteristic fat-blood interface (arrow) in a large suprapatellar effusion. Marrow fat that enters torn peripheral vessels can be trapped by the pulmonary circulation and lead to diffuse alveolar consolidation.[7]

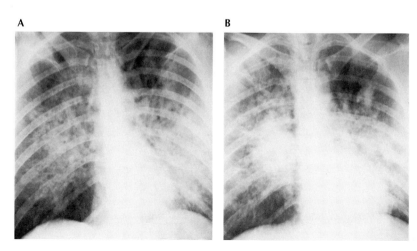

Fɪɢ C2-8. **Amniotic fluid embolism.** (A) Initial film 6 hours after the onset of acute symptoms, showing heavy bilateral perihilar infiltrate. (B) Twelve hours later, the infiltrates have become more confluent in the perihilar zones.[8]

Condition	Comments
Nontraumatic pulmonary hemorrhage (Figs C2-10 and C2-11)	Bilateral alveolar consolidation that may occur in patients with bleeding diatheses, idiopathic pulmonary hemosiderosis, Goodpasture's syndrome, polyarteritis nodosa, or Wegener's granulomatosis. There is usually clearing 2 to 3 days after a single bleeding episode, though reticular changes may persist much longer.
Acute radiation pneumonitis	Alveolar edema pattern is generally confined to the irradiated area. Rarely develops while the patient is receiving radiation therapy (radiographic changes are seldom apparent until at least 1 month after the end of treatment).
Narcotic abuse	Alveolar pulmonary edema pattern that may be unilateral due to gravitational influences. Most commonly a complication of heroin or methadone abuse. The radiographic findings may be delayed 6 to 10 hours after admission and there is usually rapid resolution (1 to 2 days). The persistence of an edema pattern after 48 hours suggests aspiration or superimposed bacterial pneumonia.
Adult respiratory distress syndrome (ARDS) or "shock lung" (Fig C2-12)	Bilateral pulmonary edema pattern that is typically delayed up to 12 hours after the clinical onset of respiratory failure. Severe, unexpected, life-threatening acute respiratory distress developing in a patient with no major underlying lung disease. Causes include sepsis, oxygen toxicity, disseminated intravascular coagulation, and cardiopulmonary bypass.
Pneumonia (Figs C2-13 and C2-14)	Bilateral alveolar infiltrates may develop after a broad spectrum of infections. The underlying organisms include bacteria, fungi, mycoplasma, viruses, malaria, and even worm infestation (almost invariably blood eosinophilia). In patients with acquired immune deficiency syndrome, a butterfly pattern sparing the periphery of the lung is highly suggestive of *Pneumocystis carinii* pneumonia.
Neoplasm	Symmetric bilateral alveolar infiltrates, usually associated with reticulonodular and linear densities, may develop in patients with alveolar cell carcinoma or lymphangitic metastases. Patients with lymphoma and leukemia may also develop bilateral alveolar infiltrates that predominantly involve the perihilar areas and lower lungs, though these findings are more often due to superimposed pneumonia, drug reaction, or hemorrhage than to the underlying malignancy itself.

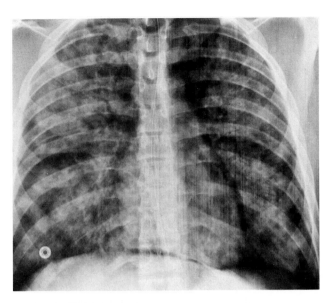

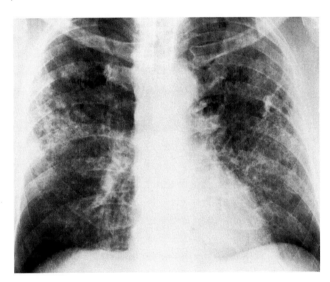

FIG C2-9. Thoracic trauma. Continuous positive-pressure ventilation has caused diffuse interstitial emphysema, pneumothorax, and pneumoperitoneum to be superimposed on a pattern of diffuse alveolar opacities.

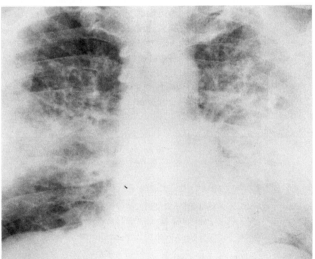

FIG C2-10. Pulmonary hemorrhage. (Left) Diffuse bilateral air-space consolidation developed in a patient receiving high-dose anticoagulant therapy. (Right) With resolution of the hemorrhage, a reticular pattern is seen in the same distribution as the alveolar infiltrate.

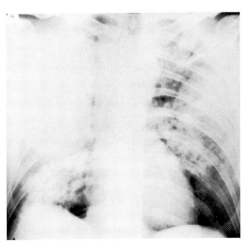

FIG C2-11. Goodpasture's syndrome. Frontal chest film in a patient with massive pulmonary hemorrhage demonstrates extensive bilateral pulmonary consolidation, which is confluent in most areas. Note the normal heart size.[6]

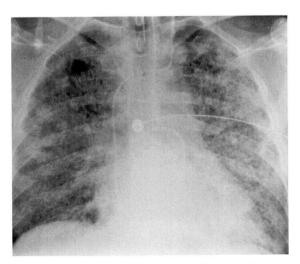

FIG C2-12. Acute respiratory distress syndrome. Ill-defined areas of alveolar consolidation with some coalescence scattered throughout both lungs.

Condition	Comments
Alveolar microlithiasis **(Fig C2-15)**	Rare disease of unknown etiology characterized by the presence of a myriad of very fine micronodules of calcific density in the alveoli of the lungs of a usually asymptomatic person. Characteristic ''black pleura'' sign (due to contrast between the extreme density of the lung parenchyma on one side of the pleura and the ribs on the other side).
Alveolar proteinosis **(Fig C2-16)**	Rare condition of unknown etiology characterized by the deposition in the air spaces of the lung of a somewhat granular material high in protein and lipid content. The bilateral and symmetric alveolar infiltrates are identical in distribution and character to those of pulmonary edema, though there is no evidence of cardiac enlargement or pulmonary venous hypertension. There is usually complete radiographic resolution, though it may occur asymmetrically and in a spotty fashion and may even be associated with the development of new foci of air-space consolidation in areas not previously affected.
Sarcoidosis **(Fig C2-17)**	Infrequent manifestation (more commonly a diffuse reticulonodular pattern). Hilar and mediastinal lymph nodes are often enlarged.
Drug hypersensitivity/ **allergy (penicillin)**	Rapid development of an alveolar edema pattern.
Pulmonary embolism with **infarction**	Bilateral alveolar consolidation, primarily involving the lower zones, is a rare manifestation of extensive thromboembolism with infarction. Associated findings include enlarged central pulmonary arteries with rapid tapering, loss of lung volume (elevated hemidiaphragms), small pleural effusions, and a prominent azygos vein. The radiographic appearance is usually rather benign, considering the severity of the clinical symptoms.

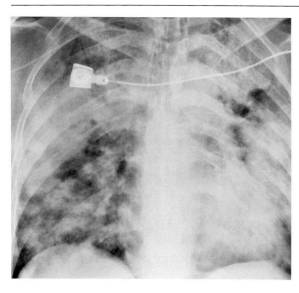

FIG C2-13. Plague pneumonia. Diffuse air-space consolidation involves both lungs.

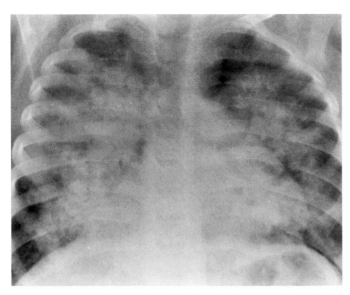

FIG C2-14. *Pneumocystis carinii* pneumonia in acquired immune deficiency syndrome. Diffuse bilateral pulmonary infiltrates.

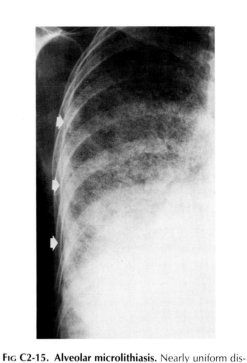

FIG C2-15. **Alveolar microlithiasis.** Nearly uniform distribution of typical fine, sandlike mottling in the lungs. The tangential shadow of the pleura is displayed along the lateral wall of the chest as a dark lucent strip (arrows).[9]

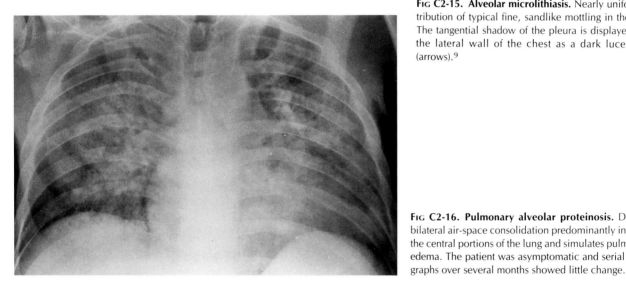

FIG C2-16. **Pulmonary alveolar proteinosis.** Diffuse, bilateral air-space consolidation predominantly involves the central portions of the lung and simulates pulmonary edema. The patient was asymptomatic and serial radiographs over several months showed little change.

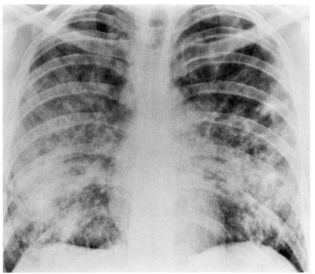

FIG C2-17. **Sarcoidosis.** Diffuse reticular nodular and alveolar infiltrates.

DIFFUSE RETICULAR OR RETICULONODULAR PATTERN

Condition	Comments
Lymphangitic metastases **(Fig C3-1)**	More prominent in the lower lung zones and often associated with pleural effusion and enlargement of hilar or mediastinal lymph nodes. Most frequent primary tumor sites are the breast, stomach, thyroid, pancreas, larynx, cervix, and lung.
Lymphoma **(Fig C3-2)**	Usually associated with hilar and mediastinal lymph node enlargement in Hodgkin's disease (often absent in non-Hodgkin's lymphoma). A similar pattern may occur in the terminal stages of leukemia.

Inorganic dust inhalation
(pneumoconiosis)
  Silicosis
  (Fig C3-3)
	Often more prominent in the middle and upper lung zones. Frequent enlargement of hilar lymph nodes (''eggshell'' calcification is infrequent but almost pathognomonic). Other radiographic patterns include well-circumscribed nodular opacities and progressive massive fibrosis. In Caplan's syndrome, silicosis is associated with rheumatoid arthritis and rheumatoid necrobiotic nodules (see Fig C6-7).

Asbestosis **(Fig C3-4)**	In the early stages, more prominent in the lower lung zones. The major radiographic abnormalities are pleural thickening, plaque formation, and calcification. A combination of parenchymal and pleural changes may partially obscure the heart border (shaggy heart sign). High incidence of mesothelioma (also bronchogenic and alveolar cell carcinoma).
Other inorganic dusts **(Figs C3-5 and C3-6)**	Numerous conditions such as talcosis, berylliosis, coal-worker's pneumoconiosis, aluminum (bauxite) pneumoconiosis, and radiopaque dust causing dense nodules (siderosis [iron], stannosis [tin], baritosis [barium], antimony, and rare-earth compounds).
Organic dust inhalation **(Fig C3-7 and C3-8)**	Late stage in such conditions as farmer's lung, bird-fancier's lung, silo-filler's disease (nitrogen dioxide), bagassosis (sugarcane), byssinosis (cotton), and mushroom-worker's lung.
Oxygen toxicity **(Fig C3-9)**	Most commonly develops in infants undergoing long-term oxygen therapy for respiratory distress (has also been described in adults). Fibrosis, atelectasis, and focal areas of emphysema produce a ''spongy'' lung.

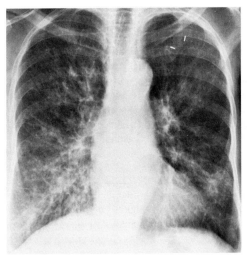

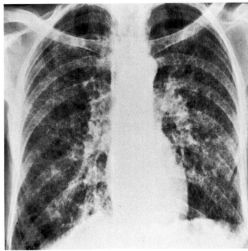

Fig C3-1. Lymphangitic metastases. (A) Coarsened bronchovascular markings of irregular contour and poor definition primarily involve the right lower lung. Note the septal (Kerley) lines and the left mastectomy in this patient with carcinoma of the breast. (B) In this patient with metastatic carcinoma of the stomach, a superimposed nodular component representing hematogenous deposits produces a coarse reticulonodular pattern.

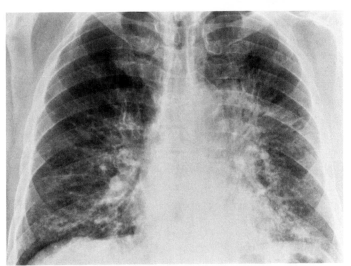

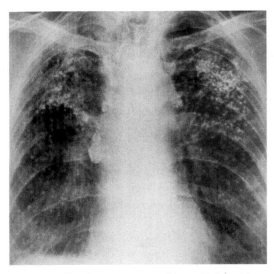

Fig C3-2. Lymphoma. Diffuse reticular and reticulonodular changes, with striking prominence of the left hilar region.

Fig C3-3. Silicosis. Prominence of interstitial markings, upward retraction of the hila, and bilateral calcific densities that tend to conglomerate in the upper lobes.

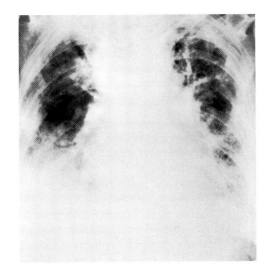

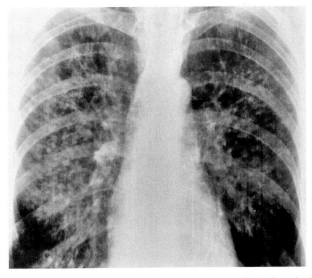

Fig C3-4. Asbestosis. Severe disorganization of lung architecture with generalized coarse reticulation, which has become confluent in the right base and obliterates the right hemidiaphragm. There is marked pleural thickening, particularly in the apical and axillary regions. A spontaneous pneumothorax is on the left.[6]

Fig C3-5. Berylliosis. Diffuse reticulonodular pattern throughout both lungs, with relative sparing of the apices and bases.

Condition	Comments
Drug-induced pulmonary disease (**Figs C3-10 and C3-11**)	Allergic reaction to the drug with associated eosinophilia (nitrofurantoin) or a toxic effect of a chemotherapeutic agent (busulfan, bleomycin, methotrexate).
Connective tissue disorders	
Scleroderma (**see Fig C4-5**)	More prominent in the lung bases. Extrapulmonary findings include abnormal peristalsis of the esophagus and small bowel, erosion of the terminal tufts, and calcification in the fingertips.
Dermatomyositis/ polymyositis	More prominent in the lung bases. May have a co-existing primary malignancy elsewhere.
Rheumatoid disease (**Fig C3-12**)	More prominent in the lung bases. Usually associated with evidence of rheumatoid arthritis.
Systemic lupus erythematosus	More prominent in the lung bases. Often has a coexisting pleural effusion.
Sjögren's syndrome	More prominent in the lung bases. Triad of keratoconjunctivitis sicca, xerostomia, and recurrent swelling of the parotid gland. Strong predominance in females. Changes in the joints resemble those of rheumatoid or psoriatic arthritis.
Chronic bronchitis (**Fig C3-13**)	Coarse increase in interstitial markings (''dirty chest'') that is often associated with emphysema and signs of pulmonary arterial hypertension.
''Small airways disease''	Inflammatory narrowing, mucous plugging, and fibrous obliteration of small airways of the lungs.
Acute bronchiolitis	More prominent in the lower lung zones and associated with severe overinflation of the lungs. Generally affects young children (under 3 years) and adults with pre-existing chronic respiratory disease. Bronchiolitis obliterans is the end stage of lower respiratory tract damage due to a variety of diseases.
Interstitial pulmonary edema (**Fig C3-14**)	Loss of the normal sharp definition of pulmonary vascular markings (especially in the lower lung zones), perihilar haze, and thickening of the interlobular septa (Kerley-B lines). Also cardiomegaly and often redistribution of pulmonary blood flow from the lower to the upper lobes. Recurrent episodes of interstitial and alveolar edema and hemorrhage in patients with chronic left heart failure may result in the development of a coarse, often poorly defined reticular pattern that predominantly involves the middle and lower lung zones.

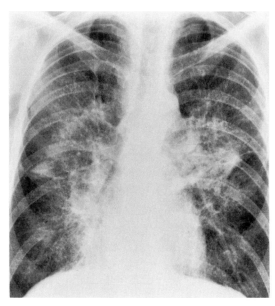

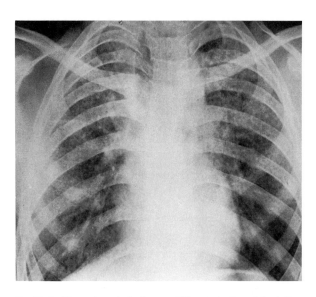

FIG C3-6. Coal-worker's pneumoconiosis. Ill-defined masses of fibrous tissue in the perihilar region extend to the right base.

FIG C3-7. Pigeon-breeder's disease. Diffuse reticulonodular infiltrate primarily involves the perihilar and upper lobe regions.

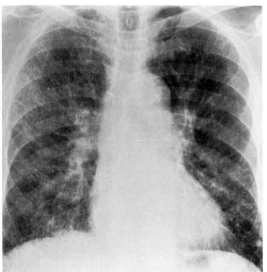

FIG C3-8. Byssinosis. Prolonged exposure has resulted in irreversible pulmonary insufficiency and a diffuse reticular pattern.

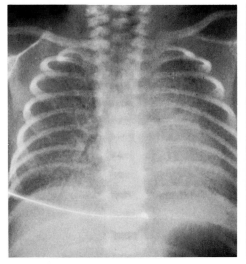

A

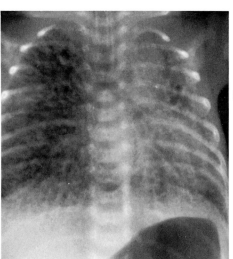

B

FIG C3-9. Oxygen toxicity. (A) Initial chest radiograph of an infant demonstrates a typical granular parenchymal pattern with air bronchograms due to hyaline membrane disease. (B) After intensive oxygen therapy, multiple small round lucencies resembling bullae have developed, giving the lungs a spongelike appearance.

Condition	Comments
Infectious agents	
Tuberculosis (Fig C3-15)	Localized or generalized prominence of interstitial structures reflects the healing phase in which tuberculous granulation tissue is replaced by fibrosis. The resulting scarring may result in considerable loss of volume.
Fungal infections (Fig C3-16)	Localized or generalized prominence of interstitial structures may develop secondary to coccidioidomycosis, cryptococcosis, blastomycosis, and histoplasmosis.
Viral pneumonia (Fig C3-17)	Generalized prominence of bronchovascular markings that may be a manifestation of various viral agents.
Mycoplasma (Fig C3-18)	More prominent in the lower lung zones. This appearance is less common than the localized form, in which a fine reticular infiltrate progresses rapidly to consolidation.
Pneumocystis carinii (Fig C3-19)	More prominent in the perihilar areas. This pattern occurs in the early stage of the disease and is followed by patchy consolidations simulating pulmonary edema.
Schistosomiasis	Probably produced by migration of ova through vessel walls with subsequent reaction to these foreign bodies. Vascular obstruction may cause pulmonary hypertension (dilatation of central pulmonary arteries with rapid peripheral tapering).
Filariasis (see Fig C17-6)	Tropical pulmonary eosinophilia. Patients with pulmonary disease usually do not have the characteristic cutaneous and lymphatic changes as in elephantiasis.
Toxoplasmosis	Early stage of the disease. Hilar lymph node enlargement is common.
Sarcoidosis (Figs C3-20 and C3-21)	Frequently associated with hilar and mediastinal lymph node enlargement, which often regresses spontaneously as the parenchymal disease develops.
Histiocytosis X (eosinophilic granuloma) (Fig C3-22)	More prominent in the upper lung zones. Most common cause of the coarse ''honeycomb'' pattern. Spontaneous pneumothorax is a frequent complication. About one third of patients are asymptomatic when initially diagnosed on a screening chest radiograph.
Cystic fibrosis (Fig C3-23)	Coarse reticular pattern with overinflation of the lungs. Often segmental areas of consolidation or atelectasis due to pneumonia or bronchiectasis. Pulmonary fibrosis along the cardiac border may produce the shaggy heart appearance.

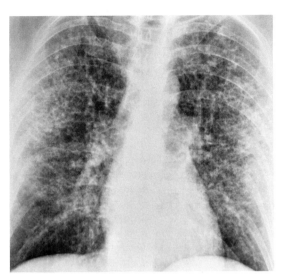

FIG C3-10. Bulsulfan-induced lung disease. Severe coarse reticular pattern.

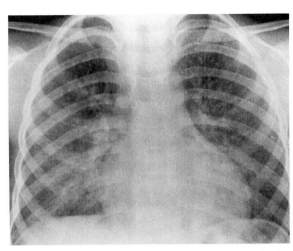

FIG C3-11. Methotrexate-induced lung disease. Diffuse interstitial pattern with patches of alveolar consolidation in a child treated for myelogenous leukemia. After methotrexate therapy ended there was rapid clinical and radiographic improvement.[10]

A

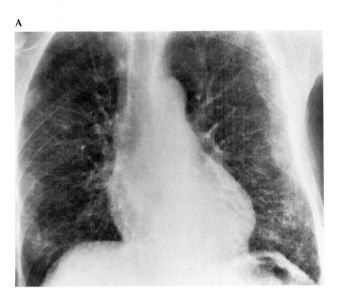

B

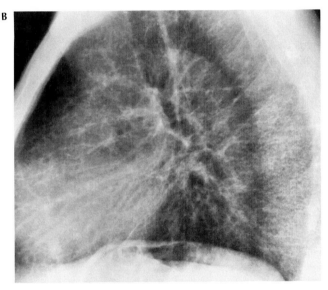

FIG C3-12. Rheumatoid lung. (A) Frontal and (B) lateral views of the chest show diffuse thickening of the interstitial structures with prominent pleural thickening.

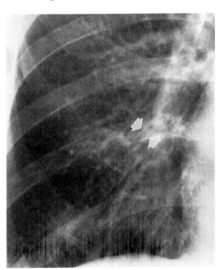

FIG C3-13. Chronic bronchitis. Coned view of the right lower lung demonstrates a coarse increase in interstitial markings. The arrows point to the characteristic parallel line shadows ("tramlines") outside the boundary of the pulmonary hilum.

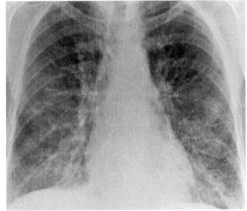

FIG C3-14. Interstitial pulmonary edema. Edema fluid in the interstitial space causes a loss of the normal sharp definition of pulmonary vascular markings and a perihilar haze. At the bases, note the thin horizontal lines of increased density (Kerley-B lines) that represent fluid in the interlobular septa.

Condition	Comments
Familial dysautonomia (Riley-Day syndrome) (Fig C3-24)	Appearance identical to that of cystic fibrosis. Often associated with patchy areas of pneumonia and atelectasis. An autosomal recessive condition, found almost exclusively in Jews, which causes widespread neurologic abnormalities.
"Usual" interstitial pneumonia (UIP) (interstitial fibrosis) (Fig C3-25)	In the early stages, more prominent in the lower lung zones. Progressive volume loss on sequential studies.
Desquamative interstitial pneumonia (DIP) (Fig C3-26)	More prominent in the lower lung zones. Progressive loss of lung volume on sequential studies. Spontaneous pneumothorax and pleural effusion may occur.
Idiopathic pulmonary hemosiderosis/ Goodpasture's syndrome	Often more prominent in the perihilar areas and the middle and lower lung zones. Initially represents a transition stage from acute air-space hemorrhage to complete resolution. Persistence of the reticular pattern after several bleeding episodes indicates irreversible interstitial fibrosis. Repeated pulmonary hemorrhage results in anemia and pulmonary insufficiency (also renal disease in Goodpasture's syndrome).
Amyloidosis (Fig C3-27)	More prominent in the lower lung zones. Hilar and mediastinal lymph nodes may be markedly enlarged (occasionally densely calcified).
Waldenström's macroglobulinemia	Rare lymphoproliferative disorder in which there is usually hepatosplenomegaly and palpable peripheral adenopathy.
Tuberous sclerosis	Diffuse interstitial fibrosis pattern with honeycombing that is more prominent in the lower lung zones. Chylous pleural effusion and pneumothorax are common. Sclerotic (occasionally lytic) bone lesions may occur.
Pulmonary lymphangiomyomatosis (Fig C3-28)	Rare condition that produces a radiographic appearance identical to that of tuberous sclerosis. Part of a generalized syndrome characterized by an excessive accumulation of muscle in relation to extrapulmonary lymphatics.
Neurofibromatosis	Additional manifestations include skin nodules, multiple bullae, scoliosis, and mediastinal neurofibromas.
Niemann-Pick disease	Also characteristic bone changes and splenomegaly.

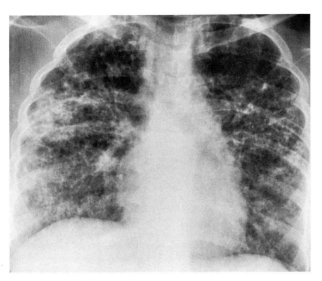

FIG C3-15. **Secondary tuberculosis.** Diffuse interstitial fibrosis pattern.

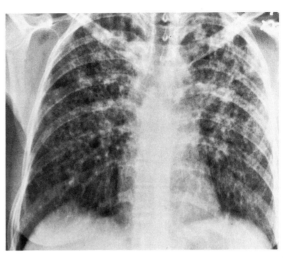

FIG C3-16. **Blastomycosis.** Diffuse interstitial disease with upper lobe predominance. Note the volume loss in the upper lobe and the overdistention of the lower lobes along with the formation of bullae at the bases.[4]

A

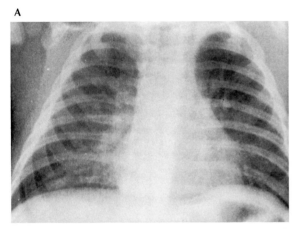

B

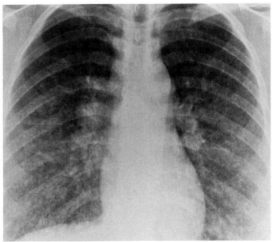

FIG C3-17. **Viral pneumonia.** Diffuse interstitial infiltrates with perihilar haze in (A) a child and (B) an adult.

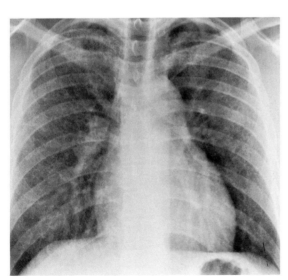

FIG C3-18. *Mycoplasma pneumoniae.* Diffuse fine reticular pattern represents acute interstitial inflammation. The radiographic pattern is indistinguishable from that of most viral pneumonias.

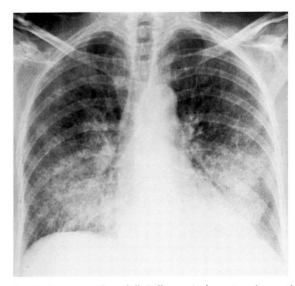

FIG C3-19. *Pneumocystis carinii.* Diffuse reticular pattern in a patient with acute myelogenous leukemia. Note the early development of alveolar consolidations at the bases. A later film showed the typical pulmonary edema pattern.

Condition	Comments
Embolism from oily contrast material	Complication of lymphography. The fine reticular pattern usually clears within 72 hours.
Interstitial fibrosis secondary to pulmonary disease (see Fig C1-26)	Common cause of localized or generalized interstitial thickening, though the offending agent is not always recognized. May be the sequela of recurrent infection, chronic aspiration, lung trauma, radiation, or thromboembolic disease.

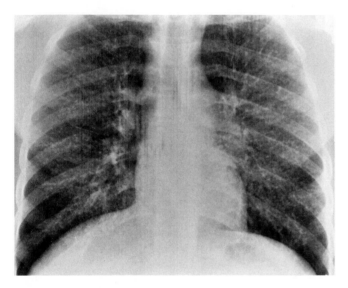

FIG C3-20. **Sarcoidosis.** Diffuse reticulonodular pattern widely distributed throughout both lungs.

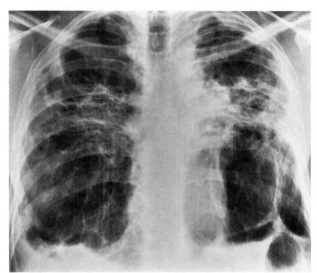

FIG C3-21. **Sarcoidosis.** In end-stage disease, there is severe fibrous scarring, bleb formation, and emphysema.

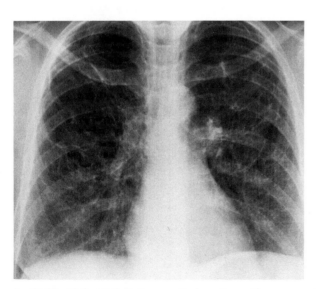

FIG C3-22. **Histiocytosis X.** Coarse reticular pattern with pronounced bleb formation in the upper zones.

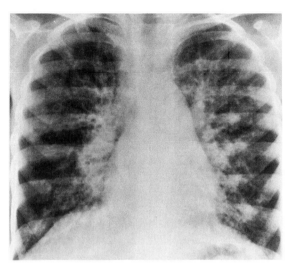

FIG C3-23. Cystic fibrosis. Diffuse peribronchial thickening appears as a perihilar infiltrate associated with hyperexpansion and flattening of the hemidiaphragms.

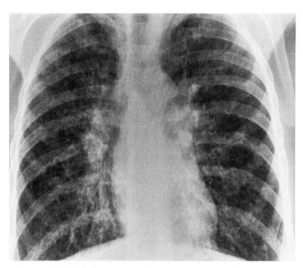

FIG C3-24. Familial dysautonomia. Pattern identical to that of cystic fibrosis.

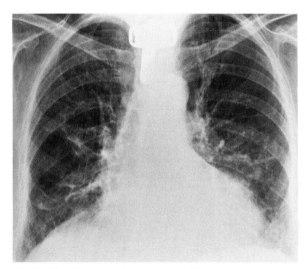

FIG C3-25. Usual interstitial pneumonia. Diffuse coarse reticulonodular pattern.

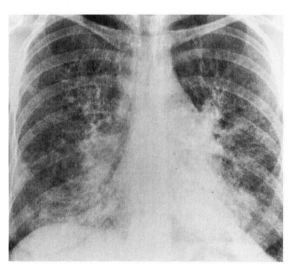

FIG C3-26. Desquamative interstitial pneumonia. Diffuse reticulonodular pattern indicating interstitial disease, combined with bibasilar air-space consolidation that obscures the borders of the heart.

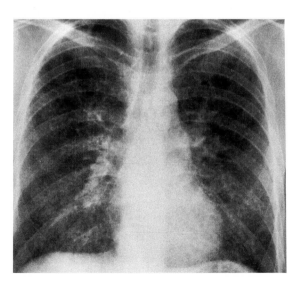

FIG C3-27. Amyloidosis. Diffuse interstitial fibrosis pattern.

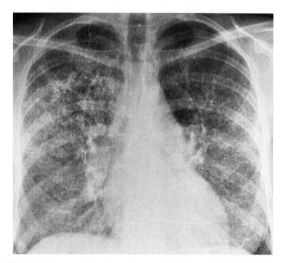

FIG C3-28. Pulmonary lymphangiomyomatosis. Diffuse reticulonodular interstitial pattern throughout both lungs.

HONEYCOMBING

Condition	Comments
Pneumoconiosis (Fig C4-1)	Silicosis, asbestosis, berylliosis, coal-miner's lung, etc. Often associated with other radiographic manifestations (nodules, eggshell calcification, and progressive massive fibrosis in silicosis; pleural plaquing and calcification in asbestosis).
Sarcoidosis (Fig C4-2)	Frequently associated with hilar and mediastinal lymph node enlargement, which often regresses spontaneously as the parenchymal disease develops.
Idiopathic interstitial fibrosis (Hamman-Rich syndrome) (Fig C4-3)	Usually most prominent at the bases and associated with progressive loss of lung volume. A similar diffuse interstitial fibrosis pattern may represent the end stage of a variety of pulmonary conditions including chronic or recurrent pulmonary edema, the inhalation of noxious gases and organic dust, and drug therapy.
Histiocytosis X (Fig C4-4)	More prominent in the upper lung zones (sparing the bases). Spontaneous pneumothorax is a frequent complication.
Tuberculosis	Bronchiectasis and fibrosis may produce a localized honeycomb pattern in the upper lobes.
Connective tissue disorders (Fig C4-5)	More prominent at the bases and usually associated with progressive loss of lung volume. Causes include scleroderma, rheumatoid lung, and dermatomyositis.
Ankylosing spondylitis	Rare manifestation that exclusively involves the upper lobes and resembles the fibrosis and bronchiectasis that may develop secondary to tuberculosis.
Desquamative interstitial pneumonia (DIP)	More prominent in the lower lung zones and associated with progressive loss of lung volume.
Amyloidosis (Fig C4-6)	More prominent in the lower lung zones and often associated with hilar and mediastinal lymphadenopathy.
Neurofibromatosis (Fig C4-7)	Additional manifestations include skin nodules, multiple bullae, scoliosis, and mediastinal neurofibromas.

A

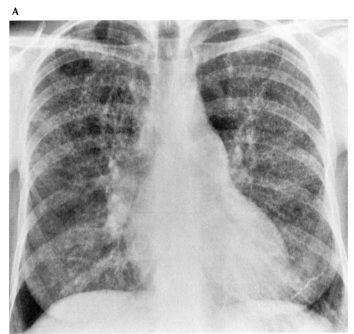

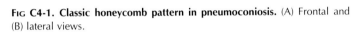

B

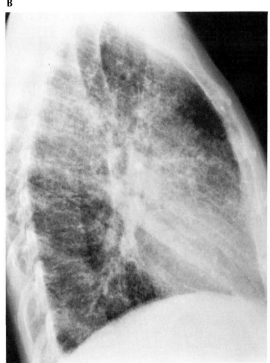

FIG C4-1. **Classic honeycomb pattern in pneumoconiosis.** (A) Frontal and (B) lateral views.

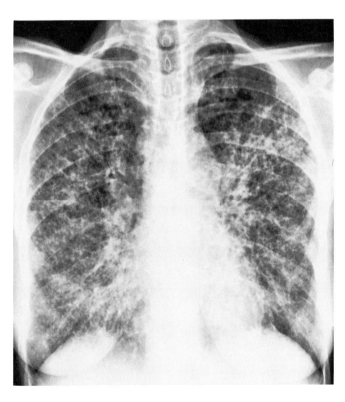

FIG C4-2. **Sarcoidosis.** Coarse honeycomb pattern.

Condition	Comments
Tuberous sclerosis	More prominent in the lower lung zones. Chylous pleural effusion and pneumothorax are common, and sclerotic (occasionally lytic) bone lesions may occur.
Niemann-Pick disease	Also characteristic bone changes and splenomegaly.
Lipoid pneumonia	Rare manifestation that usually involves a lower lobe.

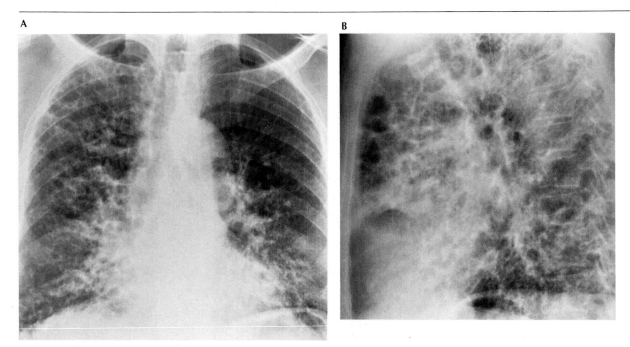

FIG C4-3. Diffuse interstitial fibrosis. (A) Frontal and (B) lateral views of the chest demonstrate a coarse reticular pattern indicating pronounced fibrosis. Intervening small areas of lucency produce the appearance of a honeycomb lung, especially in the right upper lobe.

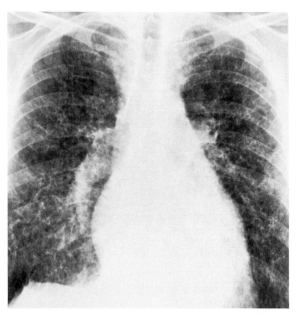

FIG C4-4. Histiocytosis X. Diffuse honeycomb pattern that is slightly more prominent in the upper lung zones.

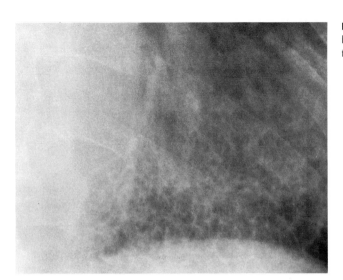

Fig C4-5. Scleroderma. Coned view of the left lower lung demonstrates a honeycomb pattern, with small emphysematous areas combined with fibrosis and fine nodularity.

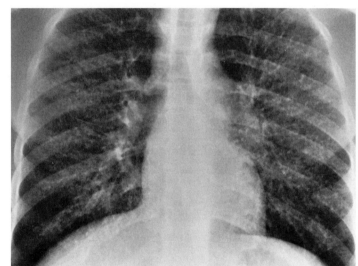

Fig C4-6. Amyloidosis.

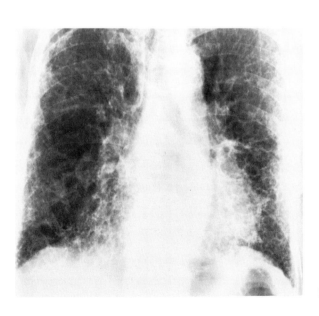

Fig C4-7. Neurofibromatosis.

SOLITARY PULMONARY NODULE

Condition	Imaging Findings	Comments
Tuberculoma (Figs C5-1 and C5-2)	Round or oval, sharply circumscribed nodule that is seldom more than 4 cm in diameter. Central calcification and "satellite" lesions are common, as is calcification of hilar lymph nodes.	Primarily involves the upper lobes (especially the right). The draining bronchus may show irregular thickening or even frank stenosis.
Histoplasmoma (Figs C5-3 and C5-4)	Round or oval, sharply circumscribed nodule that is seldom more than 3 cm in diameter. Central calcification is common and satellite lesions may occur.	Most frequently in the lower lobes. May be multiple and vary considerably in size. Often associated calcification of hilar lymph nodes.
Other fungal diseases (Fig C5-5)	Usually a single, well-circumscribed nodule (may be multiple in coccidioidomycosis).	Actinomycosis, blastomycosis, coccidioidomycosis, cryptococcosis, and nocardiosis. Cavitation is common in actinomycosis, coccidioidomycosis, and nocardiosis. Empyema may complicate actinomycosis or nocardiosis.
Echinococcal (hydatid) cyst (Fig C5-6)	Solitary, sharply circumscribed, round or oval mass that tends to have a bizarre, irregular shape. Calcification is very rare.	Predilection for the lower lobes (especially the right). Communication with the bronchial tree causes an air-fluid level in the cyst (endocyst floats on the surface to produce the "water lily" sign [see Fig C8-8] or "sign of the camalote") or the "crescent" sign (see Fig C19-3) around its periphery.
Acute lung abscess (Fig C5-7)	Round, often ill-defined mass that predominantly involves the posterior portions of the upper or lower lobes.	Bilateral in more than 60% of cases. Cavitation is very common (irregular, shaggy inner wall).
Bronchial adenoma (Fig C5-8)	Solitary, round or oval, sharply circumscribed mass. Calcification and cavitation are very rare.	About 25% appear as peripheral solitary nodules. The remaining 75% arise centrally in the bronchial lumen and cause segmental atelectasis or obstructive pneumonia. Hemoptysis occurs in more than half the patients.
Hamartoma (Figs C5-9 and C5-10)	Solitary, well-circumscribed, often lobulated mass. Popcorn calcification (multiple punctuate calcifications in the lesion) is virtually diagnostic, but occurs in less than 10% of cases.	Serial examinations may show interval growth. An endobronchial lesion (10%) may cause segmental atelectasis or obstructive pneumonia.
Bronchogenic carcinoma (Fig C5-11)	Ill-defined, lobulated, or umbilicated mass that usually exceeds 2 cm. Hilar and mediastinal lymph node enlargement is common, especially in oat cell carcinoma.	About 40% of solitary nodules are malignant. Bronchogenic carcinoma primarily involves the upper lobes with rare calcification and infrequent (2% to 10%) cavitation. Central or popcorn calcification virtually excludes a malignant lesion. The tumor almost invariably shows interval growth on serial films.

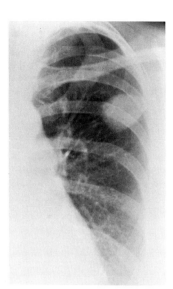

FIG C5-1. Tuberculoma. Single smooth, well-defined pulmonary nodule in the left upper lobe. In the absence of a central nidus of calcification, this appearance is indistinguishable from that of a malignancy.

A   B

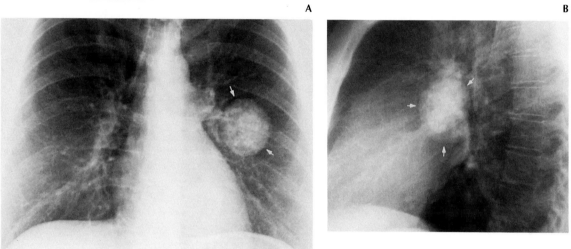

FIG C5-2. Calcified tuberculoma. (A) Frontal and (B) lateral views of the chest show a large left-lung soft-tissue mass (arrows) containing dense central calcification.

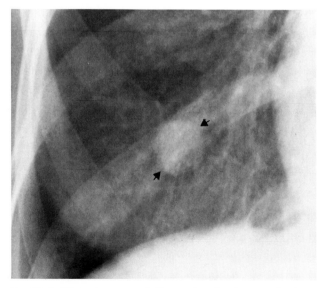

FIG C5-3. Histoplasmoma. Solitary, sharply circumscribed granulomatous nodule (arrows) in the right lower lobe.

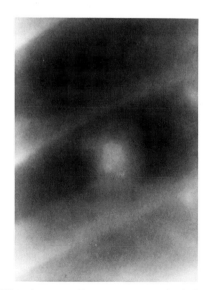

FIG C5-4. Histoplasmoma. Characteristic central calcification in a solitary pulmonary nodule.

Condition	Imaging Findings	Comments
Hematogenous metastases (Fig C5-12)	Single (25%) or multiple (75%) lesions that are generally well-circumscribed with smooth or slightly lobulated margins and a lower lobe predominance.	Represents about 5% of asymptomatic solitary pulmonary nodules. Calcification is rare (only in osteogenic sarcoma or chondrosarcoma).
Bronchioloalveolar (alveolar cell) carcinoma (Fig C5-13)	Various patterns (smooth or lobulated, sharply circumscribed or ill defined).	Characteristic findings include an air bronchogram or bronchiologram in the mass and the ''pleural tail'' sign (linear strands extending from the lesion toward the pleura). The tumor tends to grow very slowly.
Non-Hodgkin's lymphoma	Single or, more commonly, multiple nodules that often have fuzzy outlines and strands of increased density extending into the adjacent lung.	May be a manifestation of primary or secondary disease. Hilar or mediastinal adenopathy is usually associated. Because the tumor rarely obstructs the bronchial tree (unlike carcinoma), air bronchograms often occur in the mass.
Multiple myeloma (plasmacytoma) (see Fig C26-4)	Sharply circumscribed, extrapleural mass producing an obtuse angle with the chest wall.	Usually represents spread into the thorax of a primary rib lesion (therefore almost always a destructive process in one or more ribs).
Mesenchymal tumor	Usually solitary and well defined.	Rare tumor arising in a bronchial wall. May cause bronchial obstruction with peripheral atelectasis or obstructive pneumonia.
Pulmonary hematoma (Fig C5-14)	Single or multiple, unilocular or multilocular, round or oval mass that may occasionally be huge. Usually in a peripheral subpleural location deep to the area of maximum trauma.	Results from hemorrhage into a pulmonary parenchymal laceration or a traumatic lung cyst. May communicate with the bronchial tree (air-fluid level). Generally shows a slow, progressive decrease in size (may persist for several months).
Lipoid pneumonia (Fig C5-15)	Sharply circumscribed, smooth or lobulated mass that primarily occurs in the dependent portion of the lung. The lesion may have a shaggy border and simulate carcinoma.	Inflammatory reaction to aspirated oils (especially mineral oil). Characteristic streaky linear opacities may radiate outward from the periphery of the mass (interlobular septal thickening).
Wegener's granulomatosis (see Fig C8-12)	Round, solitary, or, more commonly, multiple fairly well-circumscribed nodules that may simulate metastases.	Cavitation (thick-walled with irregular shaggy inner margins) develops in about half the patients.
Rheumatoid necrobiotic nodule	Single or, more commonly, multiple smooth, well-circumscribed nodules that predominantly occur in a peripheral subpleural location.	Rare manifestation of rheumatoid lung disease that tends to wax and wane in relation to subcutaneous nodules. Cavitation is common (thick-walled with smooth inner margins).

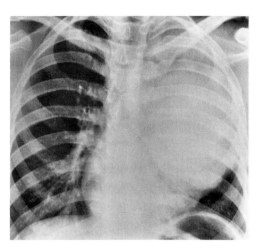

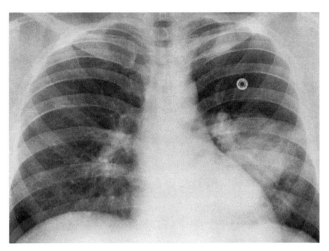

FIG C5-5. Cryptococcosis. Single fairly well-circumscribed, masslike consolidation in the superior segment of the left lower lobe.

FIG C5-6. Echinococcal cyst. Huge mass filling most of the left hemithorax.

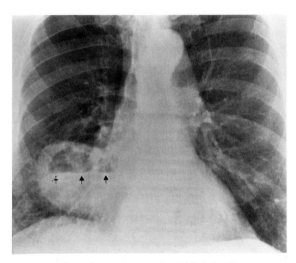

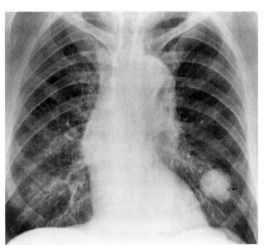

FIG C5-7. Acute lung abscess. Large right middle lobe abscess containing an air-fluid level (arrows) in an intravenous drug abuser.

FIG C5-8. Bronchial adenoma. Nonspecific solitary pulmonary nodule at the left base. Note the notched indentation of the lateral wall (arrow) of the mass. Although this "Rigler notch" sign was initially described as being pathognomonic of malignancy, an identical appearance is commonly seen in benign processes.

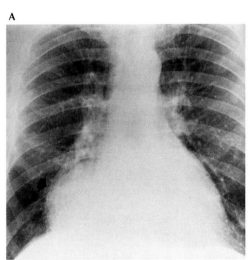

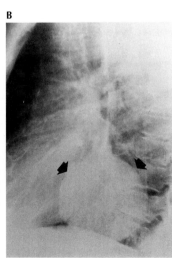

FIG C5-9. Hamartoma. (A) Frontal view of the chest shows a large mass (arrow) in the right cardiophrenic angle; the mass mimics a pericardial cyst or herniation through the foramen of Morgagni, both of which tend to occur at this site. (B) Lateral view shows the mass to be posterior (arrows), effectively excluding the other diagnostic possibilities. The mass is indistinguishable from other benign or malignant processes in the lung.

Condition	Imaging Findings	Comments
Bronchogenic cyst **(see Figs C21-3 and C21-4)**	Solitary round or oval, smooth, sharply circumscribed mass with a lower lobe predominance.	About two thirds of bronchogenic cysts are pulmonary (the rest are mediastinal). The cyst is homogeneous until a communication is established with contiguous lung (usually the result of infection).
Intralobar bronchopulmonary sequestration	Round, oval, or triangular mass that typically is well-circumscribed and contiguous with the diaphragm (two thirds of the cases are on the left).	Enclosed in visceral pleura of the affected lung. Although cystic, the mass appears homogeneous until a communication is established with contiguous lung (usually the result of infection). An intralobar sequestration is supplied by a systemic artery and drains via the pulmonary veins.
Extralobar bronchopulmonary sequestration **(Fig C5-16)**	Well-defined, homogeneous mass that is related to the left hemidiaphragm (above or below it) in about 90% of cases.	Enclosed in its own visceral pleural layer (therefore seldom infected or air-containing). An extralobar sequestration is supplied by a systemic artery (usually from the abdominal aorta) and drains via systemic veins (inferior vena cava or azygos system).
Pulmonary arteriovenous fistula **(Fig C5-17)**	Sharply defined, round or oval, often slightly lobulated lesion that predominantly involves the lower lobes.	Diagnosis requires identification of the feeding artery and the draining vein. About one third of the fistulas are multiple (arteriography of both lungs required if surgical resection is contemplated). About 50% of the patients have hereditary hemorrhagic telangiectasia (Rendu-Osler-Weber disease).
Mucoid impaction **(Fig C5-18)**	Generally a fingerlike mass, although it may have a Y- or V-shaped configuration when a bronchial bifurcation is plugged.	Affects patients with bronchospasm (plugs present in dilated proximal segmental bronchi) and a sensitivity to *Aspergillus fumigatus*. Almost always associated with asthma or pre-existing chronic bronchial disease. Usually transient, but may persist for months and even enlarge. Cavitation (lung necrosis) is rare.
Congenital bronchial atresia	Smooth, sharply defined oval mass that has a strong predilection for the apicoposterior bronchus of the left upper lobe.	The mass consists of inspissated mucus that accumulates in the bronchus immediately distal to the point of obstruction. The lung parenchyma distal to the occlusion is overinflated because of collateral air drift. This very rare anomaly is usually asymptomatic and is discovered on a screening chest radiograph.
Pulmonary vein varix	Round or oval, lobulated, well-defined mass (may be multiple) involving the medial third of the lung.	Very rare congenital or acquired tortuosity and dilatation of a pulmonary vein just before its entrance into the left atrium. On lateral view, it typically projects posterior and inferior to the hilar structures. Change in size and shape with Valsalva and Mueller maneuvers (as with arteriovenous fistulas).

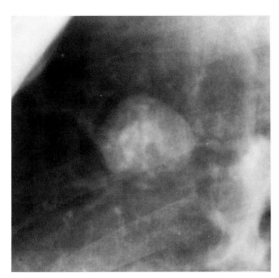

Fig C5-10. Hamartoma. Well-circumscribed solitary nodule containing characteristic irregular scattered calcifications (popcorn pattern).

Fig C5-11. Bronchogenic carcinoma. (A) Relatively well-defined mass. (B) Ill-defined solitary nodule.

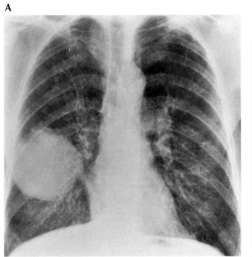

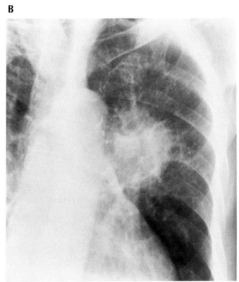

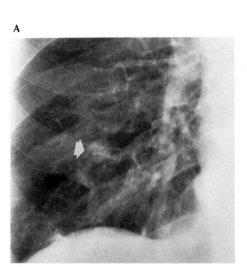

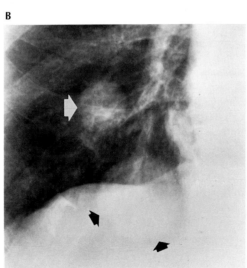

Fig C5-12. Metastases. (A) Solitary metastasis (arrow). (B) Repeat examination 5 months later shows rapid growth of the previous solitary nodule (white arrow). There is a second huge nodule (black arrows) that was not appreciated on the previous examination because it projected below the right hemidiaphragm.

Condition	Imaging Findings	Comments
Pseudolymphoma	Peripheral nodule.	Nodular lesions are less common than segmental parenchymal consolidation in this rare lesion. Closely resembles malignant lymphoma but does not involve hilar and mediastinal lymph nodes and shows no recurrence after surgical resection.
Inflammatory pseudotumor	Solitary pulmonary nodule (or homogeneous consolidation) that may mimic a primary or metastatic neoplasm.	Probably represents a reparative process secondary to an unresolved pneumonia (though there is often no history of an acute respiratory illness).
Progressive massive fibrosis (PMF) **(see Figs C6-9 and C6-10)**	Large, often bilateral (but usually asymmetric), spindle-shaped mass in the upper half of the lungs. Typically arises near the periphery of the lung, with its lateral border (paralleling the rib cage) usually better defined than the medial edge. Tends to migrate toward the hili with time.	A manifestation of pneumoconiosis (especially silicosis or coal-miner's disease). Usually of homogeneous density unless there is cavitation (caused by ischemic necrosis or superimposed tuberculosis). May occasionally contain small calcifications (unlike bronchogenic carcinoma).

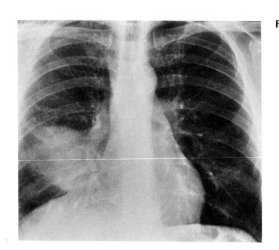

FIG C5-13. Alveolar cell carcinoma. Large, well-circumscribed tumor mass.

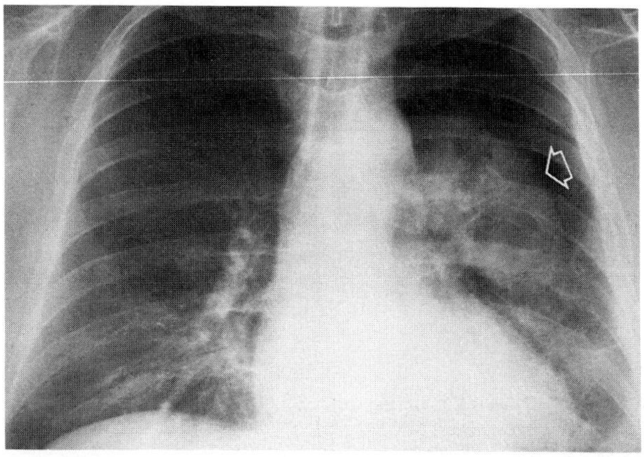

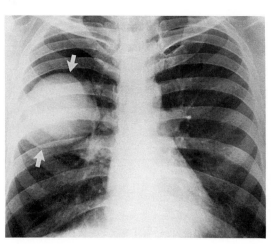

FIG C5-14. Pulmonary hematoma. After a stab wound, a homogeneous kidney-shaped opacity (arrow) developed in the superior segment of the left lower lobe. There is blunting of the left costophrenic angle.

FIG C5-15. Lipoid pneumonia. Sharply demarcated granulomatous-lipoid mass (arrows) simulating a neoplastic process.

A
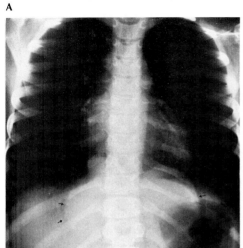

B
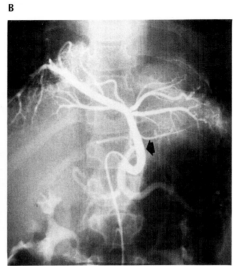

FIG C5-16. Bilateral pulmonary sequestration. (A) Frontal view of the chest shows bilateral oval, slightly lobulated paravertebral masses (arrows) in the juxtadiaphragmatic region. (B) Selective angiogram of a large anomalous artery (arrow) arising from the celiac trunk shows several branches supplying the bilateral paravertebral masses. The venous drainage was via the pulmonary veins.[11]

FIG C5-17. Pulmonary arteriovenous fistula. (A) View of the right lung shows a round soft-tissue mass (straight arrows) at the left base. Feeding and draining vessels (curved arrows) extend to the lesion. (B) An arteriogram clearly shows the feeding artery and draining veins (closed arrows) associated with the arteriovenous malformation (open arrow).

A
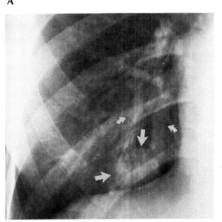

B
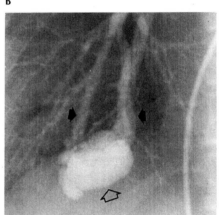

A
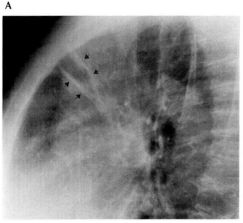

B
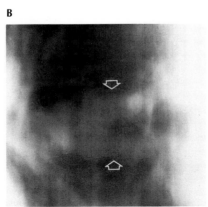

FIG C5-18. Mucoid impaction. (A) V-shaped and (B) Y-shaped masses.

MULTIPLE PULMONARY NODULES

Condition	Imaging Findings	Comments
Pyogenic abscesses (Fig C6-1)	Round, well-circumscribed masses (may have poor definition in the acute stage).	Cavitation (irregular, thick-walled) is very common. May reflect septic emboli in an intravenous drug addict.
Granulomatous infections (Fig C6-2)	Generally round or oval, well-circumscribed nodules. Irregular and poorly defined masses in *Pseudomonas*.	Histoplasmosis, tuberculosis, coccidioidomycosis, *Pseudomonas*. Calcification is common in histoplasmosis, tuberculosis, and coccidioidomycosis; cavitation is common in coccidioidomycosis and *Pseudomonas*.
Paragonimus westermani (Fig C6-3)	Well-circumscribed cystic masses that have a predilection for the periphery of the lower lobes.	Characteristic appearance of multiple ring opacities or thin-walled cysts (may mimic cystic bronchiectasis).
Hematogenous metastases (Figs C6-4 and C6-5)	Various patterns (from diffuse micronodular shadows resembling miliary disease to multiple large, well-defined "cannonballs"). Tend to be more numerous in the lower lobes.	Nodules typically vary in size in the same patient. Calcification is rare but is virtually diagnostic of osteogenic sarcoma or chondrosarcoma. Cavitation occurs in about 4% and most commonly involves squamous cell neoplasms (also adenocarcinomas of the large bowel and sarcomas).
Bronchioloalveolar (alveolar cell) carcinoma (Fig C6-6)	Poorly defined nodules scattered throughout both lungs.	Other presentations include a single well-circumscribed peripheral solitary nodule (see Fig C5-13), focal "pneumonia" (see Fig C1-25), and a miliary pattern (see Fig C7-5).
Papillomatosis of lung (see Fig C8-16)	Round, sharply circumscribed nodules that frequently cavitate (often resembling advanced cystic bronchiectasis).	Usually associated with laryngeal or tracheal papillomas. Typically obstruct the airways, resulting in peripheral atelectasis and obstructive pneumonia.
Lymphoma	Multiple nodules that often have fuzzy outlines and are most numerous in the lower lobes.	Manifestation of secondary disease. Usually associated with mediastinal and hilar lymph node enlargement. Cystlike lesions may simulate central cavitation.
Pulmonary arteriovenous fistulas (see Fig C5-17)	Sharply defined, round or oval, often slightly lobulated nodules that predominantly involve the lower lobes. The lesions may change in size between the Valsalva and the Mueller maneuvers.	Diagnosis requires identification of the feeding artery and the draining vein. About one third of the fistulas are multiple (arteriography of both lungs required if surgical resection is contemplated). About 50% have hereditary hemorrhagic telangectasia (Rendu-Osler-Weber disease).
Wegener's granulomatosis (see Fig C8-12)	Round, fairly well-circumscribed nodules that may simulate metastases.	Cavitation (thick-walled with irregular, shaggy inner margins) develops in about half the patients.

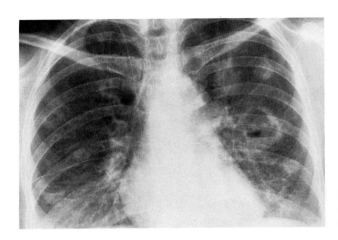

Fig C6-1. Septic pulmonary emboli. Several round lesions, many with cavitation, are seen throughout the lungs in this intravenous drug abuser with staphylococcal tricuspid endocarditis.

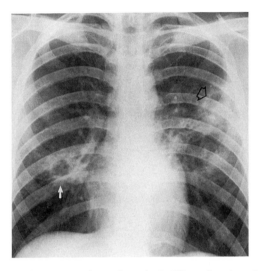

Fig C6-2. Secondary tuberculosis. Bilateral cavitary lesions (arrows) with relatively thick walls.

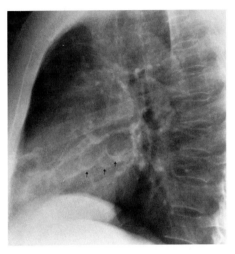

Fig C6-3. *Paragonimus westermani.* Arrows point to a few of the multiple cysts in the right middle lobe. The cysts are thin-walled and most have a prominent crescent-shaped opacity along one side of their borders, the characteristic ring shadow of paragonimiasis.

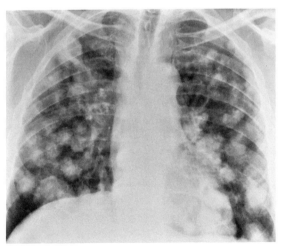

Fig C6-4. Hematogenous metastases. Multiple well-circumscribed nodules scattered diffusely throughout both lungs.

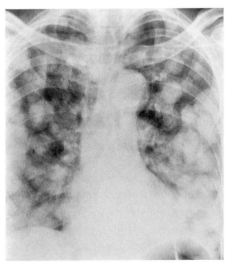

Fig C6-5. Cannonball metastases in a patient with choriocarcinoma.

Condition	Imaging Findings	Comments
Rheumatoid necrobiotic nodules (Fig C6-7)	Smooth, well-circumscribed nodules that predominantly occur in peripheral subpleural locations. Cavitation is common (thick-walled with smooth inner margins).	Rare manifestation of rheumatoid lung disease that tends to wax and wane in relation to the activity of the rheumatoid arthritis and the presence of subcutaneous nodules. May be associated with pneumoconiosis (Caplan's syndrome).
Amyloidosis	Multiple nodules that may cavitate and show calcification or ossification.	Discrete masses of amyloid may develop in the rare parenchymal form of the disease. The nodular parenchymal form of the disease has a better prognosis than the tracheobronchial (obstructive) or diffuse interstitial types (see Fig C3-27).
Pulmonary hematomas (see Fig C5-14)	Unilocular or multilocular, round or oval nodules that are occasionally huge. Usually in peripheral subpleural locations deep to areas of maximum trauma.	Result from hemorrhage into pulmonary parenchymal lacerations or traumatic lung cysts. May communicate with the bronchial tree (air-fluid level). Generally a slow, progressive decrease in size (may persist for several months).
Sarcoidosis (Fig C6-8)	Sharply circumscribed and widely distributed nodules that may simulate metastatic disease.	Rare manifestation. Usually associated with a reticulonodular pattern and often concomitant hilar and mediastinal adenopathy.
Pulmonary ossification	Small, densely calcified or ossified nodules throughout the lungs.	Primarily a manifestation of mitral stenosis (or other causes of elevated left atrial pressure).
Pneumoconiosis (progressive massive fibrosis) (Figs C6-9 and C6-10)	Conglomerate masses that predominantly involve the upper lobes and are usually irregular and ill-defined with peripheral stranding.	Masses represent confluence of individual silicotic nodules, sometimes associated with superimposed tuberculous infection. They typically develop in the mid-zone or periphery of the lung and tend to migrate toward the hilum.
Polyarteritis	Poorly defined nodules that are often associated with patchy consolidations.	The pulmonary manifestations typically show progression and regression of lesions on serial films, reflecting the appearance of new lesions and the healing of old ones. The angiographic demonstration of multiple arterial aneurysms in one or more abdominal organs is considered virtually diagnostic of this disease.
Pulmonary varices	Multiple round, well-defined opacities that most commonly appear on lateral radiographs projecting posterior and inferior to the hilar structures.	Congenital or acquired tortuosity and dilatation of pulmonary veins just before their entrance into the left atrium. The varicosities change shape and size with the Valsalva and Mueller maneuvers (similar to arteriovenous fistulas).
Mucoid impactions (see Fig C5-18)	Multiple (more commonly single) round, oval, or elliptical opacities caused by plugs in dilated bronchi.	Usually associated with hypersensitivity aspergillosis in patients with asthma or pre-existing chronic bronchial disease.

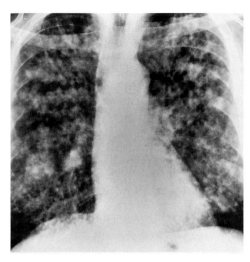

FIG C6-6. Alveolar cell carcinoma. Multiple poorly defined nodules scattered throughout both lungs.

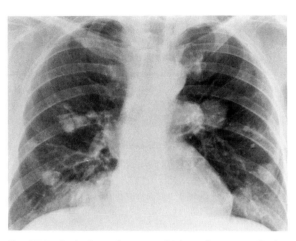

FIG C6-7. Caplan's syndrome. Multiple well-circumscribed, rounded nodules of varying size in a patient with subcutaneous rheumatoid nodules.

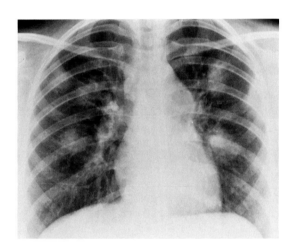

FIG C6-8. Sarcoidosis. Patchy, ill-defined areas of air-space consolidation scattered throughout both lungs.

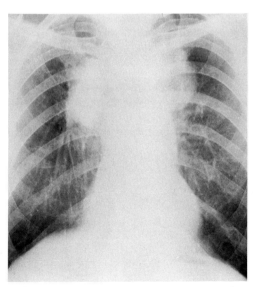

FIG C6-9. Progressive massive fibrosis in silicosis. Nonsegmental areas of homogeneous density in both upper lobes.

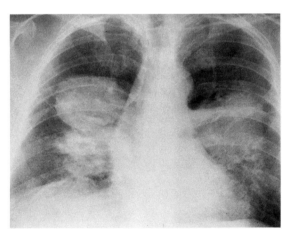

FIG C6-10. Progressive massive fibrosis in silicosis. Large, irregular nodules in both perihilar regions.

MILIARY NODULES*

Condition	Comments
Tuberculosis (Fig C7-1)	Hematogenous dissemination that almost invariably leads to a dramatic febrile response with night sweats and chills. There may be minimal symptoms in severely debilitated patients, especially the elderly and those on steroids.
Fungal diseases (Figs C7-2 and C7-3)	Hematogenous dissemination, most commonly of histoplasmosis but also coccidioidomycosis, blastomycosis, and candidiasis. May represent the healing phase of the acute epidemic form of histoplasmosis.
Disseminated hematogenous metastases (Fig C7-4)	Most commonly thyroid carcinoma ("snowstorm"), which may remain unchanged for a long time because of the very low grade of malignancy. Other causes include trophoblastic disease, bone sarcomas, renal cell carcinoma, and, infrequently, melanoma and carcinomas of the breast and gastrointestinal tract.
Bronchioloalveolar (alveolar cell) carcinoma (Fig C7-5)	Other presentations include a well-circumscribed, peripheral solitary nodule (see Fig C5-13), focal "pneumonia" (see Fig C1-25), and multiple poorly defined nodules (see Fig C6-6).
Pneumoconiosis (Figs C7-6 and C7-7)	Silicosis, coal-worker's pneumoconiosis, berylliosis. The nodules represent localized areas of fibrosis (or the summation of linear shadows).
Histiocytosis X	Early active stage of the disease. The nodules represent individual granulomatous foci.
Sarcoidosis (see Fig C11-8)	Associated bilateral and symmetric hilar adenopathy is virtually pathognomonic (though the adenopathy classically regresses as the parenchymal disease progresses).
Allergic alveolitis (farmer's lung)	Allergy involving the alveolar wall due to a variety of noninvasive fungi. Represents the subacute or chronic phase of the illness.
Viral pneumonia (Fig C7-8)	Primarily chickenpox pneumonia (adults more than children). May heal with the development of multiple calcified nodules (as in histoplasmosis).

*Diffuse fine nodules less than 5 mm in diameter.

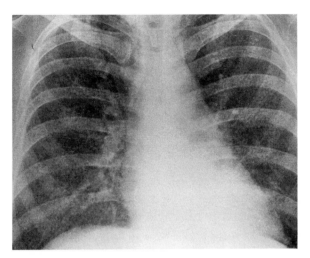

FIG C7-1. **Tuberculosis.**

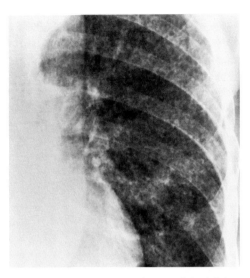

FIG C7-2. **Coccidioidomycosis.** Coned view of the left lung shows a diffuse pattern of fine nodules simulating miliary tuberculosis.

A   B

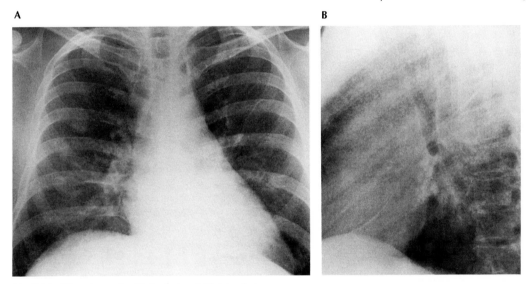

FIG C7-3. **Histoplasmosis.** (A) Frontal and (B) lateral views.

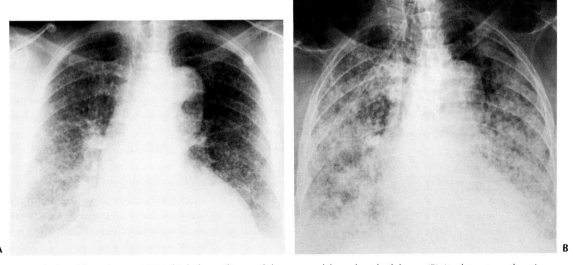

A   B

FIG C7-4. **Metastatic thyroid carcinoma.** (A) Multiple fine miliary nodules scattered throughout both lungs. (B) At a later stage, there is a more coarse miliary pattern.

Condition	Comments
Alveolar microlithiasis (see Fig C2-15)	Diffuse, very fine micronodules of calcific density that are usually asymptomatic. Characteristic black pleura sign (due to contrast between the extreme density of the lung parenchyma on one side of the pleura and the ribs on the other side).
Pulmonary hemosiderosis (Fig C7-9)	Develops in patients with long-standing severe mitral stenosis who have had multiple episodes of hemoptysis.
Amyloidosis	Rare manifestation in which amyloid infiltrates almost every alveolar septum and is deposited around capillaries and within interstitial tissue.
Bronchiolitis obliterans	End result of lower respiratory tract damage in which the bronchioles become obstructed by organizing exudate and polypoid masses of granulation tissue.
Oil embolism	Complication of lymphography (lipid material in the extravascular interstitial tissue).
Interstitial fibrosis	Early stage before the development of the more classic reticulonodular and reticular patterns.
Niemann-Pick disease	Rare lipid storage disease. The miliary nodule pattern (and early age of onset) is a differential point from Gaucher's disease.
Parasitic disease (Fig C7-10)	Schistosomiasis, filariasis.
Listeriosis (Fig C7-11)	Rare bacterial disease that primarily occurs as an intrauterine infection with a high mortality rate, or as a disease of the newborn.
Rheumatoid disease	Miliary pattern occurs in the early "subacute" stage of the disease before the development of the more characteristic diffuse interstitial pulmonary fibrosis.
Wegener's granulomatosis	Rare manifestation representing a diffuse granulomatous reaction occurring around vessels. The small fine nodules usually develop in combination with larger, more ill-defined densities that often cavitate.

Fig C7-5. Alveolar cell carcinoma. Miliary pattern diffusely involving both lungs represents bronchogenic spread.

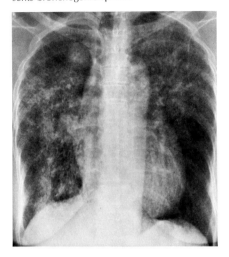

Fig C7-6. Silicosis.

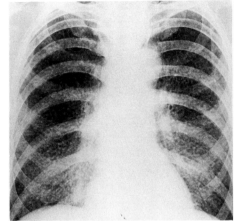

Fig C7-7. Coal-worker's pneumoconiosis.

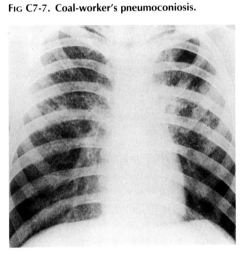

Fig C7-8. Chickenpox pneumonia. Bilateral, coarse miliary infiltrates distributed diffusely throughout both lungs.

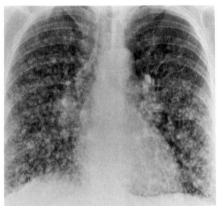

Fig C7-9. Pulmonary hemosiderosis.[12]

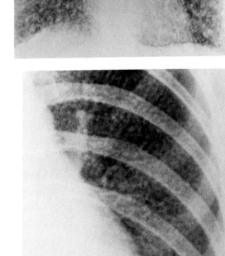

Fig C7-10. Schistosomiasis. Perivascular granulomas produce small nodular and linear densities that are distributed diffusely throughout the lungs in a miliary pattern simulating tuberculosis.

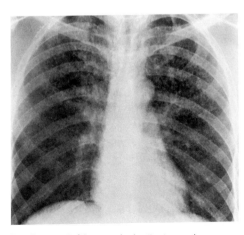

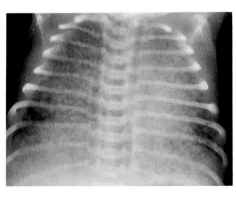

Fig C7-11. Listeriosis. Diffuse miliary pattern of coarse, irregular granular densities is distributed throughout both lungs.

CAVITARY LESIONS OF THE LUNGS

Condition	Imaging Findings	Comments
Bacterial lung abscess (Fig C8-1)	Generally a thick-walled cavity with a shaggy inner lining.	Most frequently *Staphylococcus*, *Klebsiella*, *Pseudomonas*, and *Proteus*. An empyema is commonly associated. Multiple cavities often occur with anaerobic organisms.
Pneumatocele (Fig C8-2)	Thin-walled cystic space (may be multiple).	Develops in about 50% of children with staphylococcal pneumonia. Results from a check-valve obstruction of the communication between a peribronchial abscess and the bronchial lumen.
Mycobacteria (Figs C8-3 and C8-4)	Wall of the cavity is usually of moderate thickness and has a generally smooth inner lining.	Cavitation (often multiple) tends to be a more prominent feature of atypical mycobacterial disease than of *mycobacterium tuberculosis*. Tuberculous cavities predominantly involve the apical and posterior regions of the upper lobes and the posterior segments of the lower lobes. Thin-walled cavities may persist after chemotherapy in the absence of acute disease.
Fungal lung abscess (Figs C8-5 to C8-7)	Single or multiple cavities, most of which are thick-walled (coccidioidomycosis tends to produce a very thin-walled lesion).	Pleural effusion and extension into the chest wall are common in actinomycosis and nocardiosis. Histoplasmosis typically involves the apical and posterior segments of the upper lobes (indistinguishable from tuberculosis), while coccidioidomycosis is characteristically located in the anterior segment. Candidiasis, aspergillosis, sporotrichosis, and mucormycosis are essentially limited to debilitated patients and those with underlying diseases (diabetes mellitus, lymphoma, leukemia).
Amebic lung abscess	Thick-walled cavity with a ragged inner lining.	Almost always in the right lower lobe and associated with a right pleural effusion (organisms from a liver abscess enter the thorax by direct extension via the right hemidiaphragm).
Hydatid cyst (*Echinococcus granulosus*) (Fig C8-8)	Thin-walled cavity with a lower lobe predominance.	Rupture of the cyst into a bronchus results in part or all of its liquid contents being expelled into the bronchial system, producing the characteristic ''meniscus sign'' and ''water lily sign'' (irregularity of the air-fluid layer caused by collapsed cyst membranes). A hydropneumothorax may also occur.
Paragonimus westermani (Fig C8-9)	Thin-walled cysts (ring shadows) that are generally multiple and have a predilection for the periphery of the lower lobes.	Typically a crescent-shaped opacity along one aspect of the inner lining. May mimic cystic bronchiectasis.

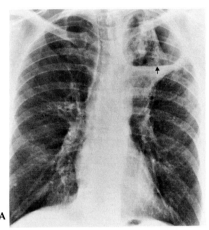

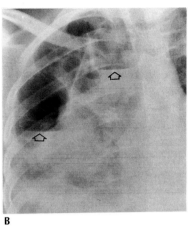

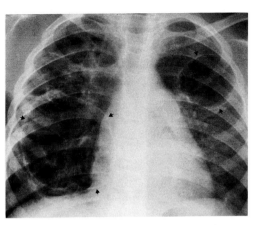

A

B

FIG C8-1. Bacterial lung abscess. (A) *Proteus* pneumonia. Large, thick-walled left upper lobe abscess with an air-fluid level (arrow) and an associated infiltrate. (B) Staphylococcal pneumonia. Multiple lung abscesses with air-fluid levels (arrows) associated with diffuse air-space consolidation and a large pleural effusion.

FIG C8-2. Pneumatocele. Residual thin-walled cystic spaces (arrows) in the pulmonary parenchyma many years after a childhood staphylococcal pneumonia.

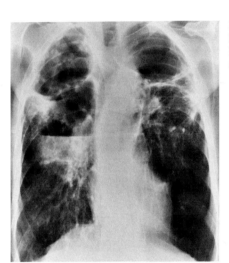

FIG C8-3. Tuberculosis. Multiple large cavities with air-fluid levels in both upper lobes. Note the chronic fibrotic changes and upward retraction of the hila.

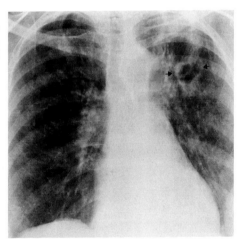

FIG C8-4. Atypical mycobacteria. Cavitary lesion (arrows) in the left upper lobe. The wall of the cavity is mildly irregular and there is minimal parenchymal disease.

A

B

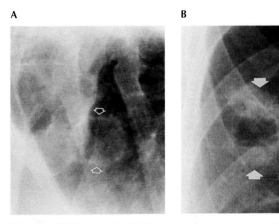

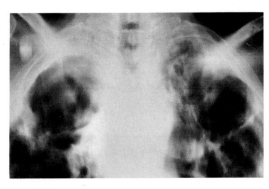

FIG C8-5. Coccidioidomycosis. (A) Thin-walled cavity (arrows). (B) Irregular, thick-walled cavity with surrounding infiltrate.

FIG C8-6. Sporotrichosis. Frontal tomogram shows extensive bilateral upper lobe cavities.[13]

Condition	Imaging Findings	Comments
Bronchogenic carcinoma (Fig C8-10)	Generally a thick-walled cavity with an irregular, nodular inner lining (occasionally a thin-walled cavity simulating a bronchogenic cyst).	Cavitation in 2% to 10% of cases, most commonly in peripheral squamous cell tumors of the upper lobes. Multiple primaries are very rare.
Hematogenous metastases	Thin- or thick-walled cavities may develop in a few or multiple metastatic nodules. Most commonly involves upper lobe lesions.	Cavitation in about 4% of cases. Most commonly involves squamous cell neoplasms (also adenocarcinomas of the large bowel and sarcomas).
Hodgkin's disease	Single or multiple thick-walled cavities with irregular inner linings.	Cavitation typically develops in peripheral parenchymal consolidations (most often in the lower lobes). Usually also enlargement of mediastinal and hilar lymph nodes.
Septic embolism (Fig C8-11)	Generally thin-walled cavities (less commonly thick-walled with shaggy inner linings).	Almost always multiple with a lower lobe predominance. A wide variation in size may reflect recurrent showers of emboli.
Silicosis	Thick-walled cavity with an irregular inner lining. Often multiple with a strong upper lobe predominance.	Generally a background of nodular or reticulonodular disease and associated hilar lymph node enlargement. Cavitation in conglomerate lesions is more often the result of superimposed tuberculosis than ischemic necrosis. Cavitation also occurs in coal-worker's pneumoconiosis.
Wegener's granulomatosis (Fig C8-12)	Usually multiple thick-walled cavities with irregular inner linings (may eventually become thin-walled cystic spaces).	Cavitation eventually occurs in about half the patients. With treatment, the cavitary lesions may disappear or heal with scar formation.
Rheumatoid necrobiotic nodule	Thick-walled cavity with a smooth inner lining (may become thin-walled and even disappear with remission of the arthritis).	Often multiple and generally in a peripheral subpleural location (most often the lower lobe). May be associated with pleural effusion or spontaneous pneumothorax.
Cystic bronchiectasis (Fig C8-13)	Multiple thin-walled cavities with a lower lobe predominance. Often a tiny air-fluid level at the bottom of the ring shadow.	Cavities represent severely dilated segmental bronchi. Generally a considerable loss of volume in the affected region.
Bleb/bulla (Fig C8-14)	Very thin-walled cystic space. Usually multiple with an upper lobe predominance.	Air-fluid levels develop with infection. Often radiographic evidence of diffuse pulmonary emphysema.
Traumatic lung cyst	Single or several thin-walled cavities that may contain air-fluid levels.	Typically occurs in a peripheral subpleural location immediately underlying the point of maximum injury.

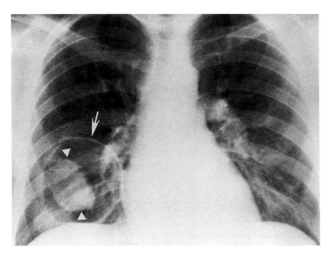

FIG C8-7. Mucormycosis. Large thin-walled cavity (arrows) containing a smooth, elliptical, homogeneous mass (arrowheads) representing a fungus ball.

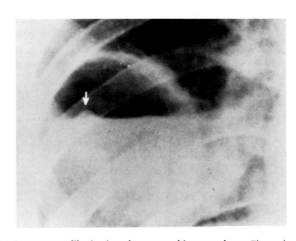

FIG C8-8. Water lily sign in pulmonary echinococcal cyst. The endocyst membranes (arrow) are floating on the surface of fluid in a ruptured hydatid cyst.[14]

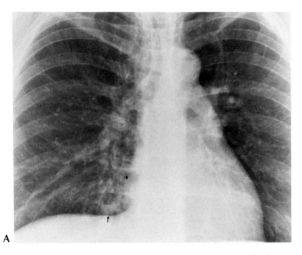

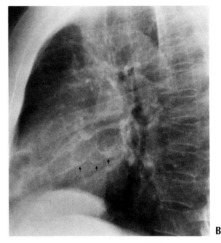

FIG C8-9. Paragonimiasis. (A) Frontal and (B) lateral chest radiographs demonstrate multiple cysts (arrows) in the right middle lobe. The cysts are thin-walled and most have a prominent crescent-shaped opacity along one side of their borders, the characteristic ring shadow of paragonimiasis.

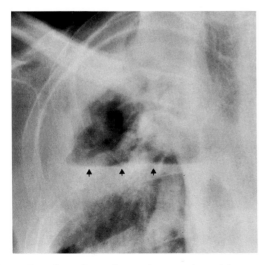

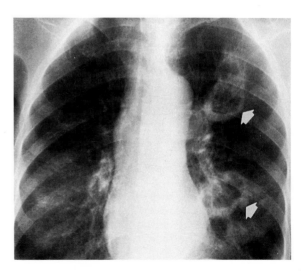

FIG C8-10. Bronchogenic carcinoma. Large cavitary right upper lobe mass with an air-fluid level (arrows) and associated rib destruction.

FIG C8-11. Septic pulmonary emboli. Large cavity lesions (arrows) in the left lung of an intravenous drug abuser with septic thrombophlebitis.

Condition	Imaging Findings	Comments
Sarcoidosis	Cystic lesions developing on a background of diffuse reticulonodular pulmonary disease.	Very uncommon manifestation (should suggest superimposed tuberculosis or fungal disease). A mycetoma may occur in a cavitary lesion.
Intralobar bronchopulmonary sequestration	Thin- or thick-walled cystic mass that is often multilocular or multiple.	Almost invariably arises contiguous to the diaphragm (two thirds are on the left). May be obscured by pneumonia in the surrounding parenchyma.
Bronchogenic cyst	Solitary thin-walled cystic mass that may contain an air-fluid level.	About 75% of bronchogenic cysts that are originally opaque and fluid-filled eventually become air-containing because of an infectious communication with the contiguous lung.
Congenital cystic adenomatoid malformation (see Fig C12-7)	Multiple air-containing cysts scattered irregularly throughout a mass of soft-tissue density.	Expands the ipsilateral hemithorax (depresses the hemidiaphragm and shifts the mediastinum to the contralateral side). May occasionally be confused with a diaphragmatic hernia containing bowel loops. The malformation can often be detected by fetal ultrasound.
Cystic fibrosis (mucoviscidosis) (Fig C8-15)	Thin-walled cystic lesions with or without air-fluid levels associated with diffuse, coarse, reticular changes, hyperinflation, and pulmonary arterial hypertension.	Ring shadows in this condition can be caused by cystic bronchiectasis, bullae, microabscesses, or honeycombing.
Papillomatosis (Fig C8-16)	Multiple thin-walled cysts.	Laryngeal papillomatosis is a common disease in children that infrequently seeds distally in the tracheobronchial tree to produce excavating lesions in the lung.
Plombage (Fig C8-17)	Plastic (lucite) spheres appear radiographically as multiple perfectly round, cavity-like lucencies.	Former therapy for pulmonary tuberculosis that consisted of filling of the extrapleural space with a sufficient volume of inert material to collapse the adjacent lung. The spheres are often not entirely watertight, so that a small amount of fluid may collect in each. On upright views, the resulting air-fluid levels can simulate cavitation and suggest the incorrect diagnosis of acute infection.

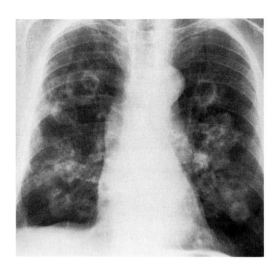

FIG C8-12. **Wegener's granulomatosis.** Multiple thick-walled cavities with irregular, shaggy inner linings.

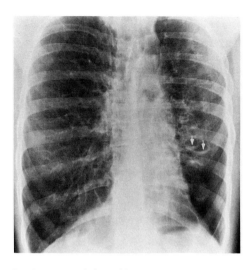

FIG C8-13. **Cystic bronchiectasis.** Multiple cystic spaces, some with air-fluid levels (arrows), predominantly involve the left lung.

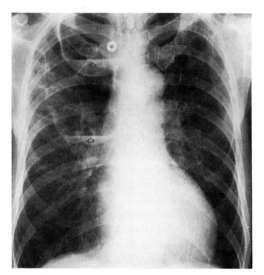

FIG C8-14. **Pulmonary emphysema.** Large bullae in the right upper lung. The presence of air-fluid levels (arrows) in the cystic spaces indicates superimposed infection.

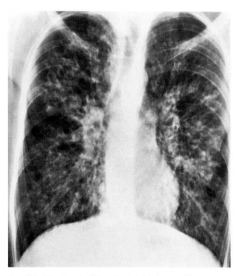

FIG C8-15. **Cystic fibrosis.** Multiple small cysts superimposed on a diffuse, coarse, reticular pattern.

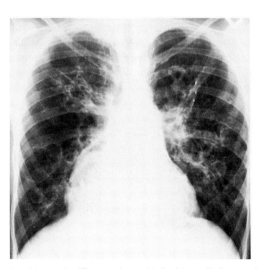

FIG C8-16. **Papillomatosis.** Multiple thin-walled cystic lesions.

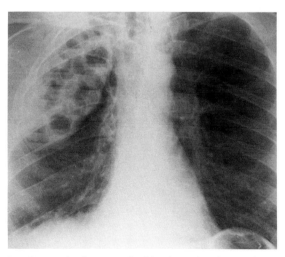

FIG C8-17. **Plombage.** Air-fluid levels in the plastic spheres simulate cavitation.

UNILATERAL HILAR ENLARGEMENT

Condition	Comments
Inflammatory lymphadenopathy (Figs C9-1 and C9-2)	Histoplasmosis, tuberculosis, coccidioidomycosis. The hilar nodes often calcify and are usually associated with ipsilateral parenchymal disease.
Intrabronchial neoplasm	Hilar mass generally represents local nodal metastases (the endobronchial lesion itself usually produces only a minimal mass effect).
Metastatic neoplasm (Fig C9-3)	Often bilateral, with involvement of mediastinal lymph nodes. In lymphangitic spread there is generally a diffuse reticular or reticulonodular pattern.
Lymphoma	Primarily Hodgkin's disease, which often produces asymmetric bilateral hilar adenopathy. There may be pulmonary involvement or pleural effusion. The nodes may calcify after mediastinal irradiation.
Valvular pulmonic stenosis (see Fig CA13-6)	Poststenotic dilatation of the left pulmonary artery. There is usually enlargement of the right ventricle. Central dilatation of the right pulmonary artery also occurs, but the dilated segment is hidden in the mediastinum (left-sided enlargement is *not* due to the direction of the jet emanating from the constricted valve).
Pulmonary embolism (Fig C9-4)	Result of vascular distension by bulk thrombus (not increased vascular resistance in the affected lung). The occluded vessel is often more sharply delineated than normal and may terminate suddenly ("knuckle" sign).
Pulmonary artery aneurysm	Congenital or post-traumatic.
Pulmonary artery coarctation	Poststenotic dilatation of the affected pulmonary artery.
Pulmonary arteriovenous fistula	Enlargement of hilar vessels is due to increased blood flow on the affected side. There is often evidence of single or multiple parenchymal nodules with characteristic feeding arteries and draining veins.
Normal variant (see Fig CA13-1)	Prominence of the left pulmonary artery occurs in adults under 30 (especially women).

Condition	Comments
Narrowed or occluded pulmonary artery	Unilateral enlargement of the opposite hilum may develop in patients with carcinoma, Swyer-James syndrome, or congenital absence of the pulmonary artery.

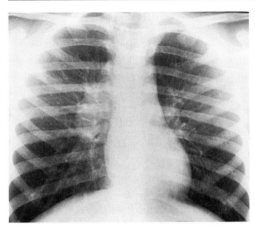

Fig C9-1. Primary tuberculosis. Enlargement of right hilar nodes without a discrete parenchymal infiltrate.

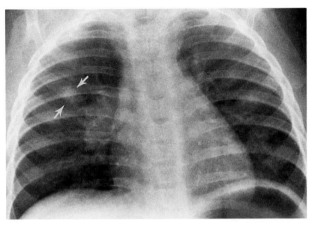

Fig C9-2. Primary tuberculosis. The combination of a focal parenchymal lesion (arrows) and enlarged right hilar lymph nodes produces the classic primary complex.

Fig C9-3. Lymphadenopathy due to oat cell carcinoma of the lung. In addition to left hilar adenopathy (open arrow), there is enlargement of anterior mediastinal lymph nodes (closed arrows).

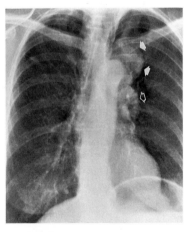

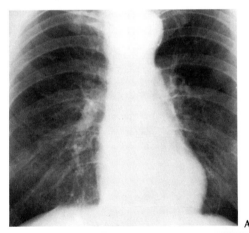

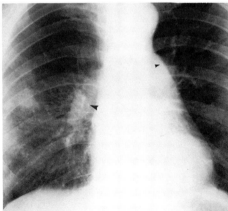

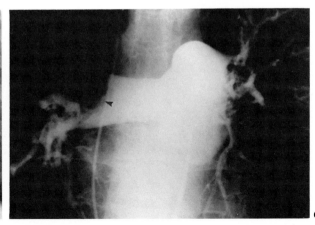

Fig C9-4. Pulmonary embolism. (A) Baseline chest radiograph demonstrates normal-sized pulmonary arteries. (B) Enlargement of the main pulmonary artery (small arrow) and right pulmonary artery (large arrow) coincides with the onset of the patient's symptoms. (C) Arteriogram demonstrates multiple bilateral pulmonary emboli and a large right saddle embolus (arrow).

BILATERAL HILAR ENLARGEMENT

Condition	Imaging Findings	Comments
Lymphadenopathy (Figs C10-1 through C10-6)	Bilateral enlargement of hilar nodes that may be associated with reticular or reticulonodular parenchymal disease.	Causes include infectious agents (especially tuberculosis, histoplasmosis, mycoplasma and viral pneumonia), malignancy (carcinoma, lymphoma), silicosis, and sarcoidosis.
Congenital heart disease (see Fig CA13-4)	Bilateral enlargement of pulmonary vessels that is usually associated with cardiomegaly.	Severe left-to-right shunts (atrial septal defect, ventricular septal defect, patent ductus arteriosus). Also cyanotic admixture lesions (transposition of great vessels, persistent truncus arteriosus).
Pulmonary arterial hypertension (Fig C10-7)	Bilateral enlargement of central pulmonary arteries with rapid tapering and small peripheral vessels. Also cardiac enlargement (especially the right ventricle).	Primary or secondary to such conditions as widespread peripheral pulmonary emboli, Eisenmenger syndrome (reversed left-to-right shunt), and chronic obstructive emphysema. Rare causes include metastases from trophoblastic neoplasms, immunologic disorders (Raynaud's phenomenon, rheumatoid disease), schistosomiasis, multiple pulmonary artery stenoses or coarctations, and vasoconstrictive diseases.
Pulmonary embolism	Bilateral enlargement of central pulmonary arteries. Usually obliteration of peripheral vessels and right-sided cardiac enlargement.	May reflect massive bilateral central emboli or widespread peripheral emboli.
Pulmonary venous hypertension	Bilateral enlargement of central pulmonary veins associated with cardiomegaly and cephalization of pulmonary blood flow.	Causes include left-sided heart failure and mitral stenosis.
Primary polycythemia	Generalized bilateral increase in central and peripheral pulmonary vascularity.	Increased blood volume produces prominence of the pulmonary vascular shadows, usually without the cardiomegaly associated with the increased pulmonary vascularity in patients with congenital heart disease. Intravascular thrombosis may cause pulmonary infarctions that appear as focal consolidations or bands of fibrosis.

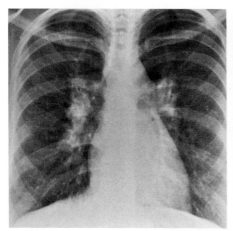
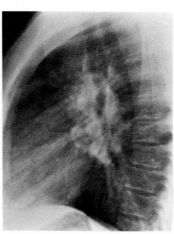

FIG C10-1. Infectious mononucleosis. (Left) Frontal and (right) lateral views of the chest demonstrate marked bilateral hilar adenopathy.

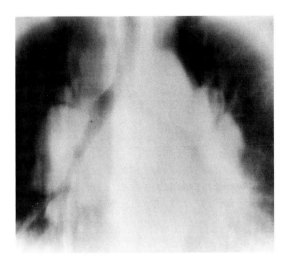

FIG C10-2. **Bronchogenic carcinoma.** Tomography demonstrates bilateral bulky hilar adenopathy typical of oat cell carcinoma.

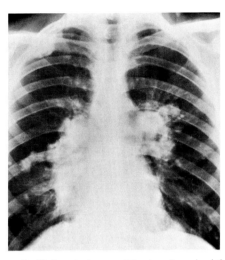

FIG C10-3. **Ossified metastases** to hilar lymph nodes bilaterally from osteogenic sarcoma. There are also multiple parenchymal metastases.

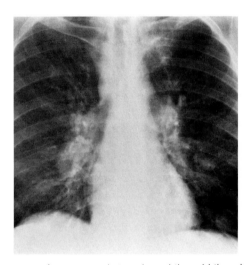

FIG C10-4. **Lymphoma.** Frontal view shows bilateral hilar adenopathy.

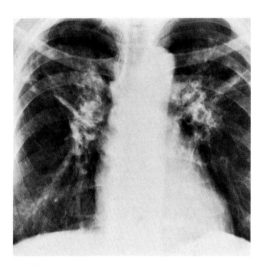

FIG C10-5. **Silicosis.** Characteristic eggshell lymph node calcification associated with bilateral perihilar masses.

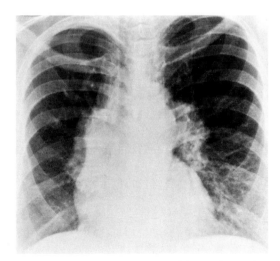

FIG C10-6. **Sarcoidosis.** Prominent bilateral hilar adenopathy with a suggestion of enlarged nodes in the right and left paratracheal regions.

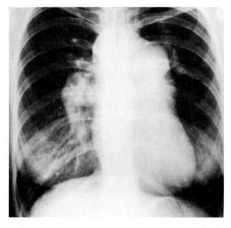

FIG C10-7. **Pulmonary arterial hypertension.** Frontal chest film in a patient with atrial septal defect and Eisenmenger physiology demonstrates a huge pulmonary outflow tract and central pulmonary arteries with abrupt tapering and sparse peripheral vasculature.[15]

HILAR AND MEDIASTINAL LYMPH NODE ENLARGEMENT

Condition	Imaging Findings	Comments
Primary tuberculosis (see Figs C9-1 and C9-2)	Enlarged hilar and paratracheal nodes that often calcify. Bilateral involvement in about 20% of cases.	Almost always associated with ipsilateral parenchymal disease (may even obscure the lymphadenopathy).
Histoplasmosis	Unilateral or bilateral enlargement of hilar, mediastinal, and occasionally intrapulmonary nodes.	Usually associated with parenchymal disease (often absent in children). The enlarged nodes may extrinsically obstruct the airways and cause distal infection or atelectasis. Calcification of nodes is common and may even lead to erosion into the bronchial lumen.
Coccidioidomycosis	Unilateral or bilateral enlargement of hilar or paratracheal nodes.	There may be associated parenchymal disease. Enlargement of paratracheal lymph nodes may indicate imminent dissemination.
Mycoplasma pneumoniae	Unilateral or bilateral enlargement of hilar nodes.	Common in children, rare in adults. Always associated with ipsilateral parenchymal disease.
Viral diseases (Fig C11-1; see Fig C10-1)	Hilar node enlargement that is often bilateral.	Psittacosis, infectious mononucleosis (also splenomegaly), rubeola, echovirus, varicella. Usually parenchymal involvement or increased bronchovascular markings.
Bacterial infections (Figs C11-2 and C11-3)	Various patterns of nodal enlargement.	Unilateral in pertussis (whooping cough) and tularemia (ipsilateral hilar enlargement in 25% to 50% of tularemic pneumonias); bilateral involvement in anthrax and plague.
Bronchogenic carcinoma (Fig C11-4)	Usually unilateral enlargement of hilar nodes.	Presenting sign in up to one third of patients (primary carcinoma arising in a major hilar bronchus or metastasis from a small primary tumor in adjacent or peripheral parenchyma). Bulky, even bilateral, nodal enlargement suggests oat cell carcinoma.
Lymphoma (Figs C11-5 and C11-6)	Enlargement of all hilar and mediastinal nodes (the anterior mediastinal and retrosternal nodes are frequently affected). Typically bilateral but asymmetric (unilateral node enlargement is very rare).	Most common radiographic finding in Hodgkin's disease (visible on the initial chest films of about 50% of patients). Pulmonary involvement or pleural effusion occurs in about 30%. Calcification may develop in intrathoracic lymph nodes after mediastinal irradiation.
Leukemia (Fig C11-7)	Symmetric enlargement of hilar and mediastinal nodes in about 25% of patients.	Lymphadenopathy occurs more commonly in lymphocytic than in myelocytic leukemia. There may also be pleural effusion and parenchymal involvement.

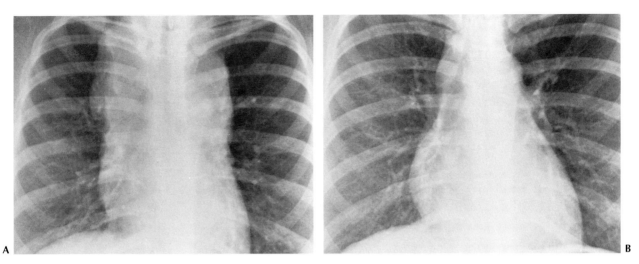

FIG C11-5. **Lymphoma.** (A) Initial chest film demonstrates marked widening of the upper half of the mediastinum due to pronounced lymphadenopathy. (B) After chemotherapy, there is a marked decrease in the width of the upper mediastinum.

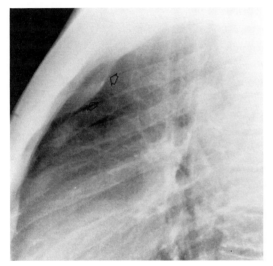

FIG C11-6. **Lymphoma.** Lateral view of the chest shows subtle enlargement of a retrosternal (internal mammary) lymph node (arrows).

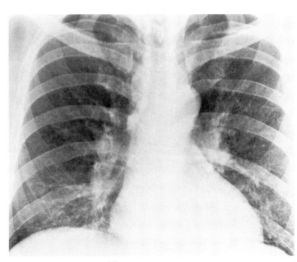

FIG C11-7. **Leukemia.** Bilateral hilar and right paratracheal lymphadenopathy.

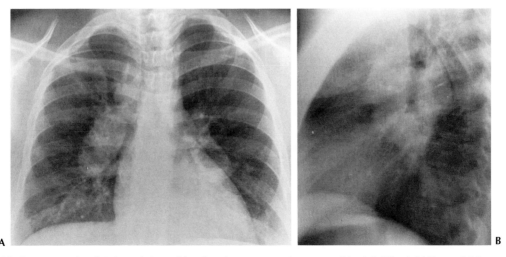

FIG C11-8. **Sarcoidosis.** (A) Frontal and (B) lateral views of the chest demonstrate enlargement of the right hilar, left hilar, and right paratracheal lymph nodes, producing the classic 1-2-3 pattern of adenopathy.

UNILATERAL, LOBAR, OR LOCALIZED HYPERLUCENCY OF THE LUNG

Condition	Imaging Findings	Comments
Local obstructive emphysema	Localized hyperlucency of the lung associated with thin, attenuated vessels (predominantly involves the lower zones).	About 50% of cases of emphysema have local rather than diffuse involvement radiographically. Affected zones show air trapping on expiration and overinflation at full lung capacity.
Bulla/bleb (Figs C12-1 and C12-2)	Sharply defined, air-containing spaces that are bounded by curvilinear, hairline shadows and vary in size from 1 cm to an entire hemithorax.	Predominantly unilateral. Unlike local obstructive emphysema, the vascular markings are absent rather than attenuated. Overinflation and air trapping usually occur.
Foreign body aspiration (see Fig C23-3)	Segmental distribution with a lower lobe predominance (especially on the right). Characteristic air trapping on expiratory films and often local oligemia.	Most common manifestation of foreign body aspiration. An opaque foreign body may be demonstrated.
Compensatory overaeration (Fig C12-3)	Overinflation and oligemia of the remaining lobe(s).	Lobar collapse or agenesis causes overdistension of the normal portions of the lung.
Pulmonary neoplasm	Segmental, lobar, or entire lung involvement. Air trapping on expiratory films.	Benign or malignant endobronchial neoplasms are a rare cause of unilateral or segmental hyperlucent lung (more commonly bronchial obstruction is complete and results in atelectasis or postobstructive pneumonia). Metastases to hilar lymph nodes occasionally compress a bronchus and cause oligemia.
Thromboembolic disease (Fig C12-4)	Affected segment often shows moderate loss of volume, but may still appear hyperlucent due to local oligemia (Westermark's sign).	Almost invariably associated with obstruction of a major lobar or segmental pulmonary artery. The affected artery is typically widened and is sharper than normal.
Unilateral or lobar emphysema (Swyer-James syndrome) (Fig C12-5)	Usually involvement of an entire lung (unilateral radiolucency), though a single lobe is occasionally affected. Air trapping during expiration (mediastinal shift toward the normal lung).	Probably results from acute pneumonia during infancy or childhood that causes bronchiolitis obliterans and an emphysema-like picture. The hilar and peripheral vessels are small.
Congenital lobar emphysema (Fig C12-6)	Severe overinflation of a pulmonary lobe (especially the right upper or the right middle lobe).	About one third of cases apparent at birth (others noted several weeks later). Severe air trapping causes marked lobar enlargement, contralateral displacement of the mediastinum, and ipsilateral depression of the diaphragm.

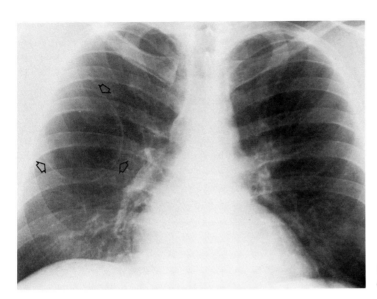

Fɪɢ C12-1. Congenital emphysematous bulla. Large thin-walled air cyst (arrows) in the midportion of the right lung.

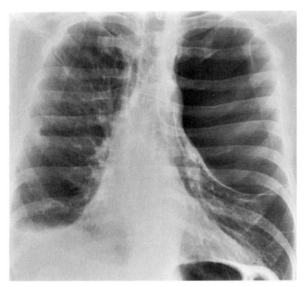

Fɪɢ C12-2. Giant emphysematous bulla. The air-containing mass fills most of the left hemithorax.

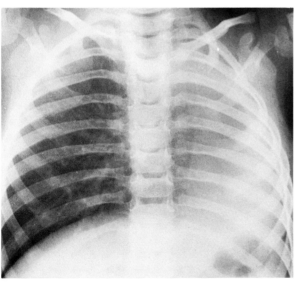

Fɪɢ C12-3. Compensatory overaeration in agenesis of the left lung. There is virtually total absence of aerated lung in the left hemithorax. The right lung is markedly overinflated and has herniated across the midline. The entire mediastinum lies within the left hemithorax. The chest wall is asymmetric and the ribs are somewhat close together on the left.

Condition	Imaging Findings	Comments
Cystic adenomatoid malformation (Fig C12-7)	Usually appears as a mass composed of numerous air-containing cysts scattered irregularly throughout a soft-tissue density in a single lobe. Occasionally a single air-filled cyst predominates, simulating infantile lobar emphysema.	Rare congenital anomaly consisting of an intralobar mass of disorganized pulmonary tissue that is classified as a hamartoma, though it is not neoplastic. If the malformation does not communicate with the bronchial tree, it contains only fluid and appears radiographically as a large pulmonary mass. The lesion expands the ipsilateral hemithorax by depressing the hemidiaphragm and shifting the mediastinum toward the contralateral side.
Hypogenetic lung syndrome (see Fig CA7-8)	Small, often hyperlucent right lung associated with a small or absent pulmonary artery. May be associated with an anomalous draining vein that forms a broad, gently curved shadow descending to the diaphragm just to the right of the heart (scimitar sign).	Very rare anomaly in which the right lung is supplied partly or completely by systemic arteries (left-to-right shunt). Other cardiopulmonary anomalies are common.
Pulmonary branch stenosis	Ipsilateral lung is hypoplastic and has reduced volume and there is an absent or diminutive hilum. No air trapping on forced expiration (unlike Swyer-James syndrome).	Very rare anomaly in which the involved lung is supplied by a hypertrophied bronchial circulation. The anomalous artery is usually on the side opposite the aortic arch (when on the left, there is a high incidence of associated cardiovascular anomalies).
Anomalous origin of left pulmonary artery from right pulmonary artery	Hyperlucent right lung due to air trapping and overinflation (anomalous vessel compresses the right main bronchus).	Very rare anomaly in which severe compression may collapse the lung. Compression of the trachea causes bilateral overinflation and air trapping on expiration. An esophagram shows pathognomonic posterior displacement of the esophagus and anterior displacement of the trachea by the interposed anomalous artery.
Congenital bronchial atresia	Characteristic elliptical mass in the hilar region representing inspissated mucus distal to the point of atresia. May have a linear or branched pattern.	Very rare anomaly that most commonly involves the apicoposterior segment of the left upper lobe (can affect various segments). The bronchial tree peripheral to the point of obliteration is patent and air enters the affected segment by collateral air drift.
Tuberculosis	Overinflation and oligemia due to partial bronchial obstruction from ipsilateral hilar lymph node enlargement.	Primarily involves the anterior segment of an upper lobe or the medial segment of the middle lobe. May be the result of bronchostenosis from a tuberculous granuloma. Complete obstruction causes atelectasis.
Staphylococcal infection (pneumatocele) (see Fig C8-2)	Characteristic thin-walled cystic spaces develop in about 50% of affected children. May be large and even fill an entire hemithorax. Often contain air-fluid levels.	Cystic spaces usually appear during the first week of a pneumonia and tend to disappear spontaneously within 6 weeks. Rare in adults. Probably results from check-valve obstruction of a communication between a peribronchial abscess and the bronchial lumen.

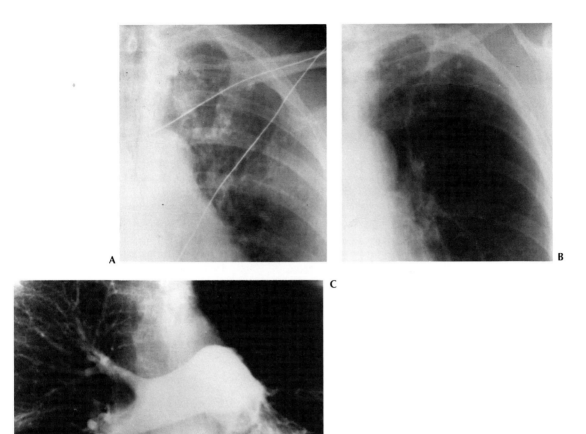

Fig C12-4. Westermark's sign of pulmonary embolism. (A) Baseline chest radiograph demonstrates normal vascularity in the left upper lobe. (B) Striking hyperlucency of the left upper lobe coincided with the onset of the patient's symptoms. (C) Arteriogram performed on the same day the film in (B) was made shows an occluding clot in the left upper lobe and multiple emboli in the right lung.

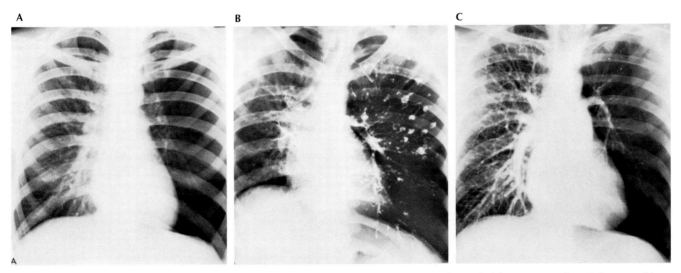

Fig C12-5. Unilateral hyperlucent lung. (A) Frontal radiograph exposed at total lung capacity reveals a marked discrepancy in the radiolucency of the two lungs, with the left showing severe oligemia but normal lung volume. (B) Frontal radiograph at residual volume after bronchography demonstrates severe air trapping in the left lung and little change in volume from total lung capacity. Since the deflation of the right lung is normal, the mediastinum has swung sharply to the right. (C) A pulmonary arteriogram shows the discrepancy in blood flow to the two lungs. The left pulmonary artery is present, though diminutive, differentiating this appearance from congenital absence of the left pulmonary artery.[6]

Condition	Imaging Findings	Comments
Hydrocarbon poisoning (Fig C12-8)	Inhalation in children can lead to the formation of pneumatoceles simulating those in staphylococcal pneumonia.	Ingestion or inhalation of hydrocarbons is the leading cause of poisoning in children. Inhaled hydrocarbon initially produces perihilar infiltrates and pulmonary edema; ingested hydrocarbon is absorbed through the gastrointestinal tract and is carried by the bloodstream to the lungs, where it adds to the pulmonary injury.
Broncholith	Overinflation and oligemia due to partial bronchial obstruction from an endobronchial calcified mass.	Erosion of a calcified lymph node (usually from histoplasmosis) into the bronchial lumen.
Sarcoidosis	Hyperlucency of the lung due to air trapping and overinflation.	Rare cause. May be due to bronchial compression from enlarged nodes, but more commonly results from endobronchial sarcoid deposits.
Nonpulmonary causes (normal vessels)		
Mastectomy	Unilateral hyperlucent lung. Absent breast shadow.	May be bilateral.
Absent pectoralis muscles (Fig C12-9)	Unilateral hyperlucent lung.	Disparity in thickness of the supraclavicular soft tissues and axillary folds.
Faulty radiographic technique	Unilateral hyperlucent lung.	Most commonly due to patient rotation, which projects the soft tissues and the spine over one side of the chest while rotating them off the opposite, more lucent side (especially prominent in women with large pendulous breasts). Another cause is improper centering of the x-ray beam.

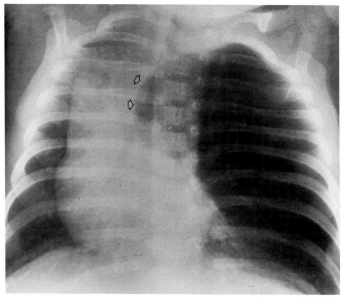

FIG C12-6. Congenital lobar emphysema. Severe overdistention of the left upper lobe causes marked radiolucency of the left hemithorax along with depression of the ipsilateral hemidiaphragm and displacement of the mediastinum into the right hemithorax. The hyperinflated left upper lobe has herniated into the right side of the chest (arrows). Note the small and widely separated bronchovascular markings in the lucent left lung.

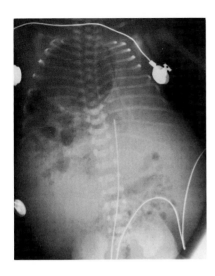

FIG C12-7. **Cystic adenomatoid malformation.** Frontal radiograph of an infant's chest and abdomen at 1 hour of age demonstrates a large lucent mass in the right hemithorax with shift of the mediastinal structures to the left. In the lower right chest, the mass appears multicystic and resembles air-filled loops of bowel. Ascites is also present.[17]

A   B

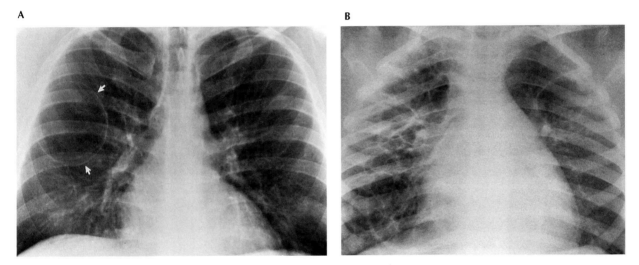

FIG C12-8. **Hydrocarbon poisoning.** (A) Large thin-walled pneumatocele (arrows). (B) Multiple thin-walled pneumatoceles bilaterally, but much more marked on the right.

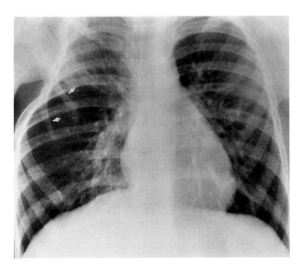

FIG C12-9. **Absence of the right pectoralis muscles.** Asymmetry of the thoracic cage with hypoplasia of the anterior ribs (arrows). The lower portion of the right lung appears hyperlucent, while the apex seems comparatively opaque.

BILATERAL HYPERLUCENT LUNGS

Condition	Imaging Findings	Comments
Chronic obstructive emphysema (Fig C13-1)	Severe hyperinflation (low, flat, or concave diaphragm; increased posteroanterior diameter of the chest; increased retrosternal space).	Marked attentuation and stretching (even virtual absence) of pulmonary vessels. Often evidence of pulmonary hypertension (enlargement of central pulmonary arteries with rapid peripheral tapering). The heart tends to be small and relatively vertical and there are often single or multiple bullae. In α_1-antitrypsin deficiency, the emphysema predominantly involves the lower lobes.
Acute asthmatic attack (Fig C13-2)	Severe overinflation of the lungs with air trapping. Characteristic tubular shadows ("tramlines") represent edema or thickening of bronchial walls.	Unlike emphysema, in this condition the vascular markings throughout the lungs are of normal caliber. Usually there is no radiographic abnormality between acute attacks.
Acute bronchiolitis	Severe overinflation of the lungs that is often associated with a reticulonodular pattern that predominantly involves the lower lobes.	Usually a viral infection of small airways that primarily affects children under age 3 and is generally self-limited. May affect adults with pre-existing respiratory disease.
Bullous disease of the lung (Figs C13-3 and C13-4)	Multiple thin-walled, sharply demarcated, air-filled avascular spaces in the lung that most commonly occur in the upper lobes and may grow. Although there is overinflation as in chronic obstructive emphysema, there is no diffuse oligemia of the remaining pulmonary parenchyma.	Generally affects males, who remain asymptomatic until there is severe compression of the uninvolved lung parenchyma. Spontaneous pneumothorax from a ruptured bulla is a common complication.
Cystic fibrosis (mucoviscidosis) (Fig C13-5)	Overinflation of the lungs associated with accentuation of interstitial markings and episodes of atelectasis and recurrent local pneumonia.	Obstruction of air passages by the tenacious mucus that is characteristic of this condition.
Diffuse infantile bronchopneumonia	Diffuse or patchy overinflation of the lungs that is usually associated with areas of consolidation and enlargement of peribronchial lymph nodes.	This pattern of bilateral pneumonia commonly complicates influenza, measles, or whooping cough. It may rarely occur with bacterial organisms.
Tracheal or laryngeal obstruction or compression	Overinflation of the lungs that may be associated with various tracheal abnormalities. Often recurrent pneumonias or evidence of parenchymal scarring from previous inflammatory disease.	Causes include vascular ring, tumor (squamous cell carcinoma, adenoid cystic carcinoma, osteochondroma, papilloma), tracheobronchomegaly (dilatation of deficient cartilage rings), relapsing polychondritis, localized tracheomalacia or stenosis (late complication of endotracheal intubation or tracheostomy), and saber-sheath trachea (narrowed coronal diameter due to chronic obstructive pulmonary disease).
Faulty radiographic technique	Bilateral "hyperlucent" lungs.	Overpenetrated film (especially portable radiographs and films on patients with very thin body habitus).

A

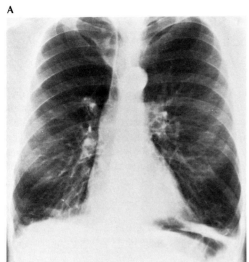

B

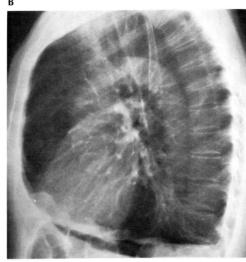

Fig C13-1. Pulmonary emphysema. (A) Frontal and (B) lateral views of the chest demonstrate severe overinflation of the lungs along with flattening and even a superiorly concave configuration of the hemidiaphragms. There is also increased size and lucency of the retrosternal air space, an increase in the anteroposterior diameter of the chest, and a reduction in the number and caliber of peripheral pulmonary arteries.

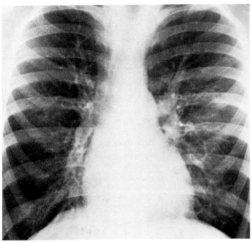

Fig C13-2. Asthma. Frontal view of the chest demonstrating hyperexpansion of the lungs with depression of the hemidiaphragms, increased anteroposterior diameter of the chest and retrosternal air space, and prominence of the interstitial structures. The heart and pulmonary vascularity are normal.

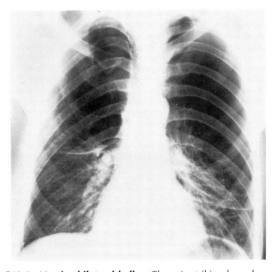

Fig C13-3. Massive bilateral bullae. There is striking hyperlucency of both lungs.

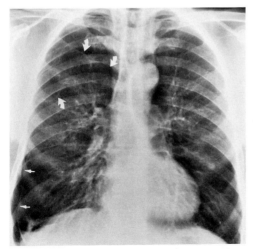

Fig C13-4. Bullous emphysema. A small right pneumothorax (straight arrows) is due to the rupture of a bullae. The curved arrows point to the walls of three of the multiple bullae in the right upper lung.

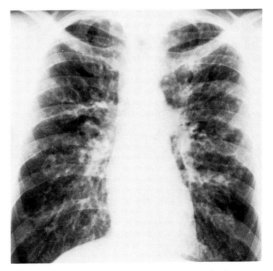

Fig C13-5. Cystic fibrosis. Bilateral overinflation of the lungs associated with coarse interstitial markings.

LOBAR ENLARGEMENT
(BULGING INTERLOBAR FISSURE)

Condition	Comments
Klebsiella pneumonia (Fig C14-1)	Tends to form a voluminous inflammatory exudate that produces a homogeneous parenchymal consolidation (containing an air bronchogram) and bulging of an interlobar fissure. High frequency of abscess and cavity formation (rare in pneumococcal pneumonia).
Pneumococcal pneumonia	Appearance similar to *Klebsiella* pneumonia, though cavitation is rare.
Hemophilus influenzae pneumonia (Fig C14-2)	Most often develops in compromised hosts (chronic pulmonary disease, immune deficiency, alcoholism, diabetes).
Plague pneumonia	Hilar and paratracheal lymph node enlargement is common.
Tuberculous pneumonia	Manifestation of primary parenchymal involvement.
Lung abscess (Fig C14-3)	Lobar expansion in an acute lung abscess (large mass, usually with cavitation) is probably related to air trapping by a check-valve mechanism in the communicating airway.
Bronchogenic carcinoma (Fig C14-4)	Any large space-occupying mass that occupies a significant volume or is contiguous with a fissure.

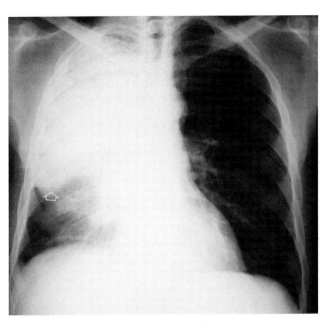

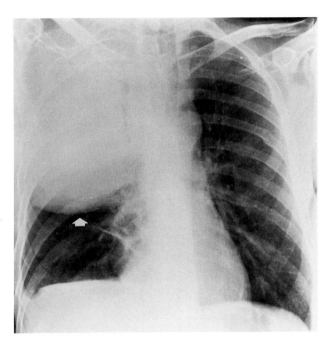

Fig **C14-1.** *Klebsiella* **pneumonia.** Downward bulging of the minor fissure (arrow) due to massive enlargement of the right upper lobe with inflammatory exudate.

Fig **C14-2.** *Hemophilus influenzae* **pneumonia.** Acute lobar consolidation with downward bulging of the minor fissure due to enlargement of the right upper lobe.[18]

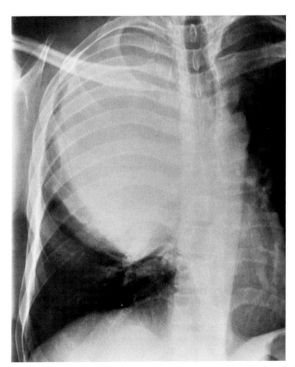

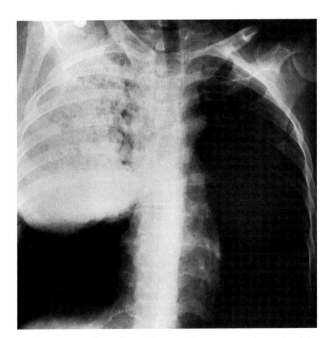

Fig **C14-3. Streptococcal pneumonia and empyema.** A large mottled opacity over the right upper lung represents an extensive empyema that obscures the underlying parenchymal pneumonia and produces an appearance indistinguishable from that of lobar enlargement. The patchy air densities in the empyema indicate communication with the bronchial tree.

Fig **C14-4. Bronchogenic carcinoma.** Appearance of massive lobar enlargement in a 30-year-old asymptomatic man.

LOBAR OR SEGMENTAL COLLAPSE*

Condition	Imaging Findings	Comments
Bronchogenic carcinoma (Fig C15-1)	Lobar collapse associated with a hilar mass (representing metastases to regional lymph nodes).	Since bronchial obstruction is a slowly progressive process, there is usually a distal infection with inflammatory exudate that prevents collapse once the bronchus is totally occluded. Characteristic Golden's S sign in right upper lobe collapse (upper laterally concave segment of the S is formed by the elevated minor fissure; lower medial convexity is caused by the tumor mass responsible for the collapse).
Bronchial adenoma (Fig C15-2)	Lobar collapse.	Most common radiographic finding of a central adenoma. Collateral air drift may prevent complete collapse.
Foreign body	Lobar or segmental collapse. An opaque foreign body may be detectable.	In adults, collapse is usually associated with aspiration of food (eg, a large piece of meat). Bizarre variety of causes in children (who more commonly present with overaeration of the lung distal to the site of obstruction due to collateral air drift).
Malpositioned endotracheal tube (Figs C15-3 and C15-4)	Usually collapse of the left lung.	Advancing the tube too far (into the bronchus intermedius) occludes the left main stem bronchus.
Mucous plug (Fig C15-5)	Primarily segmental collapse.	Most common cause of small airway obstruction. Frequent complication of abdominal and thoracic surgery, anesthesia and respiratory depressant drugs, and infectious diseases (eg, tetanus) that produce respiratory depression and impaired clearance of tracheobronchial secretions.
Mucoid impaction	Segmental or subsegmental collapse.	Develops in patients with asthma and hypersensitivity (allergic) aspergillosis.
Bronchial metastases	Lobar or segmental collapse.	Most frequently renal cell carcinoma. Also breast carcinoma and melanoma.
Chronic obstructive pulmonary disease	Segmental or subsegmental collapse (also evidence of underlying disease).	Obstruction of small airways with the formation of small intraluminal mucous plugs (most commonly in acute exacerbations of asthma, chronic bronchitis, emphysema, and bronchiolitis obliterans).

*See Figs C15-6 to C15-11.

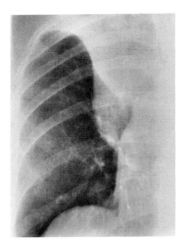

Fig C15-1. Bronchogenic carcinoma. Typical reverse S-shaped curve (Golden's sign) representing collapse of the right upper lobe associated with malignant bronchial obstruction.

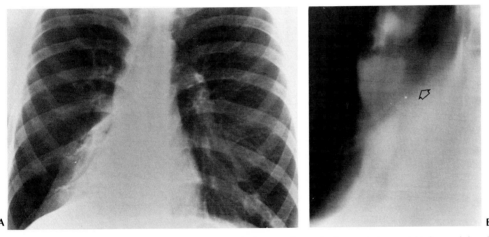

Fig C15-2. Central bronchial adenoma. (A) Frontal chest radiograph demonstrates a right lower lobe density with obscuration of the right hemidiaphragm and relative preservation of the right border of the heart, consistent with right lower lobe collapse. (B) Tomography shows an ill-defined mass causing a high-grade obstruction of the right lower lobe bronchus (arrow).

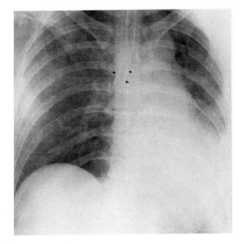

Fig C15-3. Malpositioned endotracheal tube. Collapse of the left lung, especially the left lower lobe, is due to an endotracheal tube (arrows) in the right main-stem bronchus that effectively blocks the passage of air into the left bronchial tree.

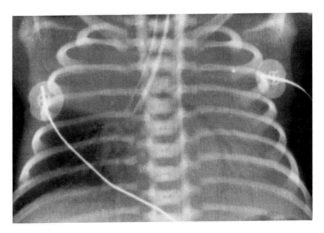

Fig C15-4. Malpositioned endotracheal tube. Inordinately low position of the endotracheal tube in the bronchus intermedius causes collapse of the right upper lobe and the entire left lung.

Condition	Imaging Findings	Comments
Pneumonia	Segmental or subsegmental collapse.	Peribronchial inflammation may lead to small airway obstruction followed by collapse. Occasionally develops in bacterial, viral, and mycoplasma pneumonias.
Cystic fibrosis	Lobar, segmental, or subsegmental collapse superimposed on a coarse interstitial pattern.	Small airway obstruction due to excessively viscous mucus that is poorly cleared from the tracheobronchial tree.
Cardiac enlargement	Usually collapse of the left lower lobe.	Dilated left atrium (mitral stenosis, atrial septal defect).
Aortic aneurysm	Lobar or segmental collapse.	Extrinsic pressure on the bronchial tree.
Mediastinal neoplasm	Lobar or segmental collapse.	Extrinsic pressure on the bronchial tree.
Inflammatory bronchial stricture	Lobar, segmental, or subsegmental collapse. Usually evidence of an alveolar or interstitial infiltrate.	Most commonly due to tuberculosis (volume loss of the upper lobe). Also histoplasmosis and other granulomatous infections.
Fractured bronchus	Lobar or segmental collapse with characteristic rounded bronchial occlusion.	Result of severe thoracic trauma. Causes a pronounced collapse because it is sudden and complete.
Pulmonary embolism	Lobar or segmental collapse.	Unusual manifestation (precise mechanism unclear).
Bronchiectasis	Lobar or segmental collapse.	Caused by retained secretions in advanced disease. More commonly, there is only moderate volume loss.
Middle lobe syndrome	Collapse of the right middle lobe. The lymph node producing the compression may contain calcium.	Chronic process caused by quiescent granulomatous lymphadenitis (histoplasmosis, tuberculosis, occasionally silicosis). A similar process may involve other lobes or segments.
Lymphadenopathy	Lobar or segmental collapse.	Hilar adenopathy is often cited as the cause of collapse, though the volume loss probably reflects the underlying pathologic process (eg, primary bronchogenic carcinoma, tuberculosis). To support this view, sarcoidosis is associated with profound hilar adenopathy yet rarely causes any volume loss.

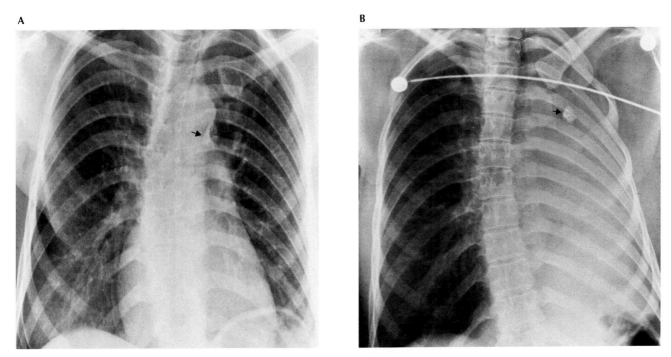

Fɪɢ C15-5. Mucous plug in a paraplegic. (A) Baseline radiograph is within normal limits. Note the calcified granuloma in the left perihilar region. (B) Complete collapse of the left lung after the lodging of a mucous plug in the left main-stem bronchus. Note the change in position of the calcified granuloma when the left lung collapses.

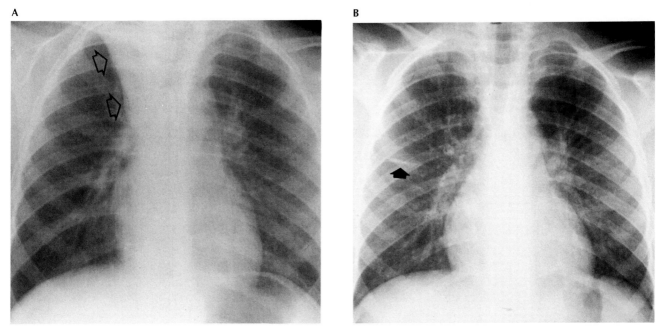

Fɪɢ C15-6. Right upper lobe collapse. (A) Initial chest radiograph demonstrates the collapsed right upper lobe, which appears as a homogeneous soft-tissue mass (arrows) in the right apex along the upper mediastinum. (B) As the collapsed lobe expands, the soft-tissue mass has disappeared and the minor fissure (arrow) has reappeared.

Condition	Imaging Findings	Comments
Radiation therapy	Lobar or segmental collapse (often a peculiar non-anatomic distribution of volume loss that coincides with the radiation port).	Late scarring may produce a substantial loss of volume superimposed on a characteristic interstitial pattern.
Broncholithiasis	Lobar or segmental collapse associated with intra-bronchial calcification.	Results from erosion of a calcified lymph node into a bronchus.

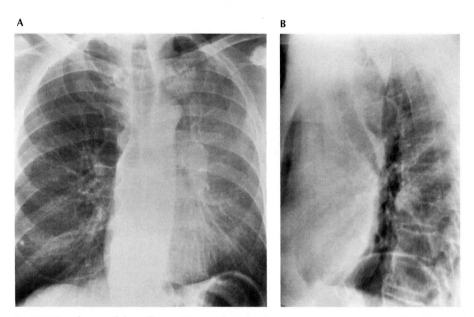

FIG C15-7. **Left upper lobe collapse.** (A) Frontal chest radiograph demonstrates a generalized increase in the density of the left hemithorax with no obliteration of the aortic knob or proximal descending aorta. The visualized vascular markings reflect lower lobe vessels. (B) A lateral view confirms the anterior position of the collapsed left upper lobe.

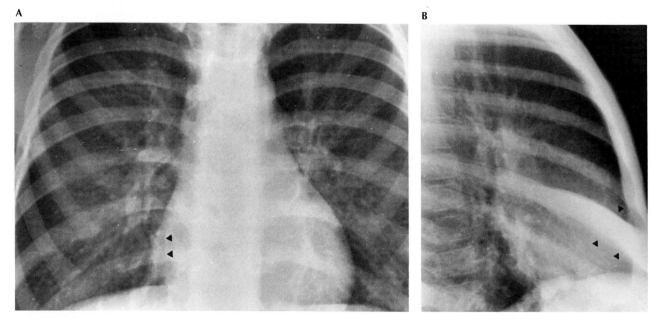

FIG C15-8. **Right middle lobe collapse.** (A) Frontal chest radiograph demonstrates minimal obliteration of the lower part of the right border of the heart (arrows). (B) Lateral view demonstrates collapse of the right middle lobe (arrows).

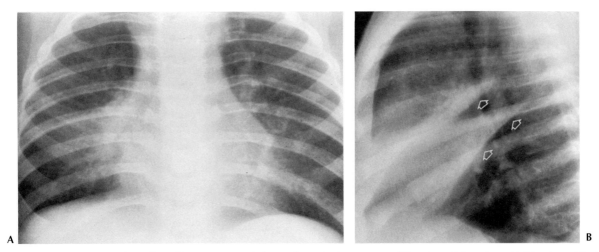

FIG C15-9. Right middle lobe and lingular collapse. (A) Frontal chest radiograph demonstrates obliteration of the right and left borders of the heart. (B) Lateral view demonstrates collapse of both the right middle lobe and the lingula (arrows).

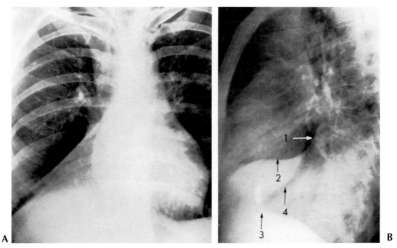

FIG C15-10. Right lower lobe collapse. (A) Frontal chest radiograph demonstrates a right lower lung density with preservation of the right border of the heart. The right hemidiaphragm is obscured. (B) Lateral view confirms the presence of right lower lobe collapse (due to bronchogenic carcinoma) with posterior displacement of the major fissure (1). The elevated right hemidiaphragm (2) is obliterated posteriorly by the airless right lower lobe, and the anterior third of the left hemidiaphragm (3) is obscured by the bottom of the heart. The overlapping shadows of the back of the heart (4), which lies in the left hemithorax, and the right hemidiaphragm simulate interlobar effusion.[19]

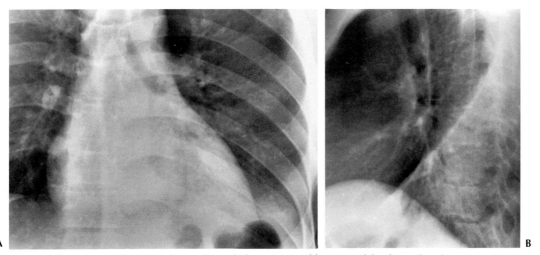

FIG C15-11. Left lower lobe collapse. (A) Frontal chest radiograph demonstrates obliteration of the descending thoracic aorta and obscuration of much of the left hemidiaphragm. (B) Lateral view confirms the posterior portion of the collapsed left lower lobe.

PULMONARY PARENCHYMAL CALCIFICATION

Condition	Imaging Findings	Comments
Histoplasmoma (Figs C16-1 and C16-2)	Central calcification that may be multiple or widespread.	Most common form of pulmonary calcification. Often associated with calcifications in regional lymph nodes and the spleen. Eccentric calcification in the mass may indicate a bronchogenic carcinoma growing around the histoplasmoma.
Other granulomatous infections (Fig C16-3)	Central calcification that may be multiple or widespread.	Tuberculosis, coccidioidomycosis. There may be calcification of regional lymph nodes. Eccentric calcification in the mass may indicate a bronchogenic carcinoma growing around the granuloma.
Fungus ball	Various patterns of calcification of the mycelial mass may occur.	Scattered small nodules of calcification, a fine rim around the periphery of the mass, or an extensive process involving most of the mycelial ball.
Chickenpox (varicella) pneumonia (Fig C16-4)	Tiny widespread calcifications.	Develops in adults one or more years after pulmonary chickenpox infection. The calcifications vary in size and number and predominate in the lower half of the lungs. No calcification of hilar lymph nodes (unlike histoplasmosis or tuberculosis).
Parasites	Multiple small pulmonary calcifications. May be solitary.	Paragonimiasis, schistosomiasis, cysticercosis, guinea worm, *Armillifer armillatus* (also in thoracic muscles or subcutaneous tissues).
Hamartoma (Fig C16-5)	Single nodule with central calcification.	Popcorn-ball calcification is pathognomonic (but occurs in less than 10%).
Silicosis (Fig C16-6)	Widespread small calcified nodules.	Punctate calcifications are reported to occur in silicotic nodules in up to 20% of cases. May also have characteristic eggshell lymph node calcification. A similar pattern may occur in coal-worker's pneumoconiosis.
Heavy metal inhalation	Widespread opaque nodules of metallic density.	Stannosis (tin), baritosis (barium), and antimony and rare-earth pneumoconioses.
Alveolar microlithiasis (see Fig C2-15)	Widespread tiny, discrete, sandlike opacities of calcific density.	Tiny spherules of calcium phosphate in myriads of alveoli and alveolar sacs. Black pleura sign (caused by the contrast between the extreme density of the lung parenchyma on one side of the pleura and the ribs on the other).

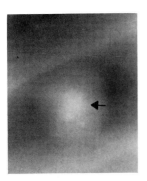

FIG C16-1. Histoplasmoma. Central calcification (arrow) in a solitary pulmonary nodule.

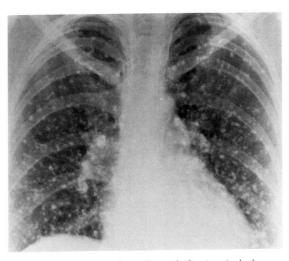

FIG C16-2. Histoplasmosis. Diffuse calcifications in the lungs produce a snowball pattern.

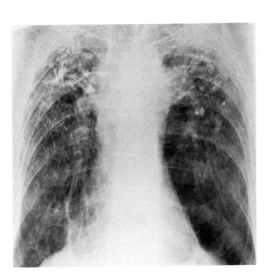

FIG C16-3. Tuberculosis. Bilateral fibrocalcific changes at the apices. There is upward retraction of the hila.

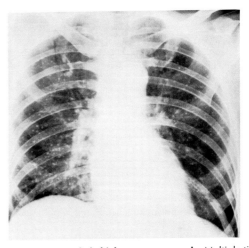

FIG C16-4. Healed chickenpox pneumonia. Multiple tiny calcific shadows are scattered widely and uniformly throughout both lungs. This 42-year-old asymptomatic man had suffered florid chickenpox with acute pneumonia 15 years earlier.[6]

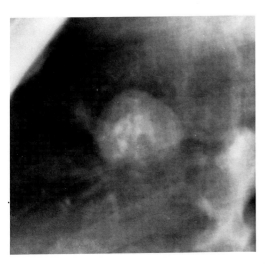

FIG C16-5. Hamartoma. Pathognomonic popcorn-ball calcification in a solitary pulmonary nodule.

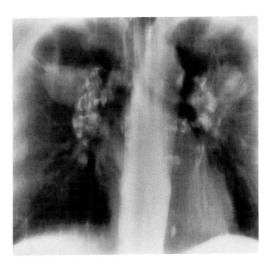

FIG C16-6. Silicosis. Tomogram of the chest demonstrates characteristic eggshell lymph node calcification associated with bilateral perihilar masses.

Condition	Imaging Findings	Comments
Pulmonary ossification	Widespread densely calcified or ossified nodules.	Manifestation of mitral stenosis (or other causes of elevated left atrial pressure). At up to 8 mm in size, usually much larger than the calcifications (up to 3 mm) of healed infectious diseases such as histoplasmosis or varicella.
Pulmonary osteopathia	Fine, branching, linear shadows of calcific density that usually involve a limited area of the lung.	Calcific density is often difficult to appreciate (since the shadows are very thin). Represents trabeculated bone along the bronchovascular distribution of the interstitial space.
Metastases (Fig C16-7)	Calcification in multiple or widespread nodules.	Rare manifestation, but virtually diagnostic of osteogenic sarcoma or chondrosarcoma. May very rarely be psammomatous calcification (thyroid, ovarian cystadenoma) or mucinous calcification (colloid carcinoma of the breast or gastrointestinal tract).
Metabolic calcification (Fig C16-8)	Widespread calcification.	Causes include primary or secondary hyperparathyroidism (especially chronic renal disease and maintenance hemodialysis), hypervitaminosis D, milk-alkali syndrome, and intravenous calcium therapy. Calcium tends to precipitate at sites of pneumonic exudation.
Broncholithiasis (Fig C16-9)	Single or multiple parabronchial or endobronchial calcifications that often occur close to the proximal margin of an area of pulmonary collapse.	Results from erosion of a calcified lymph node or parenchymal focus into a bronchus. Fragments may lodge in the bronchus and cause obstruction or be expectorated.
Bronchial adenoma	Single calcified nodule.	Calcification and ossification are rare.
Amyloidosis	Calcification or ossification in solitary or multiple masses.	Very rare manifestation. Calcification may also occur in the tracheobronchial tree.
Pulmonary thrombus	Calcification in the region of a pulmonary artery.	Thrombi in the pulmonary arteries after embolism may rarely calcify.
Pulmonary arteriovenous fistula	Single or multiple calcifications.	Rare manifestation that is probably due to phleboliths. The feeding artery and draining vein can often be detected.
Bronchogenic cyst	Curvilinear calcification about the periphery of the mass.	Cyst wall calcification is rare.

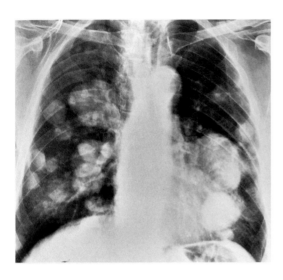

FIG C16-7. Metastases from osteosarcoma.

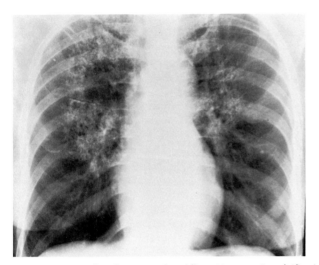

FIG C16-8. Secondary hyperparathyroidism. Heterotopic calcification in a patient with chronic renal failure.

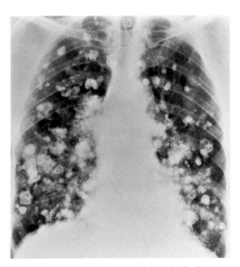

FIG C16-9. Broncholithiasis. Innumerable calcified masses scattered throughout the lungs.

PULMONARY DISEASE WITH EOSINOPHILIA

Condition	Imaging Findings	Comments
Acute idiopathic eosinophilic pneumonia (Loeffler's syndrome) (Fig C17-1)	Patchy parenchymal consolidation with blood eosinophilia.	Characteristic transitory and migratory pattern of ill-defined infiltrates that are nonsegmental in distribution and tend to involve the periphery of the lung. "Reversed pulmonary edema pattern" (involvement of the lung periphery in contrast to the perihilar or central distribution of pulmonary edema).
Chronic eosinophilic pneumonia	Patchy parenchymal consolidation with eosinophilic infiltration of the lung.	Pattern identical to that of Loeffler's syndrome, except that the lesions tend to persist unchanged for weeks unless corticosteroid therapy is instituted. Blood eosinophilia occurs in most patients, though it is not essential for the diagnosis.
Drug sensitivity (Figs C17-2 and C17-3)	Patchy nonsegmental, peripheral parenchymal consolidation with blood eosinophilia.	Sulfonamides, penicillin, isoniazid, and many other medications. Nitrofurantoin causes a diffuse reticular pattern. Withdrawal of the drug results in prompt disappearance of the clinical and radiographic manifestations.
Parasitic disease (Figs C17-4 to C17-8)	Patchy nonsegmental, peripheral parenchymal consolidation with blood eosinophilia.	Ascariasis, strongyloidiasis, tropical pulmonary eosinophilia (filariasis), ancylostomiasis (hookworm), visceral larva migrans (dog or cat roundworm), schistosomiasis. Amebiasis produces basilar consolidation (not peripheral) that may cavitate.
Hypersensitivity bronchopulmonary aspergillosis (Fig C17-9)	Round, oval, or elliptical opacities (mucous plugs) that usually develop in segmental bronchi of the upper lobes. May have homogeneous consolidation. Blood eosinophilia.	Mucous plugs contain aspergilli and eosinophils. Usually a history of long-standing bronchial asthma. Involvement of several bronchi may produce a "cluster of grapes" or Y-shaped shadows.
Asthma (Fig C17-10)	Hyperexpansion of the lungs with bronchial wall thickening (tubular shadows). Eosinophils in the sputum and slight blood eosinophilia.	Chest radiograph is often normal (especially in patients with mild disease and late age of onset). Increased incidence of pneumonia and atelectasis (mucous plugging or impaction).
Hypereosinophilic syndrome (eosinophilic leukemia)	Various patterns of eosinophilic infiltration of the pulmonary parenchyma.	Rare condition characterized by mature eosinophil infiltration of multiple organs. Occurs almost exclusively in males.
Wegener's granulomatosis (see Fig C8-12)	Patchy parenchymal consolidation with minimal blood and tissue eosinophilia.	Almost invariably multiple and frequently cavitates.
Allergic granulomatosis	Patchy parenchymal consolidation with considerable blood and tissue eosinophilia.	Granulomatous disease involving many organs and restricted to patients with a history of asthma. The consolidation is almost always multiple and frequently cavitates.

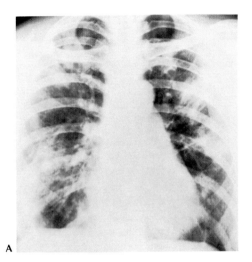

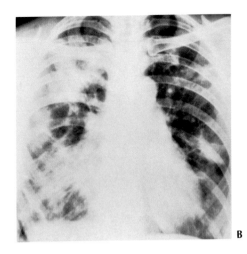

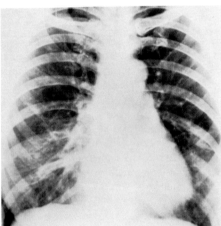

FIG C17-1. Loeffler's syndrome. (A) Initial frontal chest radiograph shows numerous bilateral areas of consolidation that have no precise segmental distribution. Note particularly the broad shadow of increased density along the lower axillary zone of the right lung. (B) One week later, the anatomic distribution of the consolidation has changed considerably, being more extensive in the right upper and lower lobes and less extensive in the left upper lobe. (C) One week later, after adrenocorticotropic hormone (ACTH) therapy, the radiographic abnormalities have completely resolved.[6]

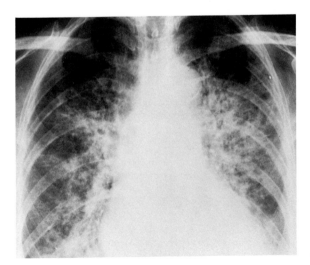

FIG C17-2. Nitrofurantoin-induced lung disease. Mixed alveolar and interstitial pattern in an elderly woman who presented with progressive cough and dyspnea after the long-term use of nitrofurantoin for recurring urinary tract infections.[10]

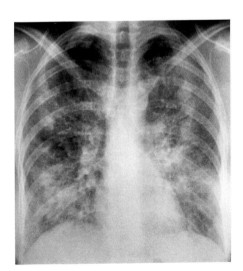

FIG C17-3. Methotrexate-induced lung disease. The diffuse, bilateral, patchy densities were changeable and fleeting during the illness. The radiographic findings cleared completely after steroid therapy.[20]

Condition	Imaging Findings	Comments
Polyarteritis nodosa	Fleeting nonsegmental patchy consolidation with tissue eosinophilia.	Hypersensitivity angiitis that typically involves the kidneys and may cause systemic hypertension. Other findings include pulmonary edema, accentuated interstitial markings, and miliary nodules.
Desquamative interstitial pneumonitis (DIP) (Fig C17-11)	Generalized reticular pattern with small numbers of eosinophils in the interstitium.	Progressive loss of lung volume on sequential studies. Spontaneous pneumothorax and pleural effusion may occur.
Coccidioidomycosis (Fig C17-12)	Various patterns of pulmonary disease, often with significant blood eosinophilia.	May produce parenchymal consolidation, nodules (single, multiple, miliary) that may cavitate, and lymph node enlargement.

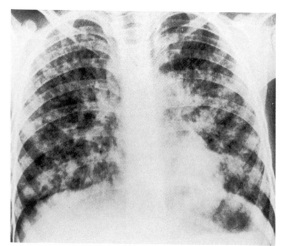

FIG C17-4. Ascariasis. Extensive pulmonary infiltrates due to the presence of *Ascaris* larvae in the lungs.[21]

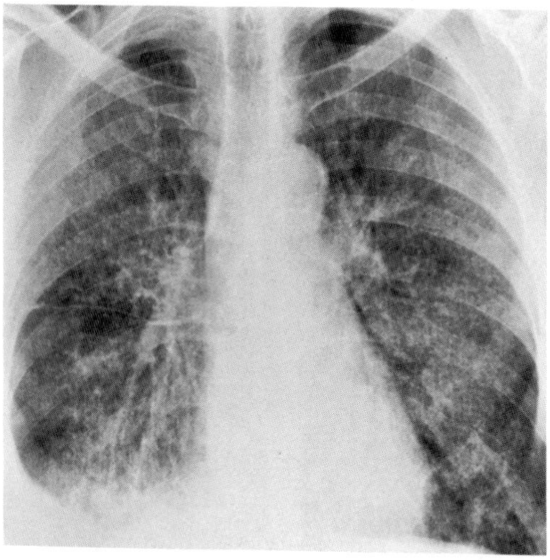

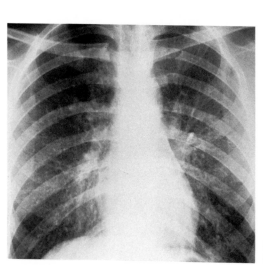

FIG C17-5. Strongyloidiasis. Chest radiograph during the stage of larval migration shows a pattern of miliary nodules diffusely distributed throughout both lungs. There is also a large right pleural effusion.

FIG C17-6. Tropical pulmonary eosinophilia. Multiple small nodules with indistinct outlines produce a pattern of generalized increase in lung markings.[22]

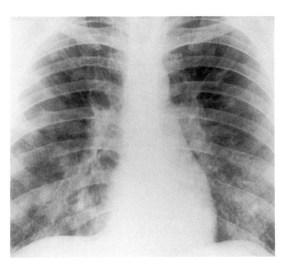

FIG C17-7. Cutaneous larva migrans. Multiple small irregular areas of air-space consolidation widely scattered throughout both lungs.[23]

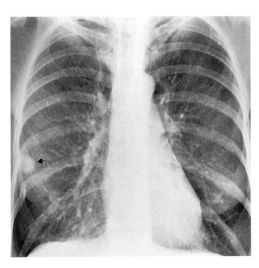

FIG C17-8. Dirofilariasis. Well-circumscribed solitary pulmonary nodule (arrow) that is indistinguishable from a malignant coin lesion.

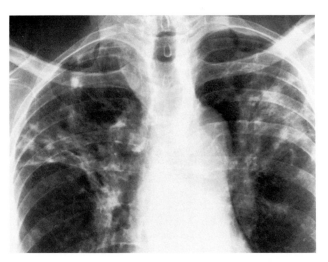

FIG C17-9. Hypersensitivity bronchopulmonary aspergillosis. Patchy opacifications in segmental bronchi of the upper lobes in a patient with asthma and pronounced peripheral eosinophilia.

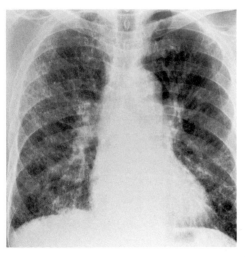

FIG C17-10. Asthma. Recurrent pulmonary infections have led to the development of diffuse pulmonary fibrosis.

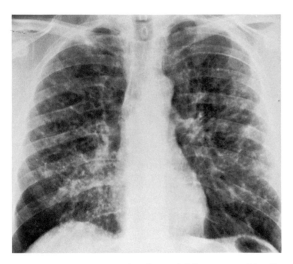

FIG C17-11. Desquamative interstitial pneumonitis. Generalized reticular pattern throughout both lungs.

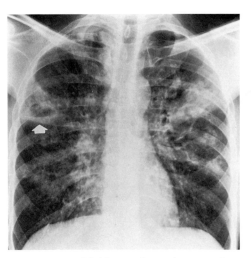

FIG C17-12. Coccidioidomycosis. Patchy areas of air-space consolidation in both lungs. There is an air-fluid level (arrow) in a right upper lobe cavity abutting the minor fissure.

SKIN DISORDER
COMBINED WITH WIDESPREAD LUNG DISEASE

Condition	Imaging Findings	Comments
Systemic lupus erythematosus (see Figs C28-4 and C29-9)	Pericardial and pleural effusions. Nonspecific, poorly defined patchy areas of parenchymal consolidation that are usually in the lung bases and situated peripherally (probably reflect acute pneumonia). Fleeting basilar atelectasis may occur.	Cutaneous manifestations (in 80% of patients) include butterfly rash, discoid lupus, alopecia, and photosensitivity. Arthritis and arthralgia occur in about 95% of cases.
Sarcoidosis (Fig C18-1)	Bilateral hilar and paratracheal adenopathy. Diffuse reticulonodular or fluffy alveolar pattern.	Cutaneous involvement (about 30% of cases) includes slightly raised, often purplish nodules (lupus pernio) that usually appear about the face, neck, shoulders, and digits. Large plaques resembling psoriasis may occur over the trunk or extremities.
Scleroderma (see Fig C4-5)	Diffuse interstitial pattern that predominantly involves the lower lung zones.	Characteristic thickened and inelastic skin. Erosion of terminal phalangeal tufts with calcification in the finger tips.
Dermatomyositis	Diffuse interstitial pattern that predominantly involves the lung bases.	Cutaneous changes include puffiness of the face and an erythematous rash involving the neck, ears, chest, and shoulders. Bilateral and symmetric muscle weakness and diffuse subcutaneous and muscular calcification. Traditionally associated with an increased incidence of malignancy.
Rheumatoid arthritis (see Fig C3-12)	Diffuse reticulonodular pattern, more prominent in the lung bases. Discrete nodular lesions (similar to subcutaneous nodules). Pleural effusion.	The hands are often cool and damp (reflecting autonomic nervous system dysfunction) and palmar erythema often occurs. In long-standing disease, the skin over the distal extremities often becomes atrophic and bruises easily. Nail-fold thrombi, small infarcts on the volar surface of the hands, digital gangrene, and ulcers of the lower part of the leg and ankle are manifestations of rheumatoid vasculitis.
Neurofibromatosis	Diffuse interstitial pulmonary fibrosis and bullae. Cutaneous nodules may project over the lungs.	Multiple fibromas and neuromas of the skin with café-au-lait spots. There may be posterior mediastinal masses and skeletal deformities (scoliosis and rib lesions).
Tuberous sclerosis (Fig C18-2)	Diffuse interstitial fibrosis with honeycombing. Pneumothorax is common.	Cutaneous manifestations include adenoma sebaceum (acneform butterfly rash on the face) and subungual fibromas. Potato-like tumor masses also involve the brain, kidneys, and eyes.
Wegener's granulomatosis (see Fig C8-12)	Multiple bilateral nodules. Thick-walled cavities in about half the cases.	Skin ulcerations and vesicular or hemorrhagic cutaneous lesions.

Condition	Imaging Findings	Comments
Measles (Fig C18-6)	Reticular pattern in primary pneumonia. Segmental consolidation and atelectasis indicate bacterial superinfection.	Red maculopapular rash that breaks out first on the forehead, spreads downward over the face, neck, and trunk, and appears on the feet on the third day. Characteristic Koplik's spots (small, red, irregular lesions with blue-white centers) appear 1 to 2 days before the onset of the rash on the mucous membranes of the mouth and occasionally on the conjunctiva or intestinal mucosa.
Acanthosis nigricans	Increased incidence of bronchogenic carcinoma.	Bilateral, symmetric hyperkeratosis and hyperpigmentation of the skin (especially in the flexural and intertriginous areas). High incidence of abdominal malignancy (especially of the stomach).
Amyloidosis (Fig C18-7)	Various patterns (intra-airway mass causing atelectasis or obstructive pneumonitis, parenchymal form with solitary or multiple masses, miliary form, lymphadenopathy, reticulonodular pattern).	Skin lesions are one of the most characteristic manifestations of amyloidosis and consist of slightly raised, waxy papules or plaques that are usually clustered in the folds of the axillary, anal, or inguinal regions; the face and neck; or mucosal areas such as the ear or tongue. Gentle rubbing may induce bleeding into the skin, leading to purpura.
Hypersensitivity reaction (Fig C18-8)	Various patterns depending on the stage of the condition.	Many forms of allergy, drug sensitivity, and parasitic infestation.
Burns	Various patterns (patchy pulmonary consolidation, atelectasis, pulmonary edema).	Cutaneous manifestations vary depending on the severity of the burn.
Bleeding disorders (see Fig C2-11)	Alveolar infiltrates that may eventually produce interstitial fibrosis after repeated episodes of bleeding.	Spectrum of appearances from extensive macules (ecchymoses) to tiny petechiae.

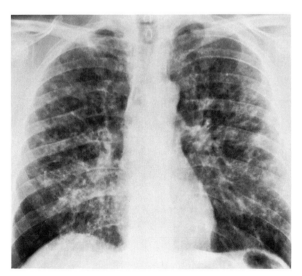

FIG C18-7. **Amyloidosis.** Diffuse reticulonodular pattern.

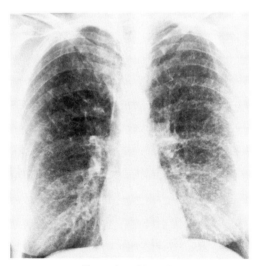

FIG C18-8. **Busulfan-induced lung disease.** Diffuse coarse reticulonodular pattern.

MENISCUS (AIR-CRESCENT) SIGN*

Condition	Comments
Aspergillus fungus ball (Figs C19-1 and C19-2)	Aspergillosis is the most common cause of this appearance. It generally develops in immunocompromised patients (especially those with disseminated malignancy).
Fungus ball of other etiology	Candidiasis, coccidioidomycosis, and nocardiosis.
Hydatid (echinococcal) cyst (Fig C19-3)	Rupture between the pericyst and the exocyst permits the entry of air between these layers.
Lung abscess with inspissated pus	Various infectious agents.
Neoplasm	Bronchogenic carcinoma, bronchial adenoma, sarcoma, and sclerosing hemangioma.
Granuloma	Tuberculous, fungal, or idiopathic.
Gangrene of lung	Large mass of necrotic lung in an abscess cavity. Most frequent in pneumococcal or *Klebsiella* pneumonia.
Intracavitary blood clot	Blood clot in a tuberculous cavity, infarct, or pulmonary laceration.

*Lucent crescent along the inner border of a cavity or between a dense parenchymal lesion and surrounding lung structures.

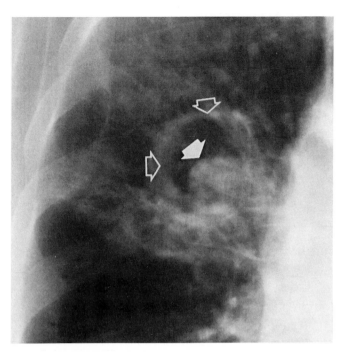

FIG C19-1. **Aspergillosis.** A mycetoma (solid arrow) appears as a homogeneous rounded mass that is separated from the thick wall of the cavity by a crescent-shaped air space (open arrows).

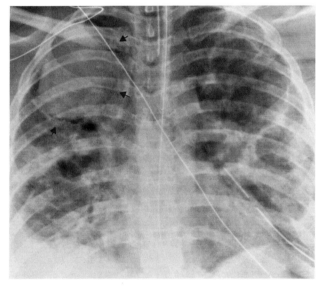

FIG C19-2. **Aspergillosis.** Multiple cavities of various sizes are superimposed on a diffuse pulmonary infiltrate. A fungus ball almost fills the large cavity in the right upper lobe (arrows). A right pleural effusion is also seen in this patient with chronic lymphocytic leukemia.

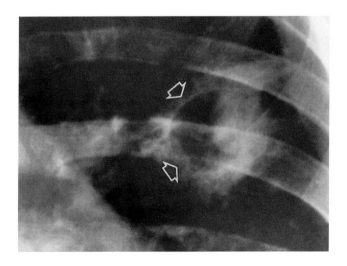

FIG C19-3. **Hydatid cyst.** A crescent of air (arrows) is seen about the periphery of the echinococcal cyst.

ANTERIOR MEDIASTINAL LESIONS

Condition	Imaging Findings	Comments
Retrosternal thyroid (Fig C20-1)	Sharply defined, smooth or lobulated mass that occurs in the superior portion of the mediastinum and may calcify.	Typically compresses the trachea or the esophagus or both. Occasionally occurs in the posterior mediastinum (almost exclusively on the right).
Thymoma (Figs C20-2 and C20-3)	Round or oval, smooth or lobulated mass that often calcifies and may protrude to one or both sides of the mediastinum. Usually arises near the junction of the heart and great vessels (displacing them posteriorly).	High fat content (relatively lucent on plain films and easily apparent on CT). Some 25% to 50% of patients have myasthenia gravis (about 15% of patients with myasthenia gravis have thymic tumors). The normal thymus appears as an anterior mediastinal mass in neonates.
Teratoma and other germinal cell neoplasms (Fig C20-4)	Round or oval, smooth or lobulated mass that may protrude to one or both sides of the mediastinum.	Calcification, bone, teeth, or fat may occur in teratomas and dermoid cysts. Benign lesions tend to be smooth and cystic, while malignant lesions are often lobulated and solid.
Lymphoma (especially Hodgkin's)/leukemia (Fig C20-5)	Enlargement of anterior mediastinal and retrosternal lymph nodes commonly occurs.	The presence of anterior mediastinal nodes in lymphoma is a differential point from sarcoidosis (which also affects hilar nodes but not nodes in the anterior compartment). There is often symmetric widening of the superior mediastinum on frontal views.
Lymphangioma (hygroma)	Smooth or lobulated mass in the superior portion of the mediastinum.	Benign or invasive lesion that is often associated with a soft-tissue mass in the neck. Chylothorax may develop.
Mesenchymal tumor (Fig C20-6)	Various patterns.	May be benign or malignant. A striking lucency suggests a lipoma or lipomatosis (steroid therapy). Phleboliths are diagnostic of a hemangioma.
Parathyroid tumor	Smooth or lobulated mass that may be too small to be detectable on plain films.	May displace the esophagus. There is often evidence of hyperparathyroidism in the thoracic spine.
Aneurysm of ascending aorta or sinus of Valsalva (Fig C20-7)	Saccular or fusiform mass that tends to extend anteriorly and to the right.	May erode the sternum. Calcification is relatively uncommon.
Morgagni's hernia (see Fig C34-7)	Round or oval lower mediastinal mass that is almost invariably on the right.	Presence of gas-filled bowel (or contrast-filled colon from an enema) in the mass is diagnostic. The hernia appears as a homogeneous opacity if it is filled with liver or omentum (mimics a fat pad or a pericardial cyst).

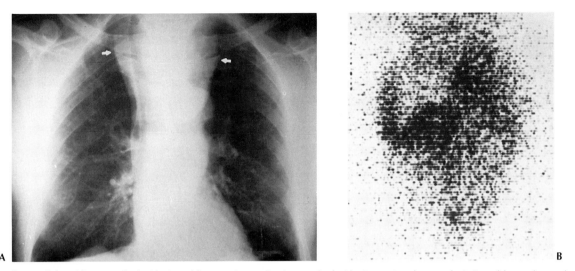

FIG C20-1. **Substernal thyroid.** (A) Marked widening of the superior mediastinum to both sides (arrows) and severe deviation of the trachea to the right. (B) Iodine-131 scan shows increased uptake of the radionuclide in the area of the mass seen on the radiograph.[24]

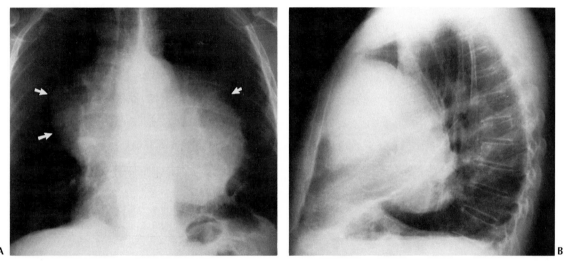

FIG C20-2. **Thymoma.** (A) Frontal view shows a large bilateral lobulated mass (arrows) extending to both sides of the mediastinum. (B) Lateral view shows filling of the anterior precardiac space by a mass and posterior displacement of the left side of the heart.

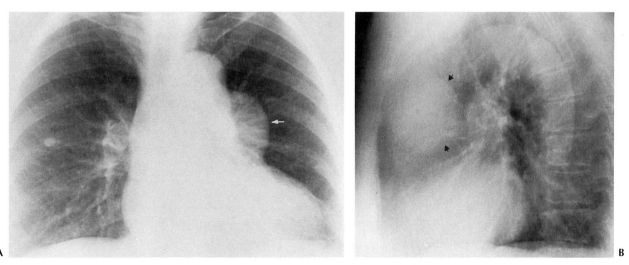

FIG C20-3. **Thymoma with myasthenia gravis.** (A) Frontal and (B) lateral views of the chest demonstrate a large mass in the anterior mediastinum (arrows).

Condition	Imaging Findings	Comments
Pericardial cyst **(Fig C20-8)**	Round or lobulated, sharply demarcated lower mediastinal mass that is usually located in the right cardiophrenic angle.	Typically touches both the anterior chest wall and the anterior portion of the right hemidiaphragm. Usually asymptomatic.
Mediastinal hemorrhage/ **hematoma**	Uniform, symmetric widening of the mediastinum, especially the superior portion.	Generally a history of trauma, surgery, or dissecting aneurysm. A discrete hematoma may compress the superior vena cava and calcify. Any mediastinal compartment may be involved.
Mediastinitis **(see Figs C21-6 and C21-7)**	Generalized widening of the mediastinum, usually most evident superiorly. A lobulated paratracheal mass predominantly projecting to the right may develop in chronic disease.	Acute mediastinitis is most often due to esophageal rupture and may be associated with mediastinal air. Chronic mediastinitis (granulomatous or sclerosing) may calcify and compress vessels (especially the superior vena cava) or a major airway.
Benign lymphoid **hyperplasia (Castleman's** **disease)**	Solitary and sharply defined mass.	Although most common in the middle and posterior compartments, in the anterior mediastinum the lesion tends to be lobulated (suggesting a thymoma or teratoma).

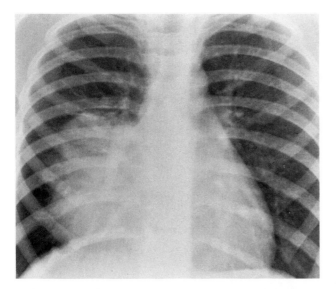

FIG C20-4. **Teratodermoid tumor.** Large lobulated mass confluent with the right border of the heart.

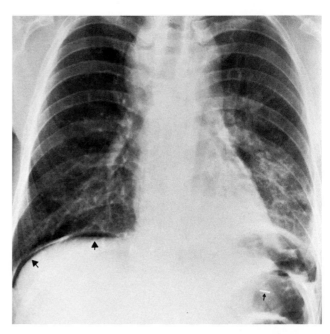

FIG C20-5. **Lymphoma.** Diffuse widening of the upper portion of the mediastinum due to lymphadenopathy. There is an ill-defined lymphomatous parenchymal infiltrate at the left base. The metallic clip overlying the region of the spleen (small arrow) and the small amount of free intraperitoneal gas seen under the right hemidiaphragm (large arrows) are evidence of a recent exploratory laparotomy and splenectomy for staging of the lymphoma.

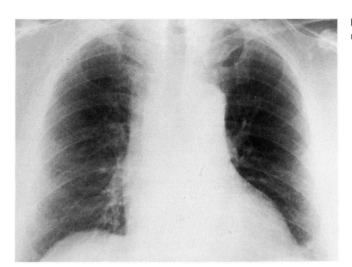

Fɪɢ C20-6. Mediastinal lipomatosis. Generalized widening of the upper mediastinum.[25]

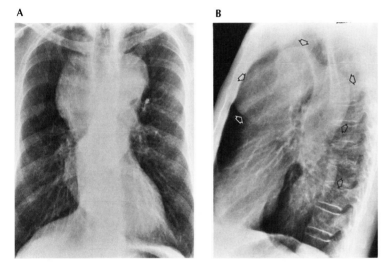

Fɪɢ C20-7. Aneurysm of the thoracic aorta. (A) Frontal and (B) lateral views of the chest demonstrate marked dilatation of both the ascending and descending portions of the thoracic aorta (arrows), producing anterior and posterior mediastinal masses, respectively.

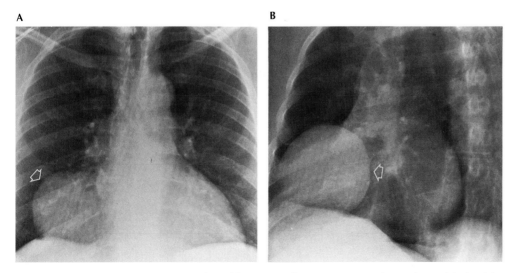

Fɪɢ C20-8. Pericardial cyst. (A) Frontal and (B) oblique views demonstrate a smooth mass (arrows) in the right cardiophrenic angle.

ANTERIOR MEDIASTINAL LESIONS
ON COMPUTED TOMOGRAPHY

Condition	Comments
Fat density **(−20 to −100 H)** **Lipomatosis**	Frequent cause of generalized mediastinal widening. Excess fat deposition in the mediastinum may be associated with moderate obesity, steroid therapy, Cushing's syndrome, or diabetes or may be a normal variant in nonobese patients. Fat deposition localized to the superior portion of the anterior compartment may simulate a mass or aortic dissection.
Lipoma	Benign collection of fatty tissue that is most common in the anterior mediastinum, though it can also occur in the middle and posterior mediastinum and adjacent to the diaphragm. Thymolipomas are anterior mediastinal masses that may be indistinguishable from lipomas. Liposarcomas are extremely rare, more commonly occur in the posterior mediastinum, generally have a higher density than benign fat, are inhomogeneous, and tend to show features of mediastinal invasion.
Omental hernia	Herniation of omental fat through a foramen of Morgagni hernia can present as a localized fatty mass virtually indistinguishable from a lipoma.

Water density
(0 to 15 H)
  Thymic cyst
  (Fig C20A-1)
	True congenital thymic cysts are rare and originate from the thymopharyngeal duct. Although usually asymptomatic, large cysts can produce tracheal or cardiac compression. They are usually round and are frequently multiloculated. Hemorrhage into the cyst is common and the cyst cavity often contains old blood, necrotic material, and cholesterol crystals so that its CT attenuation value may vary considerably from that of water. Cystic degeneration of a thymoma or thymic involvement by Hodgkin's disease or a germinoma may produce an indistinguishable CT appearance.

Soft-tissue density
(15 to 40 H)
  Thymoma
  (Figs C20A-2 and
  C20A-3)
	Wide variation of CT appearances with attenuation values varying from the low density of fat to soft-tissue density. Calcification is often visible in the mass. CT findings strongly suggestive of malignancy include extension of tumor into the mediastinum or lung parenchyma, pleural deposits (especially posteriorly and in the costophrenic angles) from transpleural seeding of tumor, and irregular pericardial thickening suggesting pericardial implants. Preservation of the low-density plane of cleavage representing fat between the tumor and mediastinal structures may be CT evidence of benignancy.

(continued page 106)

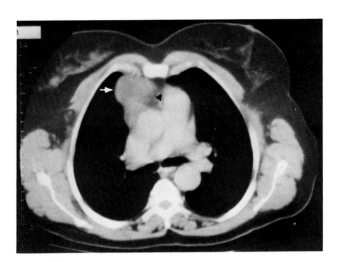

FIG C20A-1. **Thymic cyst.** Water-density mass (arrows) in the anterior mediastinum.

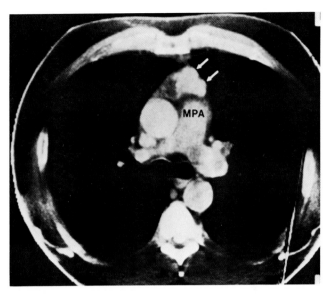

FIG C20A-2. **Thymoma.** Slightly lobulated mass (arrows) anterior to the main pulmonary artery (MPA) in a patient with myasthenia gravis.[26]

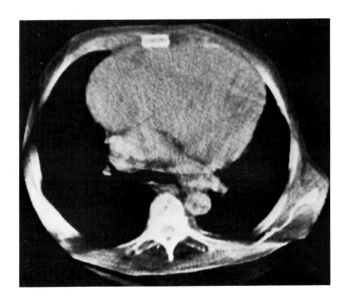

FIG C20A-3. **Thymoma.** Enormous soft-tissue mass in the anterior mediastinum with posterior displacement of other mediastinal structures. No difference in density can be seen between the mass and the heart behind it.

Condition	Comments
Thymic hyperplasia	Generalized enlargement of the thymus with preservation of its typical bilobed configuration.
Retrosternal thyroid	There is usually evidence of a connection between the mass and the thyroid gland in the neck. CT scans may show focal calcifications in the mass that are not detectable on plain chest radiographs. Multinodular goiters typically show a marked, rapid, and prolonged enhancement after the injection of intravenous contrast material.
Parathyroid tumor **(Fig C20A-4)**	Typically a small rounded mass that enhances more than muscle or lymph nodes but less than the great vessels.
Teratoma and other **germinal cell neoplasms** **(Fig C20A-5)**	Solid teratomas are indistinguishable from other soft-tissue tumors. "Cystic" teratomas are not of homogeneous water density but rather appear as complex masses with components of fat, bone, and muscle density, reflecting their varied composition of tissues from all three germ layers. Cystic teratomas often demonstrate fat-fluid interfaces and may contain calcifications and soft-tissue nodules in the mass.
Lymphoma	Involvement of anterior mediastinal lymph nodes lying ventral to the aorta and superior vena cava. The presence of enlarged nodes in this region is a differential point from sarcoidosis, which also affects hilar nodes (as does lymphoma) but not nodes in the anterior compartment.
Other neoplasms	Lymphangioma (hygroma), neurofibroma, other spindle cell tumors.
Mediastinitis/abscess	Suggested by the presence of bubbles of gas or a discrete cavity with a thick, shaggy wall.
Morgagni's hernia	A hernia containing fluid-filled bowel or part of the liver produces a mass of soft-tissue density.
Mediastinal hemorrhage/ **hematoma**	Uniform, symmetric widening of the mediastinum (especially the superior portion) in a patient with a history of trauma, surgery, or dissecting aneurysm.
Vascular/enhancing	Aneurysms, ectatic vessels.
Intrinsic high density **(more than 90 H)**	Retrosternal thyroid.

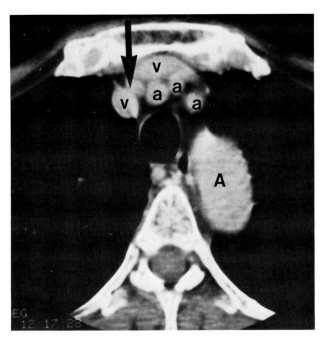

FIG C20A-4. Ectopic parathyroid adenoma. Small soft-tissue mass (arrow) in the anterior mediastinum. A, aorta; a, major branches of the aorta; and v, brachiocephalic veins.[27]

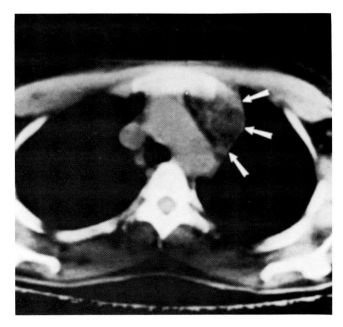

FIG C20A-5. Teratodermoid tumor. Inhomogeneous mass (arrows) lies lateral to the aortic arch and contains fat, near-water, and some tissue densities.[26]

MIDDLE MEDIASTINAL LESIONS

Condition	Imaging Findings	Comments
Lymph node enlargement (Fig C21-1)	Unilateral or bilateral hilar and paratracheal masses.	Most commonly due to metastases, tuberculosis, histoplasmosis, lymphoma, pneumoconiosis, or sarcoidosis.
Aneurysm of aorta or major branch (Fig C21-2)	Various patterns, depending on the location of the aneurysm.	Transverse arch aneurysms typically obliterate the aorticopulmonary window and are symptomatic. Mural calcification is relatively common. Mediastinal masses may also be caused by pseudocoarctation of the aorta and by dilatation of the superior vena cava or azygos vein (see pages 206 to 208)
Bronchogenic cyst (Figs C21-3 and C21-4)	Round or oval, well-defined mass that is often lobulated and tends to mold itself to surrounding structures (because of its fluid contents).	Most commonly located just inferior to the carina. Often protrudes to the right and overlaps the right hilar shadow. Rarely communicates with the tracheobronchial tree.
Mediastinal hemorrhage/ hematoma (Fig C21-5)	Uniform, symmetric widening of the mediastinum (especially the superior portion).	Generally a history of trauma, surgery, or dissecting aneurysm. A discrete hematoma may compress the superior vena cava and calcify.
Mediastinitis (Figs C21-6 and C21-7)	Generalized widening of the mediastinum, usually most evident superiorly. A lobulated paratracheal mass predominantly projecting to the right may develop in chronic disease.	Acute mediastinitis is most often due to esophageal rupture and may be associated with mediastinal air. Chronic mediastinitis (granulomatous or sclerosing) may calcify and compress vessels (especially the superior vena cava) or a major airway.
Pleuropericardial (mesothelial) cyst	Round, oval, or teardrop mass with smooth margins.	Fluid-filled cyst that is almost always asymptomatic and may change shape with respiration or alteration in body position. May also involve the anterior mediastinum.
Intrapericardial hernia (Fig C21-8)	Gas-filled loops of bowel that lie alongside the heart and remain in conformity with the heart border on multiple projections (including decubitus views).	Extremely rare congenital or posttraumatic lesion that can contain (in decreasing order of frequency) omentum, colon, small bowel, liver, or stomach. Although often asymptomatic for long periods, most patients eventually present with cardiorespiratory or gastrointestinal complaints.
Benign lymphoid hyperplasia (Castleman's disease)	Smooth or lobulated, solitary mass.	Rare condition that most often involves the posterior mediastinum.

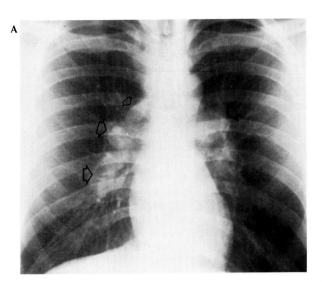

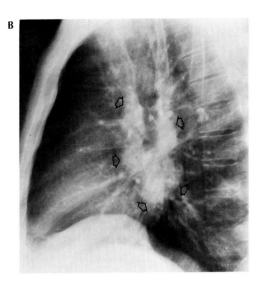

FIG C21-1. Mediastinal lymphadenopathy in sarcoidosis. (A) Frontal and (B) lateral views of the chest demonstrate enlarged mediastinal lymph nodes (arrows).

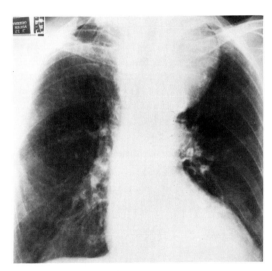

FIG C21-2. Aneurysm of the left subclavian artery. Left superior mediastinal widening in an elderly woman without chest symptoms.[25]

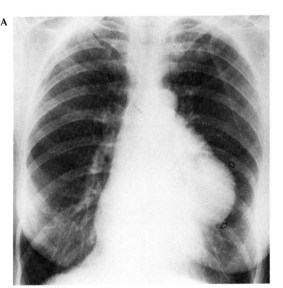

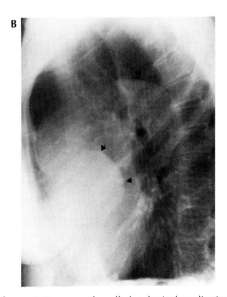

FIG C21-3. Bronchogenic cyst. (A) Frontal and (B) lateral views of the chest demonstrate a smooth-walled, spherical mediastinal mass (arrows) projecting into the left lung and left hilum.

A

B

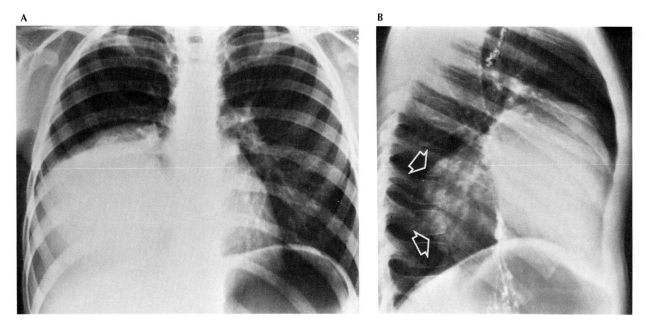

FIG C21-4. Bronchogenic cyst. (A) Frontal and (B) lateral views of the chest demonstrate a huge middle mediastinal mass (arrows) protruding to the right and filling much of the lower half of the right hemithorax. The patient was asymptomatic.

A

B

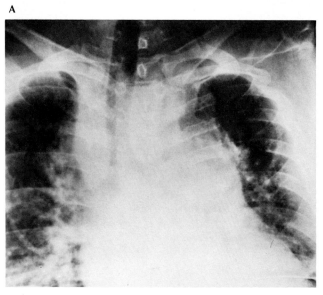

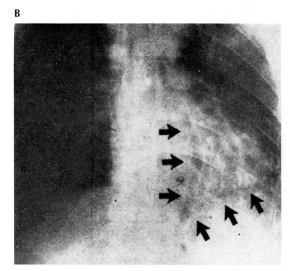

FIG C21-5. Aortic transection. Frontal chest radiograph taken immediately after trauma demonstrates mediastinal widening, obscuration of the aorta, deviation of the trachea to the right, and downward displacement of the left main-stem bronchus.[28]

FIG C21-6. Acute mediastinitis due to rupture of the esophagus. Plain radiograph demonstrates linear lucent shadows (arrows) that represent localized mediastinal emphysema and correspond to the fascial planes of the mediastinal and diaphragmatic pleurae in the region of the lower esophagus.[29]

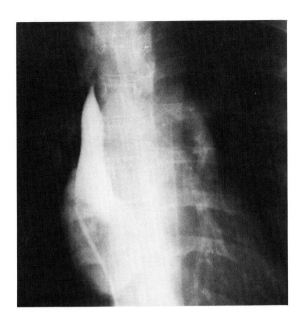

Fig C21-7. Chronic sclerosing mediastinitis. Venogram shows smooth tapering of the lower portion of the superior vena cava. This 38-year-old woman had varicosities over her upper abdomen and lower chest.[30]

A

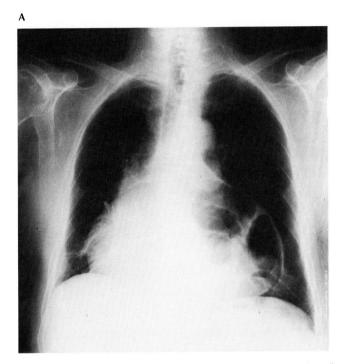

B

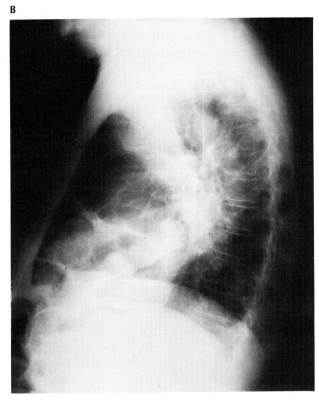

Fig C21-8. Congenital intrapericardial hernia. (A) Frontal and (B) lateral views in an asymptomatic elderly man show loops of bowel in the chest conforming to the left pericardial border.[31]

MIDDLE MEDIASTINAL LESIONS
ON COMPUTED TOMOGRAPHY

Condition	Comments
Fat density (− 20 to − 100 H)	
Lipomatosis	Extensive fat deposition in the mediastinum may be associated with moderate obesity, steroid therapy, Cushing's syndrome, or diabetes or may be a normal variant in nonobese patients.
Epicardial fat pad	Most common fatty mass in the thorax.
Pericardial lipoma	Localized collection of fat-density tissue (lipomas more commonly occur in the anterior mediastinum).
Water density (0 to 15 H)	
Pericardial cyst (Fig C21A-1)	Smooth, thin-walled mass that most commonly occurs in the right cardiophrenic angle. Malleable lesion that may change shape when the patient is scanned in the prone or decubitus position. Easily differentiated from prominent epicardial fat pads or lipomas, which also present as cardiophrenic angle masses.
Bronchogenic cyst (Fig C21A-2)	Smooth, round, homogeneous mass that usually has a thin, imperceptible rim and does not show any change in attenuation after infusion of contrast material. May contain viscous mucoid or proteinaceous material that produces a higher attenuation in the range of a solid neoplasm.
Soft-tissue density (15 to 40 H)	
Lymphadenopathy (Figs C21A-3 and C21A-4)	Most commonly due to metastases, lymphoma, granulomatous disease (tuberculosis, histoplasmosis), pneumoconiosis, or sarcoidosis.
Mediastinitis/abscess	Suggested by the presence of bubbles of gas or a discrete cavity with a thick, shaggy wall.
Mediastinal hemorrhage/ hematoma	Uniform, symmetric widening of the mediastinum (especially the superior portion) in a patient with a history of trauma, surgery, or dissecting aneurysm.
Vascular/enhancing (Figs C21A-5 and C21A-6)	Ectatic vessels, aneurysms, dissections, and congenital vascular anomalies.

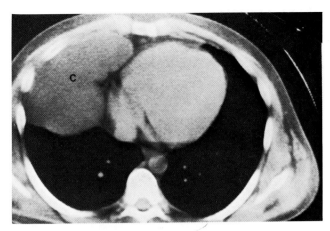

FIG C21A-1. Pericardial cyst. Large homogeneous, near-water-density mass (C) in the right cardiophrenic angle.[26]

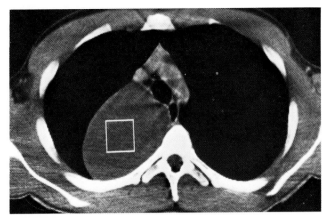

FIG C21A-2. Bronchogenic cyst. CT scan in a young man with an incidental upper respiratory infection shows a large right upper mediastinal mass extending from the right of the trachea to the posterior chest wall. The cyst had a uniform appearance and near-water density and extended vertically from the lower pole of the thyroid gland to the carina.[32]

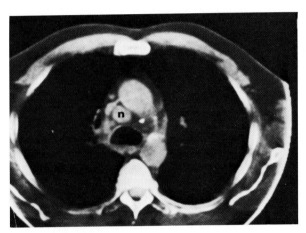

FIG C21A-3. Lymphadenopathy from spread of bronchogenic carcinoma. There is an enlarged lymph node (n) in the pretracheal region, consistent with unresectable mediastinal spread.[26]

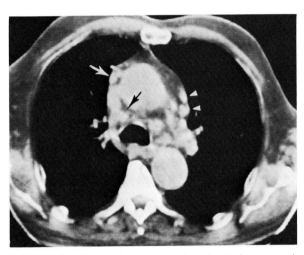

FIG C21A-4. Lymphoma. Enlarged lymph nodes in the paratracheal region (black arrow), aortopulmonary window (white arrowheads), and anterior mediastinum (white arrow) in a patient with lymphoma.[25]

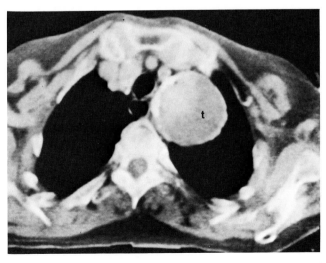

FIG C21A-5. Aneurysm of the left subclavian artery. Contrast-enhanced scan shows the large aneurysm partially filled with thrombus (t).[25]

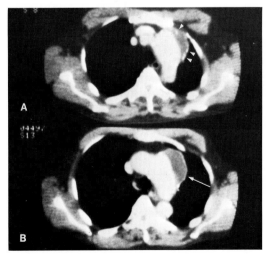

FIG C21A-6. Chronic traumatic aortic aneurysm. CT scans through (A) and slightly below (B) the aortic arch after the intravenous injection of contrast material demonstrate calcification in the wall of the aneurysm (arrowheads) and a large filling defect consisting of thrombus (arrow).

POSTERIOR MEDIASTINAL LESIONS

Condition	Imaging Findings	Comments
Neurogenic neoplasm (Fig C22-1)	Sharply circumscribed, round or oval homogeneous mass that is usually unilateral and paravertebral.	Primarily neurofibromas and neurolemmomas in adults, ganglioneuromas and neuroblastomas in children. Chemodectomas (any mediastinal compartment) and pheochromocytomas are extremely rare. There may be associated rib or vertebral erosion, calcification, and a dumbbell appearance (part of the tumor is inside and part outside the spinal canal).
Spinal neoplasm	Rounded paravertebral mass with associated bone destruction.	Tumors include osteochondroma, aneurysmal bone cyst, chondrosarcoma, osteogenic sarcoma, Ewing's tumor, myeloma, and metastases. An extraosseous soft-tissue mass is a relatively infrequent finding.
Extramedullary hematopoiesis	Single or multiple (often bilateral), lobulated or smooth mass that generally occurs in the paravertebral region in the lower half of the thorax.	Usually associated with congenital hemolytic anemia. Splenomegaly (or a history of splenectomy) is common.
Aneurysm of descending aorta (Fig C22-2)	Smooth or lobulated mass that typically projects from the posterolateral aspect of the aorta on the left side.	Frequently calcified and may become large enough to erode the vertebral column.
Bochdalek's hernia (see Fig C34-8)	Round or oval, retrocardiac mass that is usually unilateral (80% to 90% are on the left side).	Air-filled bowel loops in the mass are diagnostic. More commonly the hernia contains opaque omentum, liver, or spleen.
Hiatal hernia (Fig C22-3)	Retrocardiac mass of variable size that usually contains an air-fluid level.	Diagnosis confirmed by esophagram. Rarely completely opaque (containing only omentum or liver).
Megaesophagus (Fig C22-4)	Broad vertical opacity on the right side of the mediastinum that often contains an air-fluid level (especially in achalasia).	Causes of marked dilatation of the esophagus include achalasia, scleroderma, carcinoma, Chagas' disease, and inflammatory stenosis due to mediastinitis or recurrent esophagitis. May produce anterior bulging of the trachea.
Esophageal neoplasm	Smooth, rounded, usually unilateral mass.	Most commonly leiomyoma (may be fibroma or lipoma). Smooth compression of the esophageal lumen on barium swallow.
Mediastinal hemorrhage/ hematoma	Uniform, symmetric widening of the mediastinum.	Generally a history of trauma, surgery, or dissecting aneurysm. A discrete hematoma may calcify.
Mediastinitis (see Figs C21-6 and C21-7)	Generalized widening of the mediastinum, usually more evident superiorly.	Acute mediastinitis is most often due to esophageal rupture and may be associated with mediastinal air. Chronic mediastinitis (granulomatous or sclerosing) may calcify.

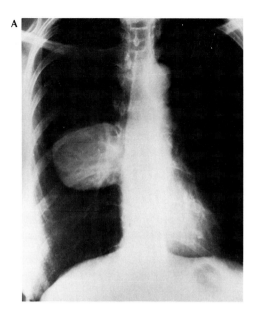

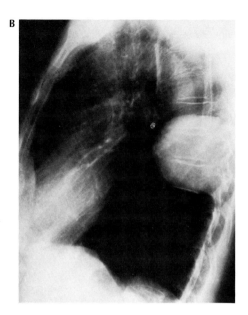

FIG C22-1. Neurogenic tumor. (A) Frontal and (B) lateral views of the chest demonstrate a large right posterior mediastinal mass.[24]

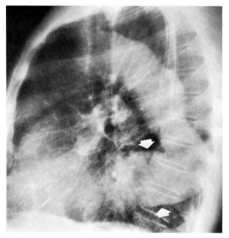

FIG C22-2. Aneurysm of the descending aorta. Lateral view of the chest demonstrates aneurysmal dilatation of the lower thoracic aorta (arrows). Note the marked tortuosity of the remainder of the descending aorta.

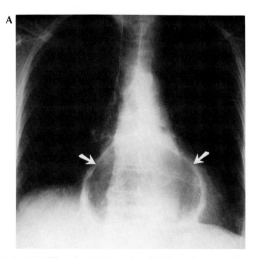

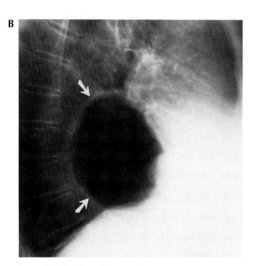

FIG C22-3. Hiatal hernia. (A) Frontal and (B) lateral views of the chest demonstrate a huge air-filled hiatal hernia that appears as a posterior mediastinal mass (arrows).

Condition	Imaging Findings	Comments
Thyroid tumor (see Fig C20-1)	Smooth or lobulated, well-defined mass that appears almost exclusively on the right.	Involves the superior portion of the mediastinum. Much more common in the anterior mediastinum.
Esophageal diverticulum (Zenker's) (see Fig GI7-2)	Cystlike structure in the superior mediastinum that often contains an air-fluid level.	Rarely large enough to be seen on chest radiographs. An esophagram is diagnostic.
Neurenteric cyst (Fig C22-5)	Sharply defined, round or oval, lobulated, homogeneous mass.	Results from incomplete separation of the endoderm from the notocordal plate during early embryonic life. Often associated with a congenital defect of the thoracic spine and symptomatic in infancy.
Gastroenteric cyst (see Fig GI6-8)	Sharply defined, round or oval mass in a paraspinal location. Tends to mold itself to the surrounding structures because of its fluid contents.	Represents failure of complete vacuolation of the originally solid esophagus to produce a hollow tube. Lined by esophageal, gastric, or small intestinal mucosa. May communicate with the gastrointestinal tract and contain air. Produces an extrinsic impression on the esophagus on barium studies.
Meningocele (meningomyelocele) (see Fig SP5-1)	Sharply defined, solitary or multiple, unilateral or bilateral mass.	Frequently associated with vertebral and rib anomalies. Usually communicates with the spinal subarachnoid space and fills on myelography.
Vertebral osteomyelitis (Fig C22-6)	Bilateral fusiform mass in the paravertebral region.	Tuberculous and pyogenic infections usually cause vertebral erosion or destruction and often abscess formation in contiguous soft tissues.
Azygos continuation of the inferior vena cava (Fig C22-7)	Irregular paravertebral mass representing the dilated azygos vein. No shadow of the inferior vena cava on lateral view.	Commonly associated with complex cardiac anomalies.

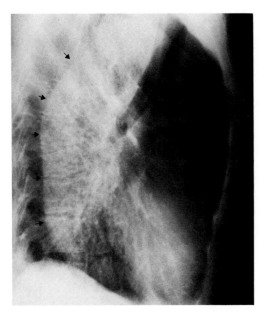

Fig C22-4. Megaesophagus. Lateral chest film in a patient with achalasia shows a mixture of fluid and air density in the dilated esophagus (arrows).

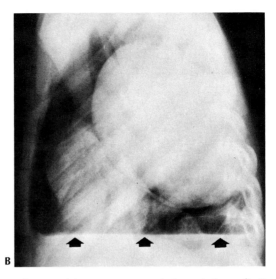

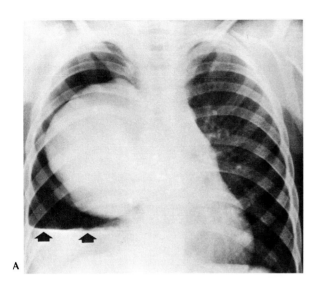

FIG C22-5. Neurenteric cyst. (A) Frontal and (B) lateral views of the chest demonstrate a large, oval, homogeneous mass in the posterior mediastinum. Note the right hydropneumothorax (arrows) with a long air-fluid level that developed as a complication of a diagnostic needle biopsy.

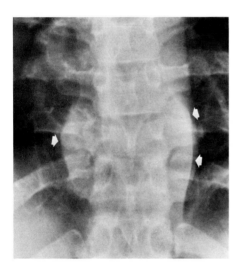

FIG C22-6. Tuberculous osteomyelitis of the spine. Large paravertebral abscess produces a fusiform soft-tissue mass about the vertebrae (arrows). There is poorly marginated destruction along with loss of the superior and inferior end plates of the T9 vertebral body.

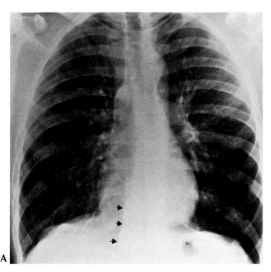

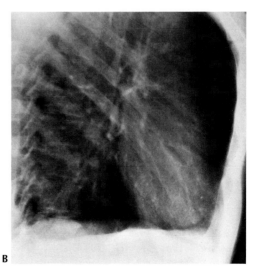

FIG C22-7. Azygos continuation of the inferior vena cava. (A) On the frontal view there is an irregular paravertebral mass (arrows). (B) Lateral view shows pulmonary vessels in the retrocardiac space but no shadow of the inferior vena cava.

POSTERIOR MEDIASTINAL LESIONS
ON COMPUTED TOMOGRAPHY

Condition	Comments
Fat density (-20 to -100 H)	
Omental hernia	Herniation of omental fat through the foramen of Bochdalek.
Liposarcoma	Rare mediastinal tumor that most commonly occurs in the posterior mediastinum. Typically has a higher density than benign fat, is inhomogeneous, and shows features of mediastinal invasion.
Lipoma/lipomatosis	Homogeneously low attenuation values.
Extramedullary hematopoiesis	Generally occurs in the paravertebral region in the lower half of the thorax. More commonly produces a soft-tissue density.
Water density (0 to 15 H)	
Neurenteric cyst	Smooth, thin-walled mass. May contain viscous fluid with a density in the range of a solid tumor. Often associated with a congenital defect of the thoracic spine.
Gastroenteric cyst	Smooth, thin-walled mass. May contain viscous fluid with a density in the range of a solid tumor.
Meningocele (meningomyelocele)	Smooth, thin-walled mass. May contain viscous fluid with a density in the range of a solid tumor. Frequently associated with vertebral and rib anomalies.
Pancreatic pseudocyst	Rarely presents as a mass in the posterior or inferior mediastinum. CT can demonstrate extension of the mass through the retrocrural portion of the diaphragm.
Soft-tissue density (15 to 40 H)	
Neurogenic tumor (Fig C22A-1)	Variable attenuation values including a fatty appearance (without the fat-fluid interfaces seen in cystic teratomas) and a mixed pattern resulting from myxoid elements and vascular lakes. More vascular neural tumors (eg, paragangliomas) show dense homogeneous contrast enhancement, while neurolemmomas enhance to a lesser degree. Neurogenic tumors often originate from or extend into the corresponding neural foramen.
Hernia	Hiatal hernia or Bochdalek's hernia (may contain an air-fluid level in the herniated bowel).
Mediastinitis/abscess	Suggested by the presence of bubbles of gas or a discrete cavity with a thick shaggy wall.

(continued page 120)

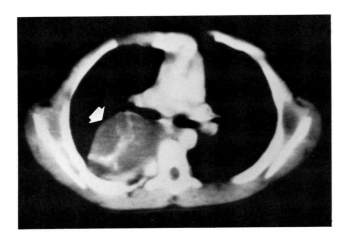

FIG C22A-1. Ganglioneuroma. Huge posterior mediastinal mass (arrow) with poor contrast enhancement.

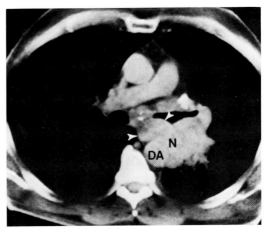

FIG C22A-2. Mediastinal spread from bronchogenic carcinoma. There is obliteration of the fat plane around the descending aorta (DA) by the adjacent neoplasm (N) in addition to extension of tumor deep into the mediastinum (arrowheads) behind the left main-stem bronchus and in front of the descending aorta.[26]

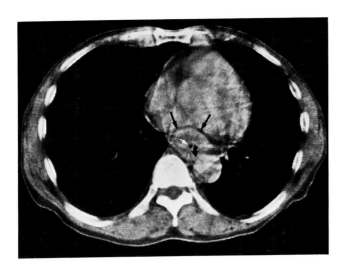

FIG C22A-3. Esophageal carcinoma. The circumferential mass of the bulky carcinoma (straight black arrows) fills the lumen of the esophagus (white arrow). Obliteration of the fat plane adjacent to the aorta (curved arrow) indicates mediastinal invasion.

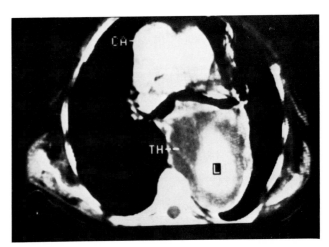

FIG C22A-4. Aneurysm of the descending aorta. Contrast-enhanced scan at a level just below the carina demonstrates a markedly dilated descending aorta (L) with a large mural thrombus (TH) surrounding the lumen of the descending aorta. Note also the markedly dilated ascending aorta (OA).

Condition	Comments
Mediastinal hemorrhage/ hematoma	Uniform, symmetric widening of the mediastinum (especially the superior portion) in a patient with a history of trauma, surgery, or a dissecting aneurysm.
Extramedullary hematopoiesis (see Fig C22A-1)	Generally occurs in the paravertebral region in the lower half of the thorax. May appear as a fat-density mass.
Lymphadenopathy (Fig C22A-2)	Posterior mediastinal (paraspinal) lymph nodes are considered enlarged if they exceed 6 mm in diameter (same criteria as for retrocrural nodes in the abdomen). Enlarged paraspinal nodes must not be mistaken for the azygos or hemiazygos veins, which are clearly tubular structures seen at multiple levels.
Bronchopulmonary sequestration	Congenital pulmonary malformation in which a portion of pulmonary tissue is detached from the remainder of the normal lung and receives its blood supply from a systemic artery. Typically appears as a sharply circumscribed mass in the posterior portion of a lower lobe (usually the left) contiguous to the diaphragm. May contain air or an air-fluid level if infection has resulted in communication with the airways or contiguous lung tissue.
Esophageal carcinoma (Fig C22A-3)	May produce a large, bulky mass outside the esophagus. The obliteration of fat planes between the esophagus and neighboring structures can be a useful sign of extraesophageal spread if these planes were intact on a previous CT scan. However, clearly defined fat planes may not be seen in thin, cachectic patients or in patients who have had previous surgery or radiation therapy. Although the lack of fat planes in these patients is of uncertain significance, the presence of a fat plane rules out extension of tumor beyond the esophagus.
Vascular/enhancing (Figs C22A-4 to C22A-6)	Aneurysm or dissection of the aorta; dilatation of the azygos vein.

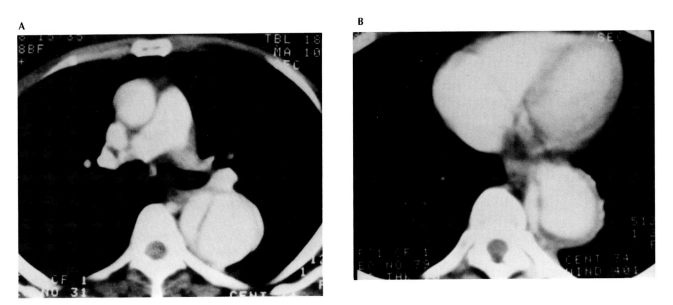

FIG C22A-5. **Dissecting aneurysm.** (A) Level of the pulmonary artery. (B) More caudal level.

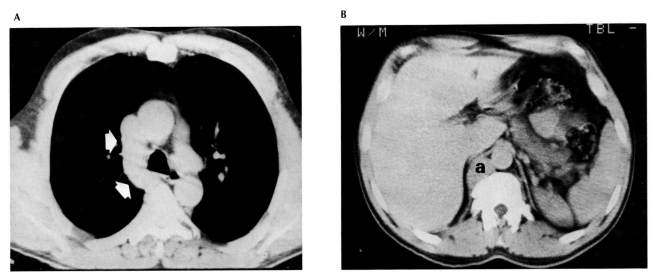

FIG C22A-6. **Azygos continuation of the inferior vena cava.** (A) The dilated azygos vein (arrows) produces a posterior mediastinal mass. (B) Upper abdominal CT scan shows the dilated azygos vein (a) in a retrocrural position adjacent to the aorta.

SHIFT OF THE MEDIASTINUM*

Condition	Comments
Decreased lung volume (shift *to* the affected side)	
Atelectasis	Increased opacification and elevation of the hemidiaphragm on the affected side.
Postoperative	Lobectomy, pneumonectomy. Elevation of the hemidiaphragm on the affected side and evidence of surgical clips.
Hypoplastic lung (see Fig C12-3)	Increased opacification and elevation of the hemidiaphragm on the affected side. Small pulmonary artery and diminished pulmonary vascularity. Often an irregular reticular vascular pattern (dilated bronchial artery collaterals).
Increased lung volume (shift *away from* the affected side)	
Foreign body obstructing main-stem bronchus (Fig C23-3)	Common cause of air trapping in children (ball-valve obstruction permits air to enter the lung but obstructs outflow). Ipsilateral hyperlucent lung with relatively opaque, but normal, contralateral lung.
Swyer-James syndrome (see Fig C12-5)	Air trapping during expiration. Probably results from acute pneumonia during infancy or childhood that causes bronchiolitis obiterans and an emphysema-like appearance. Small hilar and peripheral vessels.
Congenital lobar emphysema (see Fig C12-6)	In infants, the hyperlucent, hyperexpanded lobe frequently herniates through the mediastinum to compress normal lung and lead to serious respiratory insufficiency.
Bullous emphysema	Localized form of emphysema with characteristic large avascular lucent areas separated by thin linear densities.
Cystic adenomatoid malformation (see Fig C12-7)	Complex foregut anomaly in infants consisting of multiple cystic structures (may become overdistended with air and cause mediastinal shift).
Bronchogenic cyst	In infants, a solitary air-filled mass with a connection to a partially obstructed bronchus causing a ball-valve mechanism (massive overdistension because air can enter but not leave the cyst).
Pulmonary/mediastinal masses	Infrequent cause of mediastinal shift to or away from affected side. Very large masses may shift the mediastinum to the contralateral side. Endobronchial lesions (eg, carcinoma) may cause ipsilateral atelectasis and shift of the mediastinum to the side of the mass.

*See Figs C23-1 and C23-2.

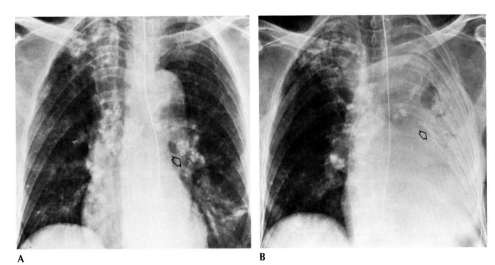

A   B

FIG C23-1. Collapse of the left lung.
(A) Initial examination showing old healed granulomatous disease. Note the position of the left infrahilar nodes (arrow). (B) Repeat chest film 2 days later shows opacification of the entire left hemithorax due to a mucous plug and a shift of the mediastinum to the affected side. Note the change in position of the left infrahilar calcifications (arrow).

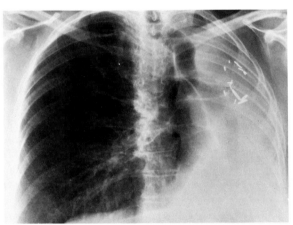

FIG C23-2. Pneumonectomy. Opacification of the left hemithorax with multiple surgical clips. The trachea and other mediastinal contents are shifted to the affected side.

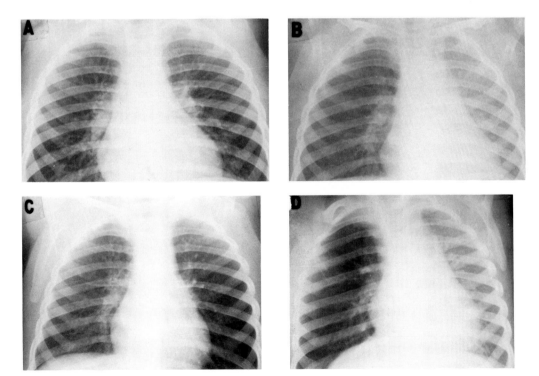

FIG C23-3. Peanut in the right main-stem bronchus. (A) During inspiration, the lungs of this 2-year-old boy are well aerated. Air trapping in the right lung is seen during expiration (B) and with the right side down (C). The normal left lung is underaerated when that side is down (D).[33]

Condition	Comments
Pleural space abnormalities (shift *away from* the affected side)	
Large unilateral pleural effusion (**Fig C23-4**)	Mediastinal shift usually occurs only after almost the entire hemithorax is opaque.
Tension pneumothorax (**Fig C23-5**)	Medical emergency that is the result of a leak of air from the lung into the pleural space. A shift of the mediastinum and depression of the diaphragm are frequently the first detectable signs. Total collapse of the lung may be a relatively late complication.
Diaphragmatic hernia (**Fig C23-6**)	Congenital or posttraumatic hernia that appears bubbly if it contains air-filled loops and opaque if it contains omentum, liver, or fluid-filled bowel.
Pleural masses	Metastatic tumor or malignant mesothelioma (ipsilateral lung may be completely opaque due to a massive pleural effusion).
Partial absence of pericardium	Striking shift of the heart to the left but no shift of other mediastinal structures (trachea, aorta).

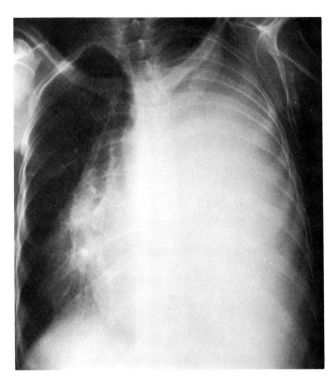

FIG **C23-4. Large unilateral pleural effusion.** The left hemithorax is virtually opaque and there is shift of the mediastinum to the right.

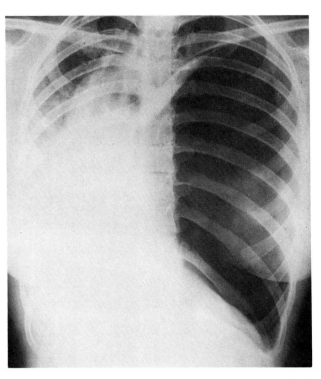

FIG **C23-5. Tension pneumothorax.** The left hemithorax is completely radiolucent and lacks vascular markings. There is a dramatic shift of the heart and mediastinum to the right. The left hemidiaphragm is markedly depressed and there is spreading of the left ribs.

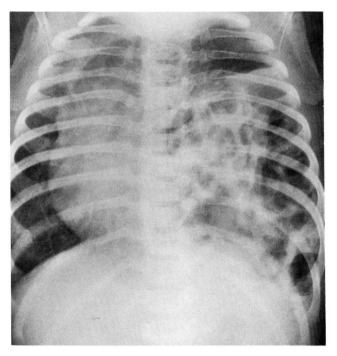

FIG **C23-6. Congenital diaphragmatic hernia.** Multiple lucencies in the left chest due to gas-filled loops of bowel. The heart and mediastinal structures are shifted to the right.

PNEUMOMEDIASTINUM

Condition	Comments
Spontaneous pneumomediastinum (Figs C24-1 and C24-2)	Caused by rupture of marginally situated alveoli with passage of air through the interstitial tissues of the lung to the hilum and the mediastinum. Many patients have no evidence of underlying lung disease. Often precipitated by a sudden increase in intra-alveolar pressure.
Trauma to chest wall	Closed-chest trauma causes an abrupt increase in intrathoracic pressure. Rupture of alveoli into the perivascular sheaths in the interstitial tissue of the lung results in the passage of air to the hilum and the mediastinum.
Rupture of the esophagus (Fig C24-3)	Most frequently occurs during episodes of severe vomiting (Boerhaave's syndrome), in which the tear involves the lower 8 cm of the esophagus (relatively unsupported by connective tissue). The tear is classically vertical and involves the left posterolateral wall of the esophagus.
Bronchial or tracheal injury (Fig C24-4)	Caused by trauma (shearing force) or a sudden increase in pressure against a closed glottis.
Iatrogenic	Surgical procedures or instrumentation of the esophagus, trachea, bronchi, or neck. Also caused by overinflation during anesthesia.
Extension of gas from below the diaphragm	Retroperitoneal rupture of the duodenum or colon. Gas extends along the aorta or esophagus into the mediastinum.
Extension of gas from the neck (Fig C24-5)	Trauma, surgical procedures, or perforating cervical lesions.
Tear of lung parenchyma	Leakage of air into the interstitial tissues followed by dissection toward the hilum and into the mediastinum. May be associated with birth trauma, anesthesia, resuscitation attempts, and the straining and coughing associated with pulmonary disease.
Hyaline membrane disease (Fig C24-6)	Frequent complication, probably related to extension of pulmonary interstitial emphysema.
Asthma	Probably related to alveolar rupture secondary to increased pressure. Pneumomediastinum is more common in children, though it can occur in adults.

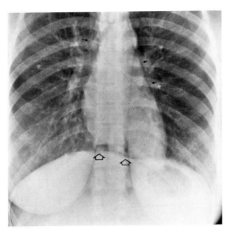

FIG C24-1. Pneumomediastinum. In addition to bilateral elevation of the mediastinal pleura (closed arrows), there is a characteristic interposition of gas between the heart and the diaphragm that permits visualization of the central portion of the diaphragm in continuity with the lateral portions (open arrows).[34]

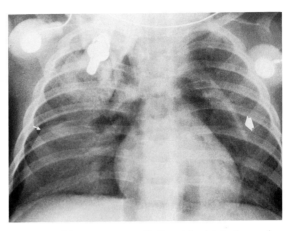

FIG C24-2. Positive-pressure ventilation. After intubation and ventilation of a child with hydrocarbon poisoning, there is the development of a pneumomediastinum (large arrow) and pneumothorax (small arrow). Note that the stiffness of the lungs has prevented substantial collapse.

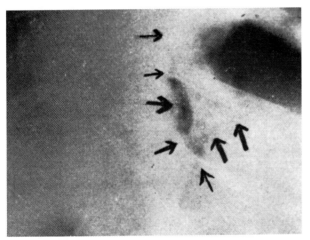

FIG C24-3. Esophageal rupture. Linear lucent shadows (arrows) represent localized mediastinal emphysema and correspond to the fascial planes of the mediastinal and diaphragmatic pleurae in the region of the lower esophagus.[29]

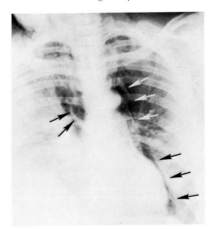

FIG C24-4. Tracheobronchial injury. Frontal chest film made after blunt trauma to the upper chest that caused transection of both main-stem bronchi demonstrates free air in the mediastinum (upper black arrows) and through the fascial planes of the neck. The lucent zone (lower black arrows) along the left cardiac border simulates the pattern produced by a pneumopericardium or pneumothorax. However, the aortic arch is sharply circumscribed by air that extends around its cephalad and right lateral margins, at a level well above the pericardial reflection (white arrows). This clearly indicates that this air also is in the mediastinum and not confined to the pericardium or pleural space.[35]

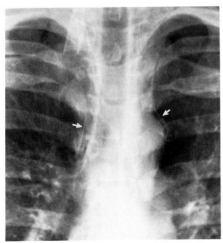

FIG C24-5. Extension of gas from the neck. Pneumomediastinum (arrows) after cervical trauma (note the overlying surgical drain on the right).

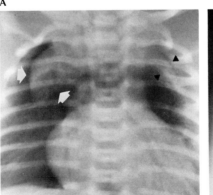
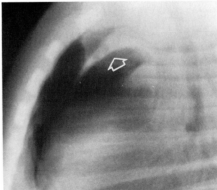

FIG C24-6. Pneumomediastinum in an infant. (A) Elevation of both thymic lobes by mediastinal air (arrows) produces the angel's-wings sign. (B) Lateral projection shows the anterior mediastinal air lifting the thymus off the pericardium and great vessels (arrow).

PLEURAL-BASED LESION

Condition	Imaging Findings	Comments
Mesothelioma **(Figs C25-1 and C25-2)**	Solitary, sharply circumscribed, homogeneous (benign); irregular, scalloped or nodular mass (malignant).	Benign tumors may often be asymptomatic and curable by surgical resection. A diffuse malignant tumor is related to asbestos exposure and is often associated with a large pleural effusion that may obscure the underlying neoplasm.
Metastases **(Fig C25-3)**	Single or multiple nodules.	Most common primaries are carcinomas of the bronchus, breast, ovary, and gastrointestinal tract. Actual metastatic deposits are often too small to be seen radiographically (CT is more sensitive). A large pleural effusion may be the only indication of pleural metastases.
Pleural fluid (loculated or interlobar) **(Figs C25-4 and C25-5)**	Smooth, sharply demarcated, homogeneous opacity.	Loculated fluid collections are caused by adhesions between contiguous pleural surfaces (tend to occur with or following pyothorax or hemothorax). An interlobar fluid collection generally results from cardiac decompensation and may simulate a neoplasm, though it tends to absorb spontaneously when the heart failure is relieved (vanishing or phantom tumor).
Pulmonary infarct	Homogeneous, wedge-shaped peripheral consolidation with its base contiguous to a visceral pleural surface.	Classic but uncommon manifestitation of an infarct. An infarct has a rounded apex, convex toward the hilum (Hampton hump), whereas pleural thickening and free pleural fluid are generally concave toward the hilum.
Rib or chest wall lesion **(see Fig C26-4)**	Extrapleural mass, often with destruction, fracture, or expansion of the underlying rib or sternum.	Primary or metastatic neoplasm, osteomyelitis, fracture with hematoma or callus.
Fibrin ball	Round, oval, or irregular mass that is most commonly located near the base of the lung.	Tumorlike collection that may develop in a serofibrinous pleural effusion and usually becomes evident after absorption of the effusion. May disappear spontaneously and rapidly or remain unchanged and mimic a solitary pulmonary nodule when viewed en face.
Pancoast tumor (superior sulcus tumor) **(Fig C25-6)**	Apical mass, often with destruction of adjacent ribs.	Site of 6% of bronchogenic carcinomas. May be associated Horner's syndrome. In the absence of bone destruction, the tumor may be identified only by asymmetry of presumed apical pleural thickening.
Lipoma	Smooth, sharply circumscribed mass.	Rare lesion that may change shape during respiration (due to its relatively fluid contents). A large tumor occasionally erodes contiguous ribs.

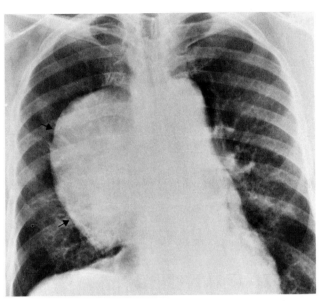

FIG C25-1. Benign localized fibrous mesothelioma. Huge, homogeneous soft-tissue mass (arrows) arising from the mediastinal pleura and projecting into the right hemithorax. The patient had only mild underlying interstitial fibrosis and no pleural plaquing.

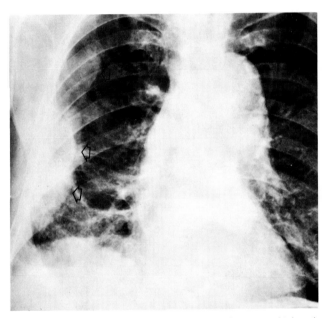

FIG C25-2. Diffuse pleural mesothelioma. Multiple masses thicken the right pleura (arrows) in an elderly man with chronic asbestos exposure.[36]

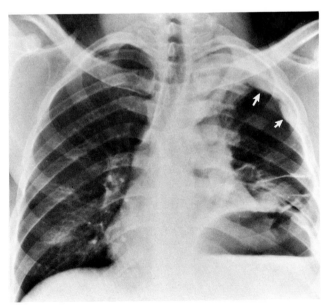

FIG C25-3. Pleural metastases (arrows) from bronchogenic carcinoma. There is also elevation of the left hemidiaphragm due to phrenic nerve involvement and postobstructive atelectatic change secondary to the left perihilar lesion.

Condition	Imaging Findings	Comments
Fungal infection (Fig C25-7)	Peripheral mass, often with cavitation. May have associated rib destruction.	Actinomycosis, nocardiosis, blastomycosis, torulosis.
Pulmonary granuloma	Smooth, sharply circumscribed mass that may contain central calcification.	Primarily histoplasmoma. Also other fungi and tuberculosis.
Rheumatoid nodule	Single or multiple nodules.	May have diffuse underlying interstitial fibrosis.

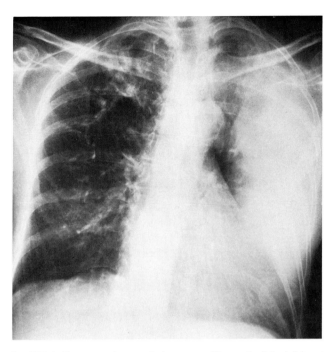

Fig C25-4. Empyema. Large soft-tissue mass fills much of the left hemithorax.

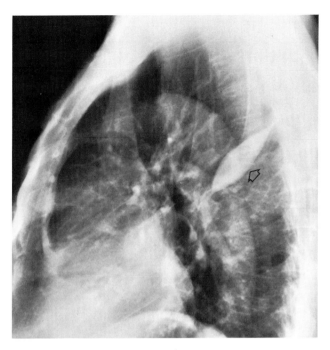

Fig C25-5. Interlobar pleural fluid. Elliptical fluid collection (arrow) in the major fissure in a patient with cardiac decompensation.

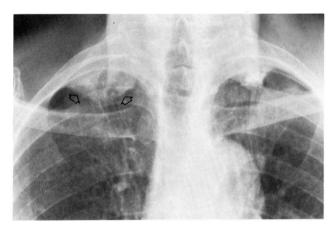

Fig C25-6. Pancoast tumor. Increased opacification in the right apex (arrows). Although this appearance may simulate benign apical pleural thickening, the marked asymmetry and irregularity of the right apical mass should suggest the diagnosis of bronchogenic carcinoma.

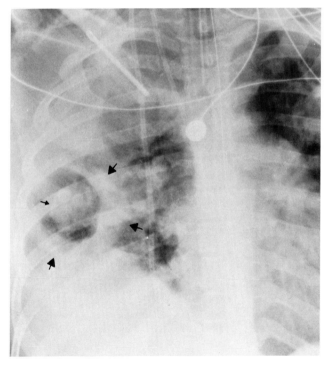

Fig C25-7. Aspergillosis. Large peripheral thick-walled cavity (large arrows) that abuts the pleura and contains an intracavitary fungus ball (small arrow).

EXTRAPLEURAL LESION

Condition	Comments
Chest wall hematoma (Figs C26-1 to C26-3)	Usually a history of trauma and often evidence of a rib fracture. May also occur with sternal fractures (hematoma best seen on lateral view). Callus formation about an old rib fracture may be mistaken for a pulmonary nodule.
Rib neoplasm (Fig C26-4)	Metastases and myeloma are the most common causes of an extrapleural mass associated with rib destruction in adults. Ewing's tumor or metastatic neuroblastoma are the most common causes in children.
Mediastinal, spinal, sternal, or subphrenic lesion (see Fig C11-6)	Tumors, cysts, and inflammatory processes may produce extrapleural masses.
Chest wall infection	An extrapleural mass with rib destruction is most commonly a manifestation of actinomycosis (often with parenchymal infiltrate, pleural effusion, and even a cutaneous fistula). A similar pattern may also be due to nocardiosis, blastomycosis, aspergillosis, or, rarely, tuberculosis.
Extrapleural lipoma	Common chest wall lesion that may grow between ribs to present as both an intrathoracic and a subcutaneous mass. Characteristic fat density on CT.
Surgery or blunt trauma	Ruptured aneurysm, partial pleurectomy, sympathectomy, plombage and mineral oil injection for the treatment of tuberculosis.
Congenital lobar agenesis	Missing lobe is often replaced by a chunk of extrapleural aureolar tissue that produces an anterior extrapleural mass paralleling the sternum. There is loss of the right heart border on frontal views.

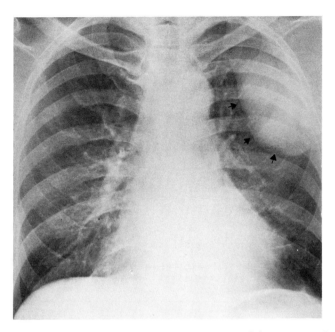

FIG C26-1. Pulmonary hematoma. Large extrapleural density (arrows) over the left upper lobe.

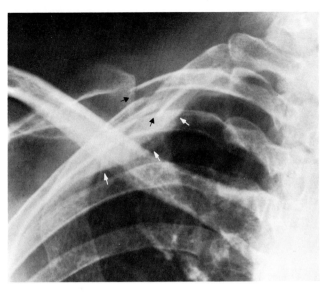

FIG C26-2. Chest trauma. Small extrapleural hematoma (white arrows) associated with fractures of the first and second ribs (black arrows).

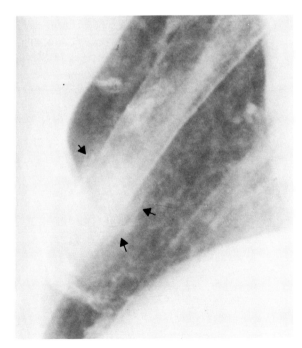

FIG C26-3. Cough fracture simulating a pulmonary nodule. A coned view of the right lower lung on a routine chest radiograph shows callus formation about a rib (arrows) in an asymptomatic person.

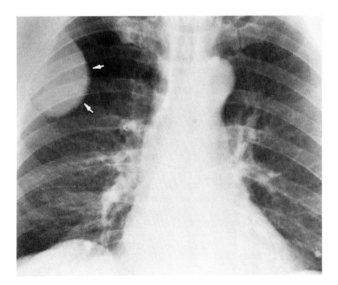

FIG C26-4. Extramedullary myeloma. Large extrapleural mass (arrows) containing a proliferation of plasma cells.

PLEURAL CALCIFICATION

Condition	Imaging Findings	Comments
Organized hemothorax	Usually unilateral calcification of the visceral pleura (Fig C27-1) in the form of a broad continuous sheet or multiple discrete plaques.	Typically extends from about the level of the mid-thorax posteriorly, coursing around the lateral lung margins in a generally inferior direction and roughly paralleling the major fissure. There is often evidence of healed rib fractures and a history of significant chest trauma.
Organized empyema (Fig C27-2)	Usually unilateral calcification of the visceral pleura in the form of a broad continuous sheet or multiple discrete plaques.	Typically extends from about the level of the mid-thorax posteriorly, coursing around the lateral lung margins in a generally inferior direction and roughly paralleling the major fissure. Usually a history of severe pulmonary infection.
Old tuberculous empyema (Fig C27-3)	Usually unilateral calcification of the visceral pleura in the form of a broad continuous sheet or multiple discrete plaques. May be bilateral (usually asymmetric).	Typically extends from about the level of the mid-thorax posteriorly, coursing around the lateral lung margins in a generally inferior direction and roughly paralleling the major fissure. Extensive apical parenchymal scarring or cavitary disease is virtually diagnostic.
Pneumoconiosis (Figs C27-4 to C27-6)	Usually bilateral plaques of calcification involving the parietal pleura, commonly along the diaphragm. There may sometimes be calcification in extensively thickened pleura along the lateral chest wall.	Most commonly caused by asbestosis. May also be due to other silicates (eg, talcosis). The diaphragmatic pleura is almost always extensively involved (unlike hemothorax or empyema). Extensive encasement of both lungs may occur. Basilar reticulonodular interstitial disease is highly suggestive, though often absent.

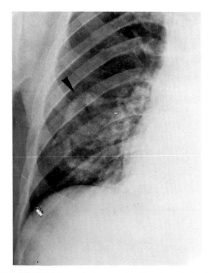
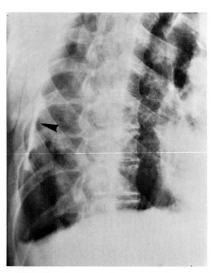

FIG C27-1. Calcified thickened pleura. (A) The density in the lower lung (arrows) has a well-defined irregular border closely resembling a cavity. (B) An oblique view, however, shows a pathognomic linear density (arrow) paralleling but separated from the chest wall.[37]

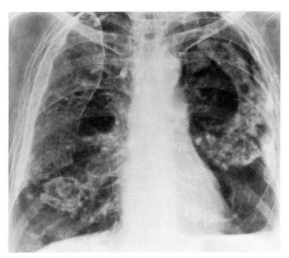

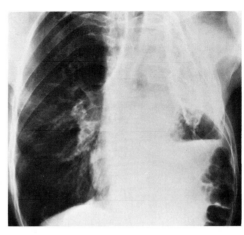

FIG C27-2. Old tuberculous empyema. Bilateral broad continuous sheets of calcification overlie much of the lung surface.

FIG C27-3. Old tuberculous empyema. Broad sheet of calcification overlies much of the left hemithorax. Note the elevation of the left hemidiaphragm and retraction of the trachea to the left, all consistent with loss of volume due to the chronic granulomatous disease.

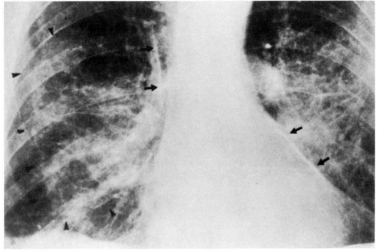

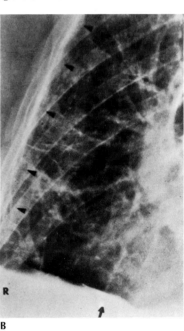

FIG C27-4. Asbestosis. (A) Frontal view shows en face calcifications on the right (arrowheads), linear calcifications in profile in the mediastinal reflection of the pleura on the right and in the pericardium on the left (transverse arrows), and linear calcification in the left diaphragmatic pleura (vertical arrow). (B) A left oblique film shows linear pleural calcification in profile in the area of the central tendon of the right hemidiaphragm (arrowheads). The en face plaques in (A) now appear in profile as extensive linear calcifications (arrowheads) adjacent to anterior ribs.[38]

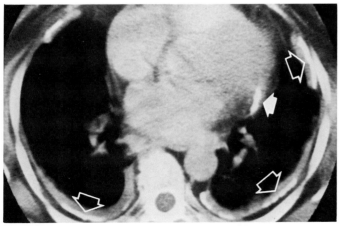

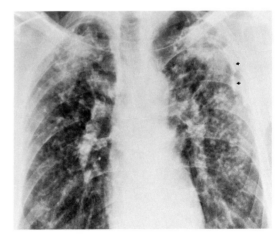

FIG C27-5. Asbestosis. CT scan shows calcified pleural plaques along the lateral and posterior chest wall (open arrows) and adjacent to the heart (closed arrow).

FIG C27-6. Coal-worker's pneumoconiosis. Bilateral fibrous masses in the apices with upward retraction of the hila. Note the pleural calcification (arrows) in the left apex.

PLEURAL EFFUSION WITH
OTHERWISE NORMAL-APPEARING CHEST

Condition	Imaging Findings and Fluid Characteristics	Comments
Tuberculosis (Fig C28-1)	Serous exudate with low glucose content and predominantly lymphocytic reaction. Almost always unilateral.	Common manifestation of primary tuberculosis in adults (about 40%), but less frequent in children (10%). The patient may have a negative tuberculin test in early stages. Active pulmonary tuberculosis often develops if the effusion is not treated.
Other infections (Fig C28-2)	Serous exudate that may be bilateral.	Bacteria, fungi (especially actinomycosis and nocardiosis), viruses, mycoplasma.
Thoracic lymphoma	Serosanguinous exudate that may be unilateral or bilateral.	Usually evidence of pulmonary or mediastinal lymph node involvement. Suggestive findings include hepatosplenomegaly and peripheral lymph node enlargement.
Metastatic carcinoma	Serous exudate with variable blood content and typically elevated glucose. Unilateral or bilateral.	Most common primary sites are breast, pancreas, stomach, ovary, and kidney. At times, a pleural effusion may be the only presenting finding.
Ovarian neoplasm (Meigs' syndrome)	Serous exudate that is more frequent on the right (may be left-sided or bilateral).	Most commonly an ovarian fibroma associated with ascites. Also can develop with other benign or malignant ovarian tumors. The effusion usually disappears after removal of the ovarian neoplasm.
Carcinoma of pancreas/ retroperitoneum	Serous exudate (pleural fluid negative for malignant cells).	Often no direct tumor involvement of the thorax. The effusion disappears after removal or treatment of the primary lesion.
Pulmonary thromboembolic disease	Serosanguinous effusion that is most often unilateral.	Effusion is infrequently the sole manifestation of pulmonary embolism (may obscure small parenchymal abnormalities). The presence of fluid almost always indicates infarction.
Subphrenic abscess	Ipsilateral serous exudate.	More commonly associated with elevation and fixation of the hemidiaphragm and basal atelectasis (see Fig C29-2). There may be gas or a mottled pattern of density in the subphrenic space.
Pancreatitis (Fig C28-3)	Serous or serosanguinous exudate with a high amylase level. Predominantly left-sided (may be bilateral).	May occur in acute, chronic, or relapsing pancreatitis or with a pancreatic pseudocyst. Other manifestations include elevation of the hemidiaphragm and basal atelectasis.

Condition	Imaging Findings and Fluid Characteristics	Comments
Trauma	Varied composition (blood, chyle, or food after esophageal rupture).	Hemothorax complicating traumatic aortic rupture and effusion after esophageal perforation are almost always left-sided. The side of a chylothorax depends on the site of the thoracic duct rupture (see Fig C30-1).
Abdominal surgery	Serous exudate.	Usually very small, but may be detected in almost half the patients if lateral decubitus views are obtained.
Postmyocardial infarction syndrome (Dressler's syndrome)	Left-sided or bilateral transudate is the most common finding (80%) and may occur alone.	Characterized by fever and pleuropericardial chest pain that begins 1 to 6 weeks after acute myocardial infarction. Pericardial effusion or pulmonary infiltrates frequently occur (see Fig CA20-2). Striking response to steroid therapy.
Cirrhosis with ascites	Transudate that is more often right-sided (may be on the left or bilateral).	Ascitic fluid probably enters the pleural space via diaphragmatic lymphatics (as in Meigs' syndrome). Usually evidence of ascites and other signs of cirrhosis.
Systemic lupus erythematosus (Fig C28-4)	Serous exudate that is bilateral in about 50% of patients. The effusion is predominantly left-sided when unilateral. Tends to be small (occasionally massive).	Pleural effusion is an isolated abnormality in about 10% of cases. It is often associated with a pericardial effusion and usually clears without residua. Nonspecific cardiomegaly and pulmonary involvement develop in most patients.
Rheumatoid disease	Serous exudate with a predominance of lymphocytes and a low glucose level. Usually unilateral.	Occurs almost exclusively in men. May antedate the signs and symptoms of rheumatoid arthritis, but usually follows them. There is often no pulmonary evidence of rheumatoid disease.
Asbestosis	Serous or blood-tinged exudate that is usually bilateral and often recurrent.	More commonly occurs in association with pleural plaques and calcification.
Renal disease (Fig C28-5)	Transudate or serous exudate.	Causes include nephrotic syndrome, acute glomerulonephritis, hydronephrosis, and uremic pleuritis.
Peritoneal dialysis	Serous exudate.	Probably the same underlying mechanism as with ascites. May be impossible to distinguish from a uremic effusion.

Condition	Imaging Findings and Fluid Characteristics	Comments
Malposition of percutaneous central venous catheter (Fig C28-6)	Unilateral collection of the fluid being instilled.	Results from perforation of the vessel either at the time of insertion of the catheter or later (gradual erosion of a relatively thin-walled intrathoracic vessel by the catheter tip).
Myxedema	Serous exudate.	More commonly causes a pericardial effusion.
Lymphedema	High protein content.	Results from hypoplasia of the lymphatic system.
Familial recurring polyserositis (familial Mediterranean fever)	Serofibrinous exudate.	Familial disorder (Armenians, Arabs, non-Ashkenazic Jews) characterized by episodic acute attacks of abdominal and chest pain. Usually associated with arthritis and arthralgia.

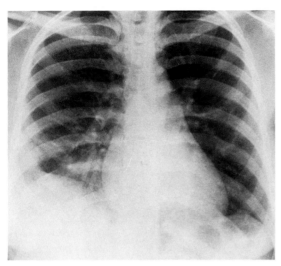

FIG C28-1. **Primary tuberculosis.** Unilateral right tuberculous pleural effusion without parenchymal or lymph node involvement.

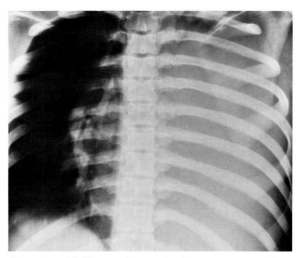

FIG C28-2. **Coccidioidomycosis.** Complete homogeneous opacification of the left hemithorax. The massive pleural effusion must be associated with virtually complete collapse of the left lung, since there is no contralateral shift of the mediastinal structures.

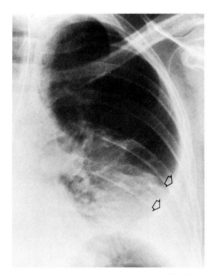

FIG C28-3. **Pancreatitis.** Blunting of the normally sharp angle between the diaphragm and the rib cage (arrows) along with a characteristic upward concave border (meniscus) of the fluid level.

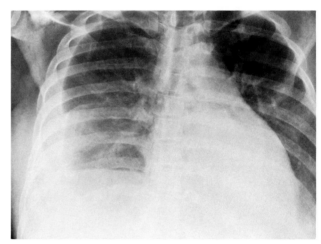

FIG C28-4. **Systemic lupus erythematosus.** Large right pleural effusion in a young woman.

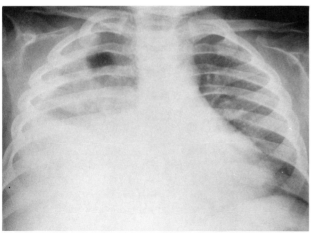

FIG C28-5. **Nephrotic syndrome.** Diffuse cardiomegaly with a large right pleural effusion, which is situated both along the lateral chest wall and in a subpulmonic location.

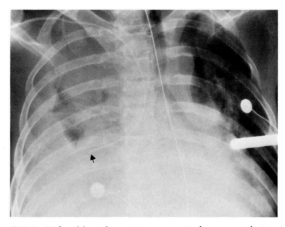

FIG C28-6. **Malposition of percutaneous central venous catheter.** A right subclavian catheter, which was introduced for total parenteral nutrition, perforated the superior vena cava and eroded into the right pleural space. Note the tip of the catheter projecting beyond the right border of the mediastinum (arrow). The direct infusion of parenteral fluid into the pleural space has led to the development of a large right hydrothorax.

PLEURAL EFFUSION
ASSOCIATED WITH OTHER RADIOGRAPHIC EVIDENCE OF CHEST DISEASE

Condition	Imaging Findings	Comments
Infectious agents (Fig C29-1)	Various patterns of effusion and associated parenchymal disease.	Bacteria (especially staphylococcus, *Klebsiella*, tularemia), fungi (especially actinomycosis and nocardiosis), viruses, mycoplasma, and parasites (primarily amebiasis with liver abscess and ruptured hydatid cyst).
Subphrenic abscess (Fig C29-2)	Ipsilateral effusion.	Usually elevation and fixation of the hemidiaphragm with basal atelectasis. There may be gas or a mottled pattern of density in the subphrenic space.
Bronchogenic carcinoma	Ipsilateral effusion in 10% to 15% of patients.	Commonly associated with obstructive pneumonia. There may be a peripheral mass (often contiguous to the visceral pleura) or hilar or mediastinal lymph node enlargement.
Lymphoma	Effusion in 15% to 30% of patients.	Typically enlargement of hilar and mediastinal nodes with single or multiple areas of consolidation. A similar pattern occurs in leukemia.
Metastases	Unilateral or bilateral effusion.	Multiple parenchymal nodules in hematogenous metastases; linear shadows in lymphangitic spread (there may also be lymph node enlargement).
Mesothelioma (Fig C29-3)	Unilateral effusion that is often massive.	Characteristic finding in the diffuse malignant type. There is usually a diffuse peripheral mass contiguous with the pleura and a history of exposure to asbestos. Pleural effusion is rare in the localized benign form of mesothelioma.
Bronchiolar (alveolar cell) carcinoma	Effusion in about 10% of patients.	Various patterns of parenchymal disease (small nodule, massive consolidation, multiple disseminated nodules). It may be difficult to differentiate from metastatic neoplasm or disseminated lymphoma.
Multiple myeloma	Effusion is uncommon.	Single or multiple soft-tissue masses protruding into the thorax and arising from the ribs (with rib destruction) is almost pathognomonic. Rare primary chest wall tumors can present a similar pattern.

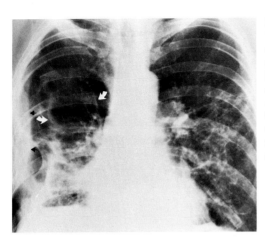

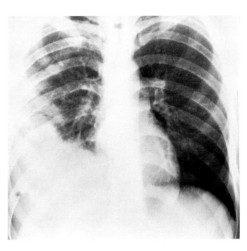

FIG C29-1. Actinomycosis. Untreated infection led to the development of a large cavity (white arrows) with extension into the pleura to produce an empyema (black arrows). The right fifth posterior rib was partially resected during surgery, which revealed thickening of the pleura circumferentially around the right lower lobe.

FIG C29-2. Subphrenic abscess. Right pleural effusion and basilar atelectasis. Note the small bubbles (arrows) in the abscess.

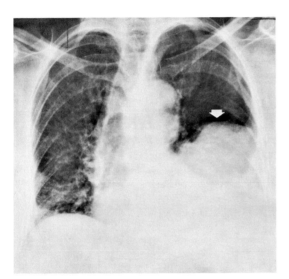

FIG C29-4. Pulmonary embolism. (A)Plain chest radiograph demonstrates right basilar atelectasis associated with elevation of the right hemidiaphragm, representing a large subpulmonic pleural effusion. (B) Pulmonary arteriogram shows virtually complete obstruction of the right pulmonary artery (arrows).

A

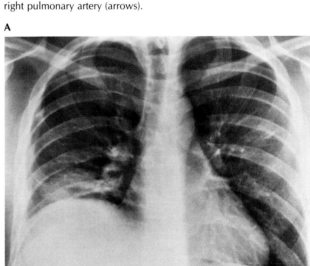

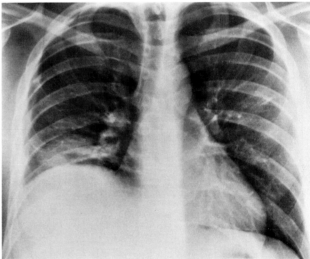

FIG C29-3. Diffuse pleural mesothelioma. After thoracentesis, the top of a large mass is evident (arrow).[36]

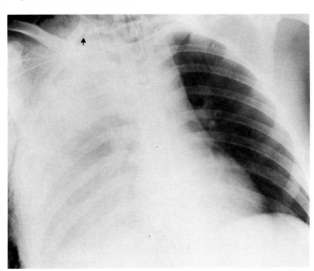

B

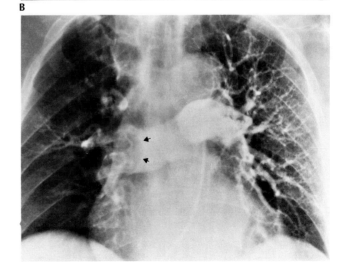

FIG C29-5. Blunt trauma. There is almost complete homogeneous opacification of the right chest, reflecting a combination of a large hemothorax and underlying pulmonary contusion. The right first rib is fractured (arrow) and subcutaneous emphysema is present in the soft tissues of the right hemithorax.

Condition	Imaging Findings	Comments
Pulmonary embolism and infarction (Fig C29-4)	Effusion is usually small and unilateral.	Pulmonary changes vary from linear shadows to segmental consolidation. There is often elevation of the hemidiaphragm with basal atelectasis.
Trauma (Fig C29-5)	Blood (hemothorax), chyle (chylothorax), ingested food (esophageal rupture).	Traumatic aortic rupture and esophageal perforation are almost always left-sided. There may be evidence of fractured ribs, pulmonary or mediastinal hemorrhage, aortic aneurysm, pneumothorax, or pneumomediastinum.
Congestive heart failure (Fig C29-6)	Effusion is frequently unilateral on the right, but rarely on the left. May be bilateral.	Usually generalized cardiomegaly and clinical signs of cardiac decompensation. There may be an associated phantom tumor (fluid localized in an interlobar pleural fissure).
Constrictive pericarditis (Fig C29-7)	Effusion is frequently unilateral on the right, but rarely on the left. May be bilateral.	Effusion develops in about 50% of cases. Characteristic pericardial calcification.
Asbestosis	Effusion occurs in 10% to 20% of cases, is usually bilateral, and is often recurrent.	Usually pleural thickening or plaques that are often calcified. High incidence of associated bronchogenic carcinoma and mesothelioma.
Sarcoidosis (Fig C29-8)	Effusion in 1% to 4% of patients.	Invariably associated with pulmonary disease. The effusion tends to clear within 2 months but may progress to chronic pleural thickening.
Systemic lupus erythematosus (Fig C29-9)	Effusion in 35% to 75% of cases. Bilateral in half the cases, and predominantly left-sided when unilateral.	Often associated with cardiac enlargement (commonly due to pericardial effusion) and nonspecific pulmonary changes (basal atelectasis or infiltrate).
Rheumatoid disease	Effusion is probably the most frequent manifestation in the thorax.	May be isolated or associated with a diffuse reticulonodular pattern that predominantly involves the bases.
Wegener's granulomatosis	Effusion is relatively common but is overshadowed by the pulmonary manifestations.	Single or multiple pulmonary nodules, often with cavitation (see Fig C8-12) and frequently associated with renal disease.
Waldenstrom's macroglobulinemia	Effusion in about 50% of patients with lung involvement.	Diffuse reticulonodular pattern. Often hepatosplenomegaly and palpable peripheral adenopathy.
Drug-induced	Unilateral or bilateral effusions may occur.	Usually associated with a diffuse interstitial pattern. Causes include nitrofurantoin, hydralazine, and procainamide.

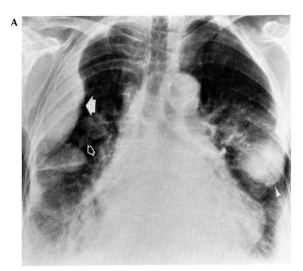 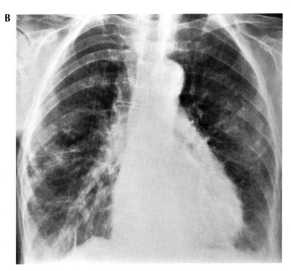

FIG C29-6. Phantom tumors. (A) Frontal chest radiograph taken during an episode of congestive heart failure demonstrates marked cardiomegaly with bilateral pleural effusions. Note the fluid collections along the lateral chest wall (closed arrow), in the minor fissure (open arrow), and in the left major fissure (arrowhead). (B) With improvement in the patient's cardiac status, the phantom tumors have disappeared. Bilateral small pleural effusions persist.

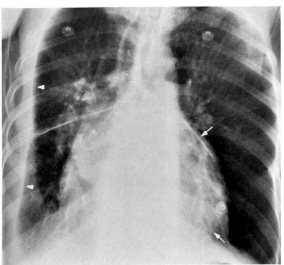 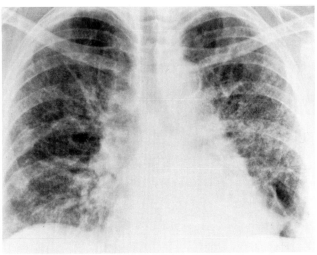

FIG C29-8. Sarcoidosis. Small left pleural effusion in a patient with diffuse interstitial lung disease.

FIG C29-7. Constrictive pericarditis. Lateral decubitus view of the chest demonstrates moderate enlargement of the cardiac silhouette and a large right pleural effusion (arrowheads). Note the calcified plaque (arrows) in the pericardium.

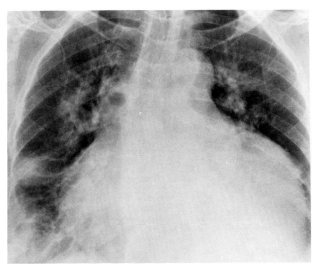

FIG C29-9. Systemic lupus erythematosus. Bilateral pleural effusions, more marked on the right, with some streaks of basilar atelectasis. The massive cardiomegaly is due to a combination of pericarditis and pericardial effusion.

CHYLOTHORAX

Condition	Comments
Iatrogenic (surgical injury to thoracic duct)	Most frequent cause of chylothorax. The thoracic duct crosses to the left of the spine between T5 and T7 and thus is particularly vulnerable to injury during surgery on the left hemithorax in the hilar region. Especially common complication in children undergoing surgery for congenital heart disease.
Trauma to thoracic duct (Fig C30-1)	Penetrating or nonpenetrating injuries (especially after a heavy meal when the duct is distended). There may be a fractured rib or vertebra, and several days may pass before the pleural fluid is detectable radiographically. An injury to the lower third of the thoracic duct produces a right-sided chylothorax. Rupture of the upper third causes left-sided fluid. Nonpenetrating trauma may be bilateral.
Tumor obstruction of thoracic duct (Fig C30-2)	Most commonly caused by lymphoma or bronchogenic carcinoma. A right-sided chylothorax develops when the lower portion of the duct is invaded; left-sided involvement occurs when the upper half is affected. May also be bilateral.
Spontaneous chylothorax	One third of the cases have no precipitating cause.
Pulmonary lymphangiomatosis	Proliferation of smooth muscle obliterates the thoracic duct, resulting in chylothorax and chylous ascites.
Intrinsic thoracic duct abnormality	Atresia, tumor, or aneurysm with rupture of the thoracic duct.
Tuberculosis	Enlarged lymph nodes or paravertebral abscess may compress or erode the thoracic duct.
Filariasis	Nematode infection causing a peripheral lymphangitis that may ascend to involve the thoracic duct and cause perforation.

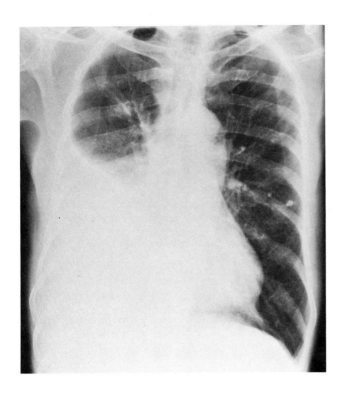

FIG C30-1. Trauma to thoracic duct. A large volume of fluid in the right hemithorax obscures fractures of several lower right ribs.

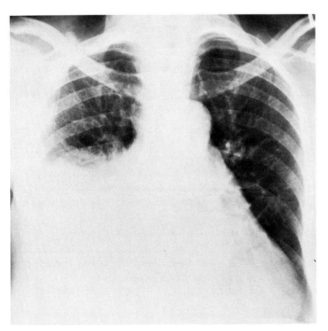

FIG C30-2. Tumor obstruction of thoracic duct. Involvement of the lower portion of the thoracic duct by bronchogenic carcinoma. The large amount of chylous fluid obscures the underlying primary tumor.

PNEUMOTHORAX

Condition	Comments
Spontaneous pneumothorax (Fig C31-1)	Occurs most commonly in men in the third and fourth decades of life. Usually due to rupture of a pleural bleb (small cystic space generally situated over the lung apex).
Iatrogenic (Figs C31-2 and C31-3)	Complication of central line insertion, thoracentesis, tracheostomy, resuscitation or artificial ventilation, or a result of thoracotomy.
Trauma (Fig C31-4)	May reflect laceration of the visceral pleura by fragments of a fractured rib.
Mediastinal emphysema	Pneumomediastinum and increased mediastinal pressure lead to the development of a unilateral or bilateral pneumothorax.
Hyaline membrane disease	Pneumothorax associated with air-space consolidation and interstitial emphysema is probably related to prolonged assisted ventilation. There may be an associated pneumomediastinum.
Interstitial lung disease (Fig C31-5)	Pneumothorax associated with a diffuse reticulonodular pattern may occur in any cause of honeycomb lung (especially eosinophilic granuloma), cystic fibrosis, hemosiderosis, and sarcoidosis.
Infectious disease (Figs C31-6 and C31-7)	Pneumothorax associated with air-space consolidation may occur in acute bacterial pneumonia or in a bronchopleural fistula from tuberculosis, fungus, or other granulomatous disease. May also be caused by a ruptured pneumatocele in staphylococcal pneumonia in children.
Catamenial pneumothorax	Pneumothorax occurring coincidentally with menses in a woman with endometriosis.
Pneumoperitoneum	Passage of air upward through the diaphragm.
Pulmonary metastases	Pneumothorax associated with parenchymal nodules. Most commonly occurs in osteogenic and other types of sarcoma. A similar pattern may occur with Wilms' tumor and carcinomas of the pancreas and adrenals.

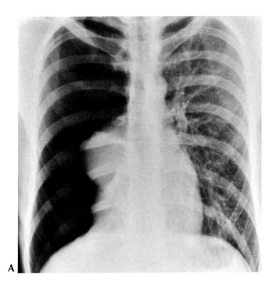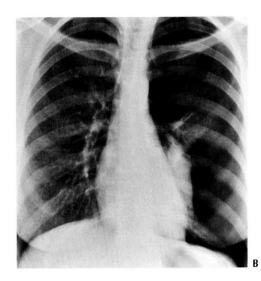

FIG C31-1. **(A and B) Spontaneous pneumothorax.** Complete collapse of the lung in two different patients.

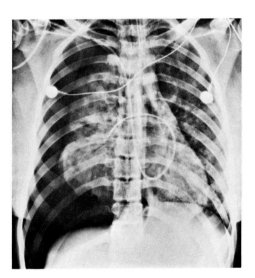

FIG C31-2. **Complication of Swan-Ganz catheter insertion.** A large right pneumothorax developed after puncture of the right pleura.[39]

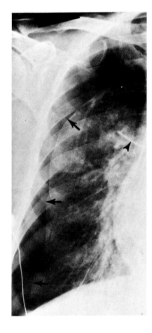

FIG C31-3. **Pneumothorax complicating nasoenteric tube placement.** Large right-sided pneumothorax (black arrows) on a radiograph obtained immediately after removal of a feeding tube (arrowhead) from the pleural space.[40]

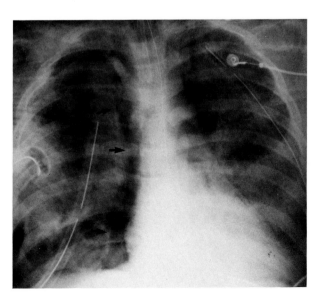

FIG C31-4. **Posttraumatic pneumothorax.** Anteromedial pneumothorax (arrows) along with extensive air-space parenchymal disease.[41]

Condition	Comments
Pulmonary infarct	Pneumothorax is a rare complication that is probably caused by intermittent positive pressure breathing or superimposed infection.
Adult respiratory distress syndrome (Fig C31-8)	Pneumothorax associated with diffuse air-space consolidation in a patient treated with prolonged artificial ventilation.
Bauxite pneumoconiosis (Shaver's disease)	Spontaneous pneumothorax is a frequent complication of this occupational disorder in workers who process bauxite in the manufacture of corundum. A diffuse interstitial pulmonary fibrosis also may develop in workers who inhale fine aluminum powder.

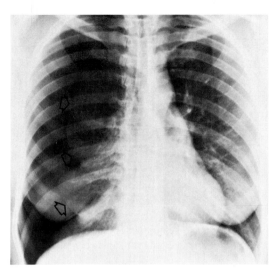

Fig C31-5. Asthma. Severe coughing and straining during an acute attack led to the development of a large pneumothorax with substantial collapse of the right lung (arrows).

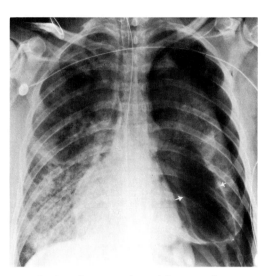

Fig C31-6. Infectious disease. Moderate left pneumothorax in a patient with severe *Pneumocystis* pneumonia. Note the air in the pulmonary ligament (arrows) and the air bronchograms in the collapsed lung.

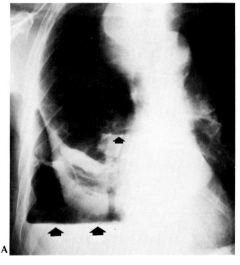

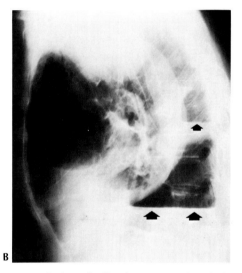

Fig C31-7. Bronchopleural fistula. (A) Frontal and (B) lateral views of the chest demonstrate multiple air-fluid levels (arrows) in the right hemithorax. The large right superior mediastinal mass represented metastatic spread from a previously resected carcinoma of the right lung.

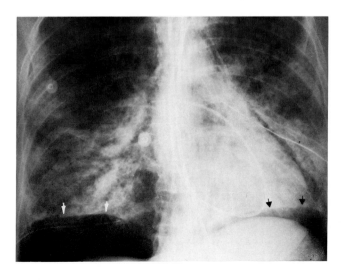

Fig C31-8. Adult respiratory distress syndrome. Bilateral subpulmonary pneumothoraxes (arrows) in this patient with severe sepsis.[41]

TRACHEAL MASS/NARROWING

Condition	Imaging Findings	Comments
Adenoma (Fig C32-1)	Round, sessile, smooth, sharply demarcated mass.	Cylindroma accounts for 40% of tracheal tumors. It tends to occur in the middle third, grows slowly, and metastasizes late (especially to bone and lung). Less frequent tumors are mucoepidermoid adenoma and carcinoid.
Tracheal carcinoma (Fig C32-2)	Irregular, lobulated, or annular lesion.	Uncommon neoplasm that is most frequently of squamous cell origin (also adenocarcinoma and oat cell). Tends to invade mediastinal soft tissues and spread to lymph nodes and the esophagus. Hematogenous metastases to lung, bone, liver, and brain.
Extramedullary myeloma (Fig C32-3)	Smooth intrinsic mass.	Abnormal plasma cell proliferation occasionally occurs outside the bone marrow. The vast majority occur in the head and neck—primarily in the nasal cavity, paranasal sinuses, and upper airway. Most patients with an extramedullary myeloma respond favorably to treatment and, even with local recurrences, may survive for many years.
Tracheal invasion from extrinsic tumor	Extrinsic mass.	Carcinomas of the thyroid, larynx, lung, and esophagus. A tracheoesophageal fistula may develop spontaneously or after radiation therapy.
Metastases	Solitary or multiple, sessile or pedunculated masses.	Metastases to the trachea are infrequent. The most common primary tumor is hypernephroma, followed by melanoma and carcinomas of the breast and colon.
Spindle cell tumor	Sessile, smooth, sharply demarcated mass.	Neurinoma, leiomyoma, fibroma, xanthoma, hemangioma. Malignant spindle cell tumors may be irregular, but cannot be differentiated from benign tumors unless metastases are demonstrated.
Cartilaginous tumor	Smooth, sessile, well-circumscribed mass.	Chondroma, hamartoma.
Papillomatosis	Innumerable small nodules that may involve the entire trachea. Rarely, a single large papilloma.	Laryngeal papillomatosis is a common disease of children that may seed distally into the tracheobronchial tree and even cause bronchial obstruction. Infrequent pulmonary nodules typically excavate to produce multiple thin-walled cystic lesions (see Fig C8-16).
Ectopic thyroid tumor	Smoothly rounded, often broad-based mass.	The ectopic thyroid tissue may undergo goitrous change or even become malignant. There may be a connecting bridge between the ectopic mass and the normally placed thyroid gland.

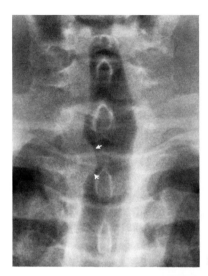

Fig C32-1. Adenoma (arrows).

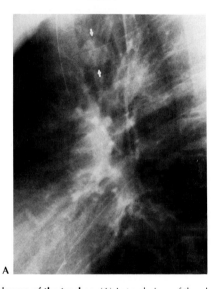

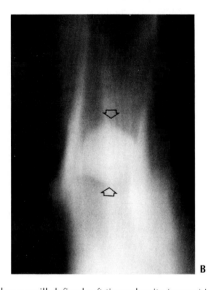

A

B

Fig C32-2. Carcinoma of the trachea. (A) Lateral view of the chest shows an ill-defined soft-tissue density (arrows) in the tracheal air column. (B) A tomogram more clearly shows the mass (arrows).

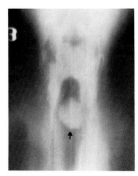

Fig C32-3. Extramedullary myeloma. Proliferation of plasma cells forms a mass in the trachea.[42]

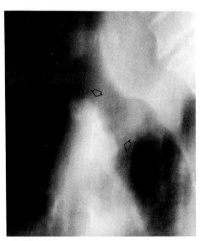

Fig C32-4. Healing of tracheostomy stoma. Lateral tomogram demonstrates thickening of the anterior tracheal wall (arrows), secondary to fibrosis and granulation tissue, at the site of the stoma. This finding was of no functional significance.[43]

Condition	Imaging Findings	Comments
Intubation stricture (Figs C32-4 and C32-5)	Luminal narrowing of variable length.	Most commonly due to tracheostomy. Also secondary to the use of endotracheal tubes (related to high-pressure cuffs).
Penetrating or blunt trauma	Often associated with subcutaneous emphysema, pneumomediastinum, pneumothorax, and fractures of the upper ribs.	If the original injury is not recognized, the healing process leads to luminal stenosis. An adjacent hematoma can cause an extrinsic impression and severely narrow the trachea.
Foreign body	Nonspecific filling defect in the airway.	Often difficult to detect and may require evidence of secondary aeration disturbances.
Amyloidosis	Diffuse narrowing of or nodular protrusions into the tracheal lumen.	Submucosal deposition of the proteinaceous amyloid material may result in obstructive hyperinflation, atelectasis, or recurrent pneumonia.
Tracheopathia osteoplastica	Multiple sessile nodular masses (often with rimming calcification).	Multiple submucosal osteocartilaginous growths along the inner surface of the trachea. The posterior membranous wall is typically spared, unlike the circumferential pattern in amyloidosis.
Rhinoscleroma	Nodular masses or diffuse symmetric narrowing.	Chronic granulomatous disorder that primarily affects the nose, paranasal sinuses, and pharynx but may extend to involve the proximal and even the entire trachea. During the healing stage, the granulation tissue is replaced by fibrous tissue with resultant stenoses of the respiratory tract.
Sarcoidosis	Luminal narrowing or discrete nodules.	Usually supraglottic, but may extend into the subglottic region or, rarely, into the distal trachea. Most patients have well-established sarcoidosis elsewhere.
Relapsing polychondritis (Fig C32-6)	Diffuse, symmetric luminal narrowing (initially involves the larynx and the subglottic trachea).	Characteristic clinical syndrome of recurrent episodes of inflammation of the pinna of the ear and the nasal, laryngeal, and tracheal cartilages. Laryngeal and tracheal involvement (in 50% of cases) may result in airway obstruction or recurrent pneumonia.
Wegener's granulomatosis	Smooth luminal narrowing of variable length.	May rarely involve the subglottic larynx and proximal trachea, though much more common in the upper or lower respiratory tract.
Chronic obstructive pulmonary disease ("saber-sheath" trachea) (Fig C32-7)	Narrowing of the coronal diameter of the intrathoracic trachea (to half that of the sagittal diameter or less).	The lateral walls of the trachea are usually thickened and there is often evidence of ossification of the cartilaginous rings. The trachea abruptly changes to a normal rounded configuration at the thoracic outlet.

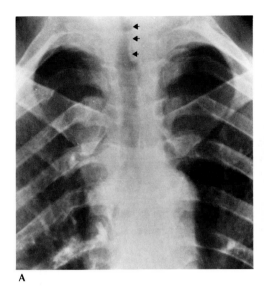

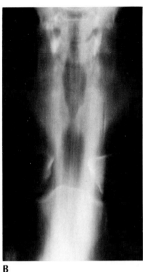

Fig C32-5. Tracheal stenosis after intubation. (A) Plain chest radiograph demonstrates narrowing of the trachea (arrows) after prolonged intubation. (B) In another patient, a frontal tomogram shows a well-defined tubular area of tracheal narrowing at the tracheostomy cuff site.

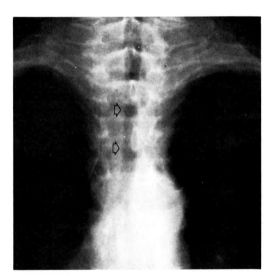

Fig C32-6. Relapsing polychondritis. Narrowing of the trachea from the subglottic region to its bifurcation (arrows) in this patient with long-standing disease.[44]

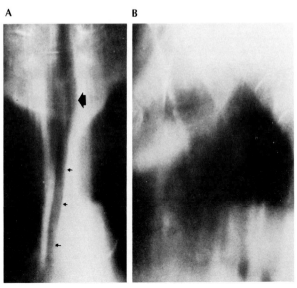

Fig C32-7. Saber-sheath trachea. (A) Frontal and (B) lateral tomographic sections in a patient with chronic obstructive pulmonary disease demonstrate severe coronal narrowing of the intrathoracic trachea (small arrows) with an abrupt change to a more rounded cross-sectional shape at the thoracic outlet (large arrow). Calcific densities are present in the tracheal rings.[45]

UPPER AIRWAY OBSTRUCTION IN CHILDREN

Condition	Imaging Findings	Comments
Croup (Fig C33-1)	Smooth tapered narrowing of the subglottic trachea.	Very common and usually mild.
Epiglottitis (Fig C33-2)	Huge swelling of the epiglottis and aryepiglottic folds (fills the entire hypopharynx).	Much more uncommon and far more dangerous condition than croup. Caused by *Hemophilus influenzae*.
Foreign body	Opaque or nonopaque lesion that may involve the pharynx, larynx, or trachea.	Foreign body at the tracheal bifurcation is difficult to diagnose (causes symptoms of both upper and lower tract obstruction; prolonged and difficult inspiration *and* expiration on fluoroscopy).
Intrinsic mass (Fig C33-3)	Single or multiple filling defects in the airway.	Tracheal hemangioma, fibroma, laryngeal papillomatosis, bronchial duplication cyst.
Extrinsic mass	Extrinsic impression on the airway.	Cystic hygroma, thyroglossal duct cyst, ectopic thyroid tissue, neoplasm.
Tracheal stricture	Diffuse or localized tracheal narrowing.	Posttraumatic, postoperative, postintubation. Primary congenital stenosis is exceedingly rare.
Vascular ring	Narrowing of the distal trachea.	Wide spectrum of anomalous vascular patterns (usually associated with a right-sided aortic arch). Often one or more impressions on the barium-filled esophagus.
Choanal atresia	Soft-tissue or bony obstruction. Usually no abnormality on plain radiographs.	Bilateral atresia causes severe respiratory distress in the newborn infant. The obstruction can be demonstrated after the introduction of a small amount of oily contrast material into the nostrils.
Enlarged tonsils and adenoids (Fig C33-4)	Soft-tissue mass narrowing the airway in the nasopharynx and oropharynx.	May be gross hypertrophy without upper airway obstruction.
Peritonsilar abscess	Soft-tissue mass in the region of the soft palate and hypopharynx.	
Pharyngeal airway obstruction by retroplaced tongue	Micrognathia associated with airway obstruction that varies between inspiratory and expiratory films.	Pierre Robin syndrome (cleft palate, micrognathia, retrodisplaced tongue); Möbius' syndrome (cranial nerve palsies often associated with micrognathia); extremely rare isolated micrognathia.

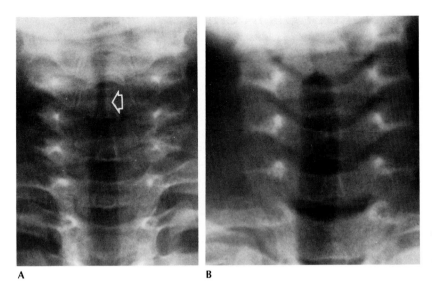

A   B

FIG C33-1. Croup. (A) Smooth, tapered narrowing of the subglottic portion of the trachea (gothic arch sign). (B) A normal trachea with broad shouldering in the subglottic region.

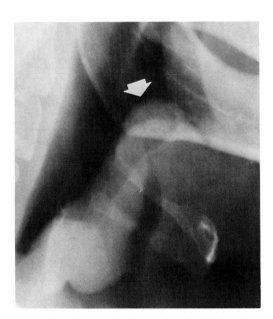

FIG C33-2. Epiglottitis. Lateral radiograph of the neck demonstrates a wide, rounded configuration of the inflamed epiglottis (arrow).[46]

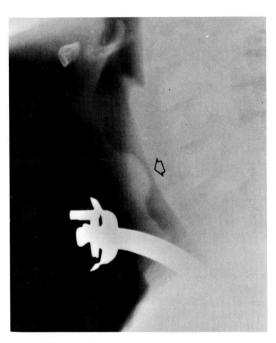

FIG C33-3. Fibroma of the cervical trachea. Lateral view of the neck shows a sharply defined homogeneous soft-tissue density (arrow) arising from the upper anterior portion of the trachea. This 11-year-old boy had experienced dyspnea and inspiratory stridor for several years.[43]

Condition	Imaging Findings	Comments
Esophageal atresia and tracheoesophageal fistula (Figs C33-5 and C33-6)	Blind air-filled upper esophageal pouch causing anterior displacement and compression of the tracheal air shadow.	Diagnosis confirmed by the looping of a radiopaque catheter (may inject a small amount of contrast material). Gas in the bowel indicates a distal tracheoesophageal fistula. Also H-type fistulas (cause recurrent aspiration).
Laryngomalacia	Downward displacement and buckling of the aryepiglottic folds in inspiration.	Aryepiglottic hypermobility (the larynx itself is structurally normal but there is excessive relaxation of the supraglottic structures). The diagnosis is made fluoroscopically with the patient in the lateral position.
Congenital vocal cord paralysis	Unilateral or bilateral absence of normal movement of the vocal cords.	Life-threatening if bilateral (vocal cords tend to remain closed).
Macroglossia	Enlarged tongue causing extrinsic impression on the airway.	May occur in hypothyroidism and in the Beckwith-Wiedemann syndrome (visceromegaly, omphalocele or umbilical hernia, pancreatic and adrenal hyperplasia, increased bone age, neoplastic disease).
Laryngeal web	Narrowing of the air column.	Membranous stenosis in a glottic, supraglottic, or infraglottic position.
Diphtheria	Narrowing of the air column.	Extension of the characteristic membrane from the pharynx into the larynx, trachea, and even the bronchial tree can lead to increasing airway obstruction, cyanosis, and finally death.
Laryngospasm	Narrowing of the air column.	Life-threatening anaphylactic reactions occur seconds to minutes after the administration of a specific antigen (generally by injection, as with radiographic contrast material, or less commonly by ingestion) and cause upper or lower airway obstruction, or both. Laryngeal edema may be experienced as a "lump" in the throat, hoarseness, or stridor, while bronchial obstruction is associated with a feeling of tightness in the chest or audible wheezing.

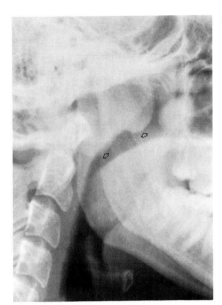

FIG C33-4. Enlarged tonsils and adenoids. Marked impressions (arrows) on the upper airway.

A   B

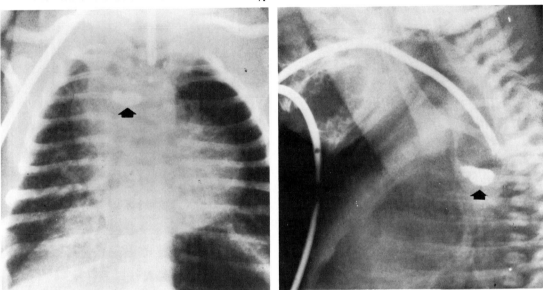

FIG C33-5. Congenital tracheoesophageal fistula. Contrast material injected through a feeding tube demonstrates occlusion of the proximal esophageal pouch (arrows) in (A) frontal and (B) lateral projections. Note the air in the stomach.

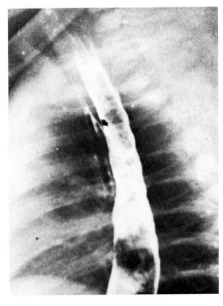

FIG C33-6. Congenital tracheoesophageal fistula (type IV, or H, fistula). Note the sharp downward course of the fistula from the trachea to the esophagus (arrow).

ELEVATED DIAPHRAGM

Condition	Comments
Normal variant	Dome of the diaphragm tends to be about half an interspace higher on the right than on the left. In about 10% of individuals, the hemidiaphragms are at the same height or the left is higher than the right.
Eventration (Figs C34-1 and C34-2)	Unilateral hypoplasia of a hemidiaphragm (very rarely both) with the thinned, weakened musculature inadequate to restrain the abdominal viscera. Localized eventration primarily involves the anteromedial portion of the right hemidiaphragm, through which a portion of the right lobe of the liver bulges. In a posterior eventration, upward displacement of the kidney can produce a rounded mass. Total eventration occurs almost exclusively on the left. Eventrations may have paradoxical diaphragmatic motion (though more commonly seen in diaphragmatic paralysis).
Phrenic nerve paralysis (Fig C34-3)	Unilateral or bilateral diaphragmatic elevation with characteristic paradoxical motion of the diaphragm (tends to ascend rather than descend with inspiration). Results from any process interfering with the normal function of the phrenic nerve (inadvertent surgical transection, primary bronchogenic carcinoma or mediastinal metastases); intrinsic neurologic disease (poliomyelitis, Erb's palsy, peripheral neuritis, hemiplegia); injury to the phrenic nerve, thoracic cage, cervical spine, or brachial plexus; pressure from a substernal thyroid or aneurysm; or lung or mediastinal infection (paralysis may be temporary).
Increased intra-abdominal volume	Unilateral or bilateral diaphragmatic elevation in patients with ascites, obesity, or pregnancy.
Intra-abdominal inflammatory disease	Unilateral or bilateral diaphragmatic elevation. Most commonly due to subphrenic abscess. Also perinephric, hepatic, or splenic abscess; pancreatitis; cholecystitis; and perforated ulcer.
Intra-abdominal mass (Fig C34-4)	Unilateral or bilateral diaphragmatic elevation caused by enlargement of the liver or spleen; abdominal tumor or cyst of the liver, spleen, kidneys, adrenals, or pancreas; or distended stomach or splenic flexure (left hemidiaphragm).
Acute intrathoracic process (splinting of diaphragm) (Fig C34-5)	Unilateral or bilateral diaphragmatic elevation due to chest wall injury, atelectasis, pulmonary infarct, or pleural disease (fibrosis, acute pleurisy).
Tumor or cyst of diaphragm	Very rare lesion that simulates unilateral diaphragmatic elevation.
Subpulmonic effusion (Fig C34-6)	Closely simulates an elevated hemidiaphragm. On frontal views, the peak of the pseudodiaphragmatic contour is lateral to that of a normal hemidiaphragm (situated near the junction of the middle and lateral thirds rather than near the center).

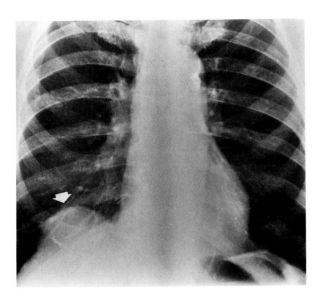

FIG C34-1. Partial eventration of the right hemidiaphragm (arrow).

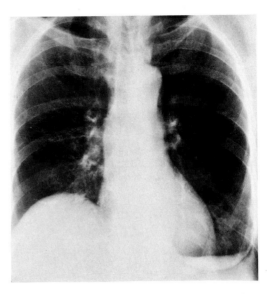

FIG C34-2. Complete eventration of the right hemidiaphragm.

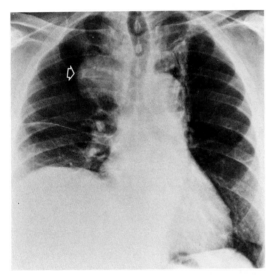

FIG C34-3. Phrenic nerve paralysis. Primary bronchogenic carcinoma (arrow) involving the phrenic nerve causes paralysis of the right hemidiaphragm.

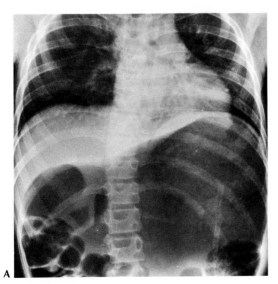

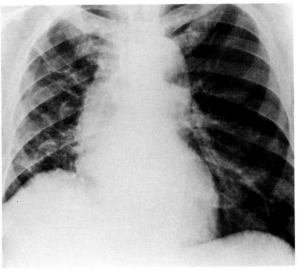

FIG C34-4. Intra-abdominal mass. (A) Acute gastric dilatation causes diffuse elevation of both leaves of the diaphragm. (B) Huge syphilitic gumma of the liver produces elevation of the right hemidiaphragm.

Condition	Comments
Altered pulmonary volume	Unilateral or bilateral diaphragmatic elevation due to atelectasis (associated pulmonary opacity); postoperative lobectomy or pneumonectomy (rib defects, sutures, shift of the heart and mediastinum); hypoplastic lung (crowded ribs, mediastinal shift, absent or small pulmonary artery, sometimes the scimitar syndrome).
Diaphragmatic hernia (Figs C34-7 and C34-8)	Mimics unilateral diaphragmatic elevation on frontal views. Lateral views show the characteristic anterior location of a Morgagni hernia or the posterior position of a Bochdalek hernia.
Traumatic rupture of diaphragm (Figs C34-9 and C34-10)	Mimics unilateral diaphragmatic elevation. Injury to the right side causes herniation of the soft-tissue density of the liver into the right hemithorax. On the left, air-containing stomach and bowel herniate into the chest (may mimic diaphragmatic elevation if the bowel loops are filled with fluid).

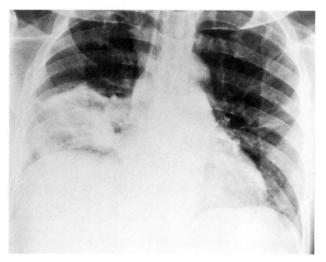

FIG C34-5. Acute pneumonia. Elevation of the right hemidiaphragm due to splinting secondary to a right lower lung infiltrate.

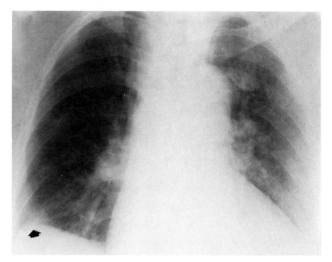

FIG C34-6. Subpulmonic effusion. The peak of the pseudodiaphragmatic contour (arrow) is lateral to that of a normal hemidiaphragm.

SOURCES

1. Reprinted with permission from ''Spherical Pneumonias in Children Simulating Pulmonary and Mediastinal Masses'' by RW Rose and BH Ward, *Radiology* (1973;106:179–182, Copyright © 1973, Radiological Society of North America Inc.

2. Reprinted with permission from ''Gram-negative Pneumonia'' by JD Unger, HD Rose, and GF Unger, *Radiology* (1973;107:283–291), Copyright © 1973, Radiological Society of North America Inc.

3. Reprinted with permission from ''Experience with Hemophilus Influenzae Pneumonia'' by M Vinick, DH Altman, and RE Parks, *Radiology* (1966;86:701–706), Copyright © 1966, Radiological Society of North America Inc.

4. Reprinted with permission from ''Pulmonary Blastomycosis'' by RA Halvorson et al, *Radiology* (1984;150:1–5), Copyright © 1984, Radiological Society of North America Inc.

5. Reprinted with permission from ''The Melting Sign in Resolving Transient Pulmonary Infarction'' by ME Woesner, I Sanders, and GW White, *American Journal of Roentgenology* (1971;111:782–790), Copyright © 1971, Williams & Wilkins Company.

6. Reprinted from *Diagnosis of Diseases of the Chest* by RG Fraser and JAP Pare with permission of WB Saunders Company, © 1979.

7. Reprinted with permission from ''The FBI Sign'' by WW Wenzel, *Colorado Medicine,* formerly *Rocky Mountain Medical Journal* (1972;69:71–72), Copyright © 1979.

8. Reprinted with permission from ''Amniotic Pulmonary Embolism'' by HR Arnold, JE Gardner, and PH Goodman, *Radiology* (1961;77:629–634), Copyright © 1961, Radiological Society of North America Inc.

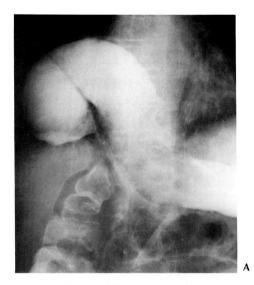 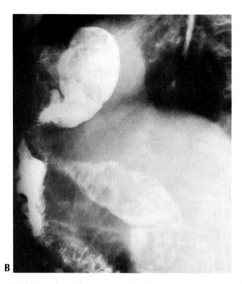

FIG C34-7. Morgagni's hernia. (A) Frontal and (B) lateral views demonstrate barium-filled bowel in a hernia sac that lies anteriorly and to the right.

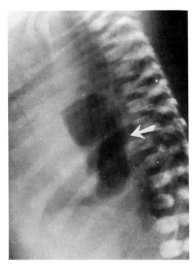 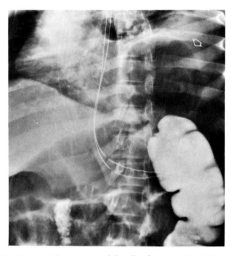

FIG C34-9. Traumatic rupture of the diaphragm. Herniation of a portion of the splenic flexure (arrow), with obstruction to the retrograde flow of barium.

FIG C34-8. Bochdalek's hernia. Gas-filled loop of bowel (arrow) is visible posteriorly in the thoracic cavity.

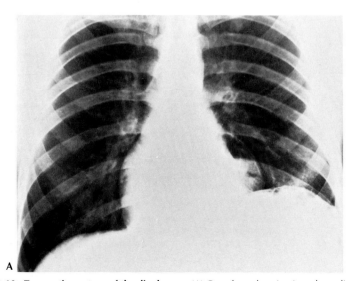 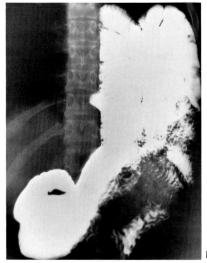

FIG C34-10. Traumatic rupture of the diaphragm. (A) On a frontal projection, the radiographic appearance simulates eventration or paralysis of the left hemidiaphragm. (B) The administration of barium clearly demonstrates the herniation of bowel contents into the chest.

9. Reprinted with permission from "An Exercise in Radiologic-Pathologic Correlation" by EG Theros, MM Reeder, and JF Eckert, *Radiology* (1968;90:784–791), Copyright © 1968, Radiological Society of North America Inc.

10. Reprinted with permission from "Pulmonary Complications of Drug Therapy" by A Brettner, RE Heitzman, and WG Woodin, *Radiology* (1970;96:31–38), Copyright © 1970, Radiological Society of North America Inc.

11. Reprinted with permission from "Bilateral Pulmonary Sequestration: CT Appearance" by KJ Wimbish, FP Agha, and TM Brady, *American Journal of Roentgenology* (1983;140:689–690), Copyright © 1983, Williams & Wilkins Company.

12. Reprinted from *Radiology of the Heart and Great Vessels* by RN Cooley and MH Schreiber, Williams & Wilkins Company, © 1978, with permission of JH Harris Jr.

13. Reprinted with permission from "Primary Pulmonary Sporotrichosis" by A Naimark and S Tiu, *Journal of Canadian Association of Radiologists* (1979;30:129–130), Copyright © 1979, Canadian Association of Radiologists.

14. Reprinted with permission from "The Ruptured Pulmonary Hydatid Cyst" by RFC Kagel and A Fatemi, *Radiology* (1961;76:60–64), Copyright © 1961, Radiological Society of North America Inc.

15. Reprinted with permission from "Eisenmenger's Syndrome" by HB Spitz, *Seminars in Roentgenology* (1968;3:373–376), Copyright © 1968, Grune & Stratton Inc.

16. Reprinted with permission from "Mediastinal Lymphadenopathy in Bubonic Plague" by VR Sites and JD Poland, *American Journal of Roentgenology* (1970;116:567–570), Copyright © 1970, Williams & Wilkins Company.

17. Reprinted with permission from "Antenatal Ultrasound Findings in Cystic Adenomatoid Malformation" by SM Donn, JN Martin, and SJ White, *Pediatric Radiology* (1981;10:180–182), Copyright © 1981, Springer-Verlag.

18. Reprinted with permission from "Bulging (Sagging) Fissure Sign in *Hemophilus Influenzae* Lobar Pneumonia" by JB Francis and PB Francis, *Southern Medical Journal* (1978;71:1452–1453), Copyright © 1978, Southern Medical Association.

19. Reprinted from *Chest Roentgenology* by B Felson with permission of WB Saunders Company, © 1973.

20. Reprinted with permission from "Diagnosis of Chemotherapy of Lung" by HD Sostman, CE Putman, and G Gamsu, *American Journal of Roentgenology* (1981;136:33–41), Copyright © 1981, Williams & Wilkins Company.

21. Reprinted from *Clinical Radiology in the Tropics* by WP Cockshott and H Middlemiss with permission of Churchill Livingstone Inc, © 1979.

22. Reprinted with permission from *British Journal of Radiology* (1963;36:889–901), Copyright © 1963, British Institute of Radiology.

23. Reprinted with permission from "Creeping Eruption with Transient Pulmonary Infiltration" by EH Kalmon, *Radiology* (1954;62:222–226), Copyright © 1954, Radiological Society of North America Inc.

24. Courtesy of the Armed Forces Institute of Pathology.

25. Reprinted with permission from "Computed Tomography in the Evaluation of Mediastinal Widening" by RL Baron et al, *Radiology* (1981;138:107–114), Copyright © 1981, Radiological Society of North America Inc.

26. Reprinted from *Computed Body Tomography* by JKT Lee, SS Sagel, and RJ Stanley (Eds) with permission of Raven Press, New York, © 1983.

27. Reprinted with permission from "Parathyroid Scanning by Computed Tomography" by DD Stark et al, *Radiology* (1983;148:297–303), Copyright © 1983, Radiological Society of North America Inc.

28. Reprinted with permission from "Laceration of the Thoracic Aorta and Brachiocephalic Arteries by Blunt Trauma" by RG Fisher, FP Hadlock, and Y Ben-Menachem, *Radiologic Clinics of North America* (1981;19: 91–112), Copyright © 1981, WB Saunders Company.

29. Reprinted with permission from "The 'V' Sign in the Diagnosis of Spontaneous Rupture of the Esophagus" by NA Naclerio, *American Journal of Surgery* (1957;93:291–298), Copyright © 1957, Yorke Medical Group.

30. Reprinted with permission from "The Multiple Roentgen Manifestations of Sclerosing Mediastinitis" by DS Feigin, JC Eggleston, and FS Siegelman, *Johns Hopkins Medical Journal* (1979;144:1–8), Copyright © 1979, Johns Hopkins University Press.

31. Reprinted with permission from "Intrapericardial Diaphragmatic Hernia" by DB Wallace, *Radiology* (1977;122:596), Copyright © 1977, Radiological Society of North America Inc.

32. Reprinted from *Computed Tomography of the Body* by AA Moss, G Gamsu, and HK Genant (Eds) with permission of WB Saunders Company, © 1983.

33. Reprinted with permission from "The Lateral Decubitus Film: An Aid in Determining Air-Trapping in Children" by MA Capitanio and JA Kirkpatrick, *Radiology* (1972;103:460–461), Copyright © 1972, Radiological Society of North America Inc.

34. Reprinted with permission from "The Continuous Diaphragm Sign: A Newly Recognized Sign of Pneumomediastinum" by B Levin, *Clinical Radiology* (1973;24:337–338), Copyright © 1973, Royal College of Radiologists.

35. Reprinted with permission from "Injuries of the Chest Wall, Pleura, Pericardium, Lungs, Bronchi, and Esophagus" by J Reynolds and JT Davis, *Radiologic Clinics of North America* (1966;4:383–398), Copyright © 1966, WB Saunders Company.

36. Reprinted with permission from "Mesotheliomas and Secondary Tumors of the Pleura" by K Ellis and M Wolff, *Seminars in Roentgenology* (1977;12:303–311), Copyright © 1977, Grune & Stratton Inc.

37. Reprinted with permission from "Roentgen Manifestations of Pleural Disease" by VA Vix, *Seminars in Roentgenology* (1977;12: 277–286), Copyright © 1977, Grune & Stratton Inc.

38. Reprinted with permission from "Pleural Plaques: A Signpost of Asbestos Dust Inhalation" by EN Sargent, G Jacobson, and JS Gordonson, *Seminars in Roentgenology* (1977;12:287–297), Copyright © 1977, Grune & Stratton Inc.

39. Reprinted with permission from "Radiologic Appearance of Compromised Thoracic Catheters, Tubes, and Wires" by RD Dunbar, *Radiologic Clinics of North America* (1984;22:699–722), Copyright © 1984, WB Saunders Company.

40. Reprinted with permission from "Pneumothorax as a Complication of Feeding Tube Placement" by GL Balogh et al, *American Journal of Roentgenology* (1983;141:1275–1277), Copyright © 1983, Williams & Wilkins Company.

41. Reprinted with permission from "Distribution of Pneumothorax in the Supine and Semirecumbent Critically Ill Adult" by IM Tocino, MH Miller, and WR Fairfax, *American Journal of Roentgenology* (1985;144:901–905), Copyright © 1985, Williams & Wilkins Company.

42. Reprinted with permission from "Plasmacytoma of the Head and Neck" by RC Gromer and AJ Duvall, *Journal of Laryngology and Otology* (1973;87:861–872), Copyright © 1973, Headley Brothers, Ltd.

43. Reprinted with permission from "Tracheal Stenosis: An Analysis of 151 Cases" by AL Weber and HC Grillo, *Radiologic Clinics of North America* (1978;16:291–308), Copyright © 1978, WB Saunders Company.

44. Reprinted with permission from "Diffuse Lesions of the Trachea" by RH Choplin, WD Wehunt, and EG Theros, *Seminars in Roentgenology* (1983;18:38–50), Copyright © 1983, Grune & Stratton Inc.

45. Reprinted with permission from "'Saber Sheath' Trachea: A Clinical and Functional Study of Marked Coronal Narrowing of Intrathoracic Trachea" by R Greene and GL Lechner, *Radiology* (1975;15:255–268), Copyright © 1975, Radiological Society of North America Inc.

46. Reprinted with permission from "The 'Thumb Sign' and 'Little Finger Sign' in Acute Epiglottitis" by JK Podgore and JW Bass, *Journal of Pediatrics* (1976;88:154–155), Copyright © 1976, The CV Mosby Company, St Louis.

Cardiovascular Patterns

2

CA1 Right atrial enlargement   **166**
CA2 Right ventricular enlargement   **168**
CA3 Left atrial enlargement   **172**
CA4 Left ventricular enlargement   **174**
CA5 Cyanotic congenital heart disease with
     increased pulmonary vascularity   **178**
CA6 Cyanotic congenital heart disease with
     decreased pulmonary vascularity   **182**
CA7 Acyanotic congenital heart disease with
     increased pulmonary blood flow   **184**
CA8 Acyanotic congenital heart disease with
     normal pulmonary blood flow   **188**
CA9 Prominent ascending aorta or aortic arch   **190**
CA10 Small ascending aorta or aortic arch   **196**
CA11 Major anomalies of the aortic arch and
     pulmonary artery   **198**
CA12 Congenital heart disease associated with
     the right aortic arch
     (mirror-image branching)   **200**
CA13 Dilatation of the main pulmonary artery   **202**
CA14 Dilatation of the superior vena cava   **206**
CA15 Dilatation of the azygos vein   **208**
CA16 Congestive heart failure in neonates
     less than 4 weeks old   **209**
CA17 High-output heart disease   **212**
CA18 Hypertensive cardiovascular disease   **214**
CA19 Cardiovascular calcification   **218**
CA20 Pericardial effusion   **224**
CA21 Constrictive pericarditis   **227**
Sources   **228**

RIGHT ATRIAL ENLARGEMENT

Condition	Imaging Findings	Comments
Left-to-right shunt	Enlarged right atrium if this chamber is the end point of a shunt.	Atrial septal defect; endocardial cushion defect; anomalous pulmonary venous return; ruptured sinus of Valsalva aneurysm into the right atrium; left ventricular–right atrial shunt.
Right ventricular enlargement/failure	Various patterns, depending on the underlying cause.	Cor pulmonale; chronic left heart failure; mitral stenosis; tetralogy of Fallot.
Tricuspid valve disease (Fig CA1-1)	Right atrial enlargement (may be extreme); often dilatation of the superior vena cava; right ventricular enlargement in tricuspid insufficiency.	Most commonly the result of rheumatic heart disease. Rarely an isolated lesion and generally associated with mitral or aortic valve disease. Tricuspid insufficiency is usually functional and secondary to marked dilatation of the failing right ventricle. Rare causes of isolated tricuspid valve disease include carcinoid syndrome, endomyocardial fibrosis, and right atrial myxoma.
Pulmonary stenosis or atresia (Fig CA1-2)	Enlargement of the right atrium and right ventricle; decreased pulmonary vascularity.	Right atrial enlargement secondary to enlargement of the right ventricle.
Hypoplastic left heart syndrome (Fig CA1-3)	Enlargement of the right atrium and right ventricle produces progressive globular cardiomegaly. Severe pulmonary venous congestion.	Consists of several conditions in which underdevelopment of left side of the heart is related to an obstructive lesion (stenosis or atresia of the mitral valve, aortic valve, or aortic arch). Causes heart failure in the first week of life.
Tricuspid atresia	Enlargement of the right atrium and left ventricle; small right ventricle; decreased pulmonary vascularity (usually some degree of pulmonary stenosis).	Right-to-left shunt at the atrial level (patent foramen ovale or true atrial septal defect). Usually also a ventricular septal defect or patent ductus arteriosus. Hypoplasia of the right ventricle and the pulmonary outflow tract. The smaller the shunt, the more marked the elevation of right atrial pressure and the more striking the enlargement of this chamber.
Ebstein's anomaly (see Fig CA6-5)	Enlargement of the right atrium causes a characteristic squared or boxed appearance of the heart. Decreased pulmonary vascularity; flat or concave pulmonary outflow tract; narrow vascular pedicle and small aortic arch.	Downward displacement of an incompetent tricuspid valve into the right ventricle so that the upper portion of the right ventricle is effectively incorporated into the right atrium. Functional obstruction to right atrial emptying produces increased pressure and a right-to-left atrial shunt (usually through a patent foramen ovale).
Uhl's disease	Radiographic pattern identical to that in Ebstein's anomaly.	Focal or complete absence of the right ventricular myocardium (the right ventricle becomes a thin-walled fibroelastic bag that contracts poorly and cannot effectively empty blood from the right side of the heart).

A B

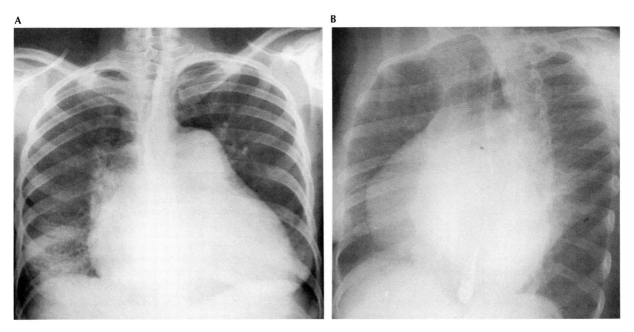

Fig CA1-1. **Tricuspid insufficiency.** (A) Frontal and (B) left anterior oblique projections show striking right atrial enlargement.[1]

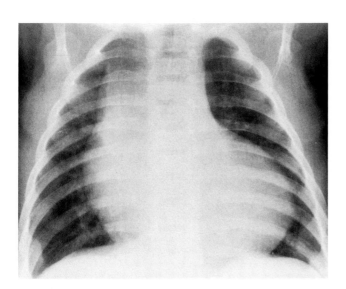

Fig CA1-2. **Pulmonary atresia.** Marked right atrial enlargement associated with decreased pulmonary vascularity.

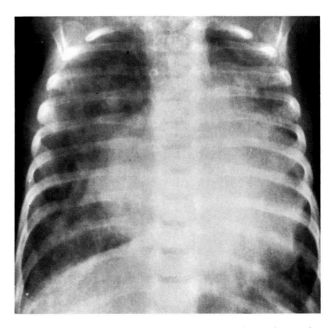

Fig CA1-3. **Hypoplastic left heart syndrome.** Globular cardiomegaly with severe pulmonary venous congestion.

RIGHT VENTRICULAR ENLARGEMENT

Condition	Imaging Findings	Comments
Tetralogy of Fallot (Fig CA2-1)	Enlargement of the right ventricle (though overall cardiac size is often normal); decreased pulmonary vascularity; flat or concave pulmonary outflow tract; right aortic arch in about 25% of patients.	Consists of (1) high ventricular septal defect, (2) obstruction to right ventricular outflow (usually infundibular pulmonary stenosis), (3) overriding of the aortic orifice above the ventricular defect, and (4) right ventricular hypertrophy. Most common cause of cyanotic congenital heart disease beyond the immediate neonatal period. If there is severe pulmonary stenosis, blood flow from both ventricles is effectively forced into the aorta, causing pronounced bulging of the ascending aorta and prominence of the aortic knob.
Pulmonary stenosis (Fig CA2-2)	Initially normal heart size; right ventricular enlargement if severe stenosis causes systolic overloading of this chamber; poststenotic dilatation of the pulmonary artery.	Common anomaly found in isolated form or in combination with other abnormalities. The stenosis is most common at the level of the pulmonary valve (supravalvular or infundibular stenosis can occur).
Mitral stenosis (Fig CA2-3)	Enlargement of the right ventricle (also the pulmonary outflow tract and central pulmonary arteries) reflects pulmonary arterial hypertension from transmitted increased pressure in the left atrium and the pulmonary veins.	Most common rheumatic valvular lesion (results from diffuse thickening of the valve by fibrous tissue or calcific deposits). Decreased left ventricular output causes a small aortic knob. Calcification of the mitral valve (best demonstrated by fluoroscopy) and pulmonary hemosiderosis may develop.
Cor pulmonale (Fig CA2-4)	Right ventricular enlargement associated with enlarged central pulmonary vessels, rapid tapering, and small peripheral vessels.	Primary or secondary to such conditions as chronic obstructive emphysema, diffuse interstitial fibrosis, widespread peripheral pulmonary emboli, and Eisenmenger's physiology (reversed left-to-right shunt). Rare causes include metastases from trophoblastic neoplasms, immunologic disease, schistosomiasis, multiple pulmonary artery stenoses or coarctations, and vasoconstrictive diseases.
Chronic left heart failure	Enlarged right ventricle associated with left ventricular enlargement and pulmonary venous congestion.	May reflect a myocardiopathy or mitral insufficiency. The transmission of increased pressure from the left side of the heart eventually leads to the development of pulmonary arterial hypertension and enlargement of the right side of the heart.
Left-to-right shunts (see Fig CA7-1)	Enlarged right ventricle and pulmonary outflow tract with increased pulmonary vascularity. The size of other structures varies depending on the specific underlying lesion.	Most commonly atrial septal defect, ventricular septal defect, or patent ductus arteriosus (for other causes see page 184).
Tricuspid insufficiency	Right ventricular enlargement that may be obscured by the often extreme enlargement of the right atrium.	Usually functional and secondary to marked dilatation of the failing right ventricle.

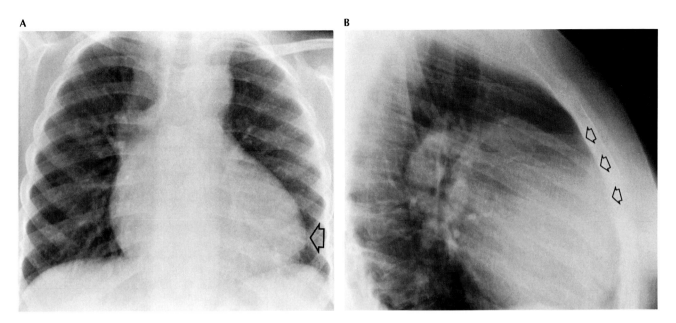

FIG CA2-1. Tetralogy of Fallot. (A) Frontal view shows right ventricular enlargement as a lateral and upward displacement of the radiographic cardiac apex (arrow). (B) On the lateral view, the enlarged right ventricle fills most of the retrosternal space (arrows).

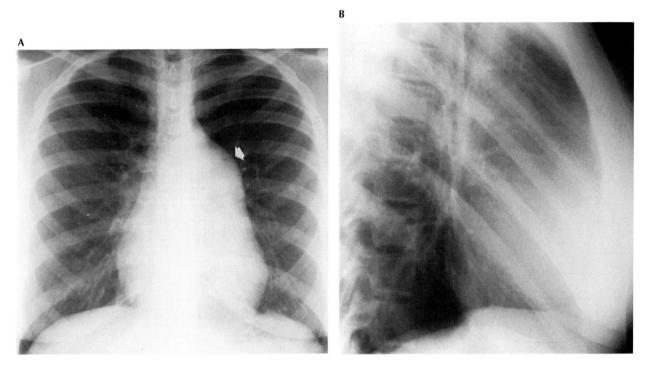

FIG CA2-2. Pulmonary stenosis. (A) Frontal and (B) lateral views show striking poststenotic dilatation of the pulmonary artery (arrow) in addition to filling of the retrosternal air space, indicating right ventricular enlargement.

Condition	Imaging Findings	Comments
Right-to-left shunts and admixture lesions	Various patterns, depending on the underlying cardiac anomaly (see pages 178 and 182).	Transposition of great vessels; trilogy of Fallot; Ebstein's anomaly; Uhl's anomaly; persistent truncus arteriosus.
Pseudotruncus arteriosus	Enlargement of the right ventricle; decreased pulmonary vascularity; flat or concave pulmonary outflow tract; right aortic arch in about 40% of patients.	Single vessel arising from the heart that is accompanied by a remnant of the atretic pulmonary artery (essentially the same as tetralogy of Fallot with pulmonary atresia).
Hypoplastic left heart syndrome	Right ventricular and right atrial enlargement cause progressive globular cardiomegaly. Severe pulmonary venous congestion.	Consists of several conditions in which underdevelopment of the left side of the heart is related to an obstructive lesion (stenosis or atresia of the mitral valve, aortic valve, or aortic arch). Causes heart failure in the first week of life.
Malformations obstructing pulmonary venous flow	Right ventricular enlargement associated with severe pulmonary venous congestion (increased pressure transmitted to the right side of the heart).	Congenital mitral stenosis; cor triatriatum (incomplete fibromuscular diaphragm dividing the left atrium); congenital pulmonary vein stenosis or atresia.
Pulmonary atresia (with tricuspid insufficiency)	Right ventricular enlargement associated with decreased pulmonary vascularity and a shallow or concave pulmonary artery segment.	May be an isolated anomaly or associated with transposition, atrial septal defect, or common ventricle.

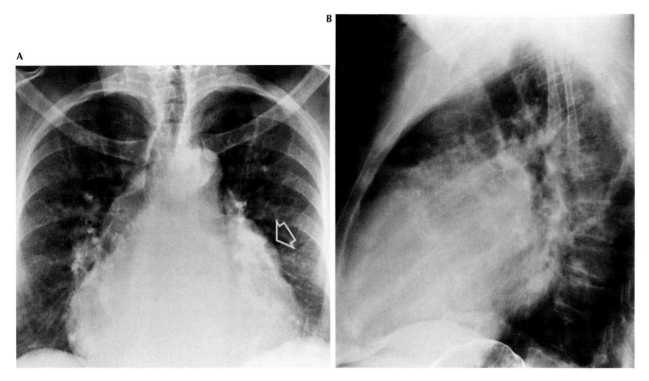

FIG CA2-3. Mitral stenosis. (A) Frontal and (B) lateral views of the chest demonstrate cardiomegaly with enlargement of the right ventricle and left atrium. The right ventricular enlargement causes obliteration of the retrosternal air space, while left atrial enlargement produces a convexity of the upper left border of the heart (arrow).

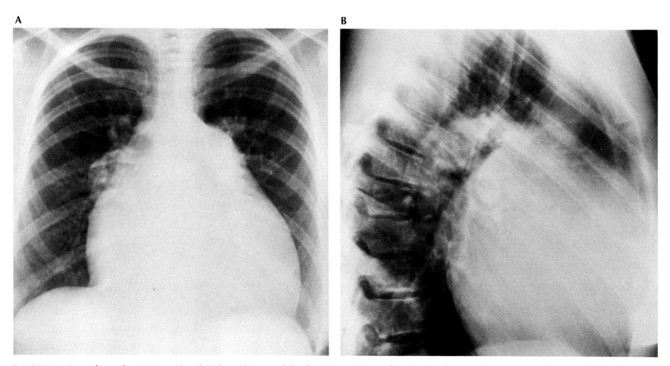

FIG CA2-4. Cor pulmonale. (A) Frontal and (B) lateral views of the chest in a patient with primary pulmonary hypertension show marked globular cardiomegaly with prominence of the pulmonary trunk and central pulmonary arteries. The peripheral pulmonary vascularity is strikingly reduced. Right ventricular enlargement has obliterated the retrosternal air space on the lateral view.

LEFT ATRIAL ENLARGEMENT

Condition	Imaging Findings	Comments
Mitral stenosis (Figs CA3-1 and CA3-2)	Left atrial enlargement; pulmonary venous congestion; enlargement of the right ventricle, pulmonary outflow tract, and central pulmonary arteries; normal-sized left ventricle; small aortic knob (decreased left ventricular output).	Most common rheumatic valvular lesion (results from diffuse thickening of the valve by fibrous tissue or calcific deposits). Obstruction of blood flow from the left atrium into the left ventricle during diastole causes increased left atrial pressure that is transmitted to the pulmonary veins and eventually to the pulmonary arteries and the right side of the heart. Calcification of the mitral valve (best demonstrated by fluoroscopy) and pulmonary hemosiderosis may develop.
Mitral insufficiency (Fig CA3-3)	Left atrial enlargement (sometimes enormous); enlargement of the left ventricle; normal-sized aortic knob.	Most often caused by rheumatic heart disease. Also rupture of chordae tendineae, papillary muscle dysfunction, or severe left ventricular dilatation that distorts the mitral annulus (congestive heart failure, aortic valve disease, coarctation of the aorta). In mitral insufficiency the left atrium is usually considerably larger than in mitral stenosis and pulmonary venous congestion is less frequent and less prominent.
Left-to-right shunts (see Fig CA7-3)	Left atrial enlargement; increased pulmonary vascularity and pulmonary outflow tract. The appearance of the right atrium, right ventricle, and aorta depends on the specific lesion (see page 184).	Ventricular septal defect, patent ductus arteriosus, and aorticopulmonary window are the most common causes. Also coronary artery fistula, persistent truncus arteriosus, and atrial septal defect with reversal of the shunt.
Myxoma of left atrium	Normal heart size and pulmonary vascularity until the tumor causes dysfunction of the mitral valve (radiographic pattern of mitral stenosis). Pathognomonic calcification is seen on fluoroscopy in about 10% of cases.	Most common primary cardiac tumor. Almost all arise in an atrium (particularly the left). The tumor is usually pedunculated and causes intermittent obstruction or traumatic injury to the mitral (or tricuspid) valve. A similar ball-valve mechanism may be produced by a left atrial thrombus. Fragmentation of the tumor may produce showers of systemic or pulmonary emboli.
Right-to-left shunts and admixture lesions	Various patterns, depending on the precise intracardiac anomaly. Left atrial enlargement may develop, though other radiographic changes are more diagnostic.	Tricuspid atresia, trilogy of Fallot, transposition of great vessels.
Endocardial fibroelastosis	Striking globular enlargement of the heart. There may be dramatic left atrial enlargement due to often-associated mitral insufficiency. Small aortic knob (decreased left ventricular output). Normal pulmonary vascularity until congestive heart failure supervenes.	Common cause of cardiac failure during the first year of life. Characterized by diffuse thickening of the left ventricular endocardium with collagen and elastic tissue.

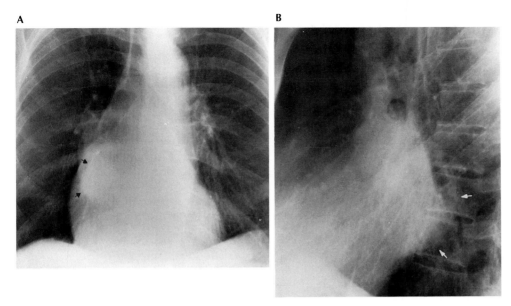

FIG CA3-1. Mitral stenosis. (A) Frontal chest radiograph demonstrates a double contour (arrows) representing the increased density of the enlarged left atrium. (B) Lateral view confirms the left atrial enlargement (arrows) in this patient with rheumatic heart disease.

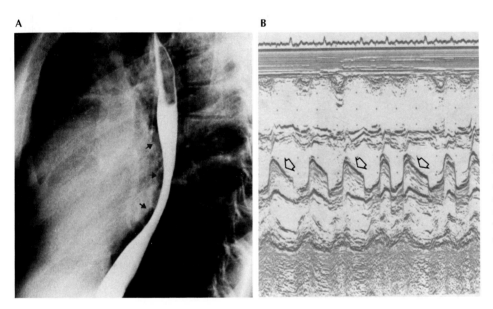

FIG CA3-2. Mitral stenosis. (A) On a lateral view, the enlarged chamber produces a discrete posterior indentation on the barium-filled esophagus. (B) Echocardiogram demonstrates thickening of the mitral valve with a decreased slope (arrows). Note that the posterior mitral valve leaflet moves anteriorly during diastole instead of posteriorly, a finding diagnostic of mitral stenosis.

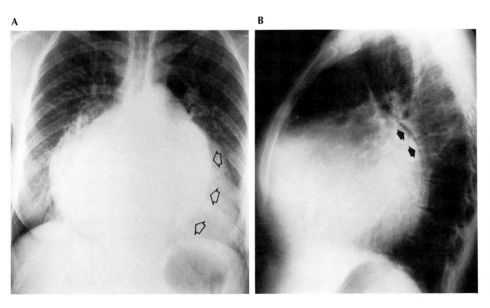

FIG CA3-3. Mitral insufficiency. (A) Frontal and (B) lateral views of the chest demonstrate gross cardiomegaly with enlargement of the left atrium and left ventricle. Note the striking double-contour configuration (open arrows) and elevation of the left main bronchus (closed arrows), characteristic signs of left atrial enlargement. The aortic knob is normal in size and there is no evidence of pulmonary venous congestion.

LEFT VENTRICULAR ENLARGEMENT

Condition	Imaging Findings	Comments
Congestive heart failure	Left ventricular enlargement with pulmonary venous congestion. Pleural effusion is common (bilateral or right-sided; unilateral left-sided effusion is rare and suggests another cause).	Precise type and degree of cardiac enlargement depend on the underlying heart disease.
High-output heart disease (see CA17)	Left ventricular enlargement associated with prominent pulmonary vascularity (both arteries and veins) and dilatation of the main pulmonary artery.	Causes include anemia, thyrotoxicosis, beriberi, hypervolemia, arteriovenous fistulas, Paget's disease, Pickwickian obesity, polycythemia vera, and pregnancy.
Arteriosclerotic heart disease (myocardial ischemia) (Fig CA4-1)	Plain chest radiograph is often normal. Left ventricular enlargement is a nonspecific finding that usually reflects the presence of a large quantity of infarcted myocardium.	Coronary artery calcification (see Fig CA19-5) strongly suggests hemodynamically significant disease. The calcification primarily involves the circumflex and anterior descending branches of the left coronary artery. Best seen with cardiac fluoroscopy (infrequently visualized on routine chest radiographs).
Acute myocardial infarction (Fig CA4-2)	Generally normal appearance. Left ventricular dilatation is usually related to superimposed pulmonary venous congestion.	Weakening of the myocardial wall at the site of an infarct may permit the development of a ventricular aneurysm, which causes focal bulging or diffuse prominence along the lower left border of the heart near the apex (located anteriorly on lateral view). Characteristic curvilinear calcification in the aneurysm wall and paradoxical or extremely limited pulsation on fluoroscopy.
Hypertension (see CA18)	Initially, increased workload causes left ventricular hypertrophy that produces no radiographic change or only rounding of the left heart border. Eventually, continued strain leads to dilatation and enlargement of the left ventricle. Aortic tortuosity with prominence of the ascending portion often occurs.	Widened superior mediastinum (increased fat deposition) and vertebral compression suggest Cushing's syndrome; figure-3 sign and rib notching indicate coarctation; paravertebral mass suggests pheochromocytoma; erosion of the distal clavicle suggests secondary hyperparathyroidism (renal disease).
Aortic insufficiency (Fig CA4-3)	Left ventricular enlargement (dilatation and hypertrophy). Dilatation of the ascending aorta and aortic knob. As the left ventricle fails, pulmonary venous congestion develops along with left atrial enlargement (due to relative mitral insufficiency).	Most commonly caused by rheumatic heart disease; also caused by infective endocarditis, syphilis, dissecting aneurysm, and Marfan's syndrome. Congenital aortic insufficiency is usually due to a bicuspid valve.
Aortic stenosis (Fig CA4-4)	Initially, concentric left ventricular hypertrophy produces only some rounding of the cardiac apex (overall heart size is normal). Left ventricular failure and dilatation develop late and are often accompanied by left atrial enlargement, pulmonary venous congestion, and prominence of the right ventricle and pulmonary artery. Poststenotic dilatation of the ascending aorta occurs with valvular stenosis.	May be due to rheumatic heart disease or a congenital valvular deformity (especially a bicuspid valve), or may represent a degenerative process of aging (idiopathic calcific stenosis). An aortic valve disorder due to rheumatic heart disease is rarely isolated and is most commonly associated with a significant lesion of the mitral valve. Aortic valve calcification (best seen with fluoroscopy) is common and indicates severe aortic stenosis.

A

B

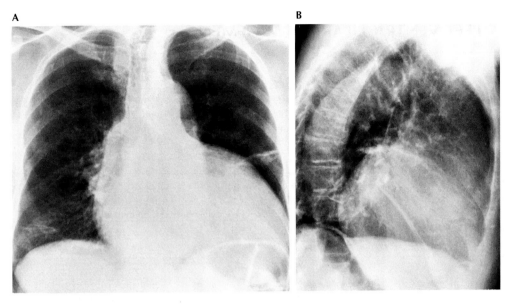

FIG CA4-1. Arteriosclerotic heart disease. (A) Frontal and (B) lateral views of the chest show marked enlargement of the left ventricle. There is also tortuosity of the aorta and bilateral streaks of fibrosis.

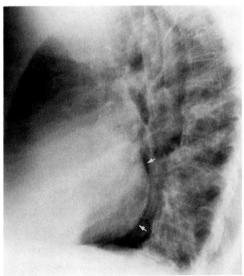

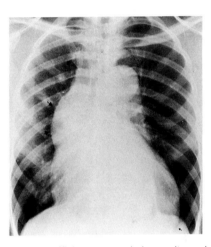

FIG CA4-2. Acute myocardial infarction. Lateral view of the chest shows marked prominence of the left ventricle (arrows).

FIG CA4-3. Aortic insufficiency. Frontal chest radiograph shows left ventricular enlargement with downward and lateral displacement of the cardiac apex. Note that the cardiac shadow extends below the dome of the left hemidiaphragm (small arrow). The ascending aorta is strikingly dilated (large arrows), suggesting some underlying aortic stenosis.

A

B

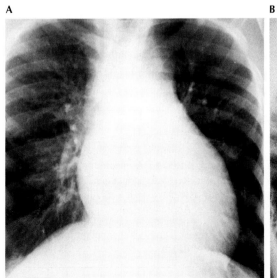

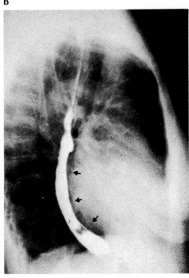

FIG CA4-4. Aortic stenosis. (A) Frontal view shows downward displacement of the cardiac apex. (B) On a lateral view, the bulging of the lower half of the posterior cardiac silhouette causes a broad indentation on the barium-filled esophagus (arrows).

Condition	Imaging Findings	Comments
Coarctation of aorta	Enlargement of the left ventricle with a characteristic double bulge in the region of the aortic knob (figure-3 sign on plain chest radiographs and reverse figure-3, or figure-E, sign on the barium-filled esophagus). There may be rib notching (usually involving the posterior fourth to eighth ribs) but rarely developing before age 6.	In the more common "adult" type, aortic narrowing occurs at or just distal to the level of the ductus arteriosus (double bulge represents prestenotic and poststenotic dilatation). In the "infantile" variety there is a long segment of narrowing lying proximal to the ductus (obligatory right-to-left shunt and early congestive heart failure). There is a relatively high incidence of coarctation in women with Turner's syndrome.
Mitral insufficiency **(Fig CA4-5)**	Enlargement (sometimes enormous) of the left ventricle and left atrium. Small or normal aortic knob. Generally normal pulmonary vascularity (there may be pulmonary venous congestion but it is much less frequent and less prominent than in mitral stenosis).	Most often caused by rheumatic heart disease; also may be due to rupture of chordae tendineae, papillary muscle dysfunction, or severe left ventricular dilatation (aortic valve disease, congestive heart failure) distorting the mitral annulus. Coexistent mitral stenosis may produce a bizarre pattern.
Myocardiopathy **(Figs CA4-6 and CA4-7)**	Generalized cardiac enlargement, often with left ventricular predominance. May mimic pericardial effusion. The development of left ventricular failure produces pulmonary venous congestion.	Causes include inflammation (rheumatic, septic, viral, toxoplasmic); infiltration (amyloidosis, glycogen storage disease, leukemia); endocrine imbalance (thyrotoxicosis, myxedema, acromegaly); ischemia; nutritional deficiency (beriberi, alcoholism, potassium or magnesium depletion); toxicity (drugs, chemicals, cobalt); collagen diseases; and postpartum heart disease.
Left-to-right shunt **(see Figs CA7-3 and CA7-5)**	Various patterns of abnormal heart size with increased pulmonary vascularity.	Ventricular septal defect (*not* atrial septal defect), patent ductus arteriosus, endocardial cushion defect, aorticopulmonary window, and, infrequently, persistent truncus arteriosus.
Right-to-left shunt or admixture lesion	Various patterns of abnormal heart size and pulmonary vascularity.	Transposition of great vessels; tricuspid atresia; pulmonary stenosis with intact ventricular septum.
Endocardial fibroelastosis **(Fig CA4-8)**	Generalized cardiac enlargement with hypertrophy and dilatation of the left ventricle and often dramatic left atrial enlargement (due to associated mitral insufficiency).	Diffuse thickening of the left ventricular endocardium with collagen and elastic tissue. A common cause of cardiac failure in the first year of life.

A

B

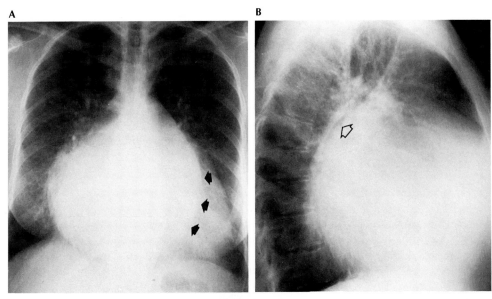

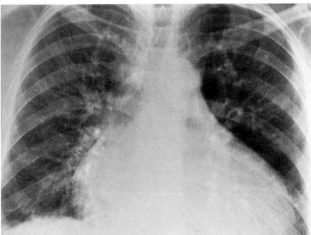

FIG CA4-5. Mitral insufficiency. (A) Frontal and (B) lateral views of the chest demonstrate cardiomegaly with enlargement of the left ventricle and left atrium. Note the striking double-contour configuration (closed arrows) and elevation of the left main-stem bronchus (open arrow), characteristic signs of left atrial enlargement.

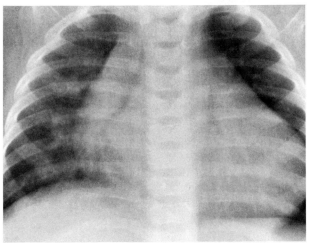

FIG CA4-6. Glycogen storage disease. Generalized globular cardiac enlargement with a left ventricular prominence.

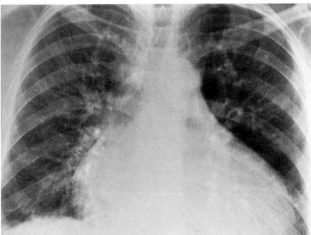

FIG CA4-7. Alcoholic cardiomyopathy. Generalized cardiac enlargement that involves all chambers but has a left ventricular predominance. There is pulmonary vascular congestion and a right pleural effusion.

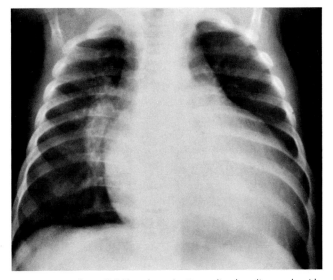

FIG CA4-8. Endocardial fibroelastosis. Generalized cardiomegaly with prominence of the left ventricle.

CYANOTIC CONGENITAL HEART DISEASE
WITH INCREASED PULMONARY VASCULARITY

Condition	Imaging Findings	Comments
Persistent truncus arteriosus (types I, II, and III) (Fig CA5-1)	Increased pulmonary vascularity; concave pulmonary outflow tract; striking enlargement of the right ventricle and eventual enlargement of the left atrium and left ventricle.	Failure of the common truncus arteriosus to divide normally into the aorta and the pulmonary artery. Results in a single large arterial trunk that receives the outflow of blood from both ventricles. Variable degree of cyanosis (more profound cyanosis if low pulmonary blood flow).
Transposition of great arteries (Figs CA5-2 and CA5-3)	Increased pulmonary vascularity (unless prominent pulmonary stenosis). Various patterns depending on the precise intracardiac anomalies (generally biventricular enlargement with an oval or egg-shaped configuration).	Reversal of the normal relation of the aorta and the pulmonary artery (the aorta arises anteriorly from the right ventricle, while the pulmonary artery originates posteriorly from the left ventricle). An intracardiac or extracardiac shunt (atrial and ventricular septal defects, patent ductus arteriosus) must be present to connect the two separate circulations. The shunts are bidirectional and permit mixing of oxygenated and unoxygenated blood (leading to cyanosis).
Taussig-Bing anomaly (Fig CA5-4)	Increased pulmonary vascularity; generalized cardiomegaly.	Aorta arises from the right ventricle while the pulmonary artery overrides the ventricular septum and receives blood from both ventricles. The pulmonary artery lies to the left of and slightly posterior to the aorta. Also a high ventricular septal defect.
Double-outlet right ventricle (Figs CA5-5 and CA5-6)	Increased pulmonary vascularity; generalized cardiomegaly; cardiac waist wider than in other types of transposition (the aorta and pulmonary artery have a more side-to-side configuration).	Both the aorta and the pulmonary artery arise from the right ventricle. A left-to-right ventricular septal defect permits oxygenated blood from the left ventricle to pass to the right ventricle and then on to the systemic circulation.
Common ventricle (Fig CA5-7)	Increased or decreased pulmonary vascularity (depending on the presence and degree of associated pulmonary stenosis); marked nonspecific globular enlargement of the heart.	Extremely large septal defect produces a functional "single ventricle." If there is associated severe pulmonary stenosis, the blood flow through the lungs is scanty and the patient has profound cyanosis.
Complete endocardial cushion defect (Fig CA5-8)	Increased pulmonary vascularity; nonspecific globular enlargement of the heart (enlargement of all cardiac chambers).	Low atrial septal defect combined with a large ventricular septal defect plus a contiguous cleft in both the mitral and the tricuspid valves (common atrioventricular canal). Bidirectional shunting with right-to-left components is responsible for producing the cyanosis.
Total anomalous pulmonary venous return (Fig CA5-9)	Increased pulmonary vascularity; "snowman" or figure-8 configuration in types I and II; characteristic indentation on the lower esophagus by the anomalous vein as it descends through the diaphragm in type III.	Pulmonary veins connect to the right atrium directly or to the systemic veins or their tributaries. Because all the pulmonary venous blood returns to the right atrium, a right-to-left shunt through an interatrial communication is necessary for blood to reach the left side of the heart and the systemic circulation (producing cyanosis).

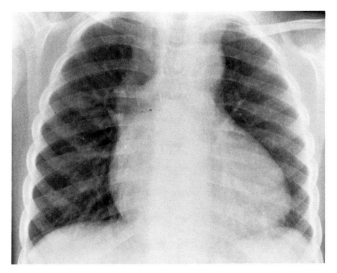

FIG CA5-1. **Persistent truncus arteriosus.** Increased pulmonary vascularity, yet typical concave appearance of the pulmonary outflow tract.

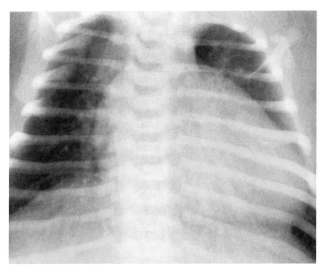

FIG CA5-2. **Transposition of the great arteries.** Biventricular enlargement produces a typical oval or egg-shaped heart. Note the narrowing of the vascular pedicle due to superimposition of the abnormally positioned aorta and pulmonary artery.

A

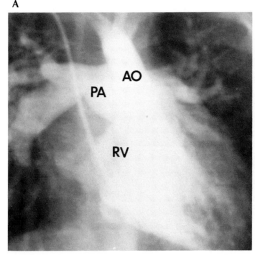

B

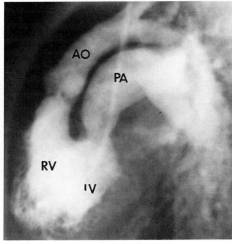

FIG CA5-3. **Transposition of the great arteries.** (A) Frontal and (B) lateral views from an angiocardiogram demonstrate contrast material in the right ventricle (RV), which is situated anteriorly and to the right. It communicates through a large ventricular septal defect with the left ventricle (LV), which is located posteriorly and to the left. The transposed aorta (AO) originates from the right ventricular infundibulum directly in front of the pulmonary artery (PA), which arises from the left ventricle.[2]

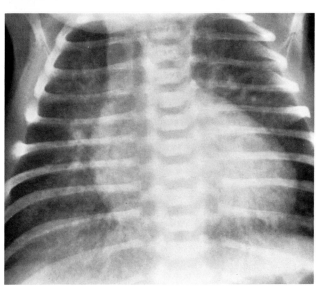

FIG CA5-4. **Taussig-Bing anomaly.** Engorged pulmonary vasculature, oval cardiomegaly, and a laterally pointing apex.

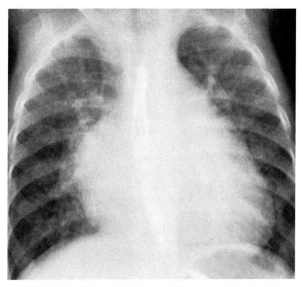

FIG CA5-5. **Double-outlet right ventricle.** Generalized cardiomegaly with increased pulmonary vascularity. Because the aorta and the pulmonary artery have a more side-to-side configuration, the cardiac waist is relatively wider than in other types of transposition.

Condition	Imaging Findings	Comments
Reversal of left-to-right shunt (Eisenmenger physiology) (Fig CA5-10)	Increased fullness of the central pulmonary arteries with abrupt narrowing and pruning of peripheral vessels.	Development of pulmonary hypertension causes reversal of the shunt leading to unoxygenated blood entering the systemic circulation (cyanosis). Most commonly develops with atrial and ventricular septal defects and patent ductus arteriosus.

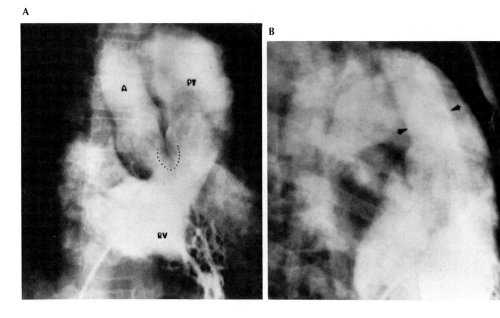

FIG CA5-6. Double-outlet right ventricle. (A) Frontal view from a selective right ventriculogram shows simultaneous and equal opacification of both great vessels from the right ventricle (RV). The ventricular septal defect was immediately beneath the crista supraventricularis (dotted line). (B) A lateral view shows the aorta (arrows) superimposed over the posterior two thirds of the pulmonary trunk. (A, aorta and PT, pulmonary trunk).[3]

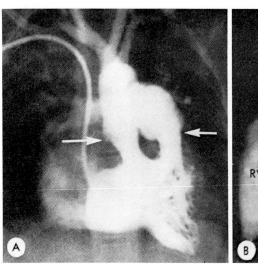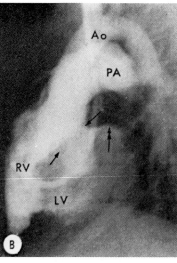

FIG CA5-7. Single ventricle. (A) Frontal view from a right ventriculogram shows muscular tracts leading from the right ventricle to both great arteries, the valves of which (arrows) are at the same horizontal level. (B) A lateral view shows the anteriorly situated right ventricle (RV) communicating with the left ventricle (LV) via a ventricular septal defect (single arrows). (PA, pulmonary artery and AO, aorta).[4]

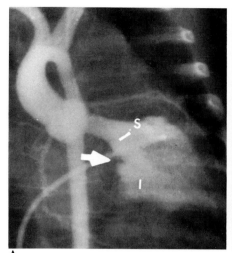

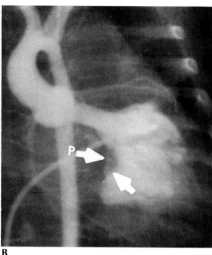

Fig CA5-8. Common atrioventricular canal.
(A) Left ventricular angiogram (frontal view) in early systole shows the cleft (arrow) between the superior (S) and inferior(I) segments of the anterior mitral leaflet located along the right contour of the ventricle. There is no evidence of mitral insufficiency or an interventricular shunt. (B) In diastole, the ventricular outflow tract is narrowed and lies in a more horizontal position than normal. The right border of the ventricle can be followed directly into the scooped-out margin (arrow) of the interventricular septum. The attachment of the posterior mitral leaflet (P) is also visible because of a thin layer of contrast material trapped between the leaflet and the posterior ventricular wall.[5]

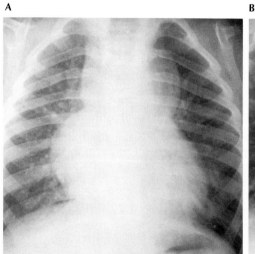

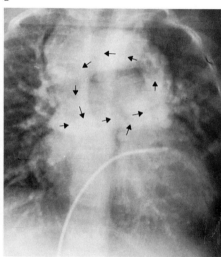

Fig CA5-9. Total anomalous pulmonary venous return (type I). (A) Frontal chest radiograph demonstrates a snowman, or figure-8, heart with right atrial and right ventricular enlargement. The widening of the superior mediastinum is due to the large, anomalous inverted-U–shaped vein. The pulmonary vascularity is greatly increased. The large pulmonary artery is hidden in the superior mediastinal silhouette. (B) Angiocardiogram demonstrates that all the pulmonary veins drain into the inverted-U–shaped vessel that eventually empties into the superior vena cava (arrows). The widening of the mediastinum produced by this vessel causes the snowman heart.[6]

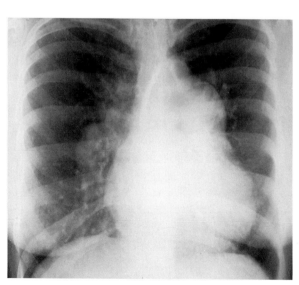

Fig CA5-10. Eisenmenger physiology in patent ductus arteriosus. There is an increased fullness of the central pulmonary arteries with an abrupt narrowing and paucity of peripheral vessels.

CYANOTIC CONGENITAL HEART DISEASE
WITH DECREASED PULMONARY VASCULARITY

Condition	Imaging Findings	Comments
Tetralogy of Fallot (Fig CA6-1)	Decreased pulmonary vascularity; flat or concave pulmonary outflow tract; enlargement of the right ventricle; right aortic arch in about 25% of cases.	Most common cause of cyanotic congenital heart disease beyond the immediate neonatal period. Consists of (1) high ventricular septal defect, (2) obstruction to right ventricular outflow (usually infundibular stenosis), (3) overriding of the aortic orifice above the ventricular defect, and (4) right ventricular hypertrophy.
Pseudotruncus arteriosus (truncus arteriosus type IV) (Fig CA6-2)	Decreased pulmonary vascularity; flat or concave pulmonary outflow tract; enlargement of the right ventricle; right aortic arch in about 40% of cases.	Single large arterial trunk receives the outflow of blood from both ventricles. The pulmonary arteries are absent, so the pulmonary circulation is supplied by bronchial or other collateral vessels.
Trilogy of Fallot (Fig CA6-3)	Decreased pulmonary vascularity; poststenotic dilatation of pulmonary artery; heart size often normal (usually some evidence of right ventricular hypertrophy).	Combination of pulmonary valvular stenosis with an intact ventricular septum and an interatrial shunt (patent foramen ovale or true atrial septal defect). Increased pressure on the right side of the heart due to pulmonary stenosis causes the interatrial shunt to be right to left.
Tricuspid atresia/stenosis (Fig CA6-4)	Decreased pulmonary vascularity (usually some degree of pulmonary stenosis); striking enlargement of the right atrium if small atrial shunt; large left ventricle; small right ventricle.	Right-to-left shunt at the atrial level (patent foramen ovale or true atrial septal defect). Usually there is also a ventricular septal defect or a patent ductus arteriosus. Hypoplasia of the right ventricle and pulmonary outflow tract is evident. The smaller the shunt, the more marked the elevation of right atrial pressure and the more striking the enlargement of this chamber. Tricuspid atresia without pulmonary stenosis produces marked cardiomegaly and increased pulmonary vascularity.
Ebstein's anomaly (Fig CA6-5)	Decreased pulmonary vascularity; flat or concave pulmonary outflow tract; characteristic squared or boxed appearance of the heart (bulging of the right heart border by the enlarged right atrium); narrow vascular pedicle and small aortic arch.	Downward displacement of an incompetent tricuspid valve into the right ventricle so that the upper portion of the right ventricle is effectively incorporated into the right atrium. The functional obstruction to right atrial emptying produces increased pressure and a right-to-left atrial shunt (usually through a patent foramen ovale).
Uhl's disease	Radiographic pattern identical to that in Ebstein's anomaly.	Focal or complete absence of the right ventricular myocardium (the right ventricle becomes a thin-walled fibroelastic bag that contracts poorly and cannot effectively empty blood from the right side of the heart).
Pulmonary atresia or severe pulmonary stenosis (Fig CA6-6)	Decreased pulmonary vascularity; shallow or concave pulmonary artery segment; variable cardiomegaly.	May be an isolated anomaly or associated with transposition, atrial septal defect, or common ventricle.

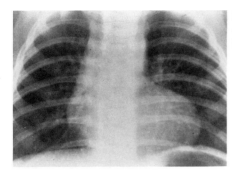

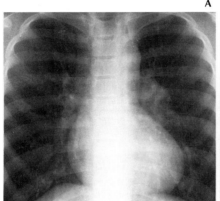

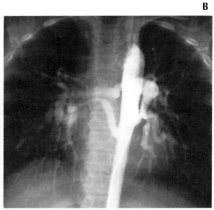

A

B

Fig CA6-1. Tetralogy of Fallot. Plain chest radiograph demonstrates decreased pulmonary vascularity and a flat pulmonary outflow tract. Note the characteristic lateral displacement and upward tilting of the prominent left cardiac apex (*coeur en sabot* appearance).

Fig CA6-2. Pseudotruncus arteriosus. (A) Plain chest radiograph shows the pulmonary vascularity to be strikingly diminished. (B) Angiogram shows that most of the blood supply to the lungs originates from two large arteries arising from the descending aorta.[1]

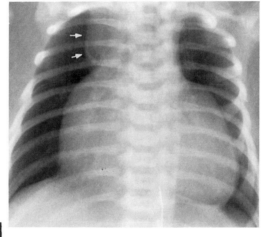

Fig CA6-5. Ebstein's anomaly. In addition to decreased pulmonary vascularity, there is enlargement of the right atrium, causing upward and outward bulging of the right border of the heart (squared appearance). Widening of the right side of the superior portion of the mediastinum (arrows) reflects marked dilatation of the superior vena cava due to right ventricular failure.

Fig CA6-3. Trilogy of Fallot. Decreased pulmonary vascularity with prominent poststenotic dilatation (arrow) of the pulmonary artery. There is enormous right atrial and moderate right ventricular enlargement.[6]

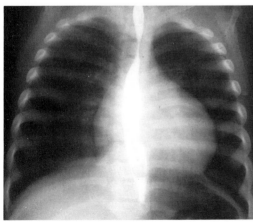

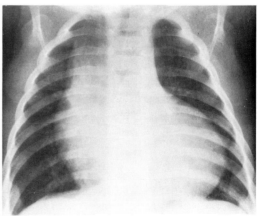

Fig CA6-4. Tricuspid atresia. Decreased pulmonary vascularity with elongation and rounding of the left border of the heart.

Fig CA6-6. Pulmonary atresia. Decreased pulmonary vascularity with a concave pulmonary outflow tract and moderate cardiomegaly.

ACYANOTIC CONGENITAL HEART DISEASE WITH INCREASED PULMONARY BLOOD FLOW

Condition	Imaging Findings	Comments
Atrial septal defect (Fig CA7-1)	Increased pulmonary vascularity; enlarged right atrium, right ventricle, and pulmonary outflow tract; normal left atrium and left ventricle; small aorta.	Most common congenital cardiac lesion. The magnitude of the shunt depends on the size of the defect, the relative compliance of the ventricles, and the difference in atrial pressure. May be combined with mitral stenosis (Lutembacher's syndrome) and cause a substantial increase in the workload of the right ventricle.
Ventricular septal defect (Fig CA7-2)	Increased pulmonary vascularity; enlarged right ventricle, pulmonary outflow tract, left atrium, and sometimes left ventricle (may be normal); normal right atrium; normal or small aorta.	Common congenital cardiac anomaly. The magnitude of the shunt depends on the size of the defect and the difference in ventricular pressure. There may also be a shunt from the left ventricle to the right atrium.
Patent ductus arteriosus (Fig CA7-3)	Increased pulmonary vascularity; enlargement of the left atrium, left ventricle, aorta, and pulmonary outflow tract; normal right atrium; enlarged or normal right ventricle.	Ductus extends from the bifurcation of the pulmonary artery to join the aorta just distal to the left subclavian artery (shunts blood from the pulmonary artery into the systemic circulation during intrauterine life). The aortic end of the ductus (infundibulum) is often dilated to produce a convex bulge on the left border of the aorta just below the knob.
Endocardial cushion defect (Fig CA7-4)	Increased pulmonary vascularity; nonspecific globular enlargement of the heart (enlargement of all cardiac chambers).	Low atrial septal defect combined with a high ventricular septal defect. Most often occurs in children with Down's syndrome.
Aorticopulmonary window (Fig CA7-5)	Increased pulmonary vascularity; enlargement of the left ventricle, left atrium, and pulmonary outflow tract (similar to patent ductus arteriosus but usually a less prominent aortic knob).	Uncommon anomaly in which a communication between the pulmonary artery and the aorta (just above their valves) is caused by a failure of the primitive truncus arteriosus to separate completely.
Ruptured sinus of Valsalva aneurysm (Fig CA7-6)	Rapid increase in pulmonary vascularity and enlargement of the right ventricle and the pulmonary outflow tract.	Rupture usually occurs into the right ventricle (occasionally the right atrium). Causes a sudden large left-to-right shunt with the acute onset of chest pain, shortness of breath, and a cardiac murmur.
Coronary artery fistula (Fig CA7-7)	Increased pulmonary vascularity; enlargement of the pulmonary outflow tract; enlargement of the right ventricle or both the right atrium and the right ventricle (depending on the site of the fistula).	Unusual anomaly in which there is a communication between a coronary artery and a cardiac chamber or the pulmonary artery. The right coronary artery most often communicates with, in order of frequency, the right ventricle, right atrium, coronary sinus, or pulmonary artery.

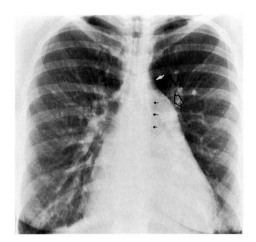

FIG CA7-1. Atrial septal defect.
Frontal view of the chest demonstrates cardiomegaly along with an increase in pulmonary vascularity reflecting the left-to-right shunt. Filling of the retrosternal space indicates enlargement of the right ventricle. The small aortic knob (white arrow) and descending aorta (small black arrows) are dwarfed by the enlarged pulmonary outflow tract (large black arrow).

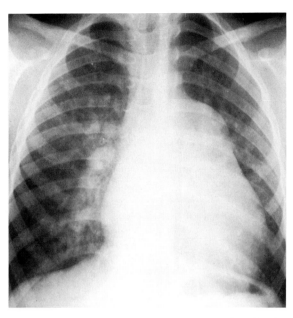

FIG CA7-2. Ventricular septal defect. The heart is enlarged and somewhat triangular and there is an increase in pulmonary vascular volume. The pulmonary trunk is very large and overshadows the normal-sized aorta, which seems small by comparison.[1]

FIG CA7-3. Patent ductus arteriosus.
(A) Preoperative frontal chest film demonstrates cardiomegaly with enlargement of the left atrium, left ventricle, and central pulmonary arteries. There is a diffuse increase in pulmonary vascularity. (B) In another patient, an aortogram shows persistent patency of the ductus arteriosus.[1]

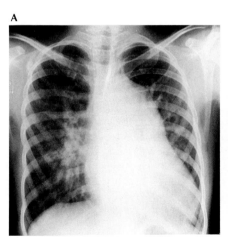

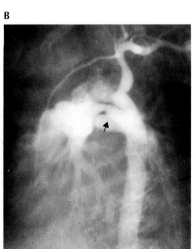

Condition	Imaging Findings	Comments
Partial anomalous pulmonary venous return (Fig CA7-8)	Increased pulmonary vascularity; enlarged right atrium, right ventricle, and pulmonary outflow tract; normal left atrium and left ventricle; small aorta.	One or more of the pulmonary veins are connected to the right atrium or its tributaries. Virtually indistinguishable from an atrial septal defect radiographically. A ''scimitar sign'' (crescent-like anomalous venous channel) on the right if associated with hypoplasia of the right lung.

FIG CA7-4. Endocardial cushion defect. Globular enlargement of the heart with increased pulmonary vascularity.

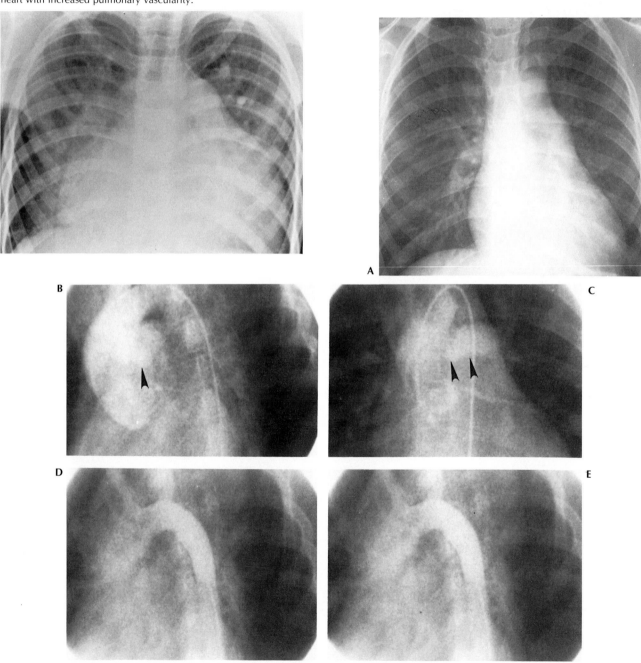

FIG CA7-5. Aorticopulmonary window. (A) Plain chest radiograph demonstrates enlargement of the left ventricle, a low position of the apex, and an increase in pulmonary vascularity. (B and C) Contrast material injected into the ascending aorta shows rapid shunting into the pulmonary arteries (arrows). (D and E) Contrast material injected into the descending aorta does not show a shunt, confirming that the shunt is in the ascending aorta.[1]

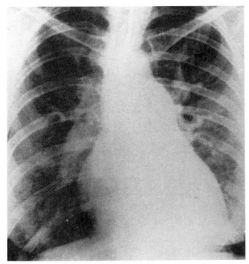

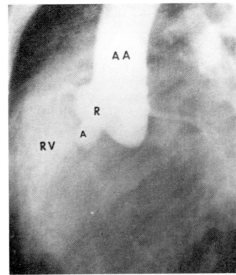

FIG CA7-6. Ruptured sinus of Valsalva aneurysm. (A) Frontal chest radiograph demonstrates cardiomegaly and increased pulmonary vascularity. (B) Lateral projection from a selective thoracic aortogram shows an aneurysm (A) of the right aortic sinus (R) projecting into the outflow tract of the right ventricle (RV). The contrast material has opacified the right ventricle through the aneurysm. (AA, ascending aorta).[7]

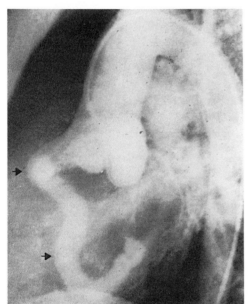

FIG CA7-7. Coronary artery fistula. Lateral view from an angiocardiogram shows a huge right coronary artery (arrows) draining into the right ventricle.[8]

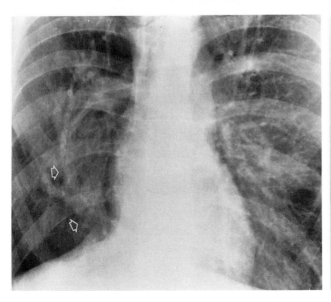

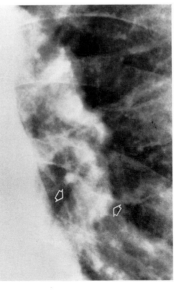

FIG CA7-8. Partial anomalous pulmonary venous return. Two examples of curvilinear venous pathways (arrows) resembling a Turkish scimitar.

ACYANOTIC CONGENITAL HEART DISEASE
WITH NORMAL PULMONARY BLOOD FLOW

Condition	Imaging Findings	Comments
Coarctation of aorta (Fig CA8-1)	Characteristic double bulge in the region of the aortic knob (figure-3 sign on plain chest radiographs and reverse figure-3, or figure-E, sign on the barium-filled esophagus). There may be rib notching (usually involving the posterior fourth to eighth ribs) but rarely developing before age 6.	In the more common "adult" type, the aortic narrowing occurs at or just distal to the level of the ductus arteriosus (double bulge represents prestenotic and poststenotic dilatation). In the "infantile" variety there is a long segment of narrowing lying proximal to the ductus (obligatory right-to-left shunt and early congestive heart failure). There is a relatively high incidence of coarctation in women with Turner's syndrome.
Aortic stenosis (Fig CA8-2)	Increased convexity or prominence of the left heart border (overall heart size often normal). Substantial cardiomegaly reflects left ventricular failure and dilatation.	Valvular, subvalvular, and supravalvular types. Bulging of the right superior mediastinal silhouette (poststenotic dilatation of the ascending aorta) is often seen with valvular stenosis.
Pulmonary valvular stenosis (see Fig CA13-6)	Poststenotic dilatation of the pulmonary artery, often associated with dilatation of the left main pulmonary artery. The heart size is initially normal (right ventricular hypertrophy and dilatation if severe pulmonary stenosis causes systolic overloading of the right ventricle).	Common anomaly found in isolated form or in combination with other abnormalities. The stenosis is most common at the level of the pulmonary valve (supravalvular or infundibular stenosis can occur). Must be differentiated from normal idiopathic poststenotic dilatation of the pulmonary artery in adolescents and young adults, especially women.
Endocardial fibroelastosis (Fig CA8-3)	Striking globular cardiac enlargement (often with left-sided prominence); small aortic knob.	Diffuse thickening of the left ventricular endocardium with collagen and elastic tissue. A common cause of cardiac failure during the first year of life. The pulmonary vascularity remains normal until congestive heart failure supervenes.
Miscellaneous lesions with normal vascularity (until left-sided failure develops in infancy) (Fig CA8-4)	Various patterns.	Includes hypoplastic left heart syndrome, mitral stenosis and insufficiency, aortic insufficiency, cor triatriatum, aberrant pulmonary origin of left coronary artery, and cardiomyopathy.

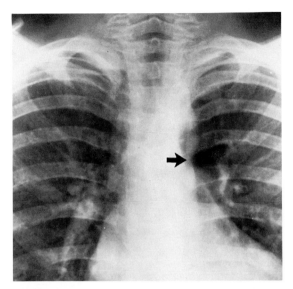

Fig CA8-1. Coarctation of the aorta. Plain chest radiograph demonstrates the figure-3 sign (arrow points to the center of the 3).

Fig CA8-2. (A) **Subvalvular aortic stenosis.** Note the muscular ridge protruding from the upper portion of the ventricular septum (arrows). The ridge is about 2 cm below the aortic valve and encroaches on the outflow tract of the left ventricle. (B) **Valvular aortic stenosis.** Irregular thickening of aortic valve leaflets and relative rigidity of the left coronary cusp. (C) **Supravalvular aortic stenosis.** Narrowed segment (arrows) located just above the coronary ostia.[9]

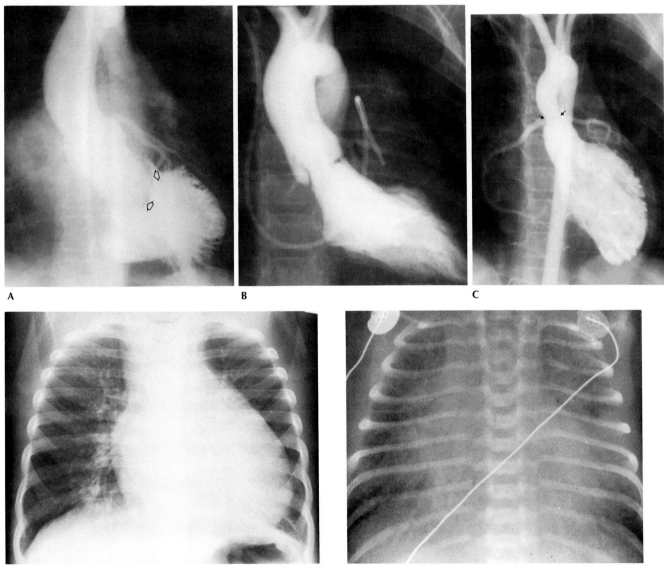

A

B

C

Fig CA8-3. Endocardial fibroelastosis. Globular enlargement of the heart.

Fig CA8-4. Hypoplastic left heart syndrome. Globular cardiomegaly with pronounced congestive failure.

PROMINENT ASCENDING AORTA OR AORTIC ARCH

Condition	Imaging Findings	Comments
Hypertensive heart disease (Fig CA9-1)	Aortic tortuosity with prominence of the ascending portion.	Increased workload of the left ventricle causes concentric hypertrophy (rounding of the left heart border). Continued strain eventually leads to dilatation and enlargement of the left ventricle.
Atherosclerosis (Fig CA9-2)	Generalized tortuosity, elongation, and moderate dilatation of the aorta. Often linear plaques of intimal calcification (especially in the aortic knob and the transverse arch).	Generally considered to be a degenerative condition of old age. However, intimal thickening, plaque formation, and vascular narrowing can develop in younger patients, especially those with diabetes mellitus, hypertension, or familial disorders of lipid metabolism.
Aortic aneurysm (see Figs C20-8 and CA19-2)	Sharply marginated, saccular or fusiform mass of homogeneous density (there may be generalized aortic dilatation). Curvilinear calcification may occur in the outer wall.	Causes include atherosclerosis, cystic medial necrosis (there may be associated Marfan's syndrome), syphilis, mycotic infection, and trauma.
Dissecting aneurysm	Progressive widening of the aortic shadow, which may have an irregular or wavy outer border. Separation (more than 4 mm) between the intimal calcification and the outer border of the aortic shadow indicates widening of the aortic wall.	Predisposing factors include atherosclerosis, hypertension, cystic medial necrosis (eg, Marfan's syndrome), trauma, aortic stenosis, coarctation of the aorta, Ehlers-Danlos syndrome, and the intramural injection of contrast material. Most dissections begin as intimal tears immediately above the aortic valve. In two thirds (type I), the dissection continues into the descending aorta. In the remainder (type II), the dissection is limited to the ascending aorta and stops at the origin of the brachiocephalic vessels. In type III the dissection begins in the thoracic aorta distal to the subclavian artery and extends proximal and distal to the original site.
Aortic valvular stenosis (Fig CA9-3)	Bulging of the ascending aorta (poststenotic dilatation). Aortic valve calcification (best seen on fluoroscopy) is common and indicates severe stenosis.	May be congenital (usually bicuspid valve) or acquired (generally on a rheumatic basis). Increased prominence of the left heart border (overall heart size is often normal). Substantial cardiomegaly reflects left ventricular failure and dilatation.
Aortic insufficiency (Fig CA9-4)	Moderate dilatation of the ascending aorta and aortic knob (marked dilatation, especially of the ascending aorta, suggests underlying aortic stenosis). Enlargement of the left ventricle.	Most commonly due to rheumatic heart disease. Other causes include syphilis, infective endocarditis, dissecting aneurysm, and Marfan's syndrome. Left ventricular failure leads to pulmonary venous congestion and left atrial enlargement (relative mitral insufficiency).
Syphilitic aortitis (Fig CA9-5)	Dilatation of the ascending aorta, frequently with mural calcification.	May cause inflammation of the aortic valvular ring that results in aortic insufficiency. About one third of patients develop narrowing of the coronary ostia that may lead to symptoms of ischemic heart disease.

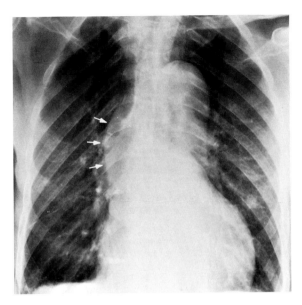

FIG CA9-1. Hypertensive heart disease. Marked dilatation (arrows) of the ascending aorta caused by increased aortic pressure.

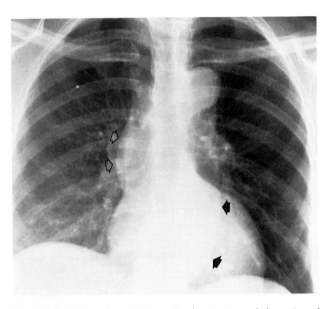

FIG CA9-2. Atherosclerosis. Generalized tortuosity and elongation of the ascending aorta (open arrows) and descending aorta (closed arrows).

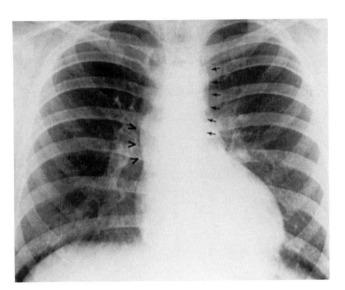

FIG CA9-3. Aortic valvular stenosis. There is prominence of the left ventricle with poststenotic dilatation of the ascending aorta (arrowheads). The aortic knob and descending aorta (arrows) are normal.[10]

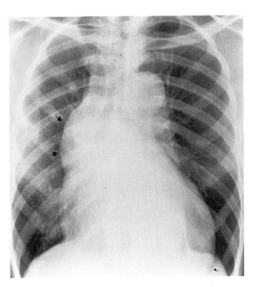

FIG CA9-4. Aortic insufficiency. Marked dilatation (large arrows) of the ascending aorta (large arrows), suggesting some underlying aortic stenosis. The left ventricle is enlarged with downward and lateral displacement of the cardiac apex. Note that the cardiac shadow extends below the dome of the left hemidiaphragm (small arrow).

Condition	Imaging Findings	Comments
Takayasu's disease ("pulseless" disease)	Widening and contour irregularity of the aorta (especially the arch). May also involve major aortic branches. Linear calcifications frequently occur.	Nonspecific obstructive arteritis, primarily affecting young women, in which granulation tissue destroys the media of large vessels. The resulting mural scarring causes luminal narrowing and occlusion. There is usually fever and constitutional symptoms. Characteristic smooth and tapering arterial narrowing on angiography.
Coarctation of aorta (see Fig CA8-1)	Prominence of the ascending aorta. Characteristic double bulge in the region of the aortic knob (figure-3 sign on plain chest radiographs and reverse figure-3, or figure-E, sign on the barium-filled esophagus). There may be rib notching (usually involving the posterior fourth to eighth ribs but rarely developing before age 6) and dilated internal mammary arteries (soft-tissue density on lateral films).	In the more common "adult" type, the aortic narrowing occurs at or just distal to the level of the ductus arteriosus. The double bulge represents prestenotic and poststenotic dilatation.
Pseudocoarctation of aorta (Fig CA9-6)	Two bulges in the region of the aortic knob mimic true coarctation. No rib notching or internal mammary collaterals (since no obstruction or hemodynamic abnormality).	Buckling or kinking of the aortic arch in the region of the ligamentum arteriosum. The bulges represent dilated portions of the aorta just proximal and distal to the kink. The upper bulge is usually higher than the normal aortic knob and can simulate a left superior mediastinal tumor.
Patent ductus arteriosus (Fig CA9-7)	Prominent aortic knob; increased pulmonary vascularity; enlargement of the left atrium, left ventricle, and pulmonary outflow tract. The aortic end of the ductus (infundibulum) is often dilated to produce a convex bulge on the left border of the aorta just below the knob.	Ductus extends from the bifurcation of the pulmonary artery to join the aorta just distal to the left subclavian artery (shunts blood from the pulmonary artery into the systemic circulation during intrauterine life). Aortic prominence is a differential point from other major left-to-right shunts (atrial and ventricular septal defects).
Tetralogy of Fallot with severe pulmonary stenosis	Pronounced bulging of the ascending aorta and prominence of the aortic knob.	Severe pulmonary stenosis effectively forces the aorta to drain both ventricles. A similar appearance occurs in pseudotruncus arteriosus (essentially tetralogy of Fallot with pulmonary atresia).
Aneurysm of sinus of Valsalva (see Fig CA7-6)	Large aneurysm produces a smooth local bulge in the right anterolateral cardiac contour (a small aneurysm is undetectable). Curvilinear calcification often occurs in the aneurysm wall.	Primarily involves the sinus above the right cusp of the aortic valve. An acute rupture (usually into the right ventricle) causes a sudden large left-to-right shunt.

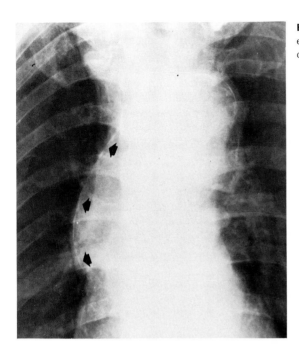

Fig CA9-5. **Syphilitic aortitis.** Aneurysmal dilatation of the ascending aorta with extensive linear calcification of the wall (arrows). Some calcification is also seen in the distal aortic arch.

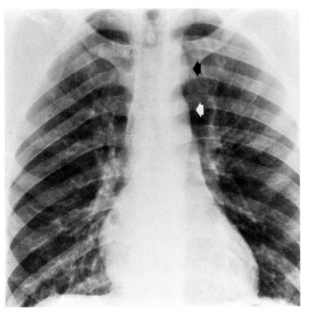

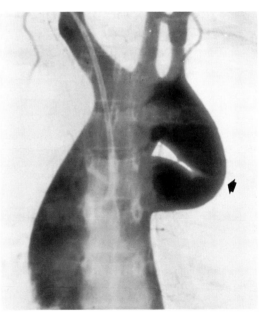

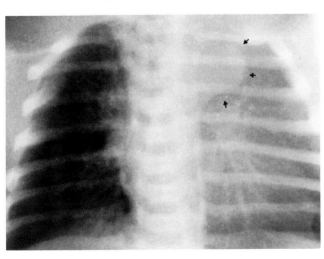

Fig CA9-6. **Pseudocoarctation of the aorta.** (A) Frontal view of the chest demonstrates two bulges (arrows) producing a well-demarcated figure-3 sign in the region of the aortic knob. The upper bulge (black arrow) is higher than the normal aortic knob and simulates a mediastinal mass. Because there is no hemodynamic abnormality, the heart is normal in size and there is no rib notching. (B) In another patient, an aortogram demonstrates extreme kinking of the descending aorta (arrow) without an area of true coarctation.

Fig CA9-7. **Patent ductus arteriosus.** A convex bulge (arrows) on the left side of the superior mediastinum represents dilatation of the aortic end of the ductus ("ductus bump").

Condition	Imaging Findings	Comments
Corrected transposition (Fig CA9-8)	Smooth bulging of the upper left border of the heart replaces the normal double bulge of the aortic knob and the pulmonary artery segment.	Combination of transposition of the origins of the aorta and the pulmonary artery and inversion of the ventricles and their accompanying atrioventricular valves. A single bulge represents the displaced ascending aorta and right ventricular outflow tract.
Persistent truncus arteriosus	Bulge in the region of the ascending aorta (represents the large single arterial trunk).	Failure of the common truncus arteriosus to divide normally into the aorta and the pulmonary artery, resulting in a single large arterial trunk that receives the outflow of blood from both ventricles.
Connective tissue disorders (Fig CA9-9)	Generalized dilatation of the aorta. Increased incidence of aneurysm and dissection.	Conditions include Ehlers-Danlos syndrome, Marfan's syndrome, osteogenesis imperfecta, and pseudoxanthoma elasticum.

A

B

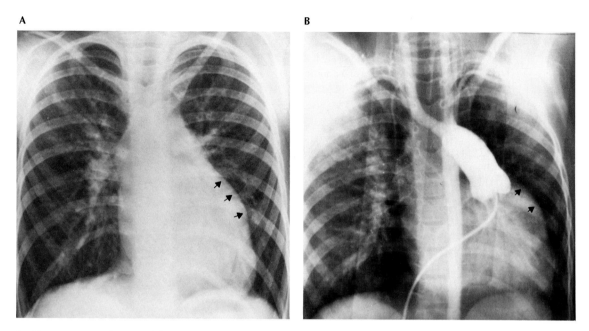

FIG CA9-8. Corrected transposition with ventricular septal defect. (A) There is fullness of the upper left border of the heart (arrows). Because of the left-to-right ventricular shunt, the pulmonary vasculature is engorged. (B) A film from an angiocardiogram demonstrates the inverted aorta and right ventricular outflow tract (arrows).[6]

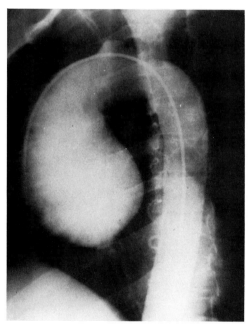

FIG CA9-9. Marfan's syndrome. Arteriogram shows enormous dilatation of the aneurysmal ascending aorta.

SMALL ASCENDING AORTA OR AORTIC ARCH

Condition	Imaging Findings	Comments
Atrial septal defect (see Fig CA7-1)	Small aorta; increased pulmonary vascularity; enlarged right atrium, right ventricle, and pulmonary outflow tract.	Shunting of blood away from the left side of the heart into the pulmonary circulation causes decreased flow through the aorta.
Ventricular septal defect (see Fig CA7-2)	Small (or normal) aorta; increased pulmonary vascularity; enlarged right ventricle, pulmonary outflow tract, and left atrium.	Shunting of blood away from the left side of the heart into the pulmonary circulation causes decreased flow through the aorta.
Infantile type of coarctation of aorta	Small (or normal) aorta; pulmonary venous congestion; cardiomegaly (biventricular but more prominent on the right).	Narrowing of a long segment of aorta proximal to the ductus arteriosus. Always a patent ductus arteriosus and often a ventricular septal defect to deliver blood from the pulmonary artery to the descending aorta and the systemic circulation. No rib notching, internal mammary collaterals, or figure-3 or figure-E signs.
Mitral stenosis	Small aorta; enlarged left atrium and increased pulmonary venous congestion; eventual enlargement of the right ventricle, pulmonary outflow tract, and central pulmonary arteries.	Decreased left ventricular output causes diminished aortic blood flow.
Decreased cardiac output	Small aorta; various patterns of heart size; usually pulmonary venous congestion, pleural effusion, and prominence of the superior vena cava.	Gross cardiomegaly in endocardial fibroelastosis and the cardiomyopathies. Normal-sized or small heart with characteristic calcification in chronic constrictive pericarditis.
Endocardial cushion defect	Nonspecific globular enlargement of the heart with increased pulmonary vascularity.	Atrial and ventricular septal defects cause shunting of blood away from the left side of the heart into the pulmonary circulation and thus decreased flow through the aorta.
Hypoplastic left heart syndrome	Small aorta; globular cardiomegaly with severe pulmonary venous congestion.	Underdevelopment of the left side of the heart is related to an obstructive lesion that causes decreased aortic blood flow.
Supravalvular aortic stenosis (Fig CA10-1)	Aortic knob is often small.	Underdevelopment and stenosis of the supravalvular portion of the aorta. Different from the poststenotic aortic dilatation that occurs with valvular aortic stenosis.
Transposition of great vessels (Fig CA10-2)	Narrowing of the vascular pedicle on frontal projection.	Caused by superimposition of the abnormally positioned aorta and pulmonary artery combined with absence of the normal thymic tissue because of stress atrophy. Widening of the vascular pedicle on lateral projection (due to the anterior position of the aorta with respect to the pulmonary artery).

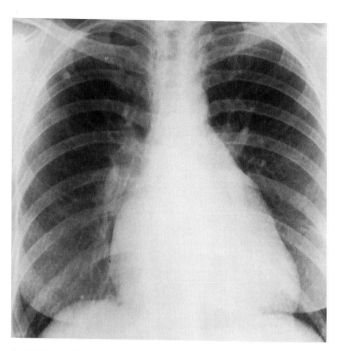

Fɪɢ CA10-1. Congenital aortic stenosis. Small aortic arch with moderate enlargement of the left ventricle.[9]

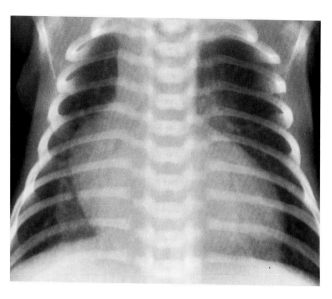

Fɪɢ CA10-2. Transposition of great vessels. Typical oval or egg-shaped heart with a small aortic arch due to narrowing of the vascular pedicle resulting from superimposition of the abnormally positioned aorta and pulmonary artery.

MAJOR ANOMALIES OF THE AORTIC ARCH
AND PULMONARY ARTERY

Condition	Imaging Findings	Comments
Right aortic arch **Mirror-image pattern** **(see Fig CA12-1)**	No indentation on the barium-filled esophagus on lateral projection.	No vessel crosses the mediastinum posterior to the esophagus. Frequently associated with congenital heart disease (tetralogy of Fallot, truncus and pseudo-truncus, tricuspid atresia, and transposition).
Aberrant left subclavian artery **(Fig CA11-1)**	Characteristic oblique posterior indentation on the barium-filled esophagus.	Left subclavian artery arises as the most distal branch of the aorta and courses across the mediastinum posterior to the esophagus to reach the left upper extremity. No associated congenital heart disease.
Isolated left subclavian artery	No esophageal impression.	Left subclavian artery is atretic at its base (totally isolated from the aorta) and receives its blood supply from the left pulmonary artery or via the ipsilateral vertebral artery (congenital subclavian steal syndrome).
Right aortic arch with left descending aorta	Prominent indentation on the posterior wall of the barium-filled esophagus.	Transverse portion of the aorta must cross the mediastinum (posterior to the esophagus) so that the aorta descends on the left.
Cervical aortic arch **(Fig CA11-2)**	Posterior impression on the esophagus (caused by the distal arch or the proximal descending aorta).	Ascending aorta extends higher than usual so that the aortic arch is in the neck. Pulsatile mass above the clavicle simulates an aneurysm. No associated congenital heart disease.
Double aortic arch **(Fig CA11-3)**	Bulges on both sides of the superior mediastinum (the right is usually larger and higher than the left). Reverse S-shaped indentation on the barium-filled esophagus.	In most patients the aorta ascends on the right, branches, and finally reunites on the left. The two limbs of the aorta completely encircle the trachea and the esophagus, forming a ring.
Aberrant right subclavian artery **(Fig CA11-4)**	Posterior esophageal indentation on lateral views. On frontal views, characteristic impression running obliquely upward and to the right.	Arises as the last major vessel of the aortic arch (just distal to the left subclavian) and must course across the mediastinum behind the esophagus to reach the right upper extremity. No associated congenital heart disease.
Aberrant left pulmonary artery (pulmonary sling) **(Fig CA11-5)**	Typical impression on the posterior aspect of the trachea just above the carina and a corresponding indentation on the anterior wall of the barium-filled esophagus.	Aberrant left pulmonary artery arises from the right pulmonary artery and must cross the mediastinum (between the trachea and the esophagus) to reach the left lung.

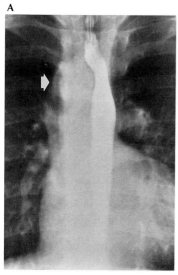

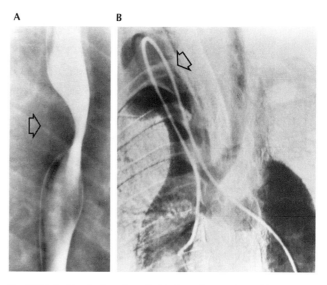

A

FIG CA11-1. Right aortic arch with aberrant left subclavian artery. (A) Frontal view from an esophagram demonstrates the right aortic arch (arrow). (B) Oblique posterior impression on the esophagus (arrow) represents the aberrant left subclavian artery as it courses to reach the left upper extremity.

FIG CA11-2. Cervical aortic arch. (A) Posterior esophageal impression (arrow) is caused by the retroesophageal course of the distal arch or the proximal descending aorta. (B) Subtraction film from an aortogram demonstrates the aortic arch extending into the neck (arrow).

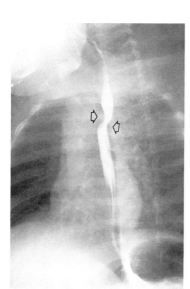

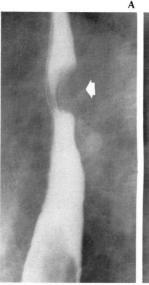

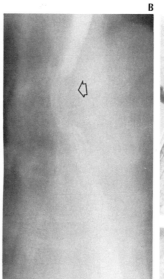

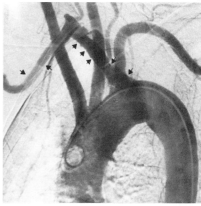

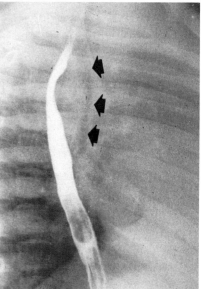

FIG CA11-3. Double aortic arch. Characteristic reverse S–shaped indentation on the esophagus (arrows). As usual, the right (posterior) arch is higher and larger than the left (anterior) arch.[6]

FIG CA11-4. Aberrant right subclavian artery. (A) Lateral view from an esophagram demonstrates a posterior esophageal impression (arrow). (B) On a frontal view, the esophageal impression runs obliquely upward and to the right. (C) Subtraction film from an arteriogram shows the aberrant vessel (arrows) arising distal to the left subclavian artery.

FIG CA11-5. Aberrant left pulmonary artery. Lateral esophagram demonstrates the characteristic indentation of the anterior wall of the esophagus. Note the posterior impression and anterior displacement of the trachea (arrows) caused by the aberrant artery.[11]

CONGENITAL HEART DISEASE
ASSOCIATED WITH THE RIGHT AORTIC ARCH
(MIRROR-IMAGE BRANCHING)

Condition	Imaging Findings	Comments
Pseudotruncus arteriosus	Decreased pulmonary vascularity; flat or concave pulmonary outflow tract; enlargement of the right ventricle.	Right aortic arch in about 40% of cases. Single vessel arising from the heart that is accompanied by a remnant of the atretic pulmonary artery (essentially the same as tetralogy of Fallot with pulmonary atresia).
Tetralogy of Fallot	Decreased pulmonary vascularity; flat or concave pulmonary outflow tract; enlargement of the right ventricle.	Right aortic arch in about 25% of cases. Consists of (1) high ventricular septal defect, (2) obstruction to right ventricular outflow (usually infundibular pulmonary stenosis), (3) overriding of the aortic orifice above the ventricular defect, and (4) right ventricular hypertrophy.
Persistent truncus arteriosus (Fig CA12-1)	Increased pulmonary vascularity; concave pulmonary outflow tract; striking enlargement of the right ventricle and eventual enlargement of the left atrium and left ventricle.	Right aortic arch in about 25% of cases. Failure of the common truncus arteriosus to divide normally into the aorta and the pulmonary artery results in a single large arterial trunk that receives the outflow from both ventricles.
Tricuspid atresia	Decreased pulmonary vascularity; striking enlargement of the right atrium if small atrial shunt; large left ventricle; small right ventricle.	Right aortic arch in about 5% of cases. An obligatory right-to-left shunt at the atrial level (there may also be a ventricular septal defect or patent ductus arteriosus). Hypoplasia of the right ventricle and pulmonary outflow tract.
Transposition of great vessels	Increased pulmonary vascularity; generally biventricular enlargement (oval or egg-shaped configuration); narrowed vascular pedicle.	Right aortic arch in about 5% of cases. Reverse of the normal relation of the aorta and the pulmonary artery (the aorta arises anteriorly from the right ventricle and the pulmonary artery originates posteriorly from the left ventricle).

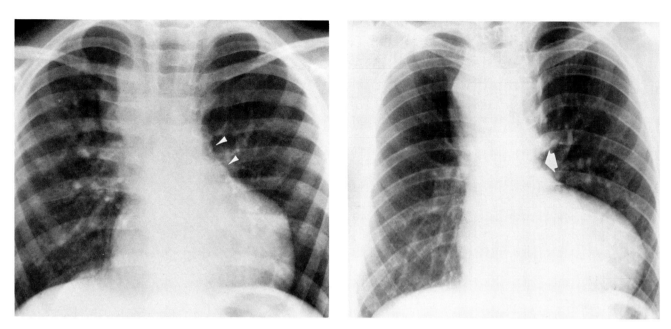

Fɪɢ CA12-1. Persistent truncus arteriosus. Two patients with the characteristic concave appearance of the pulmonary outflow tract (arrowheads) associated with a right aortic arch.

DILATATION OF THE MAIN PULMONARY ARTERY

Condition	Imaging Findings	Comments
Normal variant (Fig CA13-1)	Isolated prominence of pulmonary artery segment; normal pulmonary vascularity; no associated cardiac abnormality.	Common appearance in adolescents and adults under 30 (especially women).
Congestive heart failure	Cardiomegaly with evidence of pulmonary venous congestion. Often pleural effusion and Kerley's lines.	Failure of the left side of the heart leads to increased blood volume in the pulmonary circulation.
High-output heart disease (Fig CA13-2)	Cardiomegaly with prominent pulmonary vascularity (both arteries and veins).	Anemia; thyrotoxicosis; beriberi; hypervolemia (fluid overload, overtransfusion); peripheral arteriovenous fistulas; Paget's disease; Pickwickian obesity; polycythemia vera; pregnancy.
Cor pulmonale (Figs CA13-3 and CA13-4)	Enlargement of the main and hilar pulmonary arteries with rapid tapering and small peripheral vessels. Initially normal heart size, then right ventricular enlargement and eventually distension of the superior vena cava.	Caused by diffuse lung disease (obstructive emphysema, interstitial fibrosis); diffuse pulmonary arterial disease (thromboembolism, arteritis, primary pulmonary hypertension); chronic heart disease (reversed left-to-right shunt, left ventricular failure, mitral valve disease); and chronic hypoxia (chest deformity, neuromuscular disease, Pickwickian obesity, high-altitude dwelling).
Left-to-right shunt (Fig CA13-5)	Various patterns, depending on the level and extent of the shunt.	Most commonly atrial septal defect, ventricular septal defect, or patent ductus arteriosus (see page 184).
Pulmonary thromboembolic disease (see Fig C9-4)	Enlargement of the main pulmonary artery segment.	Caused by pulmonary hypertension or distension of the vessel by bulk thrombus. This sign is primarily of value when serial radiographs demonstrate progressive enlargement.
Pulmonary valvular stenosis (Fig CA13-6)	Prominence of the main pulmonary artery segment.	Common anomaly with poststenotic dilatation of the left pulmonary artery (central dilatation of the right pulmonary artery, but the dilated segment is hidden in the mediastinum).
Mitral stenosis or insufficiency	Enlargement of the left atrium and right ventricle; normal-sized left ventricle and small aortic arch; pulmonary vascular congestion.	Obstruction of flow from the left atrium to the left ventricle during diastole results in increased pressure and enlargement of the left atrium. The increased pressure is transmitted to the pulmonary veins and eventually to the pulmonary arteries and the right side of the heart. Usually caused by rheumatic valvular lesion; also by congenital mitral stenosis and the parachute deformity (all chordae tendineae originating from a single papillary muscle). There is a similar mechanism in the hypoplastic left heart syndrome and a large left atrial myxoma.

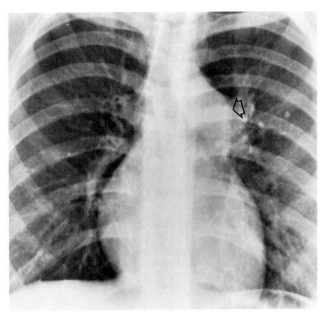

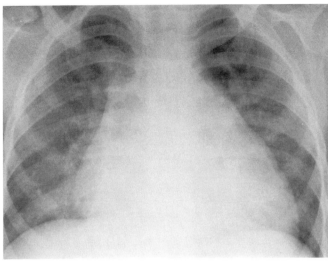

FIG CA13-2. Thyrotoxicosis. Generalized cardiomegaly with increased pulmonary vascularity.

FIG CA13-1. Idiopathic dilatation of the pulmonary artery. Plain chest radiograph in a normal young woman demonstrates prominence of the pulmonary artery (arrow) that simulates the poststenotic dilatation associated with pulmonary valvular stenosis.

A

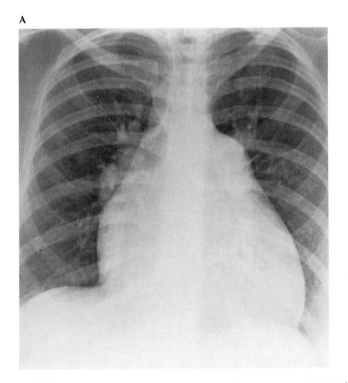

B

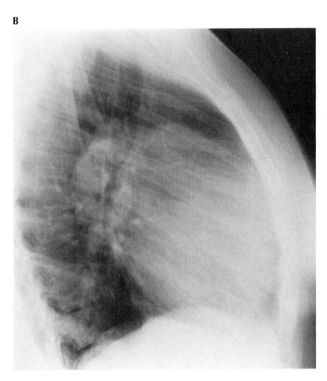

FIG CA13-3. Cor pulmonale (primary pulmonary hypertension). (A) Frontal and (B) lateral views of the chest show prominence of the pulmonary outflow tract and markedly dilated central pulmonary vessels. The lateral displacement of the cardiac apex and filling of the retrosternal air space indicate right ventricular enlargement.

Condition	Imaging Findings	Comments
Partial anomalous pulmonary venous return (see Fig CA7-8)	Increased pulmonary vascularity; enlarged right atrium, right ventricle, and main pulmonary artery segment; normal left atrium and left ventricle; small aorta.	One or more pulmonary veins connected to the right atrium or its tributaries. Virtually indistinguishable from an atrial septal defect radiographically. Scimitar sign (crescent-shaped anomalous venous channel) on the right if associated with hypoplasia of the right lung.
Trilogy of Fallot (Fig CA13-7)	Poststenotic dilatation of the pulmonary artery; decreased pulmonary vascularity; heart size often normal (usually some evidence of right ventricular hypertrophy).	Combination of pulmonary valvular stenosis with an intact ventricular septum and an interatrial shunt (patent foramen ovale or true atrial septal defect). Increased pressure on the right side of the heart due to pulmonary stenosis causes the interatrial shunt to be right to left (patient is cyanotic).
Tricuspid atresia without pulmonary stenosis	Marked cardiomegaly and increased pulmonary vascularity.	May be associated with transposition of the great vessels.
Total anomalous pulmonary venous return (see Fig CA5-9)	Increased pulmonary vascularity and enlarged main pulmonary artery segment; various patterns and characteristic "snowman," or figure-8, sign.	All pulmonary veins connect to the right atrium directly or to the systemic veins or their tributaries. Because all pulmonary venous blood returns to the right atrium, a right-to-left shunt through an interatrial communication is necessary for blood to reach the left side of the heart and the systemic circulation.

A

B

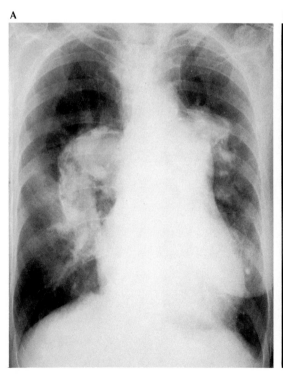
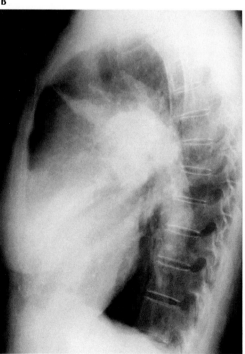

FIG CA13-4. **Eisenmenger's syndrome** in atrial septal defect. (A) Frontal and (B) lateral films demonstrate slight but definite cardiomegaly and a great increase in the size of the pulmonary trunk. The right and left pulmonary artery branches are huge, but the peripheral pulmonary vasculature is relatively sparse. Long-standing pulmonary hypertension has produced degenerative intimal changes in the pulmonary arteries, which have become densely calcified.[1]

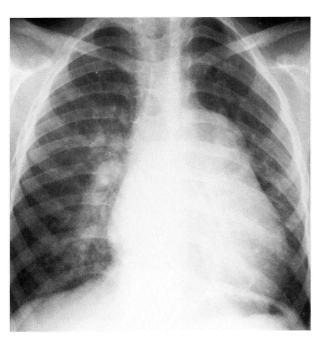

FIG CA13-5. Ventricular septal defect. The pulmonary trunk is very large and overshadows the normal-sized aorta, which seems small by comparison. The pulmonary artery branches in the hilum and in the periphery of the lung are enlarged and the pulmonary vascular volume is increased. The heart is enlarged and somewhat triangular.[1]

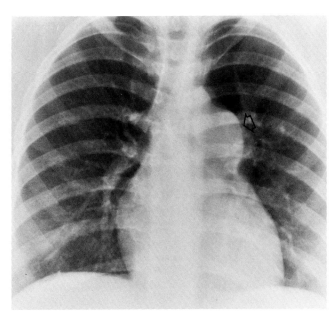

FIG CA13-6. Pulmonary valvular stenosis. Severe poststenotic dilatation of the pulmonary outflow tract (arrow). The heart size and pulmonary vascularity remain within normal limits.

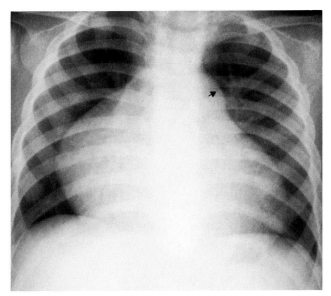

FIG CA13-7. Trilogy of Fallot. Marked poststenotic dilatation (arrow) of the pulmonary artery with decrease in overall pulmonary vascularity. There is enormous right atrial and moderate right ventricular enlargement.[6]

DILATATION OF THE SUPERIOR VENA CAVA*

Condition	Comments
Increased central venous pressure (Fig CA14-1)	In the great majority of cases this pattern is caused by congestive heart failure or by cardiac tamponade due to pericardial effusion or constrictive pericarditis.
Intrathoracic neoplasm (Figs CA14-2 to CA14-4)	There is often an associated soft-tissue mass. Primarily bronchogenic carcinoma (especially oat cell carcinoma), but also tumors of the esophagus and the mediastinum.
Mediastinal fibrosis	Idiopathic or secondary to chronic histoplasmosis, irradiation, or methylsergide ingestion.
Lymphadenopathy	Most commonly histoplasmosis or bronchogenic carcinoma.
Aneurysm of aorta or great vessels	Associated with a large soft-tissue mass representing the aneurysm. Usually due to atherosclerotic or dissecting aneurysms (syphilitic aneurysms were formally more common but are now rare).
Severe mediastinal emphysema	Striking increase in mediastinal pressure causes venous compression.
Thrombosis of superior vena cava	Reported after surgery for repair of tetralogy of Fallot and in patients with ventriculoatrial shunts for hydrocephalus.

*Pattern: Smooth, well-defined widening of the right side of the upper half of the mediastinum.

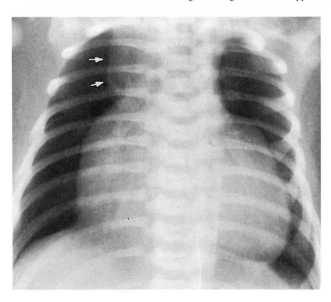

FIG CA14-1. **Right ventricular failure.** Plain chest radiograph in a patient with Ebstein's anomaly shows widening of the right side of the superior portion of the mediastinum (arrows), reflecting marked dilatation of the superior vena cava. There is enlargement of the right atrium, causing upward and outward bulging of the right border of the heart (squared appearance).

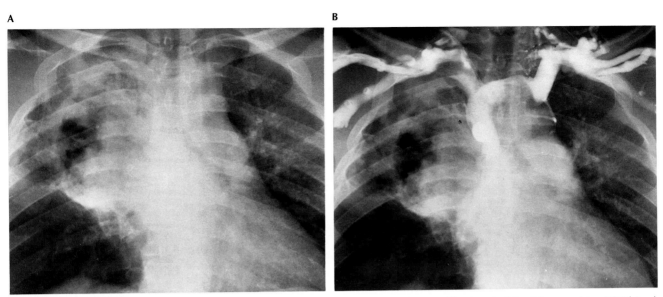

FIG CA14-2. Bronchogenic carcinoma. (A) Frontal view of the chest shows a bulky, irregular mass filling much of the right upper lobe. (B) Bilateral upper extremity venograms show almost complete occlusion of the superior vena cava by the large malignant neoplasm.

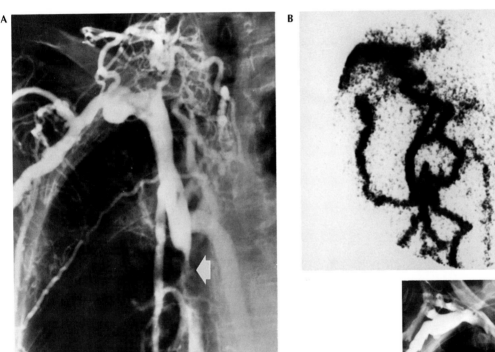

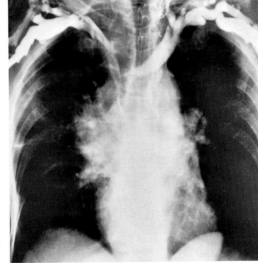

FIG CA14-3. Bronchogenic carcinoma. (A) Right upper extremity venogram shows extensive venous collaterals bypassing an obstruction of the superior vena cava (arrow). (B) Radionuclide scan in another patient shows extensive venous collaterals bypassing an obstruction of the superior vena cava.

FIG CA14-4. Bronchogenic carcinoma. Bilateral upper extremity venograms show virtual occlusion of the superior vena cava by a large oat cell tumor in the right hilar and perihilar region.

DILATATION OF THE AZYGOS VEIN*

Condition	Comments
Increased central venous pressure	Underlying causes include congestive heart failure, pericardial tamponade due to pericardial effusion, constrictive pericarditis, and tricuspid valvular lesions. Dilatation of the azygos vein may be obscured by a dilated superior vena cava. A dilated azygos vein may be differentiated from an enlarged azygos lymph node by demonstrating a marked increase in the diameter of the shadow in the supine position.
Portal hypertension	Intrahepatic or extrahepatic portal vein obstruction (tumor thrombus). Enlarged azygos and hemiazygos veins may produce widening and irregularity of the right and left paraspinal lines, respectively (this appearance also occurs with superior vena caval obstruction and congenital infrahepatic interruption of the inferior vena cava).
Occlusion of superior vena cava	Smooth, well-defined widening of the right side of the upper half of the mediastinum may obscure or obliterate the shadow of the enlarged azygos vein.
Azygos continuation of inferior vena cava	Congenital infrahepatic interruption of the inferior vena cava. Often associated with a congenital cardiac malformation, error in abdominal situs, or asplenia or polysplenia. Characteristic absence of the shadow of the inferior vena cava at the posterior border of the heart on a lateral chest radiograph.
Pregnancy	Dilatation of the azygos vein is probably secondary to generalized hypervolemia and disappears after delivery.
Traumatic aneurysm/ arteriovenous fistula	Extremely rare occurrence.

*Pattern: Round or oval shadow in the right tracheobronchial angle that measures more than 10 mm in diameter on standard upright radiographs. The azygos vein decreases in size with inspiration, upright position, and the Valsalva maneuver.

CONGESTIVE HEART FAILURE
IN NEONATES LESS THAN 4 WEEKS OLD

Condition	Imaging Findings	Comments
Hypoplastic left heart syndrome (Fig CA16-1)	Severe pulmonary venous congestion. Progressive cardiomegaly with a globular or oval heart (combination of right atrial and right ventricular enlargement).	Consists of several conditions in which underdevelopment of the left side of the heart is related to an obstructive lesion (stenosis or atresia of mitral valve, aortic valve, or aortic arch). Causes heart failure in the first week of life.
Coarctation of aorta (Fig CA16-2)	Pulmonary venous congestion. Cardiomegaly (biventricular but more prominent on the right).	"Infantile" type in which there is narrowing of a long segment of the aorta proximal to the ductus. Always a patent ductus arteriosus and often a ventricular septal defect to deliver blood from the pulmonary artery to the descending aorta and the systemic circulation. Since the shunted blood is unoxygenated, the lower half of the body is cyanotic.
Tetralogy of Fallot	Decreased pulmonary vascularity; flat or concave pulmonary outflow tract; enlargement of the right ventricle; right aortic arch in about 25% of cases.	Consists of (1) high ventricular septal defect, (2) obstruction to right ventricular outflow (usually infundibular pulmonary stenosis), (3) overriding of the aortic orifice above the ventricular defect, and (4) right ventricular hypertrophy.
Transposition of great vessels	Pulmonary vascularity and heart size are normal in the newborn. Progressive cardiac enlargement and vascular engorgement occur within a few days.	Reverse of the normal relation of the aorta and the pulmonary artery. A left-to-right shunt is required to connect the two separate circulations. The shunts are bidirectional and permit the mixing of oxygenated and unoxygenated blood.
Pseudotruncus arteriosus	Decreased pulmonary vascularity; flat or concave pulmonary outflow tract; enlargement of right ventricle; right aortic arch in about 40% of cases.	Single vessel arising from the heart that is accompanied by a remnant of the atretic pulmonary artery (essentially the same as tetralogy of Fallot with pulmonary atresia).
Large left-to-right shunt (Fig CA16-3)	Increased pulmonary vascularity; diastolic overloading and enlargement of the left atrium and the left ventricle.	Congestive heart failure may develop early in severe ventricular septal defect, patent ductus arteriosus, or common atrioventricular canal.
Persistent truncus arteriosus	Increased pulmonary vascularity; concave pulmonary outflow tract.	Early congestive heart failure if a severe left-to-right shunt. The development of pulmonary hypertension is a protective factor (reduces the pulmonary flow and the diastolic overloading of the heart).
Tricuspid atresia with transposition and no pulmonary stenosis	Increased pulmonary vascularity; marked cardiomegaly.	Because the pulmonary blood flow is exuberant there is less cyanosis, but diastolic overloading of the left side of the heart leads to early congestive heart failure.

Condition	Imaging Findings	Comments
Pulmonary atresia	Decreased pulmonary vascularity; concave pulmonary artery segment.	If the ventricular septum is intact, blood enters the pulmonary circulation via the ductus arteriosus. Once the ductus closes, the infant's condition deteriorates rapidly.
Ebstein's anomaly	Decreased pulmonary vascularity; flat or concave pulmonary outflow tract; typical squared or boxed appearance of the heart.	Downward displacement of an incompetent tricuspid valve into the right ventricle so that the upper portion of the right ventricle is effectively incorporated into the right atrium. A right-to-left atrial shunt causes cyanosis.
Uhl's disease	Radiographic pattern identical to that of Ebstein's anomaly.	Focal or complete absence of the right ventricular myocardium (the right ventricle becomes a thin-walled fibroelastic bag that contracts poorly and cannot effectively empty blood from the right side of the heart).
Common ventricle	Increased pulmonary vascularity; marked nonspecific globular enlargement of the heart.	Extremely large septal defect produces a functional ''single ventricle.'' If there is no pulmonary stenosis, there is marked diastolic overloading of the ventricular chamber and early congestive heart failure.
Premature (prenatal) closure of foramen ovale (Fig CA16-4)	Appearance identical to that of hypoplastic left heart syndrome.	Premature closure of the foramen ovale in the fetus leads to severe left-sided hypoplasia with marked elevation of pulmonary venous pressure (no possibility for left-to-right shunting).
Malformations obstructing pulmonary venous flow	Severe pulmonary venous congestion; left atrial enlargement in some conditions.	Congenital mitral stenosis; cor triatriatum (incomplete fibromuscular diaphragm dividing the left atrium); congenital pulmonary vein stenosis or atresia; total anomalous pulmonary venous return with high-grade pulmonary venous obstruction.
Myocardiopathy	Pulmonary venous congestion with striking cardiomegaly.	Endocardial fibroelastosis; glycogen storage disease (Pompe's); myocarditis (toxoplasmosis, rubella, coxsackievirus); myocardial ischemia (neonatal hypoxia; infantile coronary arteriosclerosis); anomalous left coronary artery arising from the pulmonary artery.
Arteriovenous fistula or hemangioma	High-output congestive failure.	Vein of Galen aneurysm; peripheral or pulmonary arteriovenous fistula; cutaneous or hepatic cavernous hemangioma.
Intracranial disease with increased intracranial pressure	Pulmonary venous congestion.	Cerebral birth injury.
Conduction and rhythm abnormalities	Pulmonary vascular congestion.	Tachycardia (over 200 beats per minute); complete heart block; arrhythmia.
Iatrogenic	Pulmonary venous congestion.	Fluid overload; sodium chloride poisoning.

Condition	Imaging Findings	Comments
Polycythemia	Pulmonary venous congestion.	Maternal-fetal hemorrhage; placental and twin-to-twin transfusion.
Maternal diabetes/neonatal hypoglycemia	Pulmonary venous congestion.	
High-output states	High-output congestive failure.	Severe anemia (eg, erythroblastosis); neonatal hyperthyroidism.
Asplenia or polysplenia syndrome	Pulmonary venous congestion. There may be a symmetric midline liver or a small midline stomach.	High incidence of complex congenital cardiac anomalies that may produce a bizarre configuration of the heart. The spleen may be absent or there may be multiple accessory spleens on radionuclide studies.

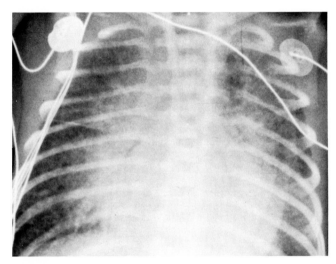

Fig CA16-1. Hypoplastic left heart syndrome.

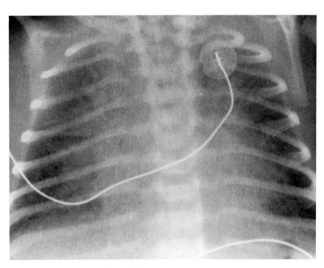

Fig CA16-2. Coarctation of the aorta.

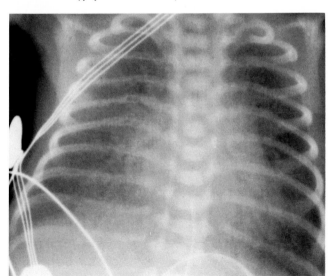

Fig CA16-3. Patent ductus arteriosus.

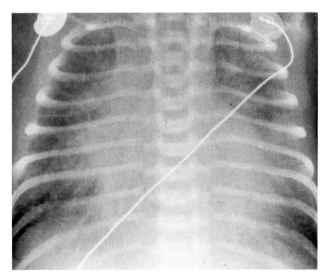

Fig CA16-4. Premature closure of the foramen ovale.

HIGH-OUTPUT HEART DISEASE

Condition	Comments
Anemia **(Fig CA17-1)**	Hemolytic anemia (eg, sickle cell disease, thalassemia) with characteristic marrow hyperplasia (widening of the medullary spaces with thinning of the cortices and coarsening of the trabecular pattern). May also occur in severe chronic blood-loss anemia. May interfere with myocardial function by producing myocardial anoxia.
Thyrotoxicosis **(Fig CA17-2)**	Direct impairment of myocardial metabolism in a patient with the characteristic clinical features of hyperthyroidism.
Beriberi **(Fig CA17-3)**	Thiamine (vitamin B_1) deficiency causes direct impairment of myocardial metabolism. The diagnosis requires a good dietary history and observation of the response to treatment.
Hypervolemia	Fluid overload; overtransfusion.
Arteriovenous fistulas	Rapid shunting of blood from the arterial to the venous system. The fistulas may be peripheral, abdominal, or cerebral.
Paget's disease	Caused by multiple microscopic arteriovenous malformations in pagetoid bone. Characteristic destructive changes are followed by an extensive reparative phase.
Polycythemia vera	Hematologic disorder characterized by hyperplasia of the bone marrow resulting in an increased production of erythrocytes, granulocytes, and platelets. The increased blood volume and viscosity cause prominence of the pulmonary vascularity, simulating congenital heart disease. Usually there is massive splenomegaly and an increased incidence of peptic ulcer disease and urate stones (secondary gout).
Pickwickian obesity **(Fig CA17-4)**	Extreme obesity causes profound hypoventilation (diffuse elevation of the diaphragm and bibasilar atelectatic changes) that results in hypoxia and secondary polycythemia.
Pregnancy	Increased blood volume and flow.

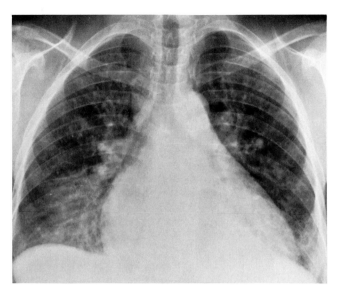

Fɪɢ CA17-1. Sickle cell anemia. Marked cardiomegaly with a generalized increase in pulmonary vascular markings.

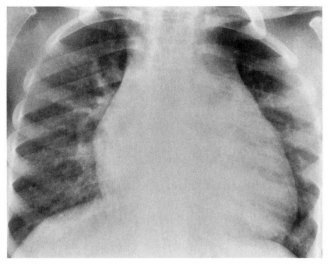

Fɪɢ CA17-2. Thyrotoxicosis. Generalized enlargement of the heart and engorged pulmonary vascularity.

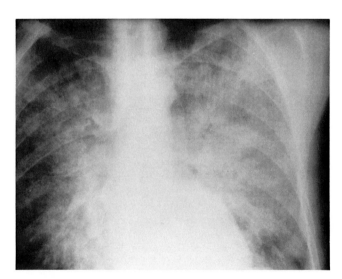

Fɪɢ CA17-3. Beriberi. Diffuse pulmonary edema due to severe high-output failure.

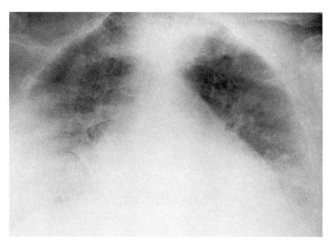

Fɪɢ CA17-4. Pickwickian syndrome. Profound obesity has led to severe hypoventilation and secondary polycythemia, causing marked cardiomegaly and engorgement of the pulmonary vessels.

HYPERTENSIVE CARDIOVASCULAR DISEASE*

Condition	Comments
Essential (idiopathic) hypertension (Fig CA18-1)	Represents the vast majority of patients with elevated blood pressure.
Renovascular disease	Suggestive findings on rapid-sequence excretory urography include (1) unilateral delayed appearance and excretion of contrast material, (2) difference in kidney size greater than 1.5 cm, (3) irregular contour of the renal silhouette (suggesting segmental infarction or atrophy), (4) indentations on the ureter or renal pelvis due to dilated, tortuous ureteral arterial collaterals, and (5) hyperconcentration of contrast material in the collecting system of the smaller kidney on delayed films. About 25% of patients with renovascular hypertension have a normal rapid-sequence excretory urogram (though this modality is also of value in detecting other causes of hypertension, such as tumor, pyelonephritis, polycystic kidneys, or renal infarction).
Renal artery stenosis (Fig CA18-2)	Most commonly due to arteriosclerotic narrowing, which tends to occur in the proximal portion of the vessel close to its origin from the aorta. Poststenotic dilatation is common. Bilateral renal artery stenoses are noted in up to one third of the patients. At times, renal artery stenosis may be detected only on oblique projections that demonstrate the vessel origins in profile.
Fibromuscular hyperplasia (Fig CA18-3)	Characteristic ''string-of-beads'' pattern, in which there are alternating areas of narrowing and dilatation (representing microaneurysms). Smooth, concentric stenoses occur less frequently. Most commonly affects young adult women and is often bilateral.
Perirenal hematoma (Page kidney)	Dense fibrous encasement of the kidney after healing of a subcapsular or perirenal hematoma compresses the renal parenchyma and causes an alteration of the intrarenal hemodynamics that produces ischemia and hypertension. The kidney is often enlarged and demonstrates a mass effect with distortion of the collecting system. Arteriography reveals splaying and stretching of the intrarenal arteries and often irregular staining in the healing portion of the hematoma. Removal of the kidney or evacuation of the offending mass may result in clearing of the hypertension.

*Pattern: The increased workload of the left ventricle due to chronic hypertension initially causes concentric hypertrophy, which produces little if any change in the radiographic appearance of the cardiac silhouette. Eventually, the continued strain leads to dilatation and enlargement of the left ventricle along with downward displacement of the cardiac apex, which often projects below the left hemidiaphragm. Aortic tortuosity with prominence of the ascending portion commonly occurs.

A

B

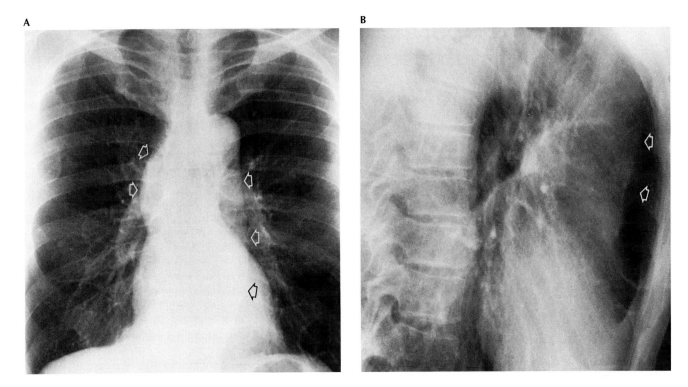

FIG CA18-1. **Essential (idiopathic) hypertension.** (A) Frontal and (B) lateral views of the chest demonstrate characteristic tortuosity of the aorta (arrows), especially the ascending portion. Because the elevated blood pressure has caused left ventricular hypertrophy without dilatation, the radiographic appearance of the cardiac silhouette remains normal.

Condition	Comments
Renal parenchymal disease	Causes include glomerulonephritis, chronic pyelone-phritis, polycystic kidney, renal tumor, and renal agenesis or hypoplasia.
Coarctation of the aorta **(see Fig CA8-1)**	Suggestive radiographic findings include inordinate dilatation of the ascending aorta, widening of the left superior mediastinum, the figure-E or figure-3 sign, and rib notching.
Adrenal disease	Causes include Cushing's syndrome (suggested by widening of the superior mediastinum due to in-creased fat deposition associated with osteoporosis and compression changes in the dorsal vertebrae), pheochromocytoma (may produce a paravertebral mass), adrenocortical adenoma, carcinoma, primary aldosteronism, and the adrenogenital syndrome.
Other endocrine disorders	Hyperthyroidism, acromegaly, and the use of estro-gen-containing oral contraceptives (this may be the most common form of secondary hypertension).
Collagen disease	Systemic lupus erythematosus; polyarteritis nodosa.
Neurogenic	Familial dysautonomia (Riley-Day syndrome); psy-chogenic.

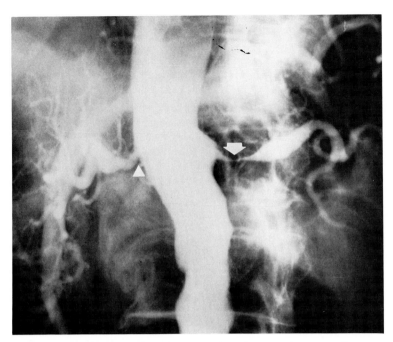

FIG CA18-2. Renovascular hypertension. Bilateral arteriosclerotic renal artery stenoses (arrows).

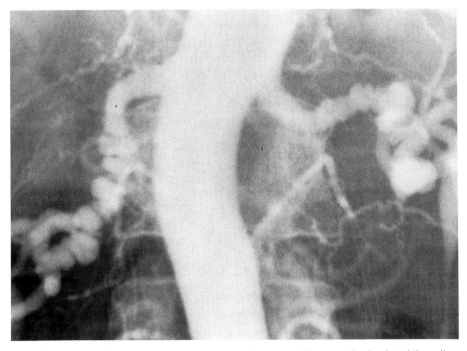

FIG CA18-3. Renovascular hypertension. String-of-beads pattern of fibromuscular dysplasia bilaterally.

CARDIOVASCULAR CALCIFICATION

Condition	Comments
Aortic wall	
Arteriosclerosis **(Fig CA19-1)**	Elongation and tortuosity of the aorta with linear plaques of calcification that most commonly occur in the aortic knob and transverse arch. In severe disease the entire aorta may be outlined by extensive calcification in its wall.
Aneurysm	An increased diameter of the aorta indicates an aneurysm, while an increased distance between intimal calcification and the outer wall of the aorta suggests a dissection.
Aortitis **(Fig CA19-2)**	Dilatation and prominence of the ascending aorta with thin, curvilinear streaks of calcification (often extensive) is characteristic of syphilitic aortitis; linear calcification also frequently occurs in patients with Takayasu's aortitis ("pulseless" disease), a nonspecific obstructive arteritis that primarily affects young women.
Valvular/annulus	
Aortic annulus or valve **(Fig CA19-3)**	Calcification of the annulus tends to be heavy and distinct, unlike valvular calcification, which is usually stippled and often not detected on plain radiographs (best demonstrated on fluoroscopic examination). Causes include arteriosclerosis, rheumatic aortic valve disease, infective endocarditis, and a congenital defect of the aortic valve.
Mitral valve	Develops in patients with long-standing severe mitral stenosis and is often indistinct and easily missed on plain radiographs (best demonstrated by fluoroscopy). The amount of calcification does not reflect the degree of functional disturbance. Multiple calcific or ossific nodules throughout the lower portions of the lungs may develop in areas of chronic interstitial edema.
Mitral annulus **(Fig CA19-4)**	Dense curved or annular calcified band around the mitral valve that usually reflects underlying arteriosclerosis. Although usually insignificant, a rigid annulus may cause functional insufficiency of the mitral valve.

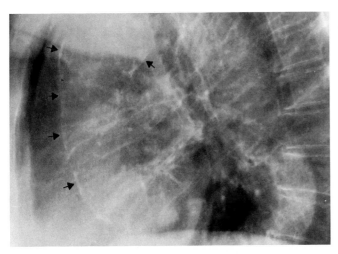

FIG CA19-1. Arteriosclerosis. Lateral view of the chest demonstrates calcification of the anterior and posterior walls of the ascending aorta (arrows). The descending thoracic aorta is tortuous.

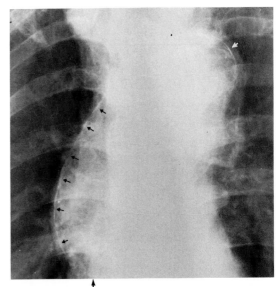

FIG CA19-2. Syphilitic aortitis. Aneurysmal dilatation of the ascending aorta with extensive linear calcification of the wall (black arrows). Some calcification is also seen in the distal aortic arch (white arrow).

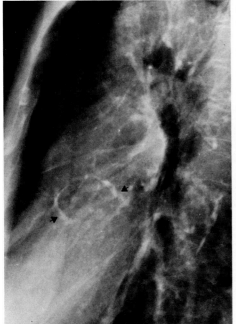

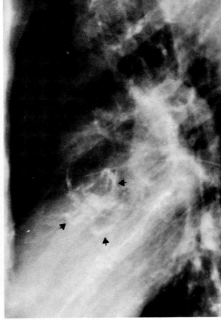

FIG CA19-3. Aortic stenosis. Calcification in (left) the aortic annulus (arrows) and (right) the three leaflets of the aortic valve (arrows).

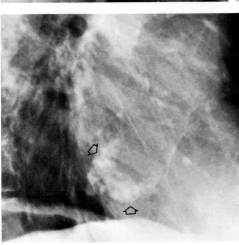

FIG CA19-4. Mitral annulus calcification (arrows) in mitral stenosis.

Condition	Comments
Coronary artery **(Fig CA19-5)**	Punctate, patchy, or tubular densities that primarily involve the circumflex and anterior descending branches of the left coronary artery and are most commonly seen along the left margin of the heart below the pulmonary artery segment. Although infrequently visualized on routine chest radiographs, calcification of a coronary artery strongly suggests the presence of hemodynamically significant arteriosclerotic coronary artery disease. Cardiac fluoroscopy is far more sensitive than plain chest radiography in demonstrating coronary artery calcification, though there is controversy about the prognostic significance of fluoroscopically identified coronary artery calcification in patients with ischemic heart disease. In patients under age 50, coronary artery calcification is a strong predictor of major narrowing in women and a moderate predictor in men. In older patients, calcification has less predictive value.
Sinus of Valsalva	Calcification primarily involves the wall of an aortic sinus aneurysm and is usually best seen on the lateral view.
Left atrium **(Figs CA19-6 and CA19-7)**	Calcification of the left atrial wall usually reflects long-standing severe mitral stenosis and appears as a thin curvilinear rim. Atrial myxomas calcify in about 10% of cases and are best seen by fluoroscopy (may present the pathognomonic appearance of a calcified mass prolapsing into the ventricle during systole). Calcification in the left atrial appendage represents a calcified thrombus.
Ventricular aneurysm **(Fig CA19-8)**	Complication of myocardial infarction in which weakening of the myocardial wall permits the development of a local bulge at the site of the infarct. Curvilinear calcification in the wall of an aneurysm is an infrequent but important finding.
Myocardium	Most commonly a manifestation of an old myocardial infarct. Rare causes include myocardial damage (trauma, myocarditis, rheumatic fever), hyperparathyroidism, and vitamin D toxicity.
Pericardium **(Fig CA19-9)**	Calcific plaques in a thickened pericardium are present in about half of patients with constrictive pericarditis. Though the heaviest deposits of calcium are located anteriorly, posterior calcification and calcification of the pericardium adjacent to the diaphragm can often be seen. At times the heart appears to be encased in a virtually pathognomonic calcific shell.

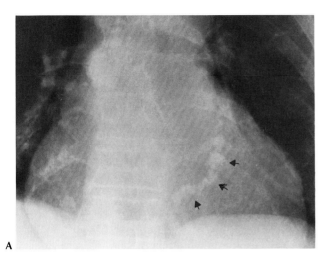

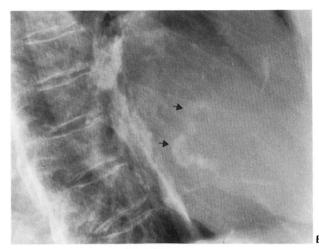

FIG CA19-5. Coronary artery calcification (arrows) in ischemic heart disease. (A) Frontal and (B) lateral views of the chest.

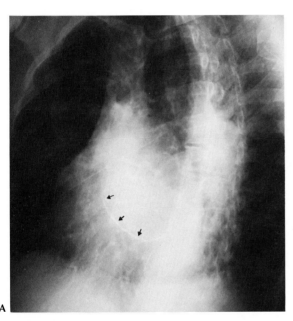

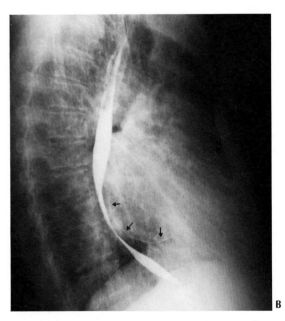

FIG CA19-6. Left atrial calcification. (A) Overpenetrated film in the left anterior oblique position and (B) lateral view with barium in the esophagus show enlargement of the left atrium and calcification of the wall of this chamber (arrows) in a patient with mitral stenosis.[12]

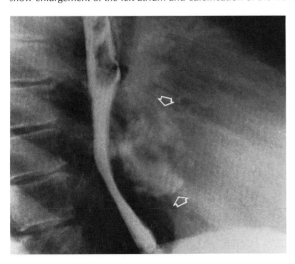

FIG CA19-7. Left atrial myxoma. The arrows point to calcification in the tumor. The myxoma has led to destruction of the mitral valve with resulting left atrial enlargement that causes an impression on the barium-filled esophagus.

Condition	Comments
Ductus arteriosus **(Fig CA19-10)**	Calcification mimicking involvement of the aortic wall may rarely occur in patients with a patent or a closed ductus arteriosus.

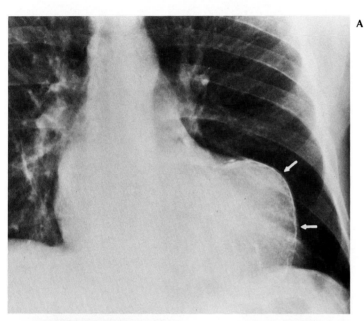

A

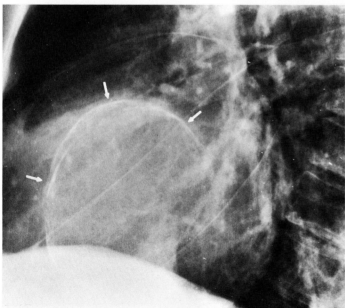

B

FIG CA19-8. **Ventricular aneurysm.** (A) Frontal and (B) lateral views of the chest demonstrate bulging and curvilinear peripheral calcification (arrows) along the lower left border of the heart near the apex. Note the relatively anterior position of the aneurysm on the lateral view.

A

B

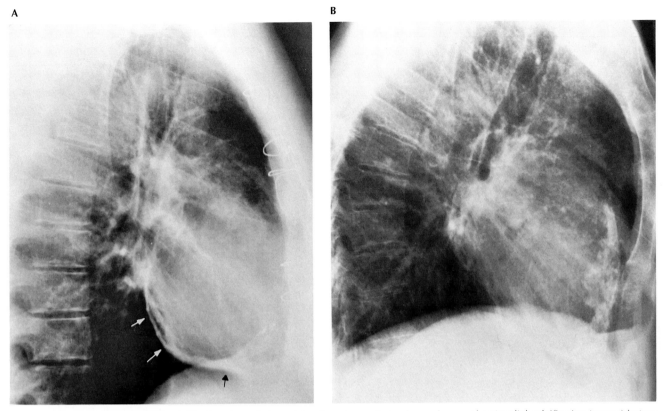

FIG CA19-9. (A and B) **Pericardial calcification.** Lateral view of the chest demonstrates dense plaques of pericardial calcification (arrows) in two patients with chronic constrictive pericarditis due to tuberculosis.

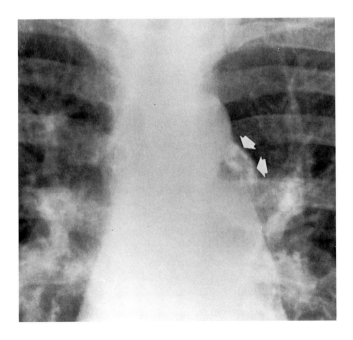

FIG CA19-10. **Ductus arteriosus calcification** (arrow).

PERICARDIAL EFFUSION

Condition	Comments
Congestive heart failure	Evidence of pulmonary venous congestion. An associated pleural effusion is common (frequently unilateral on the right, rarely on the left; may be bilateral).
Collagen disease (see Fig C19-11)	Systemic lupus erythematosus; scleroderma; polyarteritis nodosa; rheumatoid disease. There may be unilateral or bilateral pleural effusion (especially in lupus). Generalized reticulonodular disease (more prominent in the lung bases) may occur.
Infectious pericarditis (Fig CA20-1)	Most commonly coxsackievirus. Also other infections (eg, bacterial, tuberculous, histoplasmic, amebic, toxoplasmic).
Postcardiac surgery	Accumulation of fluid after pericardiotomy. Evidence of surgical clips and sutures.
Postmyocardial infarction syndrome (Dressler's syndrome) (Fig CA20-2)	Autoimmune phenomenon characterized by fever and pleuropericardial chest pain beginning 1 to 6 weeks after an acute myocardial infarction. Other manifestations include pleural effusion that is bilateral in 50% of patients (usually greater on the left) and an ill-defined pneumonia (often with atelectatic streaks) that may be bilateral or only involve the left base.
Trauma	Rapid development of a pericardial effusion may produce severe alteration of cardiac function with minimal change in the radiographic cardiac silhouette.
Tumor of pericardium or heart	Direct invasion from carcinoma of the lung or mediastinal lymphoma, or metastases from melanoma or tumors of the lung or breast. Radiation therapy may produce complete (but usually temporary) resolution of the fluid.
Uremia (Fig CA20-3)	Develops in about 15% of patients on prolonged hemodialysis. May collect rapidly and be life-threatening.
Radiation therapy	May follow the use of moderately high doses (4,000 rads in 4 to 5 weeks, as in the treatment of Hodgkin's disease or breast carcinoma).

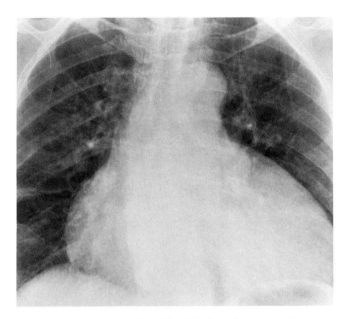

Fɪɢ **CA20-1. Infectious pericarditis.** Globular enlargement of the cardiac silhouette reflects a combination of pericarditis and pericardial effusion in a patient with coxsackievirus infection. There are small pleural effusions bilaterally.

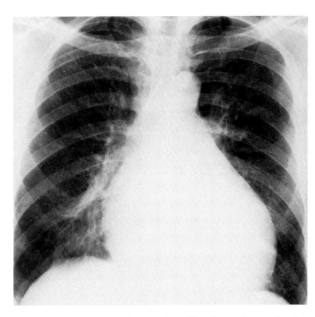

Fɪɢ **CA20-2. Dressler's syndrome.** Chest film obtained 3 weeks after an acute myocardial infarction demonstrates a large pericardial effusion appearing as a rapid increase in heart size in comparison with an essentially normal-sized heart 1 week previously.

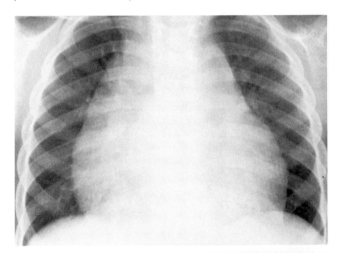

Fɪɢ **CA20-3. Uremia.** Globular enlargement of the cardiac silhouette in a child on prolonged hemidialysis.

Fɪɢ **CA20-4. Epicardial fat pad sign in pericardial effusion.** (A) In a normal person a thin, relatively dense line (arrow) representing the normal pericardium lies between the anterior mediastinal and subepicardial fat. (B) Lateral chest radiograph demonstrates a wide soft-tissue density separating the subepicardial fat stripe (arrows) from the anterior mediastinal fat. This is a virtually pathognomonic sign of pericardial effusion or thickening.

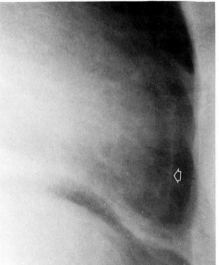

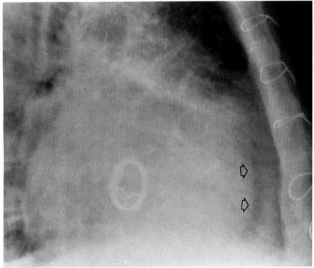

A   B

Condition	Comments
Myxedema	May cause massive chronic pericardial effusion (rarely tamponade).
Bleeding diathesis	Severe chronic anemia; erythroblastosis fetalis; excessive anticoagulant therapy.
Idiopathic	Diagnosis of exclusion for acute pericardial effusion.

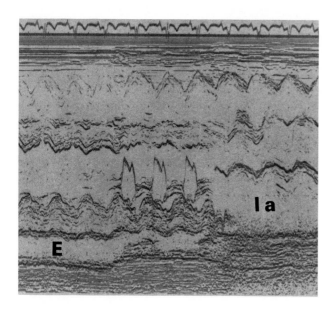

FIG CA20-5. Pericardial effusion. Echocardiogram demonstrates a large posterior effusion (E) that causes separation of the pericardium from the epicardium. Note that the effusion stops at the region of the left atrium (la), in contrast to a pleural effusion that parallels the entire cardiac silhouette.

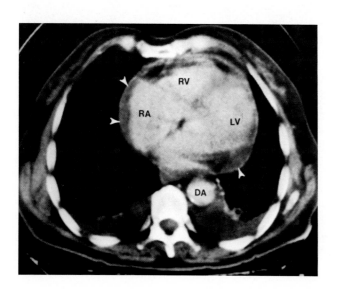

FIG CA20-6. Pericardial effusion. CT scan made after the injection of intravenous contrast material shows the pericardial effusion as a low-density area (arrowheads) that is clearly demarcated from the contrast-enhanced blood in the intracardiac chambers and descending aorta. Note the bilateral pleural effusions posteriorly. (RA, right atrium; RV, right ventricle; LV, left ventricle; and DA, descending aorta).[13]

CONSTRICTIVE PERICARDITIS

Condition	Comments
Tuberculosis (Fig CA21-1)	Etiologic agent in up to one third of older series. Now an infrequent cause.
Other infections	Pyogenic (especially staphylococcal or pneumococcal); histoplasmosis; viral (especially coxsackie B).
Radiation therapy	May follow the use of moderately high doses (4,000 rads in 4 to 5 weeks, as for the treatment of Hodgkin's disease or carcinoma of the breast).
Uremia	Relatively high incidence in patients on prolonged hemodialysis.
Trauma	Hemopericardium leading to dense fibrosis.
Idiopathic	Underlying cause of pericardial disease is often undetermined. Probably represents an asymptomatic or forgotten bout of acute pericarditis.

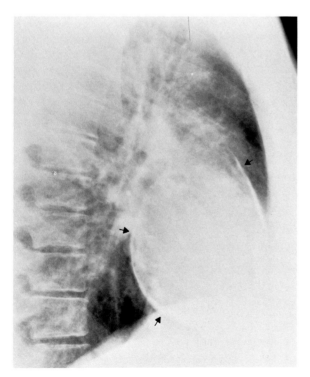

FIG CA21-1. Chronic constrictive pericarditis. Dense calcification in the pericardium (arrows) completely surrounding a normal-sized heart.

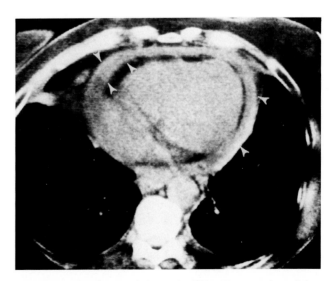

FIG CA21-2. Chronic constrictive pericarditis. CT scan performed during an infusion of contrast material shows enhancement of the soft-tissue–density pericardium (arrowheads), which is up to 6 mm thick.[13]

SOURCES

1. Reprinted from *Radiology of the Heart and Great Vessels* by RN Cooley and MH Schreiber, Williams & Wilkins Company, © 1978, with permission of JH Harris Jr.

2. Reprinted with permission from "Transposition of the Great Arteries" by A Barcia et al, *American Journal of Roentgenology* (1967;100:249–261, Copyright © 1967, Williams & Wilkins Company.

3. Reprinted with permission from "Roentgenographic Features in a Case with Origin of Both Great Vessels from the Right Ventricle without Pulmonary Stenosis" by LS Carey and JE Edwards, *American Journal of Roentgenology* (1965;93:268–287), Copyright © 1965, Williams & Wilkins Company.

4. Reprinted with permission from "Angiocardiographic and Anatomic Findings in Origin of Both Great Arteries from the Right Ventricle" by FJ Hallerman et al, *American Journal of Roentgenology* (1970;109:51–66), Copyright © 1970, Williams & Wilkins Company.

5. Reprinted with permission from "Endocardial Cushion Defects" by MG Baron, *Radiologic Clinics of North America* (1968;6:43–52), Copyright © 1968, WB Saunders Company.

6. Reprinted from *Plain Film Interpretation in Congenital Heart Disease* by LE Swischuk with permission of Williams & Wilkins Company, © 1979.

7. Reprinted with permission from "Other Forms of Left-to-Right Shunt" by LP Elliott, *Seminars in Roentgenology* (1966;1:120–136), Copyright © 1966, Grune & Stratton Inc.

8. Reprinted with permission from "Coronary Arteriovenous Fistula" by I Steinberg and GR Holswade, *American Journal of Roentgenology* (1972;116:82–90), Copyright © 1972, Williams & Wilkins Company.

9. Reprinted with permission from "Congenital Aortic Stenosis" by FB Takekawa et al, *American Journal of Roentgenology* (1966;98:800–821), Copyright © 1966, Williams & Wilkins Company.

10. Reprinted from *Diagnostic Imaging in Internal Medicine* by RL Eisenberg with permission of McGraw-Hill Book Company, © 1985. Courtesy of Marvin Belasco, MD.

11. Reprinted with permission from "Anomalous Origin of the Left Pulmonary Artery from the Right Pulmonary Artery" by KL Jue et al, *American Journal of Roentgenology* (1965;95:598–610), Copyright © 1965, Williams & Wilkins Company.

12. Reprinted with permission from "Left Atrial Calcification" by SCW Vickers et al, *Radiology* (1959;72:569–575), Copyright © 1959, Radiological Society of North America Inc.

13. Reprinted from *Computed Body Tomography* by JKT Lee, SS Sagel, and RJ Stanley (Eds) with permission of Raven Press, New York, © 1983.

Gastrointestinal Patterns

3

GI1 Esophageal motility disorders 232
GI2 Extrinsic impressions on the cervical esophagus 236
GI3 Extrinsic impressions on the thoracic esophagus 238
GI4 Esophageal ulceration 242
GI5 Esophageal narrowing 246
GI6 Esophageal filling defects 248
GI7 Esophageal diverticula 252
GI8 Gastric ulceration 254
GI9 Narrowing of the stomach 256
GI10 Filling defects in the stomach 260
GI11 Thickening of gastric folds 264
GI12 Gastric outlet obstruction 268
GI13 Gastric dilatation without outlet obstruction 272
GI14 Widening of the retrogastric space 274
GI15 Filling defects in the gastric remnant 276
GI16 Simultaneous involvement of the gastric antrum and duodenal bulb 278
GI17 Duodenal filling defects 280
GI18 Enlargement of the papilla of Vater (> 1.5 centimeters) 284
GI19 Duodenal narrowing or obstruction 286
GI20 Thickening of duodenal folds 290
GI21 Widening of the duodenal sweep 292
GI22 Adynamic ileus 294
GI23 Small bowel obstruction 297
GI24 Small bowel dilatation 300
GI25 Regular thickening of small bowel folds 303
GI26 Generalized, irregular, distorted small bowel folds 304
GI27 Filling defects in the jejunum and ileum 308
GI28 Sandlike lucencies in the small bowel 312
GI29 Separation of small bowel loops 314
GI30 Small bowel diverticula and pseudodiverticula 316
GI31 Simultaneous fold thickening of the stomach and small bowel 318
GI32 Coned cecum 320
GI33 Filling defects in the cecum 324
GI34 Ulcerative lesions of the colon 328
GI35 Narrowing of the colon 334
GI36 Filling defects in the colon 340
GI37 Thumbprinting of the colon 348
GI38 Double tracking in the colon 350
GI39 Enlargement of the retrorectal space 352
GI40 Alterations in gallbladder size 354
GI41 Filling defects in an opacified gallbladder 356
GI42 Filling defects in the bile ducts 358
GI43 Bile duct narrowing or obstruction 360
GI44 Cystic dilatation of the bile ducts 364
GI45 Pneumoperitoneum 366

GI46 Gas in the bowel wall (pneumatosis intestinalis) 368
GI47 Extraluminal gas in the upper quadrants 370
GI48 Bull's-eye lesions of the gastrointestinal tract 374
GI49 Liver calcification 376
GI50 Spleen calcification 380
GI51 Alimentary tract calcification 382
GI52 Pancreatic calcification 384
GI53 Gallbladder and bile duct calcification 386
GI54 Adrenal calcification 388
GI55 Renal calcification 390
GI56 Ureteral calcification 394
GI57 Bladder calcification 396
GI58 Female genital tract calcification 398
GI59 Widespread abdominal calcification 400
GI60 Thickened gallbladder wall (> 2 millimeters) 402
GI61 Focal anechoic (cystic) liver masses 404
GI62 Complex or solid hepatic masses 408
GI63 Focal decreased-attenuation masses in the liver 412
GI64 Generalized abnormality of hepatic attenuation 420
GI65 Generalized increased echogenicity of the liver 422
GI66 Generalized decreased echogenicity of the liver 424
GI67 Shadowing lesions in the liver 424
GI68 Pancreatic masses on ultrasound 426
GI69 Pancreatic masses on computed tomography 428
GI70 Dilatation of the pancreatic duct 432
GI71 Decreased-attenuation masses in the spleen 433
GI72 Pseudokidney sign or bull's-eye appearance in the abdomen 435
Sources 437

ESOPHAGEAL MOTILITY DISORDERS

Condition	Imaging Findings	Comments
Cricopharyngeal achalasia (Fig GI1-1)	Hemispherical or horizontal, shelflike protrusion on the posterior aspect of the esophagus at approximately the C5-C6 level.	Failure of the upper esophageal sphincter to relax. Can result in dysphagia by obstructing the passage of a swallowed bolus. In severe disease, can cause aspiration and pneumonia.
Total laryngectomy (pseudodefect)	Appearance identical to that of cricopharyngeal achalasia.	Clinically, the patient complains of dysphagia on the way down and dysphonia with esophageal speech on the way up.
Scleroderma (Fig GI1-2)	Dilated, atonic esophagus involving only the smooth muscle portion (from the aortic arch down). Normal stripping wave in the upper third of the esophagus (which is composed primarily of striated muscle). Patulous lower esophageal sphincter with gastroesophageal reflux. In the upright position, barium flows rapidly into the stomach.	Atrophy of smooth muscle with replacement by fibrosis. Often asymptomatic, though the patient may be required to eat or drink in a sitting or an erect position. High incidence of gastroesophageal reflux leading to peptic esophagitis and stricture formation.
Achalasia (Figs GI1-3 to GI1-5)	Dilatation and tortuosity of the esophagus that can produce a widened mediastinum (often with an air-fluid level) primarily on the right side adjacent to the cardiac shadow. Multiple uncoordinated tertiary contractions. Smoothly tapered, conical narrowing of the distal esophagus (beak sign). In the erect position, small spurts of barium enter the stomach (jet effect).	Incomplete relaxation of the lower esophageal sphincter related to a paucity or absence of ganglion cells in the myenteric plexuses (Auerbach's) of the distal esophageal wall. Denervation hypersensitivity response to Mecholyl (synthetic acetylcholine). A similar appearance may be produced by any generalized or localized interruption of the reflex arc controlling normal esophageal motility (eg, diseases of the medullary nuclei, abnormality of the vagus nerve, destruction of myenteric ganglion cells by inflammatory disease or carcinoma of the distal esophagus or the gastric cardia).
Chagas' disease	Pattern identical to that of achalasia.	Destruction of the myenteric plexuses by the protozoan *Trypanosoma cruzi*, which also causes megacolon with chronic constipation, ureteral dilatation, and myocarditis.
Diffuse esophageal spasm (Fig GI1-6)	Tertiary contractions of abnormally high amplitude that can obliterate the lumen. Corkscrew pattern of transient sacculations or pseudodiverticula (rosary bead esophagus).	Classic clinical triad of massive uncoordinated esophageal contractions, chest pain, and increased intramural pressure. Symptoms are frequently caused or aggravated by eating, but can occur spontaneously and even awaken the patient at night.
Presbyesophagus	Nonpropulsive tertiary contractions that are usually occasional and mild but may become frequent and strong.	Condition of aging that may be the result of a minor cerebrovascular accident affecting the central nuclei. Usually asymptomatic but can cause moderate dysphagia.

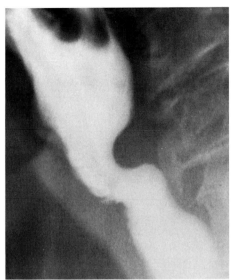

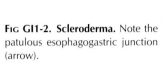

FIG GI1-1. Cricopharyngeal achalasia.

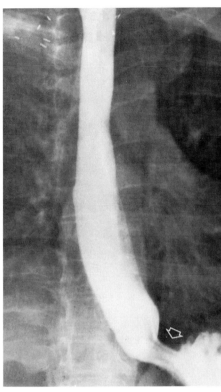

FIG GI1-2. Scleroderma. Note the patulous esophagogastric junction (arrow).

FIG GI1-3. Achalasia. The margin of the dilated, tortuous esophagus (arrows) parallels the right border of the heart.

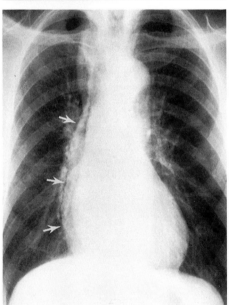

A

FIG GI1-4. Achalasia. (A) Beak sign. (B) Jet effect.

B

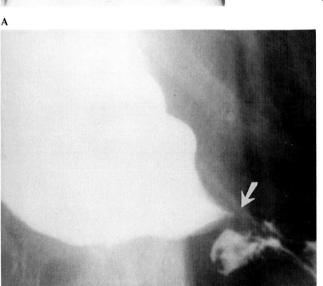

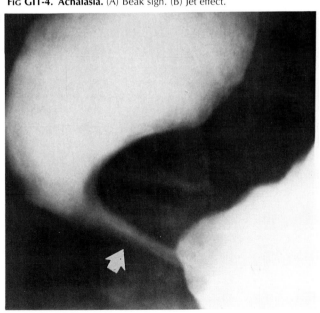

Condition	Imaging Findings	Comments
Esophagitis (Fig GI1-7)	Initially, repetitive nonperistaltic tertiary contractions occur distal to the point of disruption of the primary wave. If severe, can result in complete aperistalsis.	Disordered esophageal motility is the earliest and most frequent radiographic abnormality in esophageal inflammation, whether secondary to reflux, corrosive agents, infection, amyloidosis, or radiation injury.
Primary muscle disorders (Fig GI1-8)	Disordered peristalsis involving the upper third of the esophagus (containing striated muscle). In myasthenia gravis, the initial swallow is often normal but peristalsis weakens on repeated swallows. In myotonic dystrophy, there is reflux across the cricopharyngeus muscle (continuous column of barium extending from the hypopharynx to the cervical esophagus even when the patient is not swallowing).	Patient unable to develop a good pharyngeal peristaltic wave. In myasthenia gravis, muscular fatigue results from failure of neural transmission between the motor end-plate and the muscle fiber. In myotonic dystrophy, an anatomic abnormality of the motor end-plate leads to atrophy and an inability of the contracted muscle to relax. Other primary muscle disorders include polymyositis, dermatomyositis, amyotrophic lateral sclerosis, myopathies secondary to steroids and abnormal thyroid function, and oculopharyngeal myopathy.
Primary neural disorders	Various patterns of abnormal motility including profound motor incoordination of the pharynx and the upper esophageal sphincter, diffuse tertiary contractions, and an achalasia pattern.	Causes include peripheral or central cranial nerve palsy, cerebrovascular occlusive disease affecting the brainstem, high unilateral cervical vagotomy, bulbar poliomyelitis, syringomyelia, multiple sclerosis, and familial dysautonomia (Riley-Day syndrome).
Diabetes mellitus	Various patterns of abnormal motility including tertiary contractions and esophageal dilatation with a substantial delay in esophageal emptying when the patient is recumbent.	Markedly decreased amplitude of pharyngeal and peristaltic contractions. Primarily involves diabetics with a neuropathy of long duration.
Alcoholism	Diminished peristalsis, most pronounced in the distal portion.	Probably reflects a combination of alcoholic myopathy and neuropathy.
Drugs	Aperistalsis and dilatation of the esophagus (mimics scleroderma).	Anticholinergic agents (atropine, Pro-Banthine).
Obstructive lesions	Initially, tertiary contractions are produced in an attempt to pass the obstruction. Eventually, there may be a dilated and virtually aperistaltic esophagus.	Lesions that may cause esophageal obstruction include tumors, foreign bodies, webs, strictures, and Schatzki's rings.

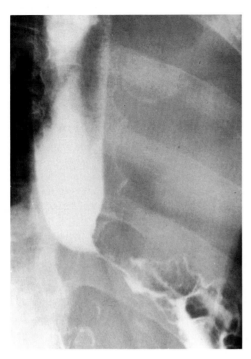

FiG GI1-5. Achalasia pattern caused by the proximal extension of carcinoma of the fundus of the stomach.

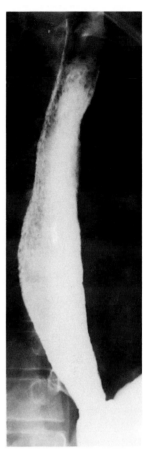

FiG GI1-6. Diffuse esophageal spasm.

FiG GI1-7. Candidiasis. Aperistalsis and esophageal dilatation are associated with diffuse ulceration.

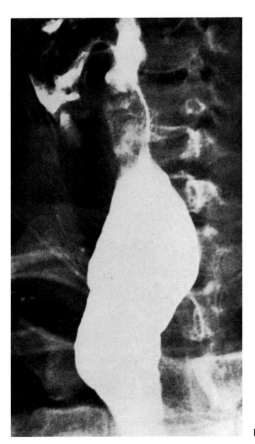

FiG GI1-8. Myotonic dystrophy.[1]

EXTRINSIC IMPRESSIONS ON THE CERVICAL ESOPHAGUS

Condition	Imaging Findings	Comments
Cricopharyngeus muscle (Fig GI2-1)	Relatively constant posterior impression on the esophagus at about the C5-C6 level.	Caused by failure of the cricopharyngeus muscle to relax. A similar posterior impression can often be observed after total laryngectomy.
Pharyngeal venous plexus (Fig GI2-1)	Anterior impression on the esophagus at about the C6 level. Appearance varies from swallow to swallow.	Caused by prolapse of lax mucosal folds over the rich central submucosal pharyngeal venous plexus. Occurs in 70% to 90% of adults and is thus considered a normal finding.
Esophageal web (Figs GI2-1 to GI2-3)	Smooth, thin lucent band (occasionally multiple) arising from the anterior wall of the esophagus near the pharyngoesophageal junction.	Usually an incidental finding of no clinical importance, but can be associated with epidermolysis bullosa, benign mucous membrane pemphigus, or the ''Plummer-Vinson syndrome.''
Anterior marginal osteophyte (Fig GI2-4)	Smooth, regular indentation on the posterior wall of the esophagus at the level of an intervertebral disk space.	Usually asymptomatic but may produce pain or difficulty in swallowing (especially with profuse osteophytosis and diffuse idiopathic skeletal hyperostosis).
Thyroid enlargement or mass (Fig GI2-5)	Smooth impression on and displacement of the lateral wall of the esophagus, usually with parallel displacement of the trachea.	Caused by localized or generalized hypertrophy of the gland, inflammatory disease, or thyroid malignancy.
Parathyroid mass	Impression on and displacement of the lateral wall of the esophagus.	Can aid in determining the site of the lesion in a patient with symptoms of hyperparathyroidism due to a functioning parathyroid tumor.
Lymphadenopathy	Smooth impression on and displacement of the esophagus.	May be calcified.
Soft-tissue abscess or hematoma	Impression on and displacement of the esophagus.	Abscess may contain gas.
Spinal neoplasm or inflammation	Posterior impression on the esophagus (may be irregular).	Suggested if there is associated destruction of a vertebral body.

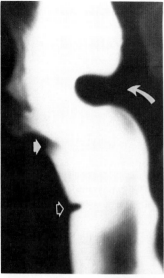

Fig GI2-1. Three impressions on the cervical esophagus: **cricopharyngeal impression** (curved arrow), **pharyngeal venous plexus** (short closed arrow), and **esophageal web** (short open arrow).[2]

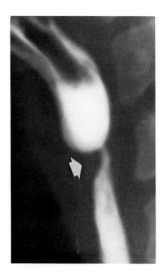

Fig GI2-2. Epidermolysis bullosa. A stenotic web (arrow) results from the healing of subepidermal blisters involving the mucous membranes.

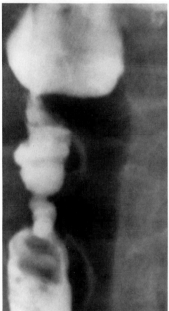

Fig GI2-3. Benign mucous membrane pemphigus. Postinflammatory scarring causes a long, irregular area of narrowing suggestive of a malignant process.

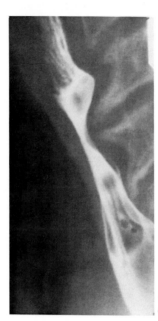

Fig GI2-4. Anterior marginal osteophytes.

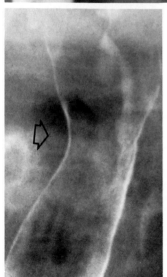

Fig GI2-5. Enlargement of the thyroid gland. Smooth impression in the cervical esophagus (arrow).

EXTRINSIC IMPRESSIONS ON THE THORACIC ESOPHAGUS

Condition	Imaging Findings	Comments
Normal structures		
Aortic knob (Fig GI3-1)	Broad impression on the esophagus at the level of the transverse arch.	More prominent as the aorta becomes increasingly dilated and tortuous with age.
Left main stem bronchus (Fig GI3-1)	Narrower impression on the esophagus at the level of the carina.	
Left inferior pulmonary vein/confluence of left pulmonary veins	Impression on the anterior aspect of the left wall of the esophagus 4 to 5 cm below the carina.	Seen in about 10% of patients [especially in a steep left posterior oblique (LPO) projection]. The vascular nature of the indentation can be confirmed by the Valsalva and Mueller maneuvers (the impression becomes smaller and more prominent, respectively).
Vascular abnormalities		
Right aortic arch (Fig GI3-2)	Impression on the right lateral wall of the esophagus at a level slightly higher than the normal left aortic knob. Deviation of the trachea to the left.	If no posterior esophageal impression (mirror-image pattern), congenital heart disease (especially tetralogy of Fallot) is frequently associated. If there is an oblique posterior indentation on the esophagus (aberrant left subclavian artery), congenital heart disease is rarely associated.
Cervical aortic arch (see Fig CA11-2)	Pulsatile mass causing a posterior impression on the esophagus above the clavicle.	Caused by the retroesophageal course of the distal arch or the proximal descending aorta. No coexistent intracardiac congenital heart disease.
Double aortic arch (see Fig CA11-3)	Reverse S–shaped impression on the esophagus. Right (posterior) arch is generally higher and larger than the left (anterior) arch. Infrequently, the two esophageal impressions are directly across from each other.	Aorta generally ascends on the right, branches, and finally reunites on the left. The two limbs of the aorta encircle the trachea and esophagus, forming a ring.
Coarctation of the aorta (see Fig CA8-1)	Characteristic figure-3 sign on plain chest radiographs. Reverse figure-3, or figure-E, impression on the barium-filled esophagus.	Usually occurs at or just distal to the level of the ductus arteriosus. Much less frequently, the area of narrowing is more proximal. The more cephalad bulge represents prestenotic dilatation, while the lower bulge reflects poststenotic dilatation. Relative obstruction of aortic blood flow leads to left ventricular hypertrophy and rib notching (collateral circulation).
Aortic aneurysm or tortuosity (Fig GI3-3)	Sickle-like deformity that typically displaces the esophagus anteriorly and to the left.	May cause esophageal symptoms ("dysphagia aortica").
Aberrant right subclavian artery (see Fig CA11-4)	Posterior impression on the esophagus that runs obliquely upward and to the right on the frontal view.	Usually asymptomatic and not associated with congenital heart disease. The aberrant artery arises as the last major vessel of the aortic arch and courses across the mediastinum behind the esophagus.
Aberrant left pulmonary artery (see Fig CA11-5)	Characteristic figure-3 sign on plain chest radiographs. Reverse figure-3, or figure-E, impression on the barium-filled esophagus.	Aberrant artery crosses the mediastinum between the trachea and the esophagus.
Anomalous pulmonary venous return (type III)	Anterior impression on the lower portion of the esophagus, just above the diaphragm but slightly below the expected site of the left atrial indentation.	Anomalous pulmonary vein travels with the esophagus through the diaphragm to insert into the portal vein or a systemic vein.

(continued page 240)

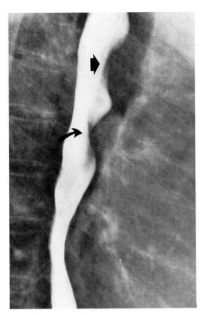

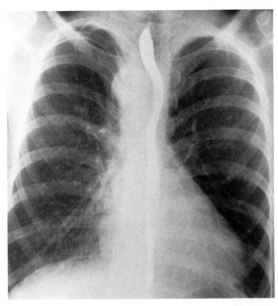

FIG GI3-2. Right aortic arch.

FIG GI3-1. Normal esophageal impressions caused by the aorta (short arrow) and left main stem bronchus (long arrow).

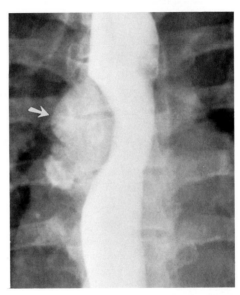

FIG GI3-4. Calcified medi-astinal lymph nodes at the carinal level (arrow) causing a focal impression on and displacement of the esophagus.

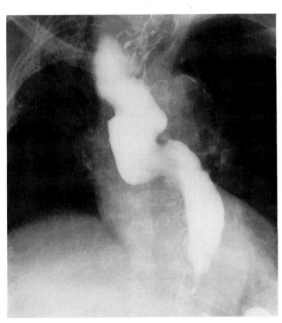

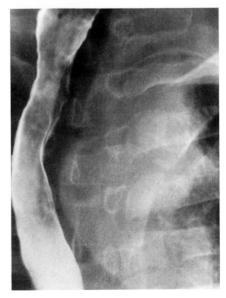

FIG GI3-3. Dysphagia aortica. Tortuosity of the descending thoracic aorta produces characteristic displacement of the esophagus to the left. Note the retraction of the upper esophagus to the right, caused by chronic inflammatory disease, which simulates an extrinsic mass arising from the opposite side.

FIG GI3-5. Squamous cell carcinoma of the lung producing a broad impression on the upper thoracic esophagus.

Condition	Imaging Findings	Comments
Persistent truncus arteriosus (type IV) (pseudotruncus arteriosus)	Discrete impression (often multiple) on the posterior wall of the esophagus that is located somewhat lower than the usual position of an aberrant left subclavian artery.	Caused by dilated bronchial artery collaterals that develop because of the absence of the pulmonary artery.
Left atrial enlargement (see CA3)	Anterior impression on and posterior displacement of the esophagus beginning about 2 cm below the carina.	Associated signs include posterior displacement of the left main stem bronchus, widening of the carina, bulging of the left atrial appendage, and a "double-density" sign on frontal views.
Left ventricular enlargement (see CA4)	Anterior impression on and posterior displacement of the esophagus at a level somewhat inferior to an enlarged left atrium.	Most often caused by aortic valvular disease or cardiac failure.
Mediastinal or pulmonary masses (Figs GI3-4 to GI3-6)	Focal or broad impression on and displacement of the esophagus. The appearance depends on the size and the position of the mass.	Most common causes are inflammatory and metastatic lesions involving lymph nodes in the carinal and subcarinal regions. Also tumors and cysts of the mediastinum, lung, and trachea.
Paraesophageal hernia (Fig GI3-7)	Usually displaces the distal esophagus posteriorly and to the right.	Extent of the impression depends on the amount of herniated stomach. The esophagogastric junction remains in its normal position below the diaphragm.
Pericardial lesions	Localized or broad impression on the anterior wall of the esophagus.	Tumors and cysts usually cause localized impressions, while effusions are generally broader.
Apical pleuropulmonary fibrosis (pseudo-impression)	Retraction of the upper thoracic esophagus toward the side of the pulmonary lesion.	Simulates the appearance of an extrinsic mass arising from the opposite side. Usually a complication of chronic inflammatory disease, especially tuberculosis.

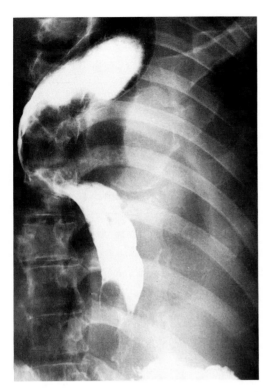

FIG GI3-6. Squamous cell carcinoma of the lung impressing and invading the midthoracic esophagus.

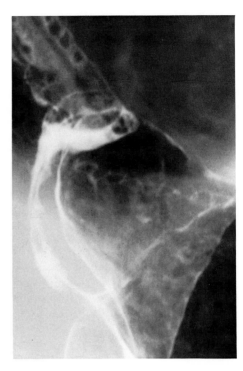

FIG GI3-7. Paraesophageal hernia impressing the distal esophagus.

ESOPHAGEAL ULCERATION

Condition	Imaging Findings	Comments
Reflux esophagitis (Figs GI4-1 to GI4-3)	Initially, superficial ulcerations or erosions appear as streaks or dots of barium superimposed on the flat mucosa of the distal esophagus. Ulcers may be linear and associated with radiating folds and slight retraction of the esophageal wall. In advanced disease, there may be deep erosions or penetrating ulcers with nodular thickening of folds.	Increased incidence with hiatal hernia, repeated vomiting, prolonged nasogastric intubation, scleroderma, and late pregnancy. Also occurs after surgical procedures in the region of the gastroesophageal junction that impair the normal function of the lower esophageal sphincter (eg, Heller procedure for achalasia). May be associated with a disorder of esophageal motility and fine transverse folds (feline esophagus).
Barrett's esophagus (Fig GI4-4)	Ulceration can occur anywhere along the columnar epithelium and tends to be deep and penetrating like peptic gastric ulcers. Postinflammatory stricture of the esophagus often develops.	Often associated with hiatal hernia and reflux, though the ulcer is generally separated from the hernia by a variable length of normal-appearing esophagus. High propensity for developing adenocarcinoma in the columnar-lined portion of the esophagus.
Infectious esophagitis *Candida* (Fig GI4-5)	Multiple ulcerations of various sizes that can involve the entire thoracic esophagus. Irregular nodular mucosal pattern with marginal serrations.	Most frequently develops in patients with chronic debilitating diseases or undergoing immunosuppressive therapy. Disordered esophageal motility (dilated, atonic esophagus) is often an early finding.
Herpetic (Fig GI4-6)	Similar to candidiasis, though the background mucosa is often otherwise normal.	Self-limited viral inflammation that predominantly affects patients with disseminated malignancy or abnormal immune systems.
Tuberculous	Single or multiple ulcers that may mimic malignancy. Sinuses and fistulous tracts are common.	Intense fibrotic response often narrows the esophageal lumen. Numerous miliary granulomas can produce multiple nodules.
Other organisms	Various patterns of ulceration, nodularity, and fistulous tracts.	Rare manifestation of syphilis and histoplasmosis.
Carcinoma of the esophagus (Figs GI4-7 and GI4-8)	Ulcer crater (often irregular) surrounded by an unchanging bulging mass projecting into the esophageal lumen.	In the relatively uncommon primary ulcerative esophageal carcinoma, virtually all of an eccentric, flat mass is ulcerated. Ulceration is an infrequent manifestation of esophageal lymphoma.
Corrosive esophagitis (Fig GI4-9)	Diffuse superficial or deep ulceration involves a long portion of the esophagus.	Most severe corrosive injuries are caused by alkali. Fibrous healing results in gradual esophageal narrowing.
Radiation injury	Multiple ulcerations of various sizes that can involve the entire thoracic esophagus. Irregular nodular mucosal pattern with marginal serrations.	Appearance indistinguishable from that of *Candida* esophagitis (which is far more common in patients undergoing chemotherapy or radiation therapy for malignant disease). Develops after relatively low radiation doses in patients who simultaneously or sequentially receive adriamycin or actinomycin D.

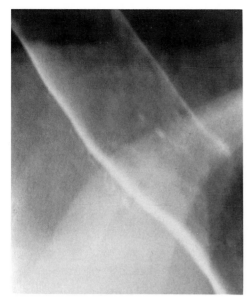

FIG GI4-1. Reflux esophagitis. Superficial ulcerations appear as streaks of contrast material superimposed on the flat mucosa of the distal esophagus.

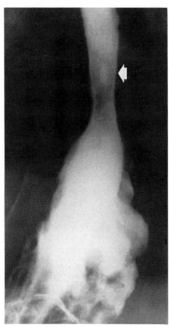

FIG GI4-2. Reflux esophagitis. Large penetrating ulcer (arrow).

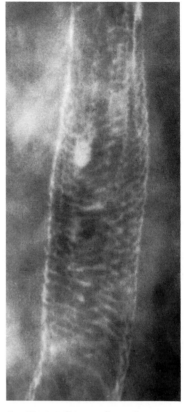

FIG GI4-3. Feline esophagus.[3]

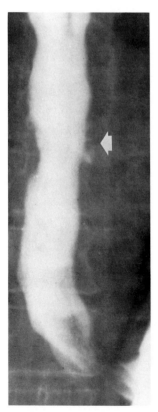

FIG GI4-4. Barrett esophagus. Ulcerations (arrow) have developed at a distance from the esophagogastric junction.

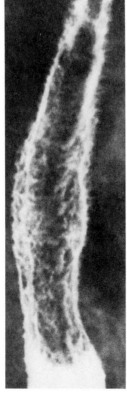

FIG GI4-5. *Candida* esophagitis. Multiple ulcers and nodular plaques produce the grossly irregular contour of a shaggy esophagus. This manifestation of far-advanced candidiasis is now infrequent because of earlier and better treatment of the disease.[4]

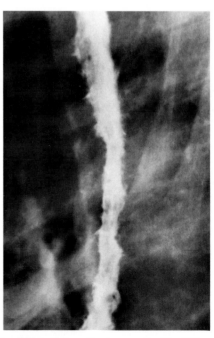

FIG GI4-6. Herpes simplex esophagitis. Diffuse irregularity and ulceration.

Condition	Imaging Findings	Comments
Crohn's disease/ eosinophilic esophagitis	Various patterns of ulceration, nodularity, and fistulous tracts.	Infrequent esophageal involvement.
Drug-induced esophagitis	Various patterns of superficial or deep esophageal ulcerations.	Primarily occurs in patients who have delayed esophageal transit time (abnormal peristalsis, hiatal hernia with reflux, or relative obstruction). Most commonly associated with potassium chloride tablets; other causes include tetracycline, emepronium bromide, quinidine, and ascorbic acid.
Intramural esophageal pseudodiverticulosis (GI4-10)	Multiple small (1 to 3 mm), ulcerlike projections arising from the esophageal wall. There is frequently an associated smooth stricture in the upper esophagus.	Rare disorder in which the pseudodiverticula represent the dilated ducts of submucosal glands. *Candida albicans* can be cultured from about half the patients, though there is no evidence suggesting the fungus as a causative agent.

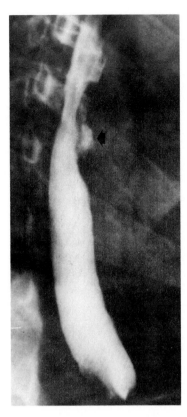

FIG GI4-7. **Squamous carcinoma** of the esophagus. On a profile view, the lesion appears as an ulcer crater (arrow) surrounded by a bulging mass projecting into the esophageal lumen.

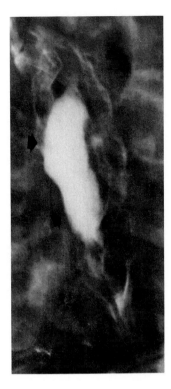

FIG GI4-8. **Primary ulcerative carcinoma.** Characteristic meniscoid ulceration (arrow) surrounded by a tumor mass.

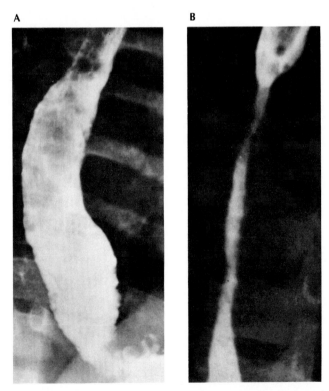

FIG GI4-9. **Corrosive esophagitis.** (A) A dilated, boggy esophagus with ulceration 8 days after the ingestion of a caustic agent. (B) Stricture formation is evident on an esophagram obtained 3 months after the caustic injury.

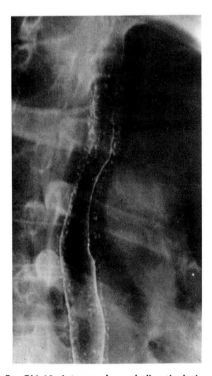

FIG GI4-10. **Intramural pseudodiverticulosis.**

ESOPHAGEAL NARROWING

Condition	Imaging Findings	Comments
Congenital esophageal web (Fig GI5-1)	Smooth, thin lucent band arising from the *anterior* wall of the esophagus near the pharyngoesophageal junction. Rarely distal or multiple.	Usually an incidental finding of no clinical importance, but can be associated with epidermolysis bullosa, benign mucous membrane pemphigus, or the "Plummer-Vinson syndrome."
Lower esophageal ring (Schatzki's ring) (Fig GI5-2)	Smooth, concentric narrowing of the esophagus arising several centimeters above the diaphragm.	Can cause dysphagia if the width of the lumen is less than 12 mm.
Carcinoma of esophagus (Fig GI5-3)	Initially, a flat plaquelike lesion on one wall of the esophagus. Later, an encircling mass with irregular luminal narrowing and overhanging margins.	Major cause of dysphagia in patients older than 40. Close association with drinking and smoking and with head and neck carcinomas. Spreads rapidly and often ulcerates.
Malignancy of fundus of the stomach (Fig GI5-4)	Irregular narrowing and nodularity of the distal esophagus.	Develops in 10% to 15% of adenocarcinomas and in 2% to 10% of lymphomas arising in the cardia.
Reflux esophagitis (Fig GI5-5)	Asymmetric, often irregular, stricture of the esophagus that usually extends to the cardioesophageal junction.	Often, but *not always*, associated with a hiatal hernia.
Barrett's esophagus (Fig GI5-6)	Smooth stricture that generally involves the midportion of the thoracic esophagus.	Usually a variable length of normal-appearing esophagus separates the stricture from the cardioesophageal junction. A technetium scan can demonstrate the columnar tissue in the lower esophagus.
Corrosive esophagitis (Fig GI5-7)	Long stricture that involves a large portion of the esophagus down to the cardioesophageal junction.	Most severe injuries are caused by the ingestion of alkali.
Prolonged nasogastric intubation	Smooth narrowing of the distal esophagus.	Caused by reflux esophagitis (tube prevents hiatal closure) or mucosal ischemia (compression effect of the tube).
Infectious or granulomatous disorders	Various patterns of esophageal narrowing.	Tuberculosis; histoplasmosis; syphilis; herpes simplex; Crohn's disease; eosinophilic esophagitis.
Motility disorders (see Fig GI1-4)	Various patterns of esophageal narrowing.	Achalasia (failure of the lower esophageal sphincter to relax, beak sign); diffuse esophageal spasm (prolonged strong contractions).
Intramural esophageal pseudodiverticulosis (Fig GI5-8)	Smooth stricture in the upper third of the esophagus associated with multiple small ulcerlike projections arising from the esophageal wall.	Dilatation of the stricture generally ameliorates the symptoms of dysphagia.

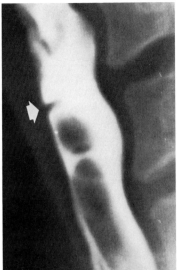

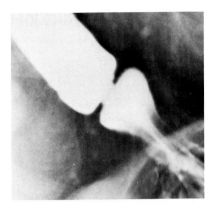

FIG GI5-2. Lower esophageal ring.

FIG GI5-1. Esophageal web.

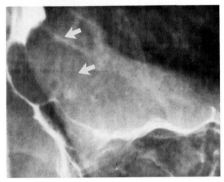

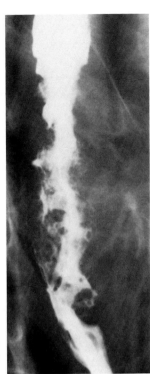

FIG GI5-3. Esophageal carcinoma. Irregular narrowing of an extensive segment of the thoracic portion of the esophagus.

FIG GI5-4. Adenocarcinoma of the fundus involving the esophagus. An irregular tumor of the superior aspect of the fundus extends proximally as a large mass (arrows) that almost obstructs the distal esophagus.

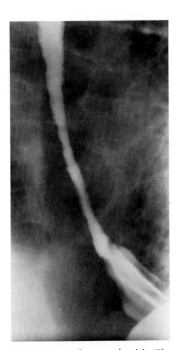

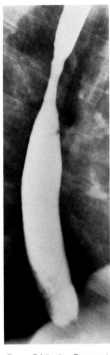

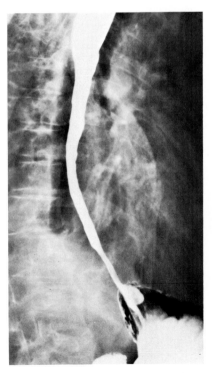

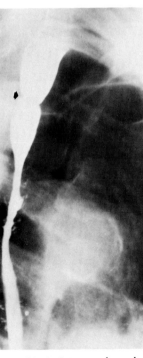

FIG GI5-5. Reflux esophagitis. The long esophageal stricture is associated with a hiatal hernia.

FIG GI5-6. Barrett esophagus. Smooth stricture in the upper thoracic esophagus.

FIG GI5-7. Extensive caustic stricture due to lye ingestion that involves almost the entire thoracic esophagus.

FIG GI5-8. Intramural esophageal pseudodiverticulosis. The arrow points to the upper esophageal stricture.

ESOPHAGEAL FILLING DEFECTS

Condition	Imaging Findings	Comments
Benign tumors		
Spindle cell tumor (Fig GI6-1)	Smooth, rounded intramural defect that is sharply demarcated from the adjacent esophageal wall. No infiltration, ulceration, or overhanging margins.	Most commonly leiomyoma, which is usually asymptomatic and rarely ulcerates, bleeds, or undergoes malignant transformation. Occasionally contains pathognomonic amorphous calcification.
Fibrovascular polyp (Fig GI6-2)	Large, oval or elongated, sausage-like intraluminal mass.	Though rare, the second most common type of benign esophageal tumor. Large polyps can locally widen the esophagus, but do not cause complete obstruction or wall rigidity as with carcinoma.
Inflammatory esophagogastric polyp (Fig GI6-3)	Filling defect in the region of the esophagogastric junction that is usually in continuity with a markedly thickened gastric fold.	Probably represents a stage in the evolution of chronic esophagitis (polyp reflects thickening of the proximal aspect of an inflamed gastric fold).
Villous adenoma	Filling defect with typical barium filling of the frondlike interstices.	Tumor of intermediate malignant potential.
Malignant tumors		
Carcinoma of esophagus (Fig GI6-4)	Irregular circumferential lesion with destruction of mucosal folds, overhanging margins, and abrupt transition to adjacent normal tissue.	Less frequently, carcinoma can present as a localized polypoid mass, often with deep ulceration and a fungating appearance.
Carcinoma or lymphoma of fundus of stomach (see Fig GI5-4)	Irregular filling defect of the lower esophagus.	Continuous with malignancy of the gastric cardia.
Sarcoma (Fig GI6-5)	Bulky mass that may ulcerate.	Rare lesions. Leiomyosarcoma; carcinosarcoma (nests of squamous epithelium surrounded by interlacing bundles of spindle-shaped cells with numerous mitoses); pseudosarcoma (low-grade nonsquamous malignancy often associated with adjacent squamous cell carcinoma).
Other malignancies (Fig GI6-6)	Variable appearance.	Rare cases of melanoma, lymphoma, metastases, or verrucous carcinoma (exophytic, papillary, or warty tumor that rarely metastasizes and has a much better prognosis than typical squamous cell carcinoma).
Lymph node enlargement (see Fig GI3-4)	Extrinsic impression simulating an intramural esophageal lesion.	Usually caused by metastases or a granulomatous process (especially tuberculosis). Occasionally due to syphilis, sarcoidosis, histoplasmosis, or Crohn's disease.
Infectious esophagitis (Fig GI6-7)	Diffuse pattern of multiple round and oval nodular defects.	Most commonly candidiasis, which is usually associated with ulceration and a shaggy contour of the esophageal wall. Rarely, herpetic esophagitis.

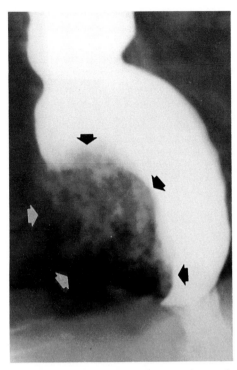

FIG GI6-1. **Leiomyoma.** Note the amorphous calcifications in this smoothly lobulated intramural tumor (arrows).[5]

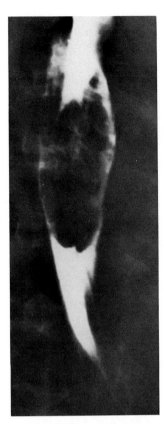

FIG GI6-2. **Fibrovascular polyp.**

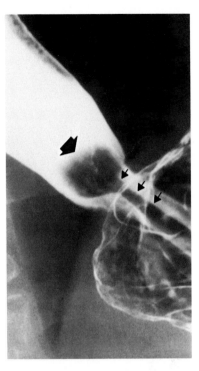

FIG GI6-3. **Inflammatory esophago-gastric polyp.** Distal esophageal filling defect (large arrow) in continuity with a thickened gastric fold (small arrows).

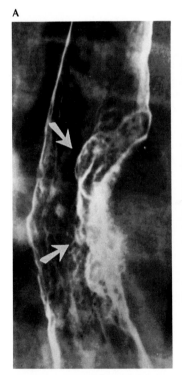

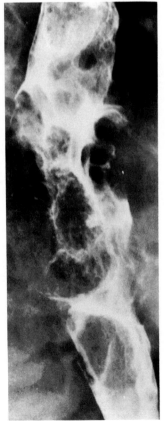

FIG GI6-4. **Carcinoma of the esophagus.** (A) Localized polypoid mass with ulceration (arrows). (B) Bulky irregular filling defect with destruction of mucosal folds.

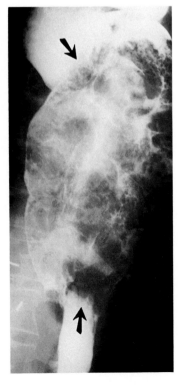

FIG GI6-5. **Carcinosarcoma.** Bulky, intraluminal, polypoid mass (arrows).

Condition	Imaging Findings	Comments
Esophageal varices (Fig GI6-8)	Diffuse round and oval filling defects reflecting serpiginous thickening of folds.	Dilated venous structures of varices change size and appearance with variations in intrathoracic pressure. Distal esophagus involved in portal hypertension. "Downhill" varices in the upper esophagus are due to superior vena cava obstruction.
Duplication cyst (Fig GI6-9)	Eccentric impression simulating an intramural mass.	Alimentary tract duplications occur least commonly in the esophagus. They rarely communicate with the esophageal lumen.
Foreign bodies (Fig GI6-10)	Various patterns depending on the material swallowed.	Usually impacted in the distal esophagus just above the level of the diaphragm. Often a distal stricture, especially if the impaction is in the cervical portion of the esophagus. Irregular margins may mimic an obstructing carcinoma.

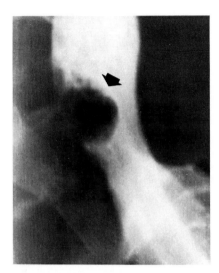

FIG GI6-6. Verrucous squamous cell carcinoma. The smooth-surfaced filling defect in the distal esophagus (arrow) has a benign appearance.

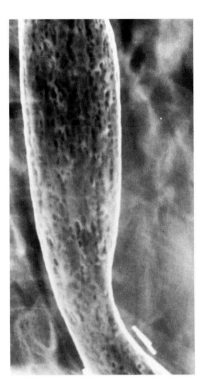

FIG GI6-7. *Candida* **esophagitis.** Numerous plaquelike defects in the middle and distal esophagus. Note that the plaques have discrete margins and a predominantly longitudinal orientation.

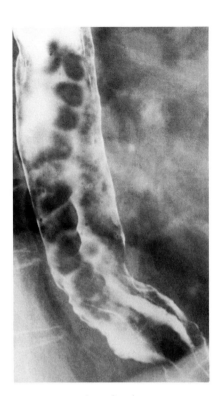

FIG GI6-8. Esophageal varices.

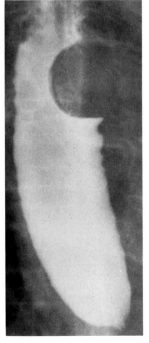

FIG GI6-9. Duplication cyst. Eccentric compression on the barium-filled esophagus simulates an intramural mass.

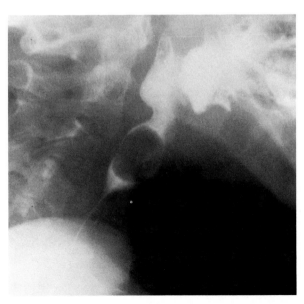

FIG GI6-10. Foreign body. Cherry pit impacted in the cervical esophagus proximal to a caustic stricture.

ESOPHAGEAL DIVERTICULA

Condition	Imaging Findings	Comments
Zenker's diverticulum (Figs GI7-1 and GI7-2)	Arises from the upper esophagus with its neck lying in the midline of the posterior wall at the pharyngoesophageal junction (approximately the C5-C6 level).	Pulsion diverticulum that is apparently related to premature contraction or other motor incoordination of the cricopharyngeus muscle. May cause dysphagia or even esophageal obstruction.
Cervical traction diverticulum (Fig GI7-3)	Variable appearance. Arises from any portion of the esophageal wall.	Rare condition resulting from fibrous healing of an inflammatory process in the neck or secondary to post-surgical changes (eg, laryngectomy).
Thoracic diverticulum (Fig GI7-4)	Arises in the middle third of the thoracic esophagus opposite the bifurcation of the trachea in the region of the hilum of the lung.	Traction diverticulum that develops in response to the pull of fibrous adhesions after mediastinal lymph node infection. There are often adjacent calcified mediastinal lymph nodes from healed granulomatous disease.
Epiphrenic diverticulum (Fig GI7-5)	Occurs in the distal 10 cm of the esophagus and tends to have a broad, short neck.	Pulsion diverticulum that is probably related to incoordination of esophageal peristalsis and relaxation of the lower sphincter. If small, can simulate an esophageal ulcer (though the mucosal pattern of the adjacent esophagus is normal).
Intramural esophageal pseudodiverticulosis (Fig GI7-6)	Multiple small (1 to 3 mm), ulcerlike projections arising from the esophageal wall. There is frequently an associated smooth stricture in the upper esophagus.	Rare disorder with pseudodiverticula (mimicking Rokitansky-Aschoff sinuses of the gallbladder) representing dilated ducts of submucosal glands. *Candida albicans* can be cultured from about half the patients, though there is no evidence suggesting that the fungus is a causative agent.

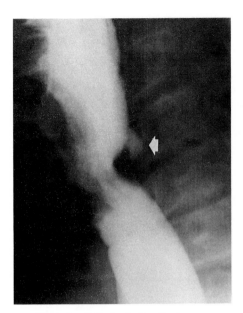

Fig GI7-1. Small Zenker's diverticulum.

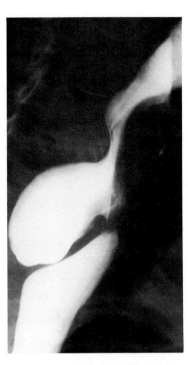

Fig GI7-2. Large Zenker's diverticulum almost occluding the esophageal lumen.

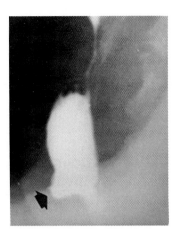

Fig GI7-3. Cervical traction diverticulum (arrow) caused by postoperative scarring after total laryngectomy.

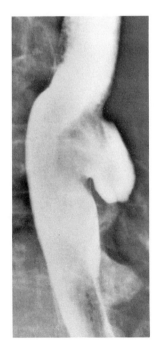

Fig GI7-4. Thoracic diverticulum.

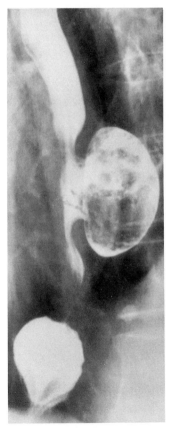

Fig GI7-5. Epiphrenic diverticulum.

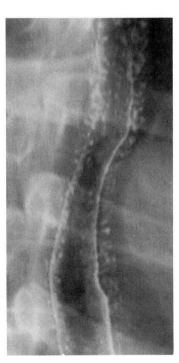

Fig GI7-6. Intramural esophageal pseudodiverticulosis.

GASTRIC ULCERATION

Condition	Imaging Findings	Comments
Peptic ulcer disease (Fig GI8-1)	Classic signs of benignancy include penetration, Hampton line, ulcer collar, ulcer mound, and radiation of smooth, slender mucosal folds to the edge of the crater.	If the ulcer crater is very shallow, a thin layer of barium coating results in a ring shadow. Irregular folds merging into a mound of polypoid tissue around the crater suggest a malignancy. Fundal ulcers above the level of the cardia are usually malignant.
Gastritis (Fig GI8-2)	Ulcers vary from superficial erosions to deep niches.	Superficial erosions occur with gastritis due to alcohol, anti-inflammatory agents, or Crohn's disease. Frank ulcerations develop in patients with corrosive gastritis or granulomatous infiltration.
Benign tumor	Central ulceration in a mass.	Predominantly spindle cell tumors, especially leiomyoma.
Radiation injury	Discrete ulcerations identical to peptic disease.	Pain is unrelenting and has no relation to meals. High incidence of perforation and hemorrhage. Healing is minimal even with intensive medical therapy.
Pseudolymphoma (Fig GI8-3)	Discrete ulcer surrounded by a mass and associated with regional or generalized enlargement of rugal folds.	Benign proliferation of lymphoid tissue that clinically and histologically simulates lymphoma and probably represents a nonspecific late reaction to chronic peptic ulcer disease.
Carcinoma (Fig GI8-4)	Ulcers vary from shallow erosions in superficial mucosal lesions to huge excavations in fungating polypoid masses.	Signs of malignant ulcer include Carman's meniscus sign (and Kirklin complex) and abrupt transition between normal mucosa and abnormal, usually nodular, tissue surrounding the ulcer. The ulcer does not penetrate beyond the normal gastric lumen.
Lymphoma (Fig GI8-5)	Irregular ulcer that often is larger than the adjacent gastric lumen. Combination of a large ulcer and an extraluminal mass may suggest extravasation of barium.	May be indistinguishable from carcinoma. Findings suggestive of lymphoma include splenomegaly and extrinsic impressions on the barium-filled stomach (due to retrogastric and other regional lymph nodes).
Sarcoma (Fig GI8-6)	Large central ulceration in a mass, which often has a prominent exophytic component.	Primarily leiomyosarcoma, which often is radiographically indistinguishable from its benign spindle cell counterpart.
Metastases (Fig GI8-7)	Single or multiple bull's-eye lesions.	Most commonly caused by malignant melanoma. An identical appearance can be due to metastases from carcinoma of the breast or lung.

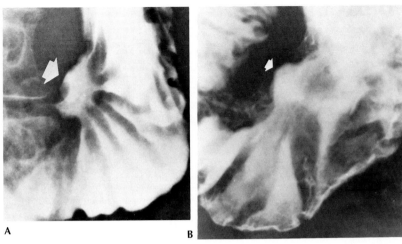

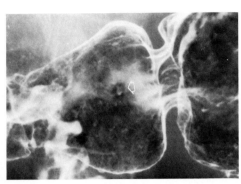

Fig GI8-2. Gastritis. Superficial gastric erosions. Tiny flecks of barium, representing erosions, are surrounded by radiolucent halos, representing mounds of edematous mucosa.

Fig GI8-1. Fold patterns in gastric ulcers (arrow). (A) Small, slender folds radiating to the edge of a benign ulcer. (B) Thick folds radiating to an irregular mound of tissue surrounding a malignant gastric ulcer (arrow).

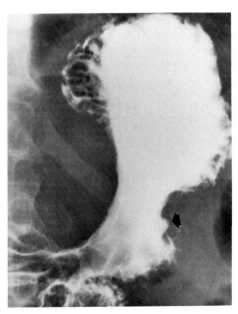

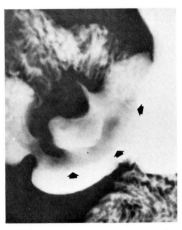

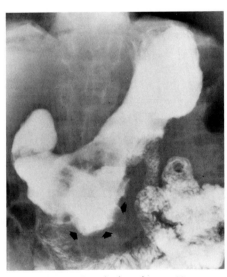

Fig GI8-3. Pseudolymphoma. Greater curvature ulcer (arrow) surrounded by a soft-tissue mass and associated with regional enlargement of rugal folds.

Fig GI8-4. Carcinoma of the stomach. Carman's meniscus sign in malignant gastric ulcer. The huge ulcer has a semicircular configuration with its inner margin convex toward the lumen. The ulcer is surrounded by the radiolucent shadow of an elevated ridge of neoplastic tissue.

Fig GI8-5. Gastric lymphoma. Huge, irregular ulcer (arrows) in a neoplastic gastric mass.

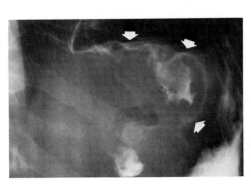

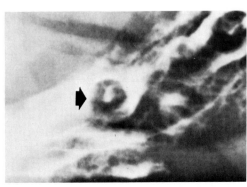

Fig GI8-6. Leiomyosarcoma of the stomach. The large fundal mass (arrows) shows exophytic extension and ulceration.

Fig GI8-7. Gastric metastases from melanoma (arrow).

NARROWING OF THE STOMACH

Condition	Imaging Findings	Comments
Carcinoma (Figs GI9-1 and GI9-2)	Thickening and fixation of the stomach wall, usually beginning near the pylorus and progressing upward.	By far the most common cause of the linitis plastica pattern. Tumor invasion of the gastric wall stimulates a strong desmoplastic response. Gastric carcinoma can also cause segmental narrowing.
Lymphoma	Luminal narrowing that primarily involves the antral region, mimicking scirrhous carcinoma.	Unlike the rigidity and fixation of scirrhous carcinoma, residual peristalsis and flexibility of the stomach wall is often preserved in Hodgkin's disease.
Metastases (Fig GI9-3)	Circumferential narrowing of the stomach, usually with more segmental involvement than in a primary gastric malignancy.	Direct extension from carcinoma of the pancreas or transverse colon or desmoplastic hematogenous metastases (eg, carcinoma of the breast).
Peptic ulcer disease (Fig GI9-4)	Antral narrowing and rigidity due to intense spasm.	Acute ulcer may not be seen because of the lack of antral distensibility. Peptic ulcer–induced rigidity usually heals with adequate antacid therapy. Midgastric ulcer in an elderly patient may heal with an hourglass deformity.
Crohn's disease (Fig GI9-5)	Smooth, tubular antrum flaring into a normal gastric body and fundus (ram's horn sign).	Often cobblestoning of antral folds with fissures and ulceration. Concomitant involvement of the adjacent duodenal bulb and proximal sweep produces the pseudo–Billroth-I pattern.
Other infiltrative disorders (Fig GI9-6)	Mural thickening and luminal narrowing predominantly involve the antrum.	Sarcoidosis; syphilis; tuberculosis; strongyloidiasis; eosinophilic gastritis; polyarteritis nodosa.
Phlegmonous gastritis (Fig GI9-7)	Diffuse irregular narrowing mimicking infiltrating carcinoma.	Extremely rare. Bacterial invasion thickens the gastric wall. The development of intramural gas bubbles is an ominous finding.
Corrosive gastritis (Fig GI9-8)	Stricturing of the antrum (within several weeks of the injury).	Acute inflammatory reaction (most severe with ingested acids) that heals by fibrosis and scarring.
Gastric irradiation or freezing (Fig GI9-9)	Various degrees of fixed luminal narrowing and mural rigidity.	Represents fibrotic healing of an acute injury. Irradiation and freezing were once used to treat intractable peptic ulcer disease.
Iron intoxication	Antral stricture (within 6 weeks of ingestion).	Ingestion of ferrous sulfate causes intense corrosion, which is often fatal.

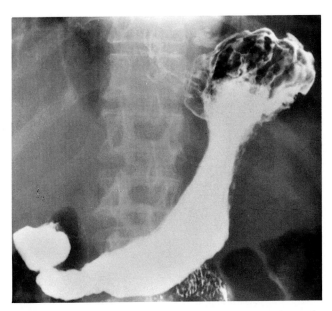

FIG **GI9-1.** **Scirrhous carcinoma** of the stomach producing a linitis plastica pattern.

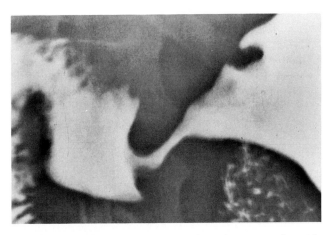

FIG **GI9-2.** **Adenocarcinoma** of the stomach causing segmental constriction of the antrum.

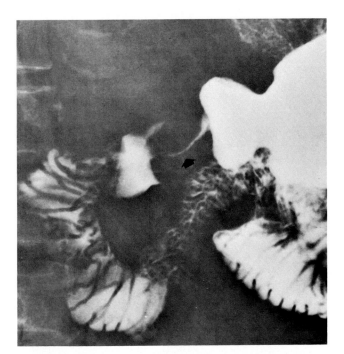

FIG **GI9-3.** **Metastatic pancreatic carcinoma.** Circumferential narrowing of the distal stomach (arrow) secondary to enlarged perigastric lymph nodes.

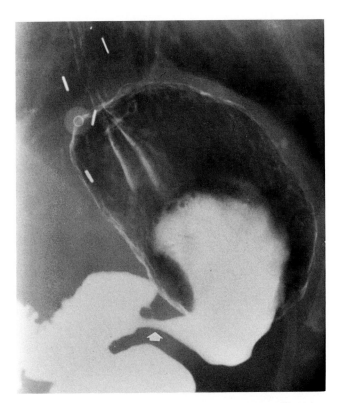

FIG **GI9-4.** **Peptic ulcer disease** causing antral narrowing and rigidity. Note the metallic clips from a previous vagotomy.

Condition	Imaging Findings	Comments
Hepatic arterial infusion chemotherapy	Narrowing and rigidity of the gastric antrum and body. Return to normal appearance after chemotherapy is discontinued.	Complications of gastroduodenal ulceration and narrowing that are probably related to leakage of the chemotherapeutic agent directly into the blood supply of nonhepatic organs.
Amyloidosis	Narrowing and rigidity that primarily involve the antrum.	Deposition of eosinophilic, extracellular protein–polysaccharide complex in the gastric wall.
Pseudolymphoma	Narrowing that usually involves a large segment of the body or antrum of the stomach.	Almost invariably associated with a large gastric ulcer crater. Benign condition mimicking lymphoma clinically and histologically.
Exogastric mass (Fig GI9-10)	Luminal narrowing due to extrinsic pressure on the stomach.	Most commonly caused by severe hepatomegaly. Also occurs with pancreatic pseudocysts or enlargement of other upper abdominal organs.
Gastroplasty	Narrowing at the operative site.	Clinical history of weight-reduction surgery and evidence of metallic suture material.
Hypertrophic pyloric stenosis (see Fig GI72-5)	Elongation and narrowing of the pyloric canal. Symmetric concave, crescentic indentation on the base of the duodenal bulb (partial invagination of the hypertrophied muscle mass into the bulb).	Histologic, anatomic, and radiographic abnormalities in adult hypertrophic pyloric stenosis are indistinguishable from those in the infantile form (may be the same entity but milder and later in its clinical appearance).

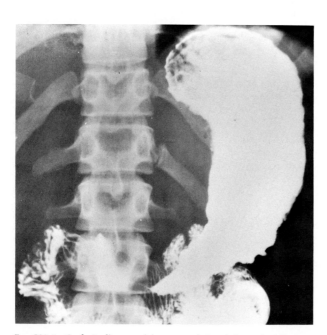

FIG GI9-5. Crohn's disease of the stomach (ram's horn sign).[6]

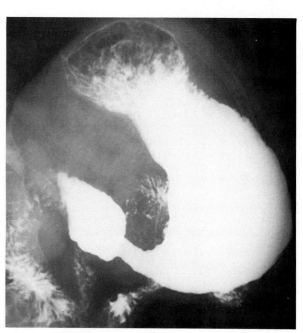

FIG GI9-6. Tuberculosis of the stomach. Fibrotic healing narrows and stiffens the distal antrum.

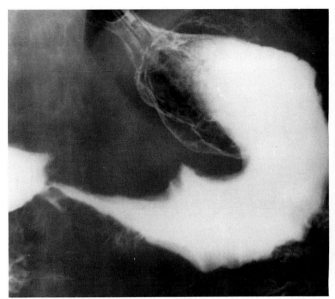

Fig GI9-7. Phlegmonous gastritis. Irregular narrowing of the antrum and distal body of the stomach with effacement of mucosal folds along the lesser curvature and marked thickening of folds along the greater curvature.[7]

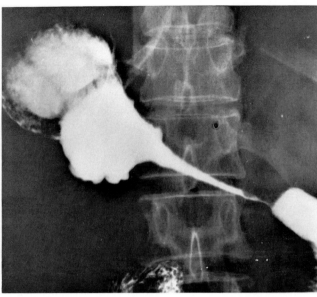

Fig GI9-8. Corrosive stricture of the antrum after the ingestion of hydrochloric acid.

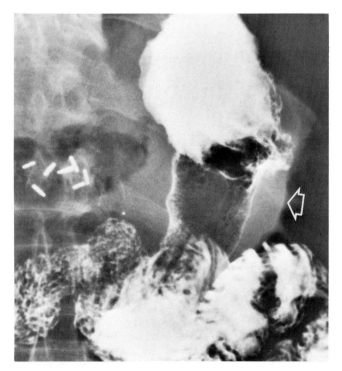

Fig GI9-9. Radiation therapy. Luminal narrowing and severe thickening of the wall of the stomach (arrow).

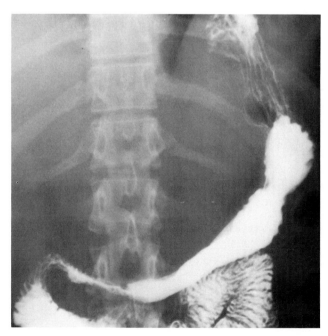

Fig GI9-10. Echinococcal cystic disease. Narrowing of the lumen of the stomach secondary to extrinsic impression by a huge liver.

FILLING DEFECTS IN THE STOMACH

Condition	Imaging Findings	Comments
Areae gastricae	Fine reticular pattern surrounded by barium-filled grooves, simulating multiple filling defects.	Represents a normal anatomic feature seen on double-contrast studies. Most commonly identified in the antrum. Prominent areae gastricae (état mamelonné) may represent nonspecific inflammation.
Benign tumors/tumorlike conditions		
Hyperplastic polyp (Fig GI10-1)	Small (1 cm), often multiple, sharply defined mass.	Most common cause of a discrete gastric filling defect. Represents excessive regenerative hyperplasia in an area of chronic gastritis rather than a true neoplasm.
Adenomatous polyp (Fig GI10-2)	Large (2 cm or more), usually single and sessile lesion with an irregular surface.	As with hyperplastic polyps, adenomatous polyps tend to develop in patients with chronic atrophic gastritis (associated with a high incidence of carcinoma). Increased incidence of gastric polyps in familial polyposis of the colon and the Cronkhite-Canada syndrome.
Hamartoma	Multiple filling defects.	No malignant potential. Occurs in Peutz-Jeghers syndrome and Cowden's disease.
Spindle cell tumor (Fig GI10-3)	Single intramural mass, often with central ulceration.	Most commonly leiomyoma. A large lesion may have an intraluminal component or produce an extensive exogastric mass mimicking extrinsic gastric compression.
Malignant tumors		
Polypoid carcinoma (Fig GI10-4)	Sessile mass that is usually relatively large, irregular, and ulcerated.	Increased incidence in patients with atrophic gastritis and pernicious anemia. May be difficult to distinguish from a benign gastric polyp.
Lymphoma (Fig GI10-5)	Large, bulky polypoid lesion that is usually irregular and ulcerated.	Factors favoring lymphoma rather than carcinoma include multiple ulcerating polypoid tumors and adjacent thickening of folds (rather than the atrophic mucosal pattern often seen in carcinoma).
Metastases (see Fig GI8-7)	Usually multiple, often ulcerated (bull's-eye appearance).	Most commonly due to malignant melanoma. Also caused by carcinomas of the breast and lung.
Sarcoma (Fig GI10-6)	Large, bulky mass that is often ulcerated.	Most are leiomyosarcomas, which are difficult to differentiate from their benign spindle cell counterparts (large exogastric mass suggests malignancy).
Villous adenoma	Characteristic barium filling of the interstices of the tumor. Often multiple.	Rare lesion with a substantial incidence of malignancy.
Ectopic pancreas (Fig GI10-7)	Smooth submucosal mass with central umbilication.	Most commonly found on the greater curvature of the distal antrum close to the pylorus. Central umbilication represents the orifice of an aberrant pancreatic duct rather than ulceration.

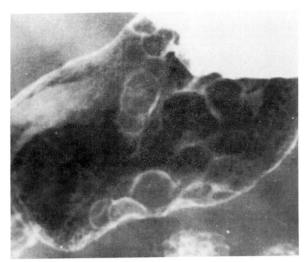

Fɪɢ GI10-1. **Hyperplastic polyps.** Multiple smooth filling defects of similar sizes.

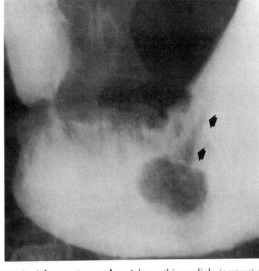

Fɪɢ GI10-2. **Adenomatous polyp.** A long, thin pedicle (arrows) extends from the head of the polyp to the stomach wall.

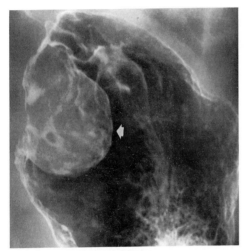

Fɪɢ GI10-3. **Leiomyoma of the fundus.**

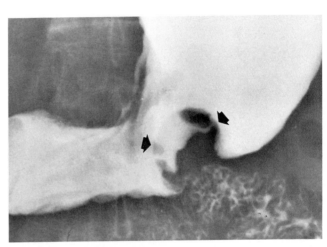

Fɪɢ GI10-4. **Carcinoma of the stomach.** A huge ulcer is evident in the smooth, fungating polypoid mass (arrows).

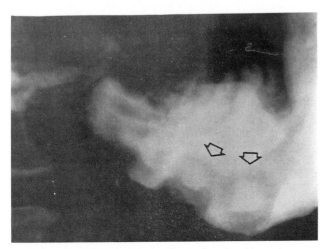

Fɪɢ GI10-5. **Lymphoma.** Multiple ulcerated, polypoid gastric masses (arrows).

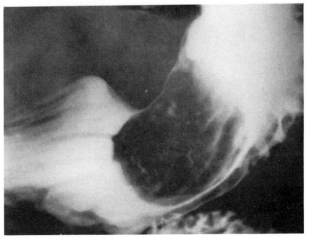

Fɪɢ GI10-6. **Leiomyosarcoma.** There is scattered ulceration in this bulky tumor.

Condition	Imaging Findings	Comments
Enlarged gastric folds (Fig GI10-8)	Multiple nodular filling defects (if viewed end-on).	Ménétrier's disease; gastric varices; Crohn's disease; sarcoidosis; tuberculosis; eosinophilic gastritis.
Bezoar (Fig GI10-9)	Large mass that may fill the entire stomach. Occasionally completely smooth (simulating an enormous gas bubble).	Contrast material coating the mass and infiltrating the interstices may produce a characteristic mottled or streaked appearance. Phytobezoars (undigested vegetable material) and trichobezoars (hairballs).
Foreign body/blood clot	Single or multiple filling defects.	Variety of ingested substances and any cause of esophageal or gastric bleeding.
Peptic ulcer disease (Fig GI10-10)	Various appearances (with or without ulceration).	Can represent a large mound of edema surrounding an acute ulcer, an incisura on the wall opposite an ulcer crater, or a double pylorus.
Eosinophilic granuloma (inflammatory fibroid polyp)	Sharply defined, smooth, round or oval mass (usually in the antrum).	Nonspecific inflammatory infiltrate that is usually asymptomatic (no food allergy or peripheral eosinophilia as in eosinophilic gastritis).
Duplication cyst	Filling defect or extrinsic mass impression.	Very rare. Tends to be asymptomatic, to involve the greater curvature, and to not communicate with the gastric lumen.
Fundoplication (Fig GI10-11)	Prominent filling defect at the esophagogastric junction. The mass is generally smoothly marginated and symmetric on both sides of the distal esophagus.	Fundal pseudotumor secondary to a surgical procedure for hiatal hernia repair. In a Nissen fundoplication, the gastric fundus is wrapped around the lower esophagus to create an intra-abdominal esophageal segment with a natural valve mechanism at the esophagogastric junction.

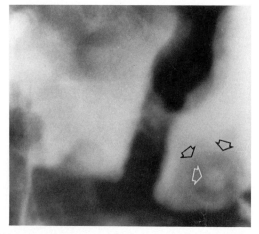

FIG GI10-7. Ectopic pancreas. Central opacification (white arrow) of a rudimentary pancreatic duct in a soft-tissue mass (black arrows) in the distal antrum.

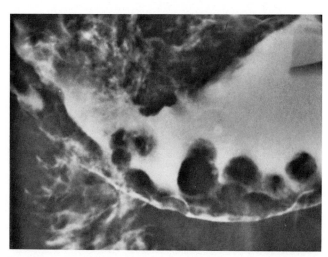

FIG GI10-8. Alcoholic gastritis. Multiple nodular filling defects (suggesting polyps) are due to enlarged gastric folds viewed on end.

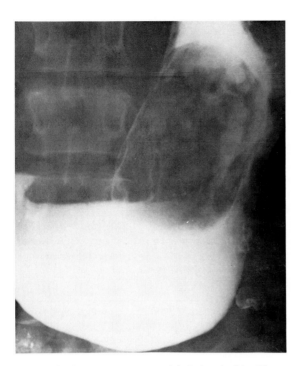

FIG GI10-9. Glue bezoar in a young model-airplane builder. The smooth mass simulates an enormous air bubble.

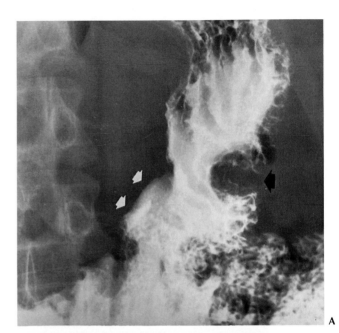

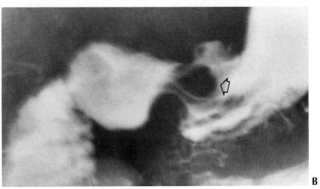

FIG GI10-10. Peptic ulcer disease. (A) Large incisura (black arrow) simulating a filling defect on the greater curvature. The incisura is incited by a long ulcer (white arrows) on the lesser curvature. (B) Double pylorus. The true pylorus and the accessory channel along the lesser curvature are separated by a bridge, or septum, that produces the appearance of a discrete lucent filling defect (arrow).

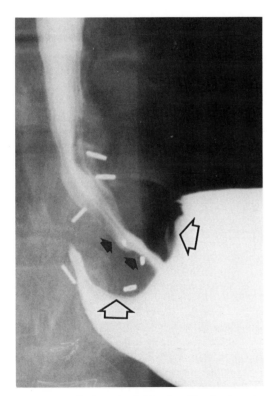

FIG GI10-11. Normal Nissen fundoplication. The distal esophagus with normal mucosal pattern (closed arrows) passes through the fundal pseudotumor (open arrows).[8]

THICKENING OF GASTRIC FOLDS

Condition	Imaging Findings	Comments
Normal variant	Apparent thickening of folds in the fundus and along the greater curvature.	Folds in the fundus and proximal body tend to be thicker and more tortuous than those in the distal stomach, especially if the stomach is partially empty or contracted.
Alcoholic gastritis (Fig GI11-1)	Generalized thickening of folds that usually subsides after withdrawal of alcohol.	Bizarre thickening may mimic malignant disease. There is a relative absence of folds in chronic alcoholic gastritis.
Hypertrophic gastritis (Fig GI11-2)	Generalized thickening of folds, more prominent proximally.	Probably reflects a hypersecretory state and is often associated with peptic ulcer disease.
Antral gastritis (Fig GI11-3)	Fold thickening localized to the antrum.	Controversial entity that most likely reflects one end of the spectrum of peptic ulcer disease. Isolated antral gastritis appears without fold thickening or acute ulceration in the duodenal bulb.
Corrosive gastritis	Predominantly distal involvement with associated ulcers, atony, and rigidity.	Ingested acids cause the most severe injury. The pylorus is usually fixed and open. Gas in the wall of the stomach is an ominous sign.
Infectious gastritis	Fold thickening may be localized or diffuse.	Due to bacterial invasion of the stomach wall or to bacterial toxins (eg, botulism, diphtheria, dysentery, typhoid fever). Gas-forming organisms can produce gas in the stomach wall.
Gastric irradiation or freezing	Generalized fold thickening.	Previous therapy for intractable gastric ulcer disease.
Peptic ulcer disease (Fig GI11-4)	Fold thickening diffusely involves the body and fundus.	Represents hypersecretion of acid and may be associated with large amounts of retained gastric fluid. Localized fold thickening with radiation of folds toward the crater is a traditional sign of gastric ulcer.
Ménétrier's disease (Fig GI11-5)	Massive enlargement of rugal folds. Classically described as a lesion of the fundus and body, but may involve the entire stomach.	Usually hyposecretion of acid, excessive secretion of gastric mucus, and protein loss into the gastric lumen. The lesser curvature of the body of the stomach is infrequently involved (different from lymphoma).
Lymphoma (Fig GI11-6)	Generalized or localized thickening, distortion, and nodularity of folds.	May mimic Ménétrier's disease, though more commonly also involves the distal stomach and lesser curvature. Splenomegaly or an extrinsic impression by enlarged nodes suggests lymphoma; lack of ulceration and rigidity or the presence of excess mucus suggests Ménétrier's disease.

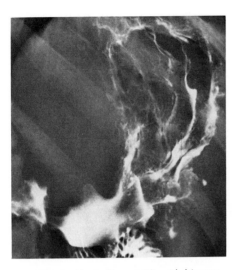

FIG GI11-1. Alcoholic gastritis with bizarre, large folds simulating a malignant process.

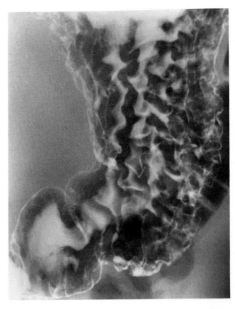

FIG GI11-2. Hypertrophic gastritis in a patient with high acid output and peptic ulcer disease.

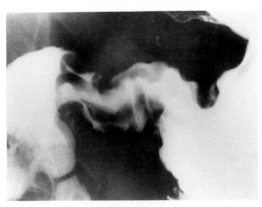

FIG GI11-3. Antral gastritis. Thickening of gastric rugal folds is confined to the antrum.

FIG GI11-4. Zollinger-Ellison syndrome. Diffuse thickening of gastric folds is associated with hypersecretion of acid and peptic ulcer disease.

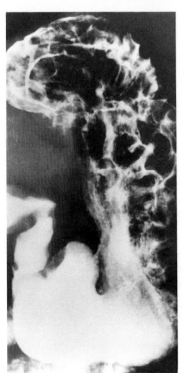

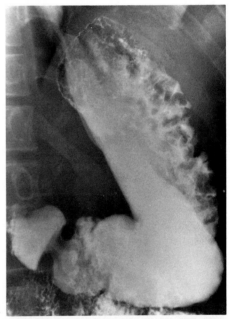

A

B

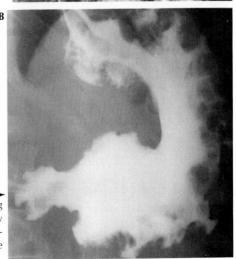

FIG GI11-5. Ménétrier's disease. (A) Fold thickening involves the greater curvature of the fundus and body and spares the lesser curvature and antrum. (B) Generalized rugal fold thickening involves the entire stomach.

Condition	Imaging Findings	Comments
Pseudolymphoma	Regional or generalized enlargement of rugal folds.	Usually associated with a large gastric ulcer and may mimic lymphoma clinically and histologically.
Carcinoma **(Fig GI11-7)**	Enlarged, tortuous, coarse gastric folds.	Carcinoma rarely produces this pattern (simulating lymphoma). Associated punctate calcification is virtually diagnostic of colloid carcinoma or mucinous adenocarcinoma of the stomach.
Gastric varices **(Figs GI11-8 and GI11-9)**	Fundal varices appear as multiple smooth, lobulated filling defects. Occasionally a single varix. Nonfundal gastric varices occasionally occur.	Usually associated with esophageal varices. Isolated gastric varices suggest splenic vein occlusion. Unlike malignancy, varices are changeable in size and shape.
Infiltrative processes **(Fig GI11-10)**	Diffuse thickening of rugal folds, especially in the distal half of the stomach.	Causes include eosinophilic gastritis, Crohn's disease, sarcoidosis, tuberculosis, syphilis, and amyloidosis.
Adjacent pancreatic disease **(Fig GI11-11)**	Fold thickening primarily involves the posterior wall and the lesser curvature.	Most commonly reflects severe acute pancreatitis.

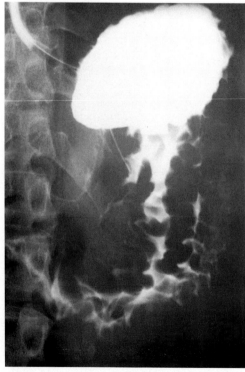

FIG GI11-6. Lymphoma. Diffuse thickening, distortion, and nodularity of gastric folds.

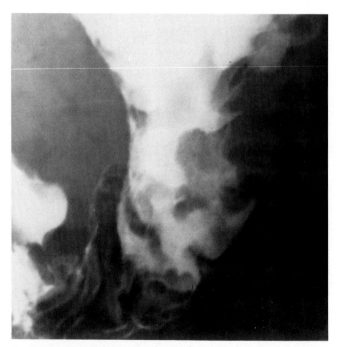

FIG GI11-7. Carcinoma of the stomach. Enlarged, tortuous, coarse rugal folds simulate lymphoma.

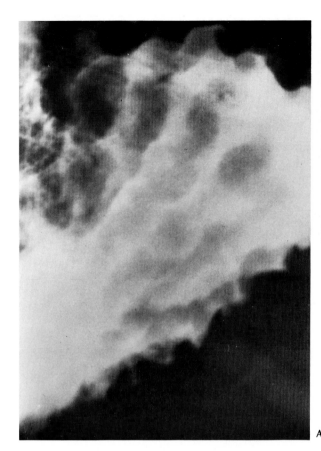

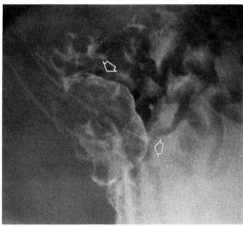

Fɪɢ GI11-8. Fundal gastric varices. (A) Multiple smooth, lobulated filling defects representing the dilated venous structures. (B) Single large gastric varix (arrows).

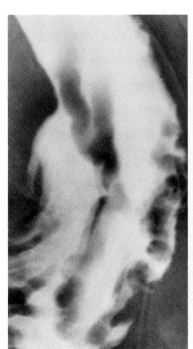

Fɪɢ GI11-9. Nonfundic gastric varices.[9]

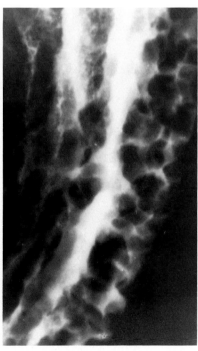

Fɪɢ GI11-10. Amyloidosis. Huge, nodular folds caused by diffuse infiltration of the stomach by amyloid.

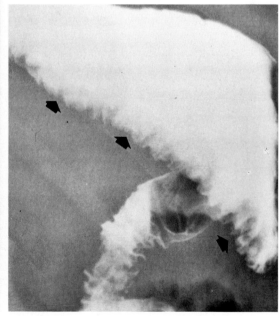

Fɪɢ GI11-11. Acute pancreatitis. Prominence of mucosal folds on the posterior wall of the stomach (arrows) and a large retrogastric mass.

GASTRIC OUTLET OBSTRUCTION

Condition	Imaging Findings	Comments
Peptic ulcer disease (Fig GI12-1)	Severe luminal narrowing resulting from spasm, acute inflammation and edema, muscular hypertrophy, or contraction of scar tissue. The obstructing lesion is usually in the duodenum, occasionally in the pyloric channel or prepyloric gastric antrum, and rarely in the body of the stomach.	By far the most common cause of gastric outlet obstruction in adults (60% to 65% of cases). Distortion and scarring of the duodenal bulb make peptic ulcer disease the most likely cause of obstruction, while a radiographically normal bulb increases the likelihood of underlying malignant disease.
Malignant tumor (Fig GI12-2)	Luminal narrowing due to an annular constricting lesion or diffuse mural infiltration by tumor.	Second leading cause of gastric outlet obstruction (30% to 35% of cases). Unlike patients with underlying peptic disease, who typically have a long history of ulcer pain, about one third of patients with obstruction due to malignancy have no pain, and most of the others have a history of pain of less than 1 year's duration.
Inflammatory disorder (Figs GI12-3 and GI12-4)	Spasm, mural infiltration, or stricture formation causing severe luminal narrowing.	Causes include Crohn's disease, pancreatitis, cholecystitis, corrosive stricture, sarcoidosis, syphilis, tuberculosis, and amyloidosis.
Congenital disorders **Antral mucosal diaphragm** (Fig GI12-5)	Persistent, sharply defined, 2- to 3-cm-wide band-like defect in the barium column that arises at a right angle to the gastric wall. Best seen when the stomach proximal and distal to is distended. The portion of the antrum proximal to the pylorus and distal to the mucosal diaphragm can mimic a second duodenal bulb.	Thin membranous septum that is usually situated within 3 cm of the pyloric canal and runs perpendicular to the long axis of the stomach. Probably a congenital anomaly resulting from failure of the embryonic foregut to recanalize. Symptoms of gastric outlet obstruction do not occur if the diameter of the diaphragm exceeds 1 cm.
Gastric duplication	Extrinsic narrowing and deformity of the antrum.	Rare manifestation (usually causes only an indentation on the stomach).
Annular pancreas	Extrinsic narrowing and deformity of the descending duodenum.	Rare manifestation (more commonly produces an extrinsic impression on the lateral aspect of the descending duodenum).
Gastric volvulus (Fig GI12-6)	Double air-fluid level on upright films, inversion of the stomach with the greater curvature above the level of the lesser curvature, positioning of the cardia and pylorus at the same level, and downward pointing of the pylorus and duodenum. Usually occurs in conjunction with a large esophageal or paraesophageal hernia that permits part or all of the stomach to assume an intrathoracic position.	Uncommon acquired twist of the stomach upon itself that can lead to gastric outlet obstruction. Organoaxial volvulus refers to rotation of the stomach upward around its long axis so that the antrum moves from an inferior to a superior position. In the mesenteroaxial type of gastric volvulus, the stomach rotates from right to left or left to right about the long axis of the gastrohepatic omentum (line connecting the middle of the lesser curvature with the middle of the greater curvature).

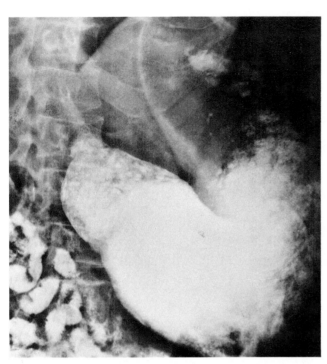

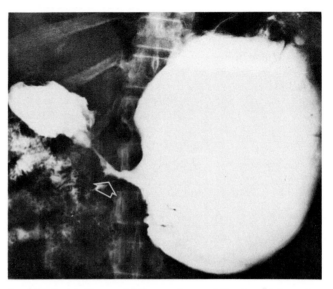

FIG GI12-2. **Annular constricting carcinoma of the stomach** (arrow).

FIG GI12-1. **Peptic ulcer disease.** The mottled density of nonopaque material represents excessive overnight gastric residue.

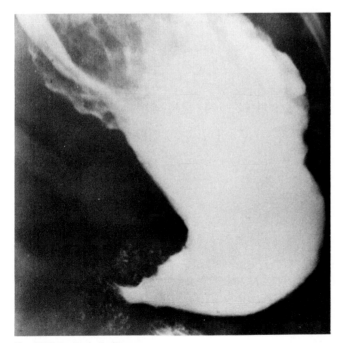

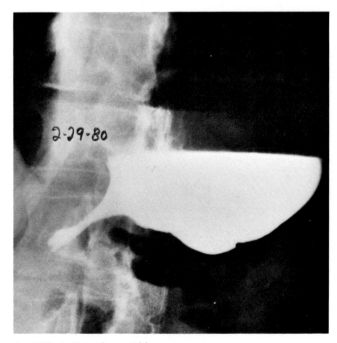

FIG GI12-3. **Crohn's disease.**

FIG GI12-4. **Corrosive gastritis.**

Condition	Imaging Findings	Comments
Hypertrophic pyloric stenosis (Fig GI12-7)	Elongation and narrowing of the pyloric canal with a characteristic symmetric, concave, crescentic indentation on the base of the duodenal bulb (presumably due to partial invagination of the hypertrophied muscle mass into the bulb).	The histologic, anatomic, and radiographic abnormalities in adult hypertrophic pyloric stenosis are indistinguishable from those in the infantile form (the disease in adults may be the same entity observed in infants and children but milder and later in clinical appearance).
Bezoar	Gastric outlet obstruction.	Masses of foreign material in the stomach are rarely of sufficient size to cause obstruction.
Prolapsed antral mucosa/ antral polyp	Intermittent pyloric obstruction.	Rare causes of intermittent gastric outlet obstruction. Prolapsed mucosa can undergo erosion or ulceration, leading to gastrointestinal bleeding and iron deficiency anemia.

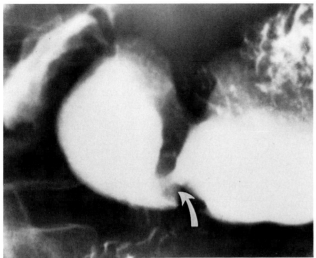

FIG GI12-5. **Antral mucosal diaphragm** (arrows).

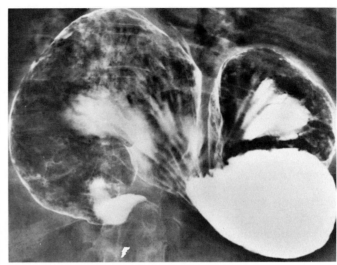

FIG GI12-6. **Organoaxial volvulus.**

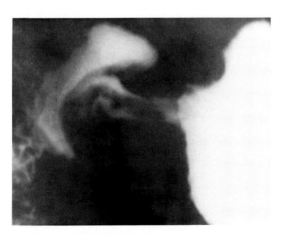

FIG GI12-7. **Adult hypertrophic pyloric stenosis.**

GASTRIC DILATATION WITHOUT OUTLET OBSTRUCTION

Condition	Comments
Acute gastric dilatation **Abdominal surgery** **(Fig GI13-1)**	The incidence of this postoperative complication has dramatically decreased with the advent of nasogastric suction, improved anesthetics, close monitoring of acid-base and electrolyte balance, and meticulous care in the handling of tissues at surgery.
Abdominal trauma **(especially involving** **the back)** **(Fig GI13-2)**	Probably caused by a reflex paralysis of the gastric motor mechanism that permits the stomach to distend abnormally as fluid and air accumulate in it.
Severe pain/abdominal **inflammation**	Reflex neurologic pathway causes acute gastric dilatation in patients with severe renal colic, biliary colic, migraine headaches, and infectious and inflammatory conditions (peritonitis, pancreatitis, appendicitis, subphrenic abscess, septicemia).
Immobilization	Patients who are immobilized (body plaster cast, paraplegia) may develop acute gastric dilatation because of difficulty in belching or because of compression of the transverse portion of the duodenum.
Chronic gastric dilatation **Diabetes mellitus** **(gastric paresis)** **(Fig GI13-3)**	Gastric motor abnormalities occur in up to 30% of diabetics, primarily those who have long-term disease under relatively inadequate control and evidence of peripheral neuropathy or other complications.
Neuromuscular **abnormalities** **(Fig GI13-4)**	Decreased peristalsis and visceral dilatation (more commonly involving the esophagus) may develop in patients with brain tumor, bulbar poliomyelitis, tabes dorsalis, scleroderma, or muscular dystrophy.
Vagotomy	Surgical or chemical (atropine or drugs with an atropine-like action).
Electrolyte or acid-base **imbalance**	Dilatation of abdominal viscera (most likely the colon) presumably develops because of alteration in muscle tone in patients with diabetic ketoacidosis, hypercalcemia, hypocalcemia, hypokalemia, hepatic coma, uremia, or myxedema.
Lead poisoning/ **porphyria**	Gastric distension reflects an alteration in muscle tone.
Emotional distress	Gastric dilatation can be due to a reflex neurologic abnormality or to hyperventilation associated with the excessive swallowing of air.

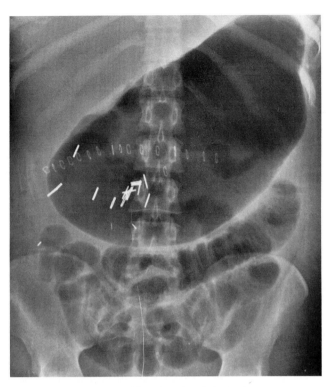

FIG GI13-1. Acute gastric dilatation after abdominal surgery.

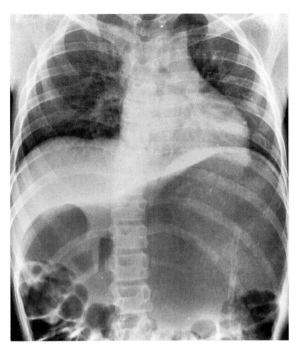

FIG GI13-2. Acute gastric dilatation after abdominal trauma.

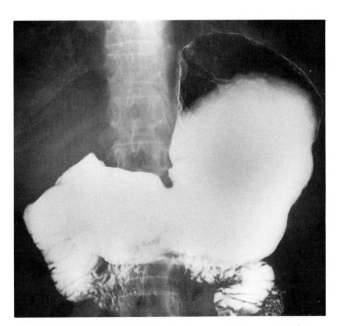

FIG GI13-3. Gastric dilatation due to chronic diabetic neuropathy.

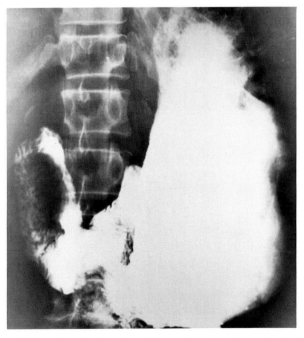

FIG GI13-4. Gastric dilatation without obstruction in a patient with scleroderma.

WIDENING OF THE RETROGASTRIC SPACE

Condition	Imaging Findings	Comments
Obesity/ascites/ previous surgery/ gross hepatomegaly (especially of caudate lobe)	Generalized widening without a discrete mass.	Anterior displacement of the stomach with no discrete posterior impression.
Pancreatic mass (Fig GI14-1)	Extrinsic impression on the antrum (head of the pancreas) or the body and fundus (body and tail of the pancreas).	Most common cause of a discrete lesion widening the retrogastric space. Causes include pancreatitis, pseudocyst, cystadenoma, and carcinoma. Findings suggesting invasive carcinoma include fixation of the gastric wall, mucosal destruction or ulceration, and a high-grade gastric outlet obstruction.
Retroperitoneal mass (Fig GI14-2)	Single or lobulated impression on the posterior wall of the stomach.	Causes include benign and malignant neoplasms, enlargement of retroperitoneal lymph nodes (lymphoma, tuberculosis), cysts, abscesses, and hematomas.
Tumor arising from posterior wall of stomach	Usually an intraluminal component in addition to the posterior impression and the widened retrogastric space.	Most commonly occurs in gastric tumors with large exogastric components (leiomyoma, leiomyosarcoma).
Aortic aneurysm/ choledochal cyst	Discrete retrogastric mass.	Diagnosis can be made by ultrasound or CT.

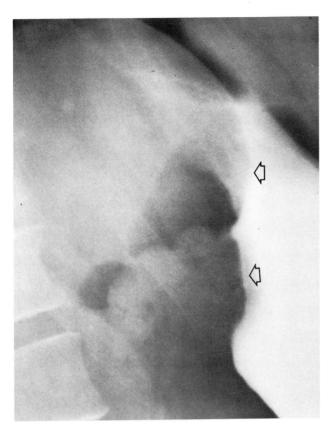

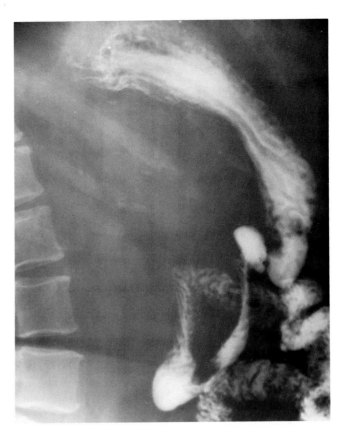

Fɪɢ **GI14-1. Pancreatic pseudocyst.** Widening of the retrogastric space with a lobulated impression (arrows) on the posterior wall of the stomach.

Fɪɢ **GI14-2. Retroperitoneal sarcoma.** Pronounced anterior displacement of the stomach and duodenum.

FILLING DEFECTS IN THE GASTRIC REMNANT

Condition	Imaging Findings	Comments
Surgical deformity	Various patterns depending on the type of surgical procedure.	Because the appearance may closely simulate a neoplastic process, a baseline upper gastrointestinal series is often obtained soon after partial gastric resection.
Suture granuloma (Fig GI15-1)	Well-defined, rounded mass at the level of the surgical anastomosis.	Can mimic a gastric neoplasm and lead to an unnecessary reoperation. Occurs only with nonabsorbable suture material.
Bezoar (Fig GI15-2)	Mottled filling defect simulating a mass of retained food.	Usually consists of the fibrous, pithy component of fruits (especially citrus) and vegetables. Can cause gastric outlet obstruction or pass into and obstruct the small bowel.
Gastric stump carcinoma (Fig GI15-3)	Irregular polypoid mass that may be ulcerated. Uniform infiltration by the tumor can narrow the gastric remnant.	Refers to a malignancy occurring in the gastric remnant after resection for peptic ulcer or other benign disease. Tends to occur 10 to 20 years after the initial surgery (after a long period of relatively good health). Must be differentiated from benign marginal ulceration, which occurs on the jejunal side of the anastomosis within 2 years of surgery (ulcer on the gastric side must be considered malignant).
Recurrent carcinoma (Fig GI15-4)	Narrowing of the stoma with local mucosal destruction or a discrete filling defect.	May be difficult to distinguish from a second primary if it occurs less than 10 years after the initial resection for malignant disease.
Bile (alkaline) reflux gastritis (Fig GI15-5)	Thickened folds, often with ulceration, on the gastric side of the anastomosis.	Reactive response of the stomach to reflux of bile and pancreatic juices from the jejunum (normally prevented by the intact pylorus).
Hyperplastic polyps	Discrete polypoid masses.	Masses developing within a few years of surgery are more likely to be hyperplastic polyps than carcinoma (but endoscopy and biopsy are essential for confirmation).
Jejunogastric intussusception (Fig GI15-6)	Spherical or ovoid intraluminal filling defect. Contrast material may outline the stretched jejunal folds.	Rare, but potentially lethal, complication of partial gastrectomy with Billroth-II anastomosis. The efferent loop alone is included in 75% of cases; the afferent loop or the afferent in combination with the efferent intussuscepts in the remaining cases. Acute intussusception is a surgical emergency.
Gastrojejunal mucosal prolapse (Fig GI15-7)	Smooth, sharply margined intraluminal mass in the efferent or afferent loop.	Antegrade prolapse occurs much more frequently than retrograde jejunogastric intussusception. Can cause partial obstruction if the anastomotic stoma is small.

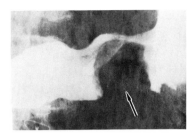

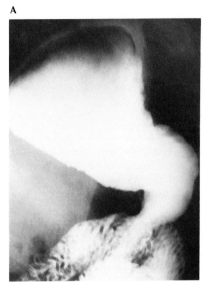

FIG GI15-1. Suture granuloma. Large mass at the greater curvature side of the antrum (arrow) projects as a smooth tumor into the gastric lumen.[10]

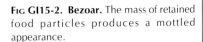

FIG GI15-2. Bezoar. The mass of retained food particles produces a mottled appearance.

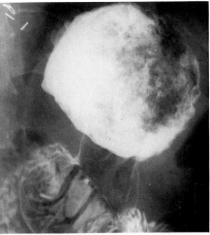

A

B

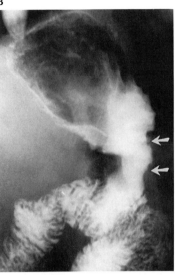

FIG GI15-3. Gastric stump carcinoma. (A) Normal gastric remnant and Billroth II anastomosis after surgery for peptic disease. (B) Irregular narrowing of the perianastomotic region (arrows) several years later represents a gastric stump carcinoma.

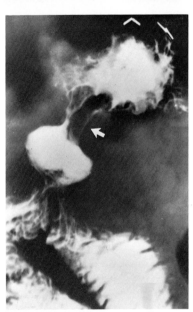

FIG GI15-4. Recurrent gastric carcinoma. Tumor infiltration narrows the gastric lumen (arrow).

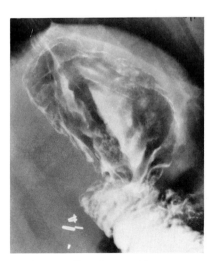

FIG GI15-5. Bile reflux gastritis.

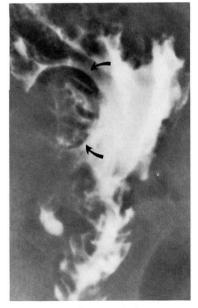

FIG GI15-6. Jejunogastric intussusception (afferent loop) producing a large, sharply defined filling defect (arrows).

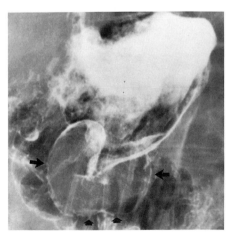

FIG GI15-7. Gastrojejunal mucosal prolapse producing a large, partially obstructing mass in the efferent loop (arrows).

SIMULTANEOUS INVOLVEMENT
OF THE GASTRIC ANTRUM AND DUODENAL BULB

Condition	Imaging Findings	Comments
Lymphoma **(Fig GI16-1)**	Contour deformities, polypoid filling defects, and ulceration.	Transpyloric extension of tumor seen in up to 33% of patients.
Carcinoma **(Fig GI16-2)**	Narrowing and irregularity, polypoid filling defects, and ulceration.	Radiographically detectable invasion of the duodenum in 5% of patients with antral carcinoma. Because carcinoma of the stomach is 50 times more frequent than gastric lymphoma, transpyloric extension of tumor in an individual patient makes carcinoma the more likely diagnosis.
Peptic ulcer disease	Mucosal thickening or ulceration of both areas.	Fibrotic healing can produce narrowing and deformity involving both the antrum and bulb.
Crohn's disease **(Fig GI16-3)**	Blending of the antrum, pylorus, and duodenal bulb into a single tubular or funnel-shaped structure.	Pylorus and duodenal bulb lose their identity as anatomic features between the antrum and the second portion of the duodenum. Simulates the radiographic appearance after a Billroth-I anastomosis.
Tuberculosis	Mural nodularity and ulceration of the pyloroduodenal area.	Rare. Duodenal involvement occurs in 10% of patients with gastric tuberculosis and in half of those in whom the pylorus is involved.
Strongyloidiasis	Nodular intramural defects, ulceration, and luminal narrowing.	Rare appearance seen only in advanced cases.
Eosinophilic gastroenteritis **(Fig GI16-4)**	Mural narrowing and mucosal fold thickening.	Associated with specific food allergies and peripheral eosinophilia.

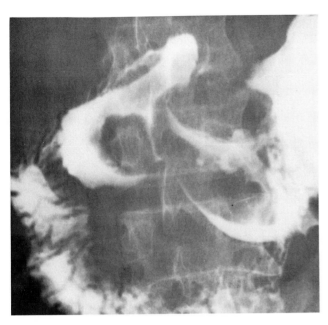

FIG GI16-1. Gastric lymphoma. There are large lymphomatous masses in the distal stomach and duodenal bulb with irregular ulceration.

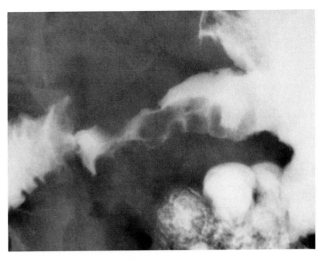

FIG GI16-2. Gastric carcinoma. Rigid, abnormal folds in the distal stomach extend to involve the base of the duodenal bulb.

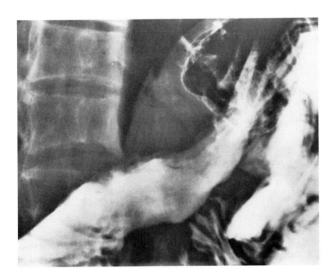

FIG GI16-3. Crohn's disease (pseudo–Billroth-I pattern). There are no recognizable anatomic landmarks between the antrum and the second portion of the duodenum.

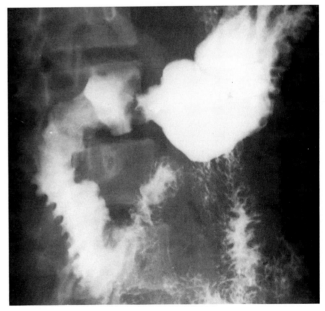

FIG GI16-4. Eosinophilic gastroenteritis. Irregular fold thickening involves the antrum and proximal duodenum.

DUODENAL FILLING DEFECTS

Condition	Imaging Findings	Comments
Pseudotumors (Figs GI17-1 and GI17-2)	Intraluminal filling defects or extrinsic impressions.	Prominent gallbladder; severe edema surrounding a small ulcer crater; retained blood clot; ingested foreign body; gallstone; prolapsed gastrostomy tube; stitch abscess; pylorus seen on end; gas-filled duodenal diverticulum.
Flexure defect	Pseudodefect on the inner margin of the junction between the first and second portions.	Acute change in the axis of the duodenum at this point causes heaping up of redundant loose mucosa and an apparent filling defect.
Ectopic pancreas (see Fig GI10-7)	Smooth, round or oval, well-demarcated filling defect.	Usually asymptomatic. Typically contains a central collection of barium representing filling of ductal structures (mimics an ulcerated mass).
Prolapsed antral mucosa	Mushroom-, umbrella-, or cauliflower-shaped mass at the base of the duodenal bulb.	Active peristalsis causes prolapse of redundant antral folds through the pylorus. As the wave relaxes, the mucosal folds tend to return into the antrum and the defect at the base of the bulb diminishes or disappears.
Brunner's gland hyperplasia (Fig GI17-3)	Multiple nodular filling defects, primarily in the bulb and the proximal half of the second portion.	Probably represents a response of the duodenal mucosa to peptic ulcer disease. May present as a large discrete filling defect (Brunner's gland "adenoma").
Benign lymphoid hyperplasia (Fig GI17-4)	Innumerable tiny nodular defects evenly scattered throughout the duodenum.	No clinical significance. Unlike Brunner's gland hyperplasia associated with peptic disease, there is normal distensibility of the duodenal bulb.
Heterotopic gastric mucosa (Fig GI17-5)	Multiple abruptly marginated, angular filling defects scattered over the surface of the duodenal bulb.	Smaller and less uniform than Brunner's gland hyperplasia. Unlike benign lymphoid hyperplasia, heterotopic gastric mucosa is more irregular and involves only the duodenal bulb.
Papilla of Vater (Fig GI17-6)	Normal "filling defect" on the medial wall of the midportion of the descending duodenum.	Situated on or immediately below the promontory, just above the straight segment. For the differential diagnosis of enlargement of the papilla (>1.5 cm), see page 284.
Choledochocele (Fig GI17-7)	Well-defined, smooth filling defect on the medial wall of the descending duodenum.	Cystic dilatation of the intraduodenal portion of the common bile duct in the region of the ampulla of Vater. This bulbous terminal portion of the common bile duct fills at cholangiography.

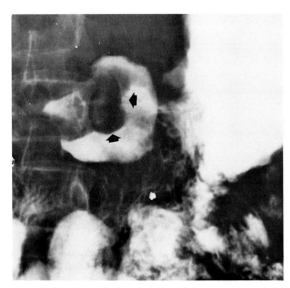

FIG GI17-1. Large blood clot (arrows) in a giant ulcer of the duodenal bulb.

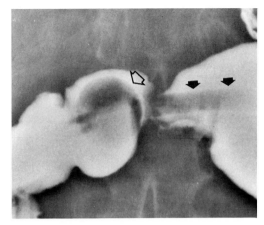

FIG GI17-2. Feeding gastrostomy tube (open arrow) prolapsed into the duodenal bulb. The tube could be mistaken for a polyp on a large stalk (solid arrows).

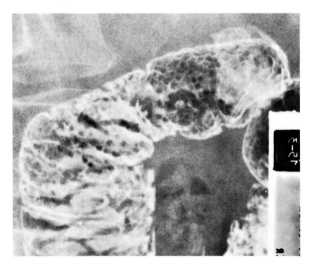

FIG GI17-4. Benign lymphoid hyperplasia.[11]

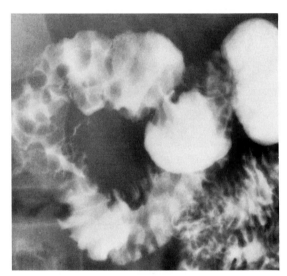

FIG GI17-3. Brunner's gland hyperplasia.

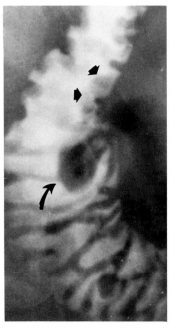

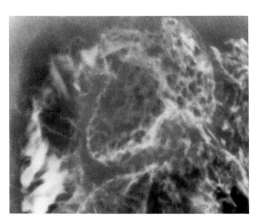

FIG GI17-5. Heterotopic gastric mucosa.

FIG GI17-6. Papilla of Vater (straight arrows). Note the large benign polyp (curved arrow) that is clearly separate from the papilla.

Condition	Imaging Findings	Comments
Duplication cyst	Sharply defined intramural defect (usually in the concavity of the first and second portions of the duodenum).	Because the cyst is fluid-filled, it may change shape with compression and on serial films. Communicates with the duodenal lumen in 10% to 20% of cases.
Pancreatic pseudocyst (Fig GI17-8)	Intramural duodenal filling defect.	Pseudocyst may rarely extend into the duodenal wall and even cause various degrees of duodenal obstruction.
Duodenal varices or mesenteric arterial collaterals (Fig GI17-9)	Solitary or, more commonly, diffuse serpiginous thickening of duodenal folds.	Duodenal varices are almost always associated with esophageal varices and are often complicated by gastrointestinal bleeding. Enlarged mesenteric arterial collaterals develop secondary to occlusion of the celiac trunk or the superior mesenteric artery.
Intramural hematoma (Fig GI17-10)	Sharply defined intramural mass that usually causes stenosis or even complete obstruction of the duodenum.	Develops in patients receiving anticoagulant therapy or with congenital bleeding diatheses, or after blunt abdominal trauma (the retroperitoneal portion of the duodenum is the most fixed part of the small bowel).
Benign tumors	Single or multiple filling defects that may ulcerate.	Adenoma; leiomyoma; lipoma; hamartoma; prolapsed antral polyp. Approximately 90% of bulb tumors are benign, while most tumors in the fourth portion of the duodenum are malignant. Equal frequency of benign and malignant tumors in the second and third portions.
Villous adenoma (Fig GI17-11)	Often-irregular filling defect with barium coating the interstices between the frondlike projections of the tumor.	Variable malignant potential. No definite radiographic criteria to differentiate benign from early malignant lesions.
Carcinoid-islet cell tumor	Solitary (occasionally multiple) submucosal filling defect, usually arising proximal to the papilla.	High endocrine activity (serotonin, insulin, gastrin). May be associated with multiple endocrine adenomatosis. There is usually progressive and intractable peptic ulceration or severe diarrhea.
Malignant tumors	Various appearances (annular constricting lesion with mucosal destruction; ulcerating intraluminal polypoid mass).	Approximately 80% to 90% are adenocarcinomas, most of which occur at or distal to the papilla. Sarcomas (mainly leiomyosarcomas) and primary lymphoma are rare. Metastases involve the duodenum by direct invasion (gastric carcinoma or lymphoma; carcinoma of the pancreas, gallbladder, colon, or kidney). Hematogenous metastases (primarily melanoma) are rare.

A

B

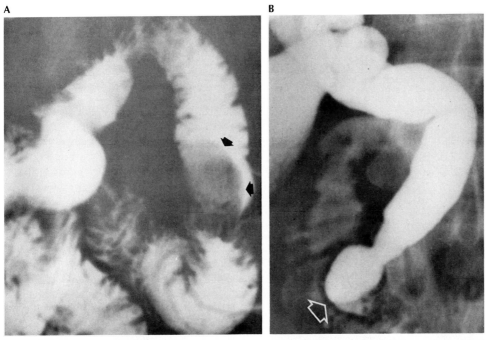

FIG GI17-7. Choledochocele.
(A) Barium study. (B) Cholangiogram.

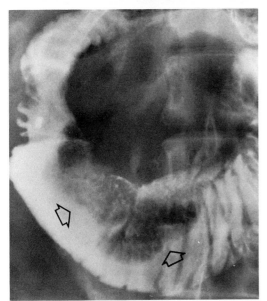

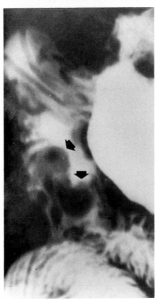

FIG GI17-10. Intramural duodenal hematoma.
The sharply defined intramural mass (arrows) obstructs the lumen in the immediate postbulbar area.

FIG GI17-8. Pancreatic pseudocyst extending into the wall of the duodenum and producing a large intramural filling defect (arrows).

FIG GI17-9. Duodenal varices (arrows).

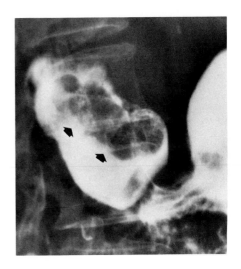

FIG GI17-11. Villous adenoma (arrows). Barium enters the interstices of this bulky mass.

ENLARGEMENT OF THE PAPILLA OF VATER
(>1.5 CENTIMETERS)

Condition	Imaging Findings	Comments
Normal variant (Fig GI18-1)	Smooth enlargement.	Found in 1% of normal examinations and is a diagnosis of exclusion (if all other causes ruled out).
Impacted stone in distal common bile duct	Papillary edema (smooth enlargement).	Typical symptoms of acute biliary colic. The papilla may rarely be irregular and mimic a perivaterian neoplasm.
Acute pancreatitis (Fig GI18-2)	Papillary edema (smooth enlargement).	Very early sign (Poppel's) that is usually present before pancreatic enlargement can be detected. There may be pancreatic calcification if the acute process represents a subacute exacerbation of disease.
Acute duodenal ulcer disease (Fig GI18-3)	Papillary edema (smooth enlargement).	Papillary fold participates in the generalized duodenal edema. There is almost invariably diffuse enlargement of folds and an acute ulcer crater in the duodenal bulb.
Perivaterian neoplasm (Fig GI18-4)	Irregular enlargement, often with ulceration.	Collective term for malignancies arising in the duodenum, head of the pancreas, distal common bile duct, and ampulla of Vater. There is usually a history of progressive jaundice and no thickening of the surrounding duodenal folds.
Papillitis	Polypoid enlargement.	Periductal inflammatory reaction rather than a true neoplasm. Exuberant fibrosis may eventually produce sphincter stenosis.
Lesions simulating enlarged papilla	Variable appearance.	Benign spindle cell tumor or ectopic pancreatic tissue on the inner aspect of the second portion of the duodenum can mimic papillary enlargement unless the papilla itself is clearly demonstrated. Central barium collection (ulcer or rudimentary duct) in an apparently enlarged papilla suggests a spindle cell tumor (especially leiomyoma) or ectopic pancreas.

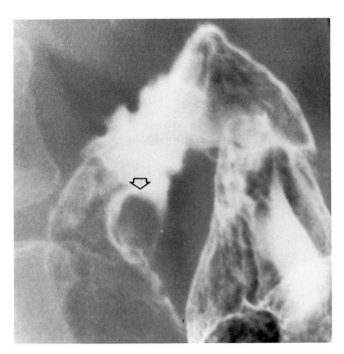

FIG GI18-1. Normal variant.

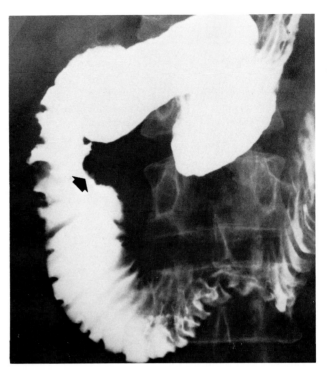

FIG GI18-2. Acute pancreatitis.

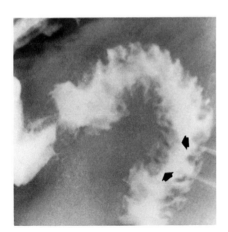

FIG GI18-3. Diffuse peptic ulcer disease.

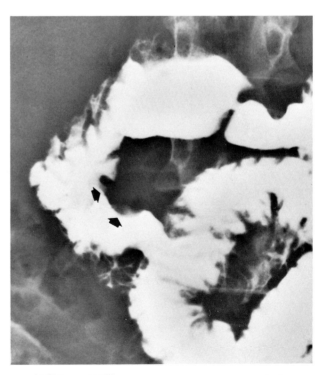

FIG GI18-4. Adenocarcinoma of the duodenum.

DUODENAL NARROWING OR OBSTRUCTION

Condition	Imaging Findings	Comments
Congenital anomalies **Duodenal atresia** **(Fig GI19-1)**	Double bubble sign. Absence of gas in the small and large bowel.	Complete obliteration of the duodenal lumen is the most common cause of congenital duodenal obstruction. Relatively high incidence in infants with Down's syndrome.
Duodenal stenosis **(Fig GI19-2)**	Double bubble sign. Some gas in the bowel distal to the obstruction.	High-grade but incomplete congenital stenosis of the duodenum.
Annular pancreas	In infants, double bubble sign with some gas in the distal bowel. In adults, a notchlike defect on the lateral wall of the duodenum causing eccentric luminal narrowing.	Incomplete obstruction with gas in the bowel distal to the level of the high-grade duodenal stenosis. Relatively high incidence in infants with Down's syndrome.
Duodenal diaphragm **(web)** **(Fig GI19-3)**	Thin lucent line across the lumen, often with proximal duodenal dilatation.	Usually involves the second part of the duodenum. May balloon out distally, producing a rounded, barium-filled, comma-shaped sac (intraluminal diverticulum).
Midgut volvulus	High-grade duodenal obstruction. Spiral course of bowel loops on the right side of the abdomen.	Occurs with incomplete rotation of the bowel. The duodenojejunal junction (ligament of Treitz) is located inferiorly and to the right of its expected position.
Congenital peritoneal **(Ladd's) bands** **(Fig GI19-4)**	Intermittent partial duodenal obstruction. Symptoms often increase with standing (bands tighten) and decrease when lying down (bands relax).	Dense fibrous bands extending from an abnormally placed, malrotated cecum or hepatic flexure over the anterior surface of the second or third portion of the duodenum to the right gutter and the inferior surface of the liver.
Duodenal duplication **cyst**	Intramural or extrinsic duodenal mass.	Usually asymptomatic. Rarely causes high-grade stenosis or complete obstruction.
Postbulbar ulcer **(Fig GI19-5)**	Eccentric duodenal narrowing (spasm or fibrosis) or a ring stricture.	Incisura represents indrawing of the lateral wall of the duodenum. Often appears similar to annular pancreas, though granular mucosa in the narrowed segment suggests healed ulceration.
Crohn's disease **(Fig GI19-6)**	Fusiform and concentric narrowing of the duodenum.	Usually evidence of Crohn's disease elsewhere. Crohn's disease of the duodenal bulb and antrum produces tubular narrowing (pseudo–Billroth-I appearance).
Tuberculosis	Appearance indistinguishable from that of Crohn's disease.	Extremely rare. Almost always associated with antropyloric disease. There may be fistulas and sinus tracts.

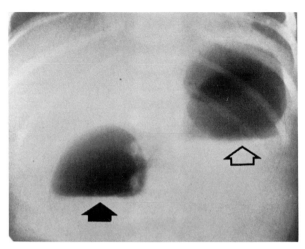

FIG GI19-1. Duodenal atresia with double-bubble sign. The left bubble (open arrow) represents air in the stomach; the right bubble (solid arrow) reflects duodenal gas. There is no gas in the small or large bowel distal to the level of the complete obstruction.

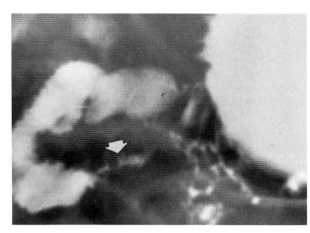

FIG GI19-4. Ladd's bands. Obstruction of the third portion of the duodenum (arrow) in a newborn infant, due to dense fibrous bands.

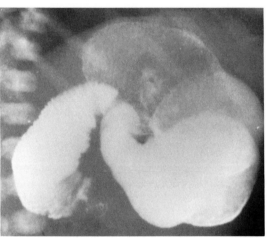

FIG GI19-2. Congenital duodenal stenosis. The presence of small amounts of gas distal to the obstruction indicates that the stenosis is incomplete.

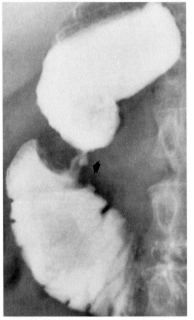

FIG GI19-5. Postbulbar ulcer. The deep incisura associated with the medial wall postbulbar ulcer (arrow) causes severe narrowing of the second portion of the duodenum.

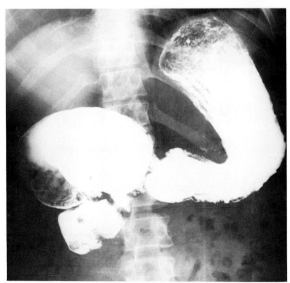

FIG GI19-3. Duodenal diaphragm. The presence of gas in the bowel distal to the diaphragm indicates that the high-grade obstruction is not complete.

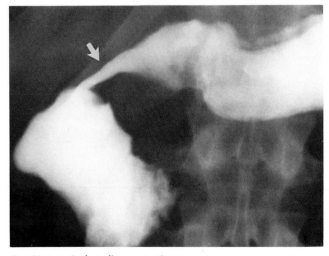

FIG GI19-6. Crohn's disease. Fusiform, concentric narrowing of the apical and postbulbar areas.

Condition	Imaging Findings	Comments
Strongyloidiasis/sprue	Single or multiple areas of stenosis of the duodenum.	Strongyloidiasis is indistinguishable from Crohn's disease. In long-standing nontropical sprue, narrowing represents healing of ulceration.
Pancreatitis/cholecystitis (Fig GI19-7)	Narrowing and deformity of the duodenum with fold thickening and spiculation.	May represent irritability and spasm due to severe acute inflammation or postinflammatory fibrotic healing.
Pancreatic pseudocyst (Fig GI19-8)	Extrinsic compression of the duodenal sweep.	Mucosal folds of the duodenum may be thickened, splayed, and distorted, but are not destroyed as with pancreatic cancer.
Pancreatic carcinoma (Fig GI19-9)	Extrinsic impression and double-contour effect. Often associated with ulceration and mucosal destruction.	May be difficult to distinguish from pancreatitis. Duodenal mucosal destruction suggests malignancy, though some pancreatic tumors can infiltrate the submucosa and produce stenosis without mucosal destruction.
Duodenal carcinoma	Annular constricting lesion with overhanging edges, nodular mucosal destruction, and ulceration.	Approximately 90% are adenocarcinomas, which usually arise at or distal to the ampulla of Vater. May be impossible to differentiate from secondary neoplastic invasion of the duodenum due to extension of tumors of the pancreas, gallbladder, or colon.
Metastatic malignancy	Irregular narrowing of the duodenum associated with mass effect and ulceration.	Primarily metastases to lymph nodes (peripancreatic, celiac, para-aortic) along the second and third portions of the duodenum.
Intramural duodenal hematoma (Fig GI19-10)	Tumorlike intramural mass causing narrowing of the duodenal lumen.	Secondary to anticoagulant therapy, abnormal bleeding diathesis, or blunt trauma (the duodenum is the most fixed portion of the small bowel).
Aorticoduodenal fistula	Extrinsic mass compressing and displacing the third portion of the duodenum.	Often fatal complication of an abdominal aortic aneurysm or the placement of a prosthetic graft.
Radiation injury	Smooth stricture, primarily involving the second portion of the duodenum.	Infrequent complication after radiation therapy to the upper abdomen.
Superior mesenteric artery syndrome (Fig GI19-11)	Narrowing or obstruction of the third portion of the duodenum with proximal dilatation.	Controversial entity referring to compression of the transverse duodenum between the aorta and the superior mesenteric artery due to any process that decreases duodenal peristalsis or thickens the bowel wall or the root of the mesentery.

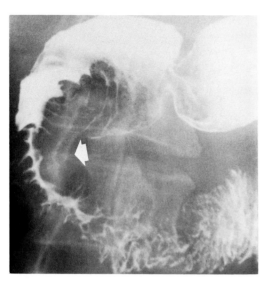

FIG GI19-7. Chronic pancreatitis with acute exacerbation. The inflammatory mass narrows the second portion of the duodenum and causes marked mucosal edema and spiculation (arrow).

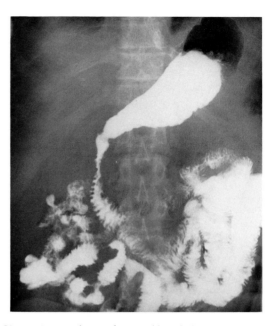

FIG GI19-8. Pancreatic pseudocyst. Although there is narrowing of the second portion of the duodenum with widening of the duodenal sweep, the mucosal folds are intact.

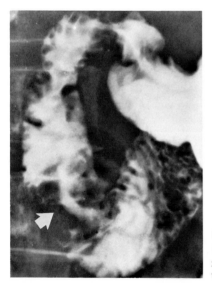

FIG GI19-9. Carcinoma of the pancreas producing an annular constricting lesion. The radiographic appearance is indistinguishable from that of primary duodenal carcinoma.

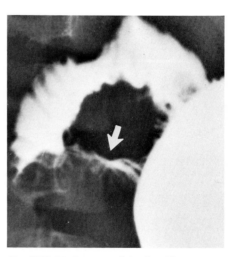

FIG GI19-10. Intramural duodenal hematoma. High-grade stenotic lesion (arrow) that developed in a young child who had been kicked in the abdomen.

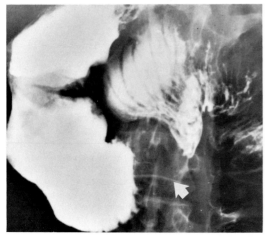

FIG GI19-11. Superior mesenteric artery syndrome in scleroderma. There is severe atony and dilatation of the duodenum proximal to the aorticomesenteric angle (arrow).

THICKENING OF DUODENAL FOLDS

Condition	Imaging Findings	Comments
Peptic ulcer disease (see Fig GI17-3)	Diffuse fold thickening, primarily involving the bulb and proximal sweep.	Most common cause. Nodular, cobblestone appearance suggests Brunner's gland hyperplasia (response of the duodenal mucosa to an ulcer diathesis).
Zollinger-Ellison syndrome (Fig GI20-1)	Diffuse fold thickening.	Associated findings include ulcerations in atypical positions (third and fourth portions of the duodenum, proximal jejunum) and a chemical enteritis of the proximal jejunum.
Pancreatitis (Fig GI20-2)	Thickened folds in the second portion.	Associated findings include mass impression and elevated serum amylase.
Uremia (chronic dialysis)	Nodular fold thickening, primarily involving the bulb and second portion.	Simulates the appearance of pancreatitis, which frequently complicates prolonged uremia and may be responsible for producing the radiographic pattern.
Crohn's disease/ tuberculosis (Fig GI20-3)	Diffuse fold thickening, often with ulceration and luminal narrowing.	In Crohn's disease, usually involvement of the terminal ileum. In tuberculosis, the antrum and pylorus are generally affected.
Parasitic infestation (see Fig GI26-6)	Nodular fold thickening.	Giardiasis (increased secretions causing a blurred appearance) and strongyloidiasis (ulcerations and luminal stenosis).
Nontropical sprue	Bizarre nodular thickening of folds.	Early manifestation of the disease.
Neoplastic disorders (Fig GI20-4)	Various patterns of fold thickening.	Lymphoma (coarse, nodular, irregular folds) and metastases to peripancreatic lymph nodes (localized duodenal impressions simulating thickened folds).
Infiltrative disorders	Diffuse fold thickening (usually generalized involvement of the small bowel).	Whipple's disease; amyloidosis; mastocytosis; eosinophilic enteritis; intestinal lymphangectasia.
Duodenal varices (Fig GI20-5)	Nodular or serpiginous fold thickening.	Esophageal varices are almost always also present.
Mesenteric arterial collaterals	Serpiginous, nodular filling defects simulating thickened folds.	Collateral vessels of the pancreaticoduodenal arcade due to occlusion of the celiac axis or the superior mesenteric artery.
Cystic fibrosis (Fig GI20-6)	Coarse thickening of folds.	Probably related to the lack of pancreatic bicarbonate, which results in inadequate buffering of normal amounts of gastric acid.

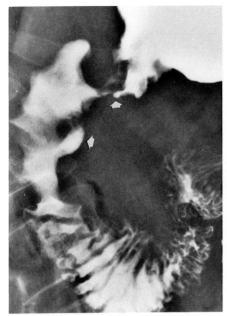

FIG GI20-1. **Zollinger-Ellison syndrome.** Diffuse thickening of folds in the proximal duodenal sweep is associated with bulbar and postbulbar ulceration (arrows).

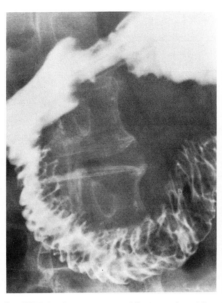

FIG GI20-2. **Acute pancreatitis.** Note the widening of the duodenal sweep, double-contour effect, and sharp spiculations.

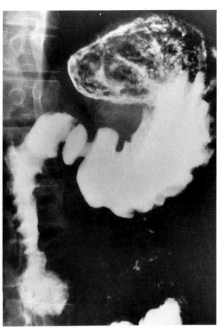

FIG GI20-3. **Tuberculosis.** Diffuse fold thickening, spasm, and ulceration of the proximal duodenum.

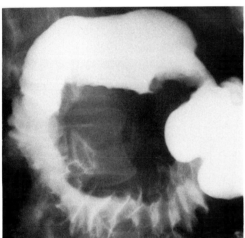

FIG GI20-4. **Metastases** to peripancreatic lymph nodes causes localized impressions on the duodenum simulating thickened folds.

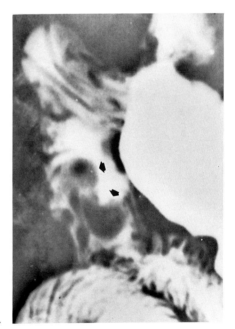

FIG GI20-5. **Duodenal varices.**

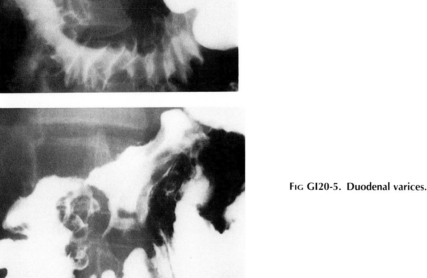

FIG GI20-6. **Cystic fibrosis.**

WIDENING OF THE DUODENAL SWEEP

Condition	Imaging Findings	Comments
Normal variant	Illusion of generalized widening.	Especially in an obese patient with a high transverse stomach and a long vertical course of the descending duodenum.
Acute pancreatitis **(Fig GI21-1)**	Generalized widening with mucosal ulcerations, fold thickening, and mass effect.	Associated radiographic findings include elevation of a hemidiaphragm, basilar atelectasis, pleural effusion (left side), colon cutoff sign, and sentinel loop.
Chronic pancreatitis	Generalized widening with fold effacement and spiculation. Pancreatic calcification is often visible radiographically.	History of alcoholism in more than half the patients. Biliary tract disease (usually with gallstones) in about one third.
Pancreatic pseudocyst **(Fig GI21-2)**	Generalized widening and compression of the duodenal sweep.	Common complication of pancreatitis. May also develop after pancreatic injury.
Pancreatic malignancy **(Fig GI21-3)**	Diffuse widening with mass impression, spiculation, and double-contour effect.	Often difficult to distinguish radiographically from benign pancreatic disease. A similar pattern may be produced by cystadenocarcinoma and metastatic lesions.
Lymph node enlargement	Generalized widening.	Lymphadenopathy due to lymphoma, metastases to lymph nodes, or inflammatory disease.
Cystic lymphangioma of mesentery **(Fig GI21-4)**	Generalized widening.	Benign cystic structure containing serous or chylous fluid resulting from the congenital obliteration of draining lymphatics or an acquired lymphatic obstruction.
Retroperitoneal mass	Generalized widening.	Primary or metastatic neoplasm; cyst.
Aortic aneurysm	Downward displacement of the third portion of the duodenum.	Definitive diagnosis made on ultrasound or CT.
Choledochal cyst	Generalized widening of the duodenal sweep or a localized impression near the papilla.	Definitive diagnosis made on ultrasound or CT.

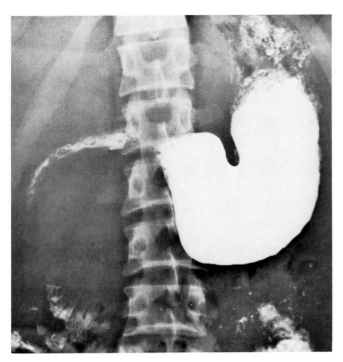

FIG GI21-1. Acute pancreatitis. Severe inflammation causes widening of the sweep and a high-grade duodenal obstruction.

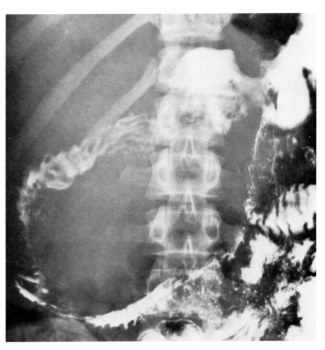

FIG GI21-2. Pancreatic pseudocyst.

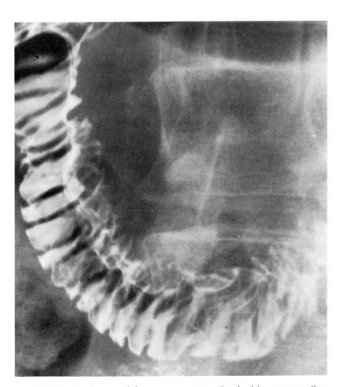

FIG GI21-3. Carcinoma of the pancreas. Note the double-contour effect along the medial aspect of the duodenal sweep.

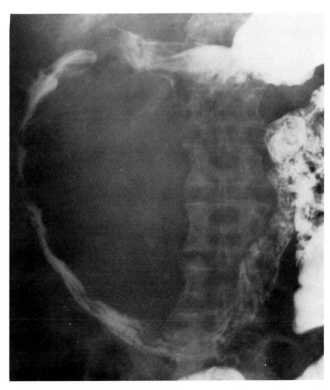

FIG GI21-4. Cystic lymphangioma of the mesentery. Scattered clumps of calcification are present in the lesion.

ADYNAMIC ILEUS*

Condition	Imaging Findings	Comments
Surgical procedure	Generalized ileus.	Usually resolves spontaneously or clears with the aid of intubation and suction. If progressive, can cause intestinal rupture and pneumoperitoneum.
Peritonitis	Generalized ileus, often with blurring of the mucosal pattern and intestinal edema.	Suggestive findings include free peritoneal fluid, restricted diaphragmatic movement, and pleural effusion. Gastroenteritis or enterocolitis *without* peritonitis can also present as generalized adynamic ileus.
Medication	Generalized ileus.	Drugs with atropine-like effects (morphine, Lomotil, L-dopa, barbiturates, and other sympathomimetic agents).
Electrolyte imbalance/ metabolic disorder	Generalized ileus.	Most commonly hypokalemia, but also occurs with hypochloremia, calcium or magnesium abnormalities, and hormonal deficits (hypothyroidism, hypoparathyroidism).
Other abdominal or chest conditions	Generalized ileus.	Abdominal trauma; retroperitoneal hemorrhage; spinal or pelvic fractures; generalized gram-negative sepsis; shock; acute pulmonary disease; mesenteric vascular occlusion.
Sentinel loop (Fig GI22-2)	Localized distended loop of small or large bowel (associated with an adjacent acute inflammatory process).	Portion of bowel involved can suggest the underlying disease (jejunum or transverse colon in acute pancreatitis, hepatic flexure in acute cholecystitis, terminal ileum in acute appendicitis, descending colon in acute diverticulitis).
Colonic ileus (Fig GI22-3)	Disproportionate gaseous distension of the large bowel without organic obstruction. Massive distension of the cecum (often horizontally oriented).	Usually related to abdominal surgery or acute inflammation. The clinical presentation simulates mechanical obstruction.
Chronic idiopathic intestinal pseudo-obstruction (Fig GI22-4)	Distension of the small bowel mimicking intestinal obstruction, but without any demonstrable obstructive lesion.	Episodic symptoms of intestinal obstruction. Recognition of the true nature of this nonobstructive condition is essential to prevent the patient from undergoing unnecessary laparotomies.
Pelvic surgery	Mimics small bowel obstruction.	Develops between the second and fifth postoperative days, especially if there was manipulation of the small bowel. Self-limited and rarely requires surgery.

*Pattern: The entire small and large bowel appears almost uniformly dilated with no demonstrable point of obstruction (Fig GI22-1).

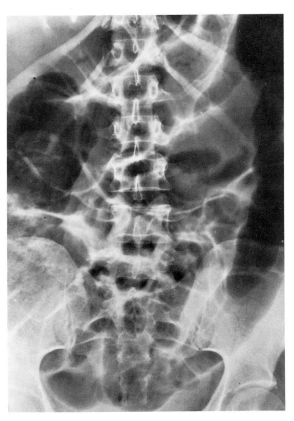

FIG GI22-1. **Adynamic ileus pattern.**

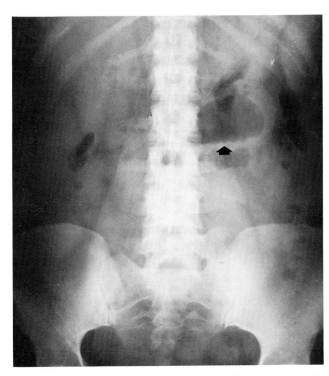

FIG GI22-2. **Sentinel loop** (arrow) in a patient with acute pancreatitis.

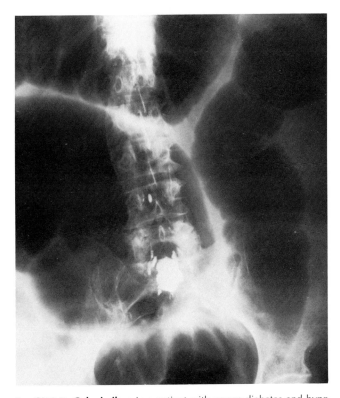

FIG GI22-3. **Colonic ileus** in a patient with severe diabetes and hypokalemia.

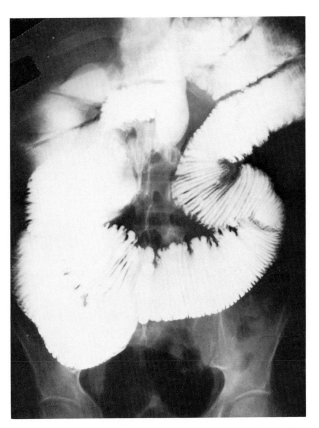

FIG GI22-4. **Chronic idiopathic intestinal pseudo-obstruction.** Diffuse small bowel dilatation simulates mechanical obstruction.[12]

Condition	Imaging Findings	Comments
Urinary retention	Mimics small bowel obstruction.	Symptoms often completely disappear after emptying of the distended bladder.
Acute intermittent porphyria (Fig GI22-5)	Mimics small bowel obstruction.	Familial metabolic disease. The diagnosis is suggested by the characteristic neurologic symptoms or the urine becoming dark on exposure to light.
Ceroidosis	Mimics small bowel obstruction.	Diffuse accumulation of a brown lipofuscin pigment in the muscularis due to long-standing malabsorption and prolonged depletion of vitamin E. May lead to unnecessary bowel resection for nonexistent obstruction.
Neonatal adynamic ileus	Mimics small bowel obstruction.	Causes include septicemia, hormonal or chemical deficits, hypoxia-induced vasculitis, respiratory distress syndrome, intestinal infection, peritonitis, and mesenteric thrombosis.

A

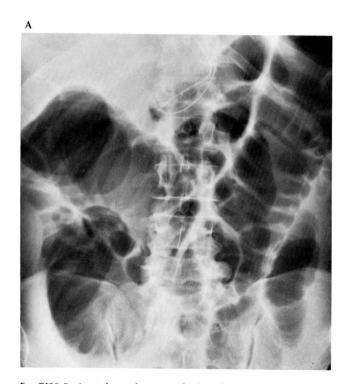

B

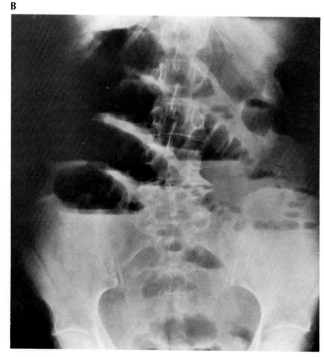

FIG GI22-5. Acute intermittent porphyria. Adynamic ileus simulating mechanical obstruction on (A) supine and (B) upright views.

SMALL BOWEL OBSTRUCTION

Condition	Imaging Findings	Comments
Fibrous adhesions (Fig GI23-1)	Most frequently involves the ileum (site of most abdominal inflammatory processes and operative procedures).	Fibrous adhesions caused by previous surgery or peritonitis account for almost 75% of all small bowel obstructions.
External hernias	May have gas or excessive soft-tissue density on the affected side.	External hernias (inguinal, femoral, umbilical, incisional) are the second most frequent cause of small bowel obstruction.
Internal hernias	Various patterns.	Results from congenital abnormalities or surgical defects in the mesentery. More than half are paraduodenal (mostly on the left).
Volvulus/congenital bands	Duodenal obstruction.	Usually associated with malrotation anomalies.
Neoplasms (Fig GI23-2)	Luminal occlusion or extrinsic impression.	Can be caused by benign or malignant neoplasms and involve any level of the small bowel.
Gallstone ileus (Fig GI23-3)	Classic triad of jejunal or ileal filling defect, gas or barium in the biliary tree, and small bowel obstruction.	Caused by a large gallstone entering the small bowel via a fistula from the gallbladder or the common bile duct to the duodenum. Usually occurs in elderly women.
Bezoar (Fig GI23-4)	Filling defect on barium studies.	Primarily seen in patients who are mentally retarded or edentulous or who have undergone partial gastric resection.
Intussusception (Fig GI23-5)	May produce the classic coiled-spring appearance (barium trapped between the intussusceptum and the surrounding portions of bowel).	A major cause of small bowel obstruction in children (much less common in adults). The leading edge of an intussusception (usually a pedunculated polypoid tumor) can be demonstrated in 80% of adults. In children, there is infrequently any apparent anatomic etiology.
Meconium ileus (Fig GI23-6)	Infant with a bubbly or frothy pattern superimposed on dilated loops of small bowel.	Caused by thick and sticky meconium due to the absence of normal pancreatic and intestinal gland secretions during fetal life. Often occurs with cystic fibrosis. A microcolon is seen on barium enema examination.
Congenital intestinal atresia or stenosis (Fig GI23-7)	Double bubble (duodenal atresia) or triple bubble (proximal jejunal atresia) signs, or a typical obstructive pattern.	Barium enema may be required to distinguish small from large bowel in a low ileal obstruction. Microcolon in ileal atresia; normal-caliber colon in duodenal atresia. Meconium peritonitis (often calcified) is a complication of small bowel atresia.

Condition	Imaging Findings	Comments
Stricture of bowel wall	May involve any level of the small bowel.	Causes include neoplasm, inflammation (Crohn's disease, tuberculosis, parasitic infections), chemical irritation (medicines such as enteric-coated potassium chloride tablets), radiation therapy, massive deposition of amyloid, and intestinal ischemia (arterial or venous occlusion).

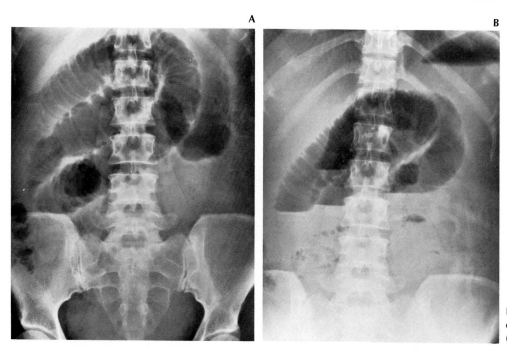

Fig GI23-1. Typical small bowel obstruction on (A) supine and (B) upright projections.

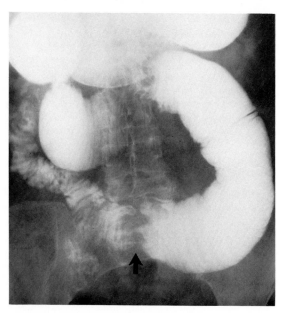

Fig GI23-2. Carcinoma of the jejunum causing small bowel obstruction. There is pronounced dilatation of the duodenum and proximal jejunum to the level of the annular constricting tumor (arrow).

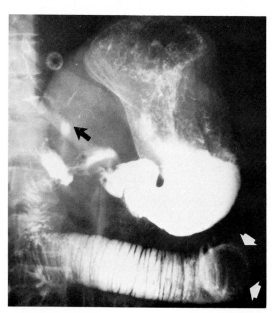

Fig GI23-3. Gallstone ileus. Upper gastrointestinal series demonstrates the obstructing stone (white arrows) and barium in the biliary tree (black arrow).

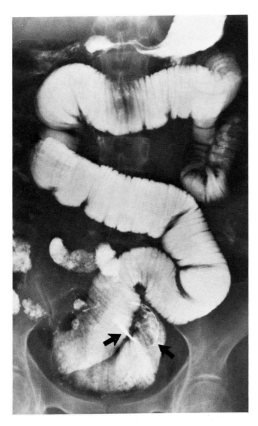

FIG GI23-4. **Impacted bezoar** (arrows) causing small bowel obstruction.

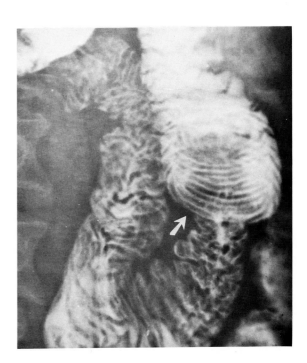

FIG GI23-5. **Intussusception.** Coiled-spring appearance in jejunojejunal intussusception.

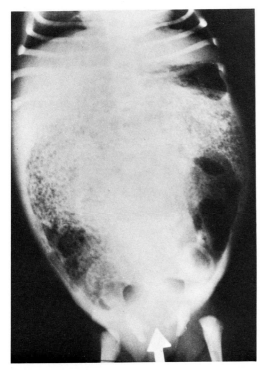

FIG GI23-6. **Meconium ileus**. Massive small bowel distension with a profound soap-bubble effect of gas mixed with meconium.[13]

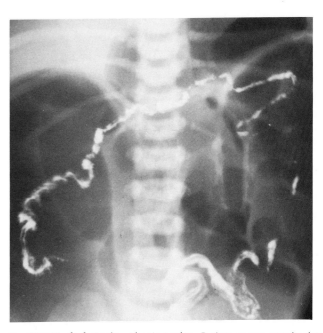

FIG GI23-7. **Ileal atresia** with microcolon. Barium enema examination shows the colon to be thin and ribbonlike. Note the markedly distended loops of small bowel extending to the point of obstruction in the lower ileum.

SMALL BOWEL DILATATION

Condition	Imaging Findings	Comments
Mechanical obstruction (see GI23)	Dilatation proximal to the level of the obstruction.	Distinct difference in caliber between loops proximal and distal to the point of the obstruction. Generally a paucity of colonic gas.
Adynamic ileus (see GI22)	Generalized dilatation of the small (and large) bowel.	No point at which the caliber of the bowel dramatically changes.
Vagotomy (surgical or chemical) (Fig GI24-1)	Generalized dilatation of the small bowel.	Vagotomy clips or a history of previous ulcer surgery; atropine-like medications (morphine, L-dopa, Lomotil, barbiturates).
Sprue (Fig GI24-2)	Generalized dilatation, but often most marked in the mid and distal jejunum. Excessive amount of fluid in the bowel lumen (coarse, granular appearance of the barium). Moulage sign and frequent transient intussusception.	Classic disease of malabsorption that includes idiopathic (nontropical) sprue, tropical sprue, and celiac disease of children. Diagnosis is made by jejunal biopsy (flattening or atrophy of intestinal villi). Nontropical sprue is treated with a gluten-free diet, tropical sprue with antibiotics or folic acid.
Lymphoma	Occasionally has an appearance indistinguishable from that of sprue.	Rare manifestation of intestinal lymphoma. More commonly thickening of the bowel wall, displacement of intestinal loops, and extraluminal masses.
Scleroderma (Fig GI24-3)	Dilatation that is usually most marked in the duodenum proximal to the aorticomesenteric angle. The entire small bowel can be diffusely involved.	"Hidebound" sign of folds abnormally packed together despite bowel dilatation. Hypomotility of the small bowel with extremely prolonged transit time. There may be pseudosacculations simulating small bowel diverticula. Similar findings occasionally occur with dermatomyositis.
Lactase deficiency (Fig GI24-4)	Generalized dilatation with dilution of barium, rapid transit time, and reproduction of symptoms after the administration of lactose.	Most common of the disaccharidase-deficiency syndromes; especially frequent in North American blacks, Mexicans, and Chinese. Patients experience abdominal discomfort, cramps, and watery diarrhea 30 minutes to several hours after ingesting milk or milk products.
Diabetes with hypokalemia	Generalized dilatation of the small bowel.	Small bowel is usually normal in patients with diabetes mellitus unless complicated by hypokalemia (probably represents a visceral neuropathy).
Vascular insufficiency/ vasculitis (Fig GI24-5)	Generalized dilatation of the small bowel.	Occasional manifestation of mesenteric ischemia (if a disturbance of intestinal motility, rather than intramural bleeding, is the major abnormality). Also occurs with the vasculitis due to systemic lupus erythematosus or massive amyloid deposition.

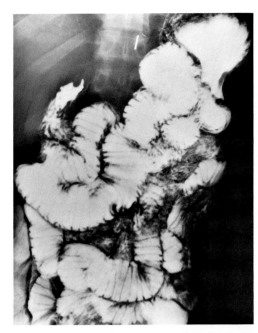

FIG GI24-1. Surgical vagotomy with partial gastrectomy and Billroth-II anastomosis.

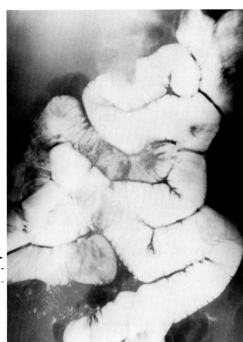

FIG GI24-2. Idiopathic (nontropical) sprue. Note the pronounced hypersecretion.

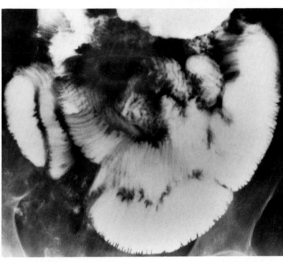

FIG GI24-3. Scleroderma. For the degree of dilatation, the small bowel folds are packed remarkably close together (hidebound pattern).

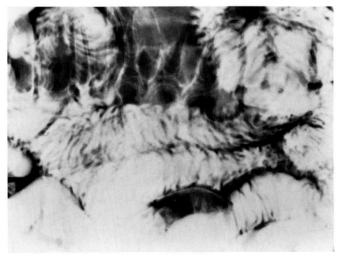

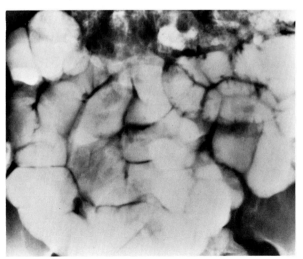

FIG GI24-4. Lactase deficiency. (Left) Normal conventional small bowel examination. (Right) After the addition of 50 g of lactose to the barium mixture, there is marked dilatation of the small bowel with dilution of barium, rapid transit, and reproduction of symptoms.

Condition	Imaging Findings	Comments
Chronic idiopathic intestinal pseudo-obstruction (see Fig GI22-4)	Small bowel obstruction pattern.	Episodic signs and symptoms of mechanical obstruction without any organic lesion. Recognition of this condition may prevent unnecessary laparotomies.
Chagas' disease	Generalized dilatation of the small bowel.	Trypanosomes extensively invade the smooth muscle and destroy intrinsic neurons and ganglion cells in the bowel wall.

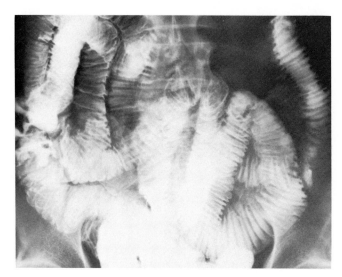

FIG GI24-5. Systemic lupus erythematosus.

REGULAR THICKENING OF SMALL BOWEL FOLDS

Condition	Comments
Hemorrhage into bowel wall (Fig GI25-1)	Usually segmental involvement of the small bowel (especially the jejunum) with scalloping and thumb-printing. Concomitant bleeding into the mesentery often results in separation of bowel loops and even an eccentric mass simulating malignancy. Causes include anticoagulant therapy, ischemic bowel disease, vasculitis (connective tissue diseases, Buerger's disease, Henoch-Schönlein purpura), hemophilia, idiopathic thrombocytopenic purpura, trauma, and coagulation defects secondary to other diseases (hypoprothrombinemia, leukemia, multiple myeloma, lymphoma, metastatic carcinoma, disorders of the fibrinogen system).
Intestinal edema (Fig GI25-2)	Generalized involvement of the small bowel. Causes include hypoproteinemia (cirrhosis, nephrotic syndrome, protein-losing enteropathies), lymphatic blockage (especially tumor infiltration), and angioneurotic edema (tends to be episodic and more localized).
Intestinal lymphangiectasia	Generalized small bowel involvement. Occurs in primary and secondary forms. Regular thickening represents a combination of intestinal edema (lymphatic obstruction or severe protein loss) and lymphatic dilatation.
Abetalipoproteinemia	Generalized small bowel involvement. Extremely rare disease manifested clinically by malabsorption of fat, progressive neurologic deterioration, and retinitis pigmentosa. Acanthocytosis (thorny appearance of red blood cells) is a characteristic finding. The small bowel folds may also be irregular or nodular.
Eosinophilic enteritis/ amyloidosis	Generalized regular thickening of small bowel folds may occur at an early stage before the development of the more characteristic irregular thickening of folds.

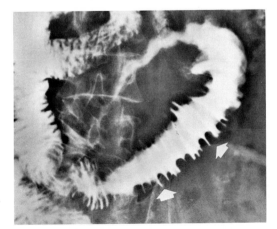

Fig GI25-1. **Small bowel ischemia** producing a segmental picket-fence pattern of regular thickening of small bowel folds (arrows).

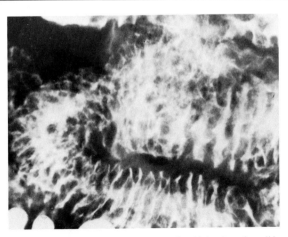

Fig GI25-2. **Hypoproteinemia** causing regular thickening of small bowel folds in a patient with cirrhosis.

GENERALIZED, IRREGULAR, DISTORTED SMALL BOWEL FOLDS

Condition	Imaging Findings	Comments
Whipple's disease (Fig GI26-1)	Most frequently involves the duodenum and proximal jejunum. Small bowel appearance may revert to normal after antibiotic therapy.	Infiltration of the lamina propria by large macrophages containing multiple glycoprotein granules that react positively to the periodic acid–Schiff (PAS) stain. Clinically, malabsorption syndrome and often extraintestinal symptoms (arthritis, fever, lymphadenopathy).
Giardiasis (Fig GI26-2)	Primarily involves the duodenum and jejunum. Small bowel pattern returns to normal after treatment with Atabrine or Flagyl.	Usually a history of travel to areas where the parasite is endemic (eg, Leningrad, India, or the Rocky Mountains of Colorado). May complicate an immune deficiency state (especially nodular lymphoid hyperplasia).
Lymphoma (Fig GI26-3)	Localized, multifocal, or diffuse. Most commonly involves the ileum (site of the greatest amount of lymphoid tissue).	May be primary or secondary (25% of patients with disseminated lymphoma have small bowel involvement at autopsy).
Amyloidosis (Fig GI26-4)	Generalized involvement of the small bowel.	Small intestinal involvement occurs in at least 70% of cases of generalized amyloidosis. May be primary or secondary to a chronic inflammatory or necrotizing process (eg, tuberculosis, osteomyelitis, ulcerative colitis, rheumatoid arthritis, malignant neoplasm), multiple myeloma, or familial Mediterranean fever.
Eosinophilic enteritis (Fig GI26-5)	Primarily involves the jejunum, though the entire small bowel is sometimes affected.	There is often concomitant eosinophilic infiltration of the stomach. Typical food allergies and peripheral eosinophilia.
Crohn's disease	Most often involves the terminal ileum, but can affect any part of the small bowel.	Characteristic findings include skip lesions, string sign, severe narrowing, separation of bowel loops, and fistula formation.
Tuberculosis	Radiographic pattern indistinguishable from that of Crohn's disease.	Tends to be more localized than Crohn's disease and predominantly affects the ileocecal region.
Histoplasmosis	Generalized involvement of the small bowel.	Fungal disease that rarely affects the gastrointestinal tract. Folds seen end-on may appear as innumerable small filling defects. Focal stenotic lesions may mimic neoplastic disease.
Mastocytosis	Generalized involvement of the small bowel.	Systemic mast cell proliferation in the reticuloendothelial system and the skin. Often lymphadenopathy and hepatosplenomegaly and occasionally sclerotic bone lesions. High incidence of peptic ulcers and episodic pruritis, flushing, tachycardia, asthma, and headaches.

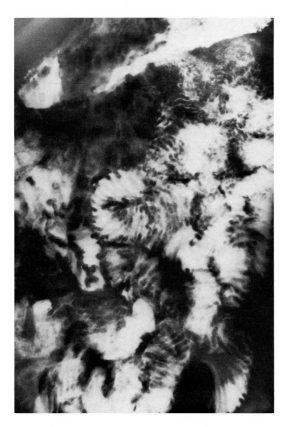

Fɪɢ **GI26-1. Whipple's disease.**

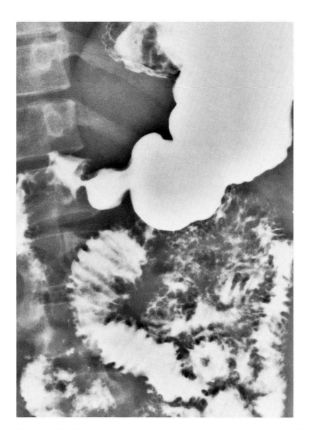

Fɪɢ **GI26-2. Giardiasis.** Irregular fold thickening is most prominent in the proximal small bowel.

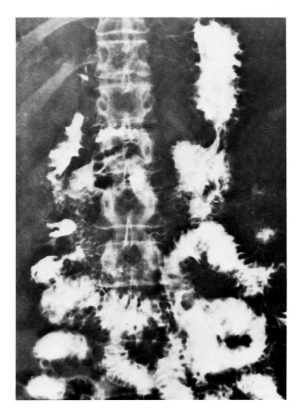

Fɪɢ **GI26-3. Lymphoma.** In addition to diffuse, irregular thickening of the small bowel folds, there is mesenteric involvement causing separation of bowel loops.

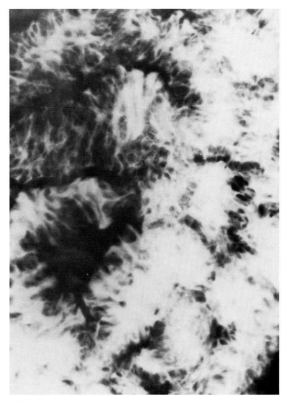

Fɪɢ **GI26-4. Amyloidosis.**

Condition	Imaging Findings	Comments
Strongyloidiasis (**Fig GI26-6**)	Predominantly involves the proximal small bowel (a severe infestation can affect the entire alimentary tract).	Roundworm that lives in warm, moist climates where there is frequent fecal contamination of the soil.
Yersinia **enterocolitis**	Predominantly a focal disease involving short segments of the terminal ileum. Infrequently affects the colon and rectum.	Gram-negative rod that causes an acute enteritis with fever and diarrhea in children and an acute terminal ileitis or mesenteric adenitis (simulating appendicitis) in adolescents and adults.
Typhoid fever	Involvement limited to the terminal ileum.	Caused by *Salmonella typhosa*. Mimics Crohn's disease, though in typhoid fever the ileal involvement is symmetric, skip areas and fistulas do not occur, and there is usually evidence of splenomegaly.
Alpha-chain disease	Generalized involvement of the small bowel.	Disorder of immunoglobulin peptide synthesis that probably permits bacterial overgrowth.
Abetalipoproteinemia	Generalized involvement of the small bowel.	Rare inherited disease manifested clinically by malabsorption of fat, progressive neurologic deterioration, and retinitis pigmentosa. The folds may be regularly thickened.

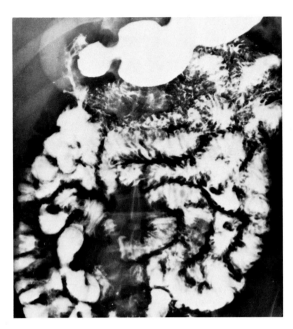

FIG GI26-5. Eosinophilic enteritis. The irregular thickening of folds primarily involves the jejunum. There is no concomitant involvement of the stomach.

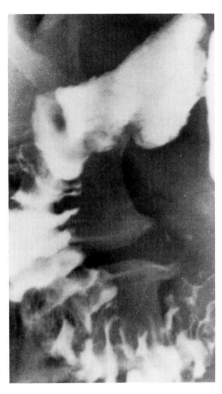

FIG GI26-6. Strongyloidiasis. Predominant involvement of the duodenal sweep.

FILLING DEFECTS IN THE JEJUNUM AND ILEUM

Condition	Imaging Findings	Comments
Benign spindle cell tumor (Fig GI27-1)	Usually a single, well-circumscribed filling defect that may ulcerate. Pedunculated tumor may cause intussusception.	Leiomyomas are most common in the jejunum; adenomas most frequently involve the ileum; lipomas primarily affect the distal ileum and the ileocecal valve area.
Hemangioma (Fig GI27-2)	Usually multiple, but often small and frequently missed on barium studies.	Combination of phleboliths and multiple filling defects in the small bowel is pathognomonic of multiple hemangiomas.
Polyposis syndrome (Fig GI27-3)	Multiple filling defects, often associated with colonic and even gastric tumors.	In Peutz-Jeghers syndrome, hamartomas are associated with mucocutaneous pigmentation. In Gardner's syndrome, adenomatous polyps are associated with osteomas and soft-tissue tumors.
Adenocarcinoma of small bowel (Fig GI27-4)	Usually a single broad-based intraluminal mass. Pedunculated polyp is extremely rare.	Most common malignant tumor of the small bowel. The tumor is usually aggressively invasive and causes luminal narrowing that soon produces obstruction.
Lymphoma (Fig GI27-5)	Discrete polypoid mass that is often large and bulky with irregular ulcerations.	Relatively infrequent manifestation of lymphoma. Multiple small or large masses can occur.
Sarcoma (Fig GI27-6)	Usually a single, large, bulky, irregular lesion, often with central ulceration.	Most tumors primarily project into the peritoneal cavity so that their major manifestation is displacement of adjacent, uninvolved barium-filled loops of small bowel.
Metastases	Usually multiple filling defects, often with central ulceration (bull's-eye appearance).	Most commonly due to melanoma and carcinomas of the breast and lung. Other tumors include Kaposi's sarcoma and primary neoplasms of the ovary, pancreas, kidney, stomach, and uterus.
Carcinoid tumor (Fig GI27-7)	Initially a small, sharply defined filling defect (often missed radiographically).	Most common primary neoplasm of the small bowel. Rule of one third (frequency of metastases, second malignancy, and multiplicity). Most often occurs in the ileum. Carcinoid syndrome (liver metastases) is infrequent.
Gallstone ileus	Single filling defect (lucent or opaque).	Classic triad of small bowel filling defect, mechanical small bowel obstruction, and gas or barium in the biliary tree.
Parasites (Fig GI27-8)	Usually multiple linear intraluminal defects. A clump of coiled worms can produce a single intraluminal filling defect.	Most commonly *Ascaris lumbricoides* (barium can fill the intestinal tract of the worm). Other parasites include *Strongyloides stercoralis*, *Ancylostoma duodenale* (hookworm), and *Taenia solis* (tapeworm).

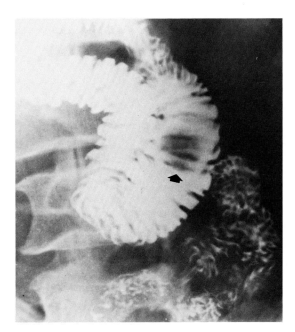

FIG GI27-1. Leiomyoma of the jejunum (arrow).[14]

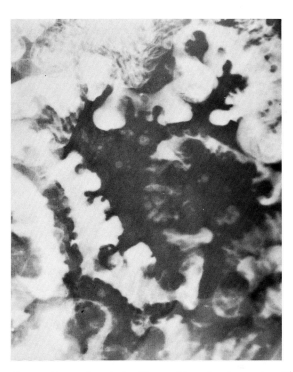

FIG GI27-2. Hemangiomatosis of the small bowel and mesentery. Characteristic phleboliths are associated with multiple filling defects in the small bowel.

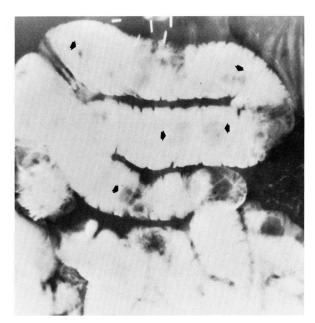

FIG GI27-3. Peutz-Jeghers syndrome. Multiple small bowel hamartomas are present in a patient with mucocutaneous pigmentation. The arrows point to a few of the many filling defects in the barium column.

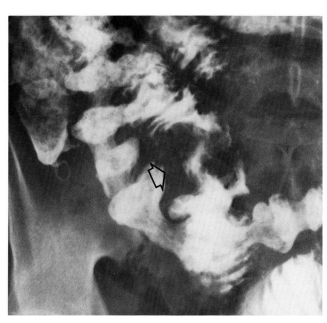

FIG GI27-4. Primary adenocarcinoma of the ileum (arrow) appearing as an annular constricting lesion.

Condition	Imaging Findings	Comments
Endometrioma	Single filling defect.	In premenopausal women with associated pelvic endometriosis.
Duplication cyst	Single filling defect.	Typically changes contour with external pressure and rarely communicates with the small bowel lumen.
Nodular lymphoid hyperplasia	Single filling defect or multiple nodules diffusely scattered through the small bowel.	Larger filling defects may mimic polypoid masses.
Ingested material	Single or multiple filling defects.	Food particles, fruit pits, foreign bodies, bezoars, and pills.

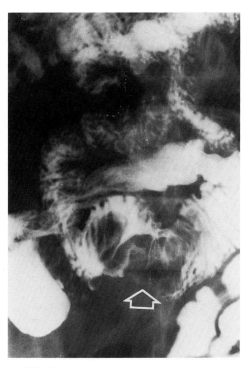

FIG GI27-5. **Lymphoma.** Large, bulky, irregular lesion.

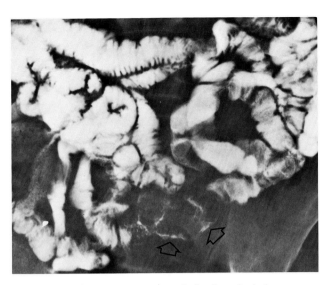

Fɪɢ GI27-6. Leiomyosarcoma. Large, bulky, irregular lesion.

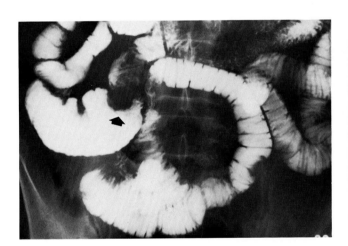

Fɪɢ GI27-7. Carcinoid tumor (arrow).

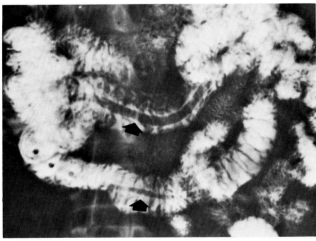

Fɪɢ GI27-8. *Ascaris lumbricoides.* On barium studies the worms appear as elongated, radiolucent filling defects (arrows).

SANDLIKE LUCENCIES IN THE SMALL BOWEL

Condition	Imaging Findings	Comments
Macroglobulinemia (Waldenström's disease) (Fig GI28-1)	Generalized involvement of the small bowel.	Plasma cell dyscrasia with a highly elevated level of immunoglobulin M (IgM) in the serum. Insidious onset in late adult life. Characterized by anemia, bleeding, lymphadenopathy, and hepatosplenomegaly.
Mastocytosis	Generalized involvement of the small bowel.	Sandlike lucencies superimposed on a generally irregular, thickened fold pattern.
Nodular lymphoid hyperplasia (Figs GI28-2 to GI28-4)	Primarily involves the jejunum, but can occur throughout the entire small bowel.	In adults, almost invariably associated with late-onset immunoglobulin deficiency. Frequently associated with *Giardia lamblia* infection and irregular thickening of folds. In children, a pattern of multiple small symmetric nodules in the terminal ileum is a normal finding and there is usually no immune deficiency.
Intestinal lymphangiectasia (Fig GI28-5)	Generalized involvement of the small bowel.	Usually the early onset of massive edema, hypoproteinemia, and lymphocytopenia.
Whipple's disease	Primarily involves the duodenum and the proximal jejunum.	Extensive infiltration of the lamina propria by large macrophages with a positive periodic acid-Schiff (PAS) reaction.
***Yersinia* enterocolitis**	Primarily involves the ileum.	Healing stage of the disease (follicular ileitis) that can persist for many months.
Histoplasmosis (Fig GI28-6)	Generalized involvement of the small bowel.	Rarely involves the gastrointestinal tract. May be superimposed on irregular, distorted folds.
Miscellaneous causes	Generalized involvement of the small bowel.	Sandlike pattern reported in eosinophilic enteritis (often with gastric involvement), Cronkhite-Canada syndrome (associated with colonic polyposis), and cystic fibrosis.

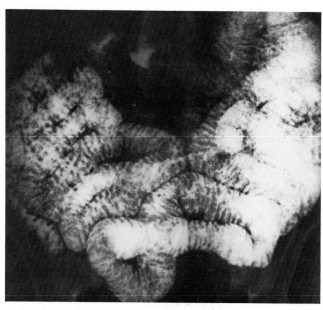

FIG GI28-1. **Waldenström's macroglobulinemia.**

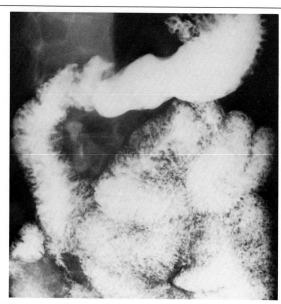

FIG GI28-2. **Nodular lymphoid hyperplasia.** Innumerable tiny polypoid masses are uniformly distributed throughout the involved segments of small bowel. The underlying fold pattern is normal. The patient showed no evidence of associated disease.

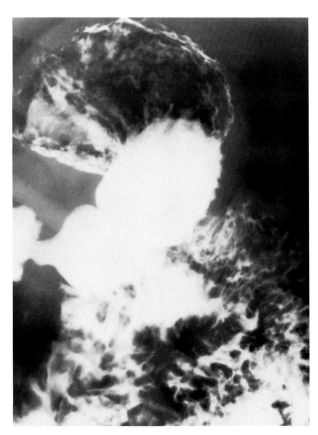

FIG GI28-3. **Nodular lymphoid hyperplasia** in a patient with an immune deficiency and *Giardia lamblia* infestation. The relatively larger nodules are superimposed on an irregularly thickened and grossly distorted underlying fold pattern.

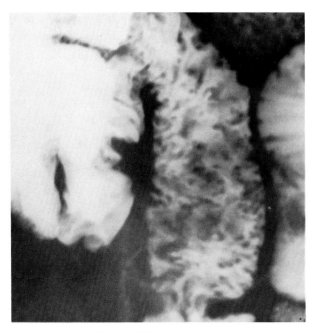

FIG GI28-4. **Normal terminal ileum in an adolescent**. The multiple small nodules represent normal prominence of lymphoid follicles.

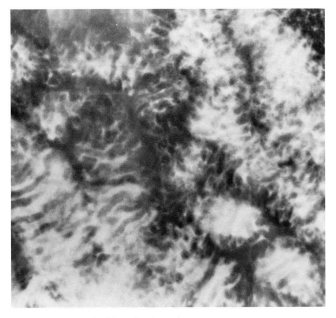

FIG GI28-5. **Intestinal lymphagiectasia.**

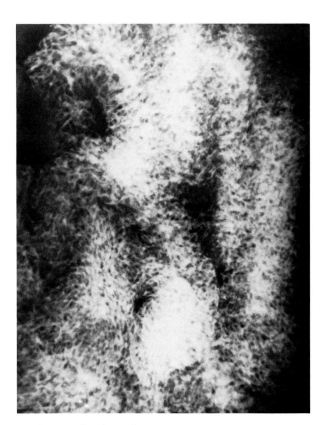

FIG GI28-6. **Histoplasmosis.**

SEPARATION OF SMALL BOWEL LOOPS

Condition	Imaging Findings	Comments
Thickening or infiltration of bowel wall or mesentery (Figs GI29-1 and GI29-2)	May be associated with extrinsic masses, luminal narrowing, and regular or irregular thickening of folds.	Causes include Crohn's disease, tuberculosis, intestinal hemorrhage or mesenteric vascular occlusion, Whipple's disease, amyloidosis, and lymphoma.
Radiation injury	May be associated with shallow mucosal ulceration, irregular fold thickening, and nodular filling defects.	Probably secondary to an endarteritis with vascular occlusion and bowel ischemia.
Carcinoid tumor (Figs GI29-3 and GI29-4)	Localized or generalized separation of loops.	Severe desmoplastic response typically produces one or several intramural nodules coexisting with a bizarre pattern of severe intestinal kinking and angulation.
Ascites	General abdominal haziness (ground-glass appearance).	Causes include hepatic cirrhosis, peritonitis, congestive failure, constrictive pericarditis, peritoneal carcinomatosis, and primary or metastatic disease of the lymphatic system.
Neoplasms	Often single or multiple mass impressions or angulated segments of small bowel.	Causes include metastases (peritoneal carcinomatosis) and primary tumors of the peritoneum and mesentery. Stretching and fixation of mucosal folds transverse to the long axis of the bowel lumen is an important sign.
Intraperitoneal abscess	Soft-tissue mass often associated with extra-luminal bowel gas (multiple small lucencies ["soap bubbles"] or linear lucencies following fascial planes).	Localized collection of pus after generalized peritonitis or a more localized intra-abdominal disease process or injury. May have adjacent localized ileus (sentinel loop).
Retractile mesenteritis (Fig GI29-5)	Bizarre pattern of diffuse separation of loops.	Fibroadipose thickening and sclerosis of the mesentery. If there is prominent fibrosis, the bowel tends to be drawn into a central mass with kinking, angulation, and conglomeration of adherent loops.
Retroperitoneal hernia (Fig GI29-6)	Separation of normal loops from loops of bowel crowded closely together in the hernia sac.	Occurs in fossae formed by peritoneal folds in para-duodenal, paracecal, or intrasigmoidal locations. The normal small bowel remains free in the peritoneal cavity.

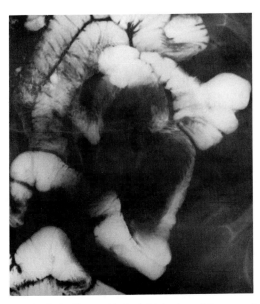

FIG GI29-1. **Crohn's disease.** Marked thickening of the mesentery and mesenteric nodes produces a lobulated mass that widely separates small bowel loops.

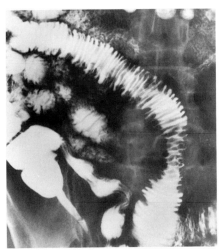

FIG GI29-2. **Intestinal hemorrhage** with bleeding into the bowel wall and mesentery.

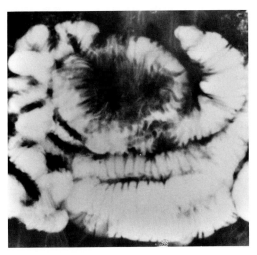

FIG GI29-3. **Carcinoid tumor.** Localized separation of bowel loops with luminal narrowing and fibrotic tethering of mucosal folds.

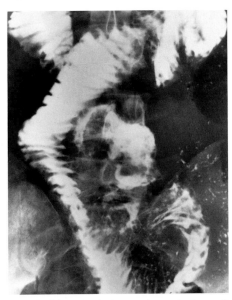

FIG GI29-4. **Carcinoid tumor.** An intense desmoplastic reaction incited by the tumor causes kinking and angulation of the bowel and separation of small bowel loops in the mid-abdomen.

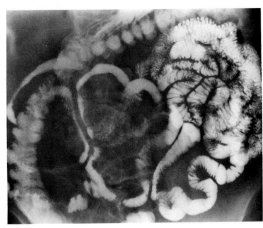

FIG GI29-5. **Retractile mesenteritis.**[15]

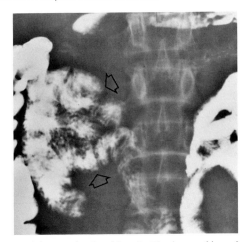

FIG GI29-6. **Right paraduodenal hernia.** The loops of bowel crowded together in the hernia sac (arrows) are widely separated from other segments of small bowel that remain free in the peritoneal cavity.

SMALL BOWEL DIVERTICULA AND PSEUDODIVERTICULA

Condition	Imaging Findings	Comments
Duodenal diverticulum	Smooth rounded shape with normal mucosal folds. Generally changes configuration during the study. Often multiple.	Incidental finding in 1% to 5% of barium examinations. Most commonly found along the medial border of the descending duodenum in the periampullary region; 30% to 40% arise in the third and fourth portions. Anomalous insertion of the common bile duct and pancreatic duct into a duodenal diverticulum can promote retrograde inflammation.
Giant duodenal ulcer (Fig GI30-1)	Rigid-walled cavity that lacks a normal mucosal pattern and remains constant in size and shape throughout the study.	Usually there is narrowing of the pylorus proximal to the giant ulcer and of the duodenum distal to the ulcer (may be severe enough to produce gastric outlet obstruction). Great propensity for perforation and massive hemorrhage (high mortality rate) unless there is a prompt diagnosis and the institution of appropriate therapy.
Pseudodiverticulum of duodenal bulb	Deformity representing spasm or fibrosis.	Exaggerated outpouchings of the inferior and superior recesses at the base of the bulb related to duodenal ulcer disease.
Intraluminal duodenal diverticulum (Fig GI30-2)	Fingerlike sac separated from contrast material in the duodenal lumen by a lucent band representing the diverticular wall (halo sign).	Related to forward pressure by food and strong peristaltic activity on a congenital duodenal web originating near the papilla of Vater.
Jejunal diverticulum (Fig GI30-3)	Usually multiple and with a wider neck than a colonic diverticulum.	May produce the blind loop syndrome with bacterial overgrowth and folic acid deficiency. A major cause of pneumoperitoneum without peritonitis or surgery. Diverticulitis is a rare complication.
Pseudodiverticula of jejunum or ileum (Fig GI30-4)	Simulate intestinal diverticula.	Occur in scleroderma (sacculations resulting from smooth muscle atrophy and fibrosis), Crohn's disease (strictures and characteristic mucosal changes), and lymphoma (fusiform aneurysmal dilatation of the bowel).
Meckel's diverticulum (Fig GI30-5)	Arises on the antimesenteric side of the ileum within 100 cm of the ileocecal valve.	Most frequent congenital anomaly of the intestinal tract. An outpouching of the rudimentary omphalomesenteric duct (embryonic communication between the gut and yolk sac that is normally obliterated in utero). May be inflamed and simulate acute appendicitis or may contain heterotopic gastric mucosa (seen on a technetium scan).
Ileal diverticulum (Fig GI30-6)	Small, often multiple, and situated in the terminal portion near the ileocecal valve.	Least common of the small bowel diverticula. Ileal diverticulitis mimics acute appendicitis.

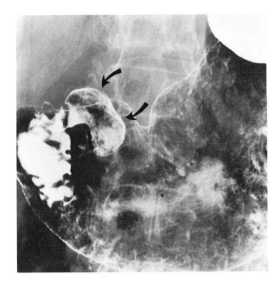

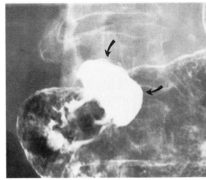

FIG GI30-1. Giant duodenal ulcer. There is little change in the appearance of the rigid-walled cavity (arrows) in air-contrast (A) and barium-filled (B) views.[16]

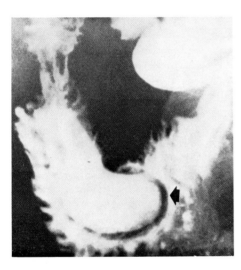

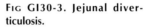

FIG GI30-2. Halo sign of intraluminal duodenal diverticulum.[17]

FIG GI30-3. Jejunal diverticulosis.

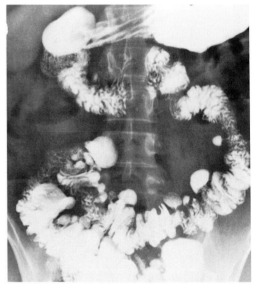

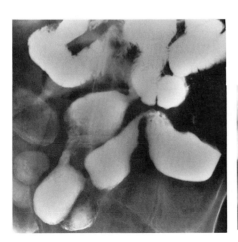

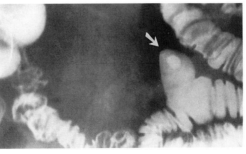

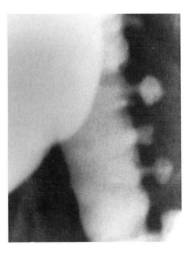

FIG GI30-4. Pseudodiverticula in Crohn's disease.

FIG GI30-5. Meckel's diverticulum (arrow) with a small diverticulum (area of increased density) arising from it.

FIG GI30-6. Ileal diverticula. Note that these diverticula are near the ileocecal valve, unlike Meckel's diverticula, which are situated more proximally.

SIMULTANEOUS FOLD THICKENING
OF THE STOMACH AND SMALL BOWEL

Condition	Imaging Findings	Comments
Lymphoma (see Figs GI16-1 and GI26-3)	Generalized, irregular fold thickening.	May also be a discrete mass or malignant ulceration in the stomach and an ulcerated filling defect, extrinsic impressions, or separation of loops in the small bowel.
Crohn's disease (see Figs GI16-3 and GI29-1)	Generalized, irregular fold thickening.	Narrowing and pseudo–Billroth-I deformity in the stomach; strictures, ulceration, cobblestoning, fistulas, and sinus tracts in the small bowel.
Eosinophilic gastroenteritis (see Fig GI26-5)	Generalized, irregular fold thickening.	Characteristic clinical pattern of food allergies and peripheral eosinophilia.
Zollinger-Ellison syndrome (Fig GI31-1)	Extreme prominence of gastric rugae, irregular thickening of folds in the proximal small bowel, and often ulcerations in unusual locations in the distal duodenum or jejunum.	Hyperrugosity reflects a hypersecretory state in response to a gastrin-secreting islet cell tumor of the pancreas. An excessive volume of acidic gastric secretions floods the small bowel and produces a chemical enteritis.
Ménétrier's disease (see Fig GI11-5)	Giant hypertrophy of gastric rugae and diffuse regular thickening of small bowel folds.	Protein-losing enteropathy associated with giant gastric folds. Hypoproteinemia results in regular thickening of small bowel folds.
Gastric varices with hypoproteinemia (see Figs GI11-8 and GI11-9)	Gastric varices with diffuse regular thickening of small bowel folds.	Gastric varices (prominent rugae or nodular fundal masses) reflect severe liver disease, which causes hypoproteinemia that results in regular thickening of small bowel folds.
Amyloidosis/ Whipple's disease (Fig GI31-2)	Generalized, irregular fold thickening.	Both conditions can also infiltrate the wall of the distal stomach and narrow the antrum.

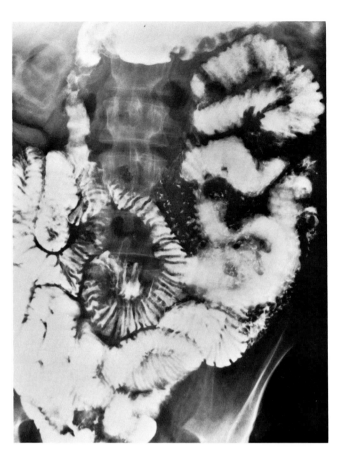

FIG GI31-1. Zollinger-Ellison syndrome. In addition to prominent thickening of gastric and duodenal folds, there is dilatation of the small bowel with excessive secretions causing the barium to have a granular, indistinct quality.

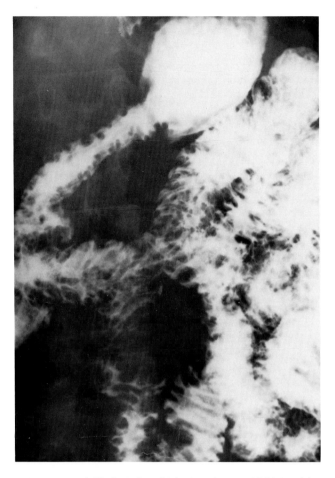

FIG GI31-2. Amyloidosis. Diffuse thickening of mucosal folds involving the stomach, duodenum, and visualized small bowel. Infiltration of amyloid into the wall of the distal stomach narrows the antrum.

CONED CECUM

Condition	Imaging Findings	Comments
Amebiasis (Fig GI32-1)	Initially, small shallow ulcers produce a finely granular mucosa and an irregular bowel margin. Eventually, the ileocecal valve is thickened, rigid, and fixed in an open position.	Cone shape represents fibrotic narrowing of the cecum, which is involved in about 90% of cases of chronic amebiasis. Terminal ileum is *not* involved (unlike Crohn's disease or tuberculosis). Rapid return to normal appearance after antiamebic therapy.
Crohn's disease (Fig GI32-2)	Narrowing and rigidity of the cecum.	Terminal ileum almost invariably involved, often with a thin, linear collection of barium (string sign) representing incomplete filling due to the irritability and spasm accompanying the severe ulceration.
Tuberculosis	Shortening and narrowing of the purse-shaped cecum.	Usually there is involvement of the terminal ileum, which may appear to empty directly into the stenotic ascending colon with nonopacification of the fibrotic, contracted cecum (Stierlin's sign).
Ulcerative colitis (Fig GI32-3)	Cecal narrowing usually limited to a short segment.	Terminal ileum involvement (backwash ileitis) in 10% to 25% of cases. Gaping ileocecal valve.
Appendicitis (see Fig GI33-1)	Eccentric defect at the base of the cecum, most commonly on its medial aspect.	Appendiceal abscess can impress the cecum and produce a cone-shaped appearance.
Carcinoma of cecum	Stiffness and rigidity of the cecal wall.	Cecum may be narrowed because of either the tumor itself or an inflammatory reaction from necrosis and perforation of the tumor.
Perforated cecal diverticulum (Fig GI32-4)	Extrinsic impression narrowing the cecum.	Walled-off pericecal abscess (mimicking acute appendicitis) from a perforated cecal diverticulum (which is uncommon, frequently solitary, and usually situated within 2 cm of the ileocecal valve).
Actinomycosis	Inflammatory narrowing of the cecum.	Uncommon infection. The combination of a palpable abdominal mass and an indolent sinus tract draining through the abdominal wall is highly suggestive of this condition.

A

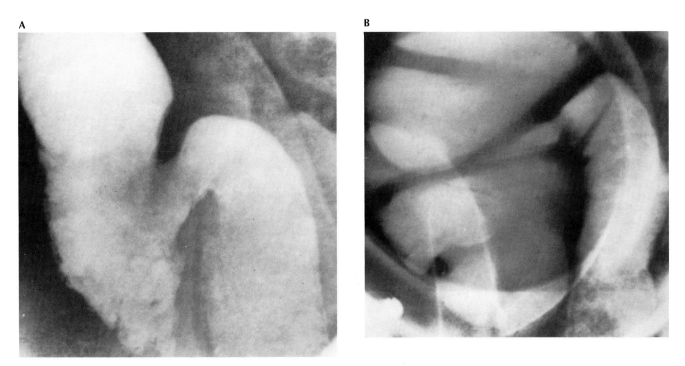

B

FIG GI32-1. Amebiasis. (A) The small, shallow ulcers produce an irregular bowel margin and finely granular mucosa. The terminal ileum is not involved. (B) After a course of antiamebic therapy, the cecum returns to a normal appearance.

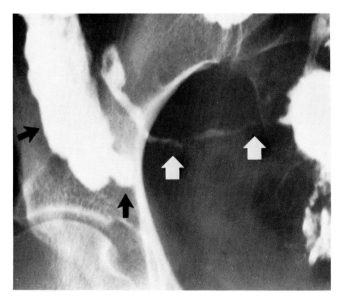

FIG GI32-2. Crohn's disease. In addition to rigid narrowing of the cecum (black arrows), there is incomplete filling of the terminal ileum (string sign; white arrows).

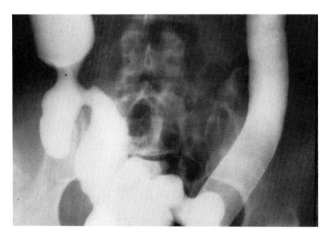

FIG GI32-3. Ulcerative colitis. Concentric narrowing of the cecum with a gaping ileocecal valve.

Condition	Imaging Findings	Comments
South American blastomycosis	Narrowing and rigidity of the cecum.	Granulomatous fungal disease caused by *Paracoccidioides brasiliensis* that also usually involves the terminal ileum (mimics Crohn's disease).
Anisakiasis (Fig GI32-5)	Narrowing and rigidity of the cecum.	Caused by an ascarislike nematode in patients eating raw fish (especially in Japan, Holland, and Scandinavia). Terminal ileum often involved.
Typhoid fever/ *Yersinia* enterocolitis (Figs GI32-6 and GI32-7)	Narrowing and irregularity of the cecum.	Most severe inflammatory changes usually involve the terminal ileum.
Treated leukemia/ lymphoma	Irritability and distortion of the cecum.	Rare, but well-recognized, complication (especially in children). Most cases are probably related to progressive ulceration and infection by enteric organisms after potent antimetabolite therapy.

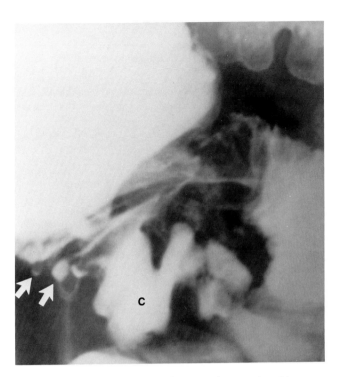

FIG GI32-4. Cecal diverticulitis. Deformity and contraction of the cecum on a barium enema examination performed about 3 weeks after the onset of symptoms in a 27-year-old man. Several diverticula (arrows) are seen along the lateral wall of the cecum (C).[18]

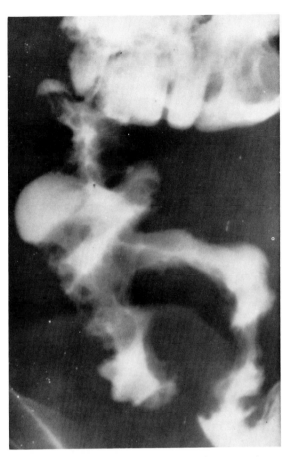

FIG GI32-5. Anisakiasis. Severe inflammatory changes in the cecum, ascending colon, and ileocecal valve in a patient who developed severe abdominal pain after eating raw fish.

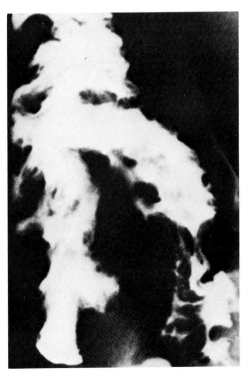

FIG GI32-6. Typhoid fever. Nodularity and irregularity of the terminal ileum with deformity of the cecum. There was a rapid return to a normal appearance after appropriate therapy.[19]

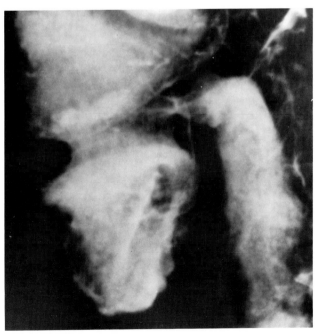

FIG GI32-7. *Yersinia* enterocolitis. Conical narrowing and irregular margins of the cecum are present with mild inflammatory changes in the terminal ileum.

FILLING DEFECTS IN THE CECUM

Condition	Imaging Findings	Comments
Appendicitis/appendiceal abscess (Figs GI33-1 and GI33-2)	Irregular extrinsic impression at the base of the cecum associated with the failure of barium to enter the appendix. If the appendix is retrocecal, the cecal impression is more proximal and is usually on its lateral aspect.	Appendicolith is virtually diagnostic and is associated with a high incidence of complications (especially perforation and abscess formation). Failure of barium to fill the appendix is *not* a reliable sign of appendicitis (occurs in 20% of normal patients).
Crohn's disease	Large extrinsic mass impinging on the cecal tip and the medial cecal wall.	Crohn's disease is rarely limited to the appendix with no evidence of terminal ileal involvement.
Inverted appendiceal stump (Fig GI33-3)	Smooth filling defect at the base of the cecum in the expected site of the appendix.	Often very prominent for several weeks after surgery until the postoperative edema and inflammation subside. May be indistinguishable from a neoplasm, especially if lobulated or irregular.
Mucocele of appendix (Fig GI33-4)	Sharply outlined, smooth-walled, broad-based filling defect indenting the lower part of the cecum. Usually on the medial side and associated with nonfilling of the appendix.	May result from proximal luminal obstruction or represent a mucinous cystadenoma. May have a mottled or rimlike calcification around the periphery. Rupture of a mucocele of the appendix (or ovary) can lead to the development of pseudomyxoma peritonei.
Myxoglobulosis	Smooth extramucosal mass impressing the cecum that is associated with the failure of barium to enter the appendix.	Rare type of mucocele composed of multiple round or oval translucent globules mixed with mucus. Characteristic finding is a calcified rim about the periphery of individual globules.
Intussusception of appendix (Fig GI33-5)	Oval, round, or fingerlike filling defect projecting into the medial wall of the cecum. Appendix is not visible.	Invagination of the appendix into the cecum that simulates a cecal tumor. Can present as an acute surgical emergency or as a subacute recurring condition.
Benign neoplasm of appendix	Small filling defect (rarely diagnosed radiographically).	About 90% are carcinoids (almost always benign; rarely metastasize or cause the carcinoid syndrome). Others are spindle cell tumors.
Malignant neoplasm of appendix (Fig GI33-6)	Extrinsic mass deforming and displacing the cecum.	Most appendiceal malignancies are adenocarcinomas. Extensive tumor may form an acute angle between the mass and the adjacent cecal wall and mimic an intramural or even an intraluminal cecal mass.

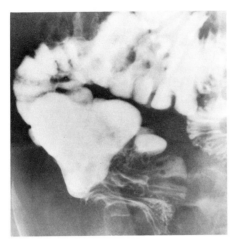

FIG GI33-1. **Periappendiceal abscess.** There is fixation and a mass effect at the base of the cecum with no filling of the appendix.

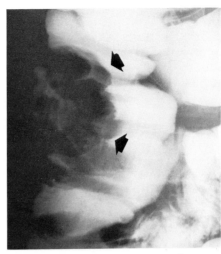

FIG GI33-2. **Periappendiceal abscess.** Severe inflammatory mucosal changes and a mass effect on the lateral aspect of the ascending colon (arrows) in a patient with a ruptured retrocecal appendix.

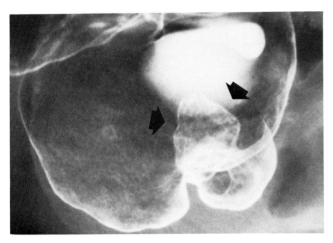

FIG GI33-3. **Inverted appendiceal stump.** In this example the mass (arrows) is large and irregular, simulating a neoplasm at the base of the cecum.

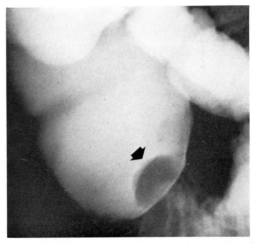

FIG GI33-4. **Mucocele of the appendix.** Smooth, broad-based filling defect (arrow) indents the lower medial part of the cecum. There is no filling of the appendix with barium.

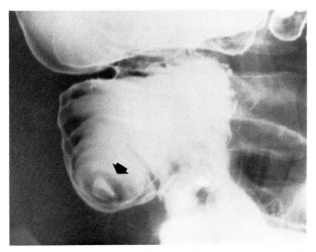

FIG GI33-5. **Intussusception of the appendix** (arrow). After reduction, the cecum and appendix appeared normal on another barium enema examination.

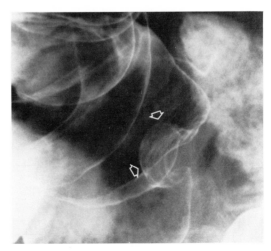

FIG GI33-6. **Adenocarcinoma of the appendix.** The extensive tumor produces a large mass (arrows) that mimics an intraluminal cecal neoplasm.

Condition	Imaging Findings	Comments
Metastases (Fig GI33-7)	Localized defect on the medial aspect of the cecum below the ileocecal valve.	Primary pancreatic carcinoma typically spreads along the mesentery to this region. Intraperitoneal seeding from carcinoma of the ovary, colon, or stomach can cause an extrinsic impression in the region of the ileocecal junction or on the lateral and posterior aspects of the cecum.
General colonic lesions	Various patterns of filling defects.	Inflammatory masses (especially ameboma), benign and malignant primary cecal neoplasms, and ileocecal intussusception.
Ileocecal diverticulitis (see Fig GI32-4)	Smooth eccentric mass that is sharply demarcated from the adjacent colonic wall.	Localized mural abscess in the wall of the colon that often occurs in young patients (unlike colonic diverticulitis) and mimics acute appendicitis. There may be extraluminal barium in a fistula or abscess cavity.
Solitary benign cecal ulcer	Filling defect simulating a discrete tumor mass.	Mass represents granulation tissue caused by the healing of a solitary benign ulcer of the cecum (the ulcer itself is infrequently detected).
Adherent fecalith (Fig GI33-8)	Persistent tumorlike mass in the cecum.	Sticky fecal material that is most commonly found in patients with cystic fibrosis and simulates a colonic neoplasm.
Endometriosis	Intramural, extramucosal lesion with a smooth surface and sharp margins.	Rarely associated with the fibrotic compression and kinking of the colon that are characteristic of the disease in the sigmoid region.
Burkitt's lymphoma (Fig GI33-9)	Large mass in the ileocecal area.	Childhood tumor of the reticuloendothelial system that may cause intussusception or obstruction (primarily reported in the North American variety).

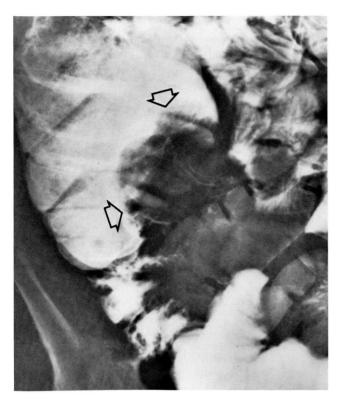

FIG GI33-7. Carcinoma of the pancreas metastatic to the cecum. There is a localized extrinsic pressure defect (arrows) on the medial and inferior aspects of the cecum and no filling of the appendix.

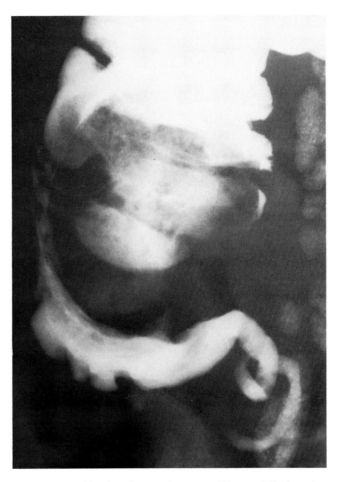

FIG GI33-9. Burkitt's lymphoma. A huge mass fills essentially the entire cecum.

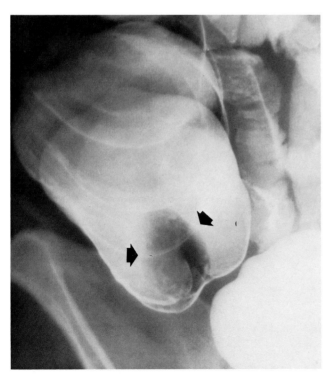

FIG GI33-8. Adherent fecalith (arrows) in cystic fibrosis.

ULCERATIVE LESIONS OF THE COLON

Condition	Imaging Findings	Comments
Ulcerative colitis (Fig GI34-1)	Initially, fine mucosal granularity. Later, discrete ulcers of various sizes symmetrically distributed around the bowel wall.	Primarily involves the rectosigmoid, though pancolitis can occur. Mild involvement of the terminal ileum (backwash ileitis) in 10% to 25% of cases. Complications include colon carcinoma, stricture formation, perforation, and toxic megacolon.
Crohn's colitis (Fig GI34-2)	Initially, aphthous ulcers on a background of normal mucosa. Later, random and asymmetric distribution of deep, irregular ulcers.	Primarily affects the proximal colon. Terminal ileal involvement in about 80% of cases. Noncontinuous skip lesions are common (never occur in ulcerative colitis) and fistulas and sinus tracts are characteristic.
Ischemic colitis (Fig GI34-3)	Initially, fine superficial ulceration. Later, deep penetrating ulcers may occur.	Characteristic clinical presentation (abrupt onset of lower abdominal pain and rectal bleeding). Most patients are over age 50 (except women taking birth control pills). Usually involves a relatively short segment (pancolitis can occur) and returns to a normal appearance (postischemic strictures can develop).
Infectious colitides **Amebiasis** (Fig GI34-4)	Initially, superficial ulcerations especially involving the cecum. Later, deep penetrating ulcers may produce a bizarre appearance.	May present as a segmental process with skip lesions (simulating Crohn's disease) or as a diffuse colitis mimicking ulcerative colitis. The terminal ileum is virtually never involved.
Schistosomiasis	Diffuse granular pattern of tiny ulcerations simulating ulcerative colitis.	Primarily involves the descending and sigmoid colon (adult worms have a predilection for invading the inferior mesenteric vein). Multiple small filling defects constitute a more characteristic appearance.
Shigellosis/ salmonellosis	Initially, diffuse fine ulcerations. Later, deep ulceration.	Frequently it is impossible to distinguish the colonic involvement of shigellosis (bacillary dysentery) from salmonellosis (food poisoning, typhoid fever). Involvement of the terminal ileum strongly suggests salmonellosis.
Tuberculous colitis	Appearance virtually indistinguishable from that of Crohn's disease.	Predominantly involves the cecum with concomitant disease in the distal ileum. May extend to affect the ascending and transverse colon. There is rarely segmental involvement in the sigmoid region.
Gonorrheal proctitis	Rectal ulceration and mucosal edema.	Barium enema examination is usually normal.
Staphylococcal colitis	Generalized ulcerating colitis.	Cause of postantibiotic diarrhea after orally administered broad-spectrum antibiotics (usually tetracycline).

(continued page 330)

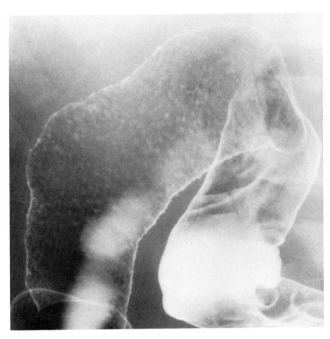

FIG GI34-1. **Early ulcerative colitis.** Fine granularity of the mucosa reflects the hyperemia and edema that are seen endoscopically.

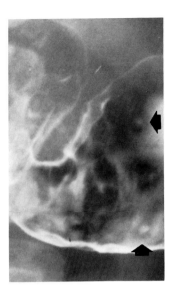

FIG GI34-2. **Aphthoid ulcers of early Crohn's colitis.** Punctate collections of barium are surrounded by lucent halos of edema (arrows).

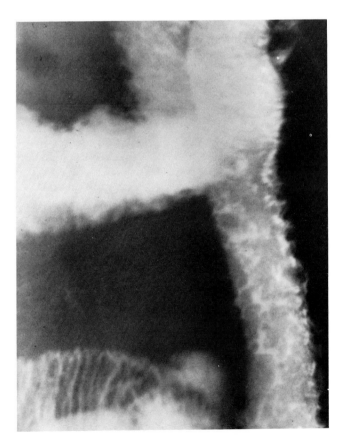

FIG GI34-3. **Ischemic colitis.** Superficial ulcers and inflammatory edema produce a serrated outer margin of the barium-filled colon simulating ulcerative colitis.

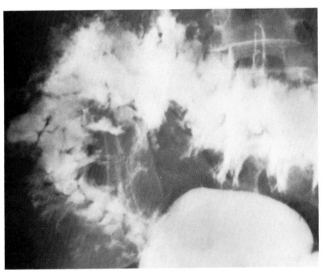

FIG GI34-4. **Amebic colitis.** Deep, penetrating ulcers produce a bizarre appearance.

Condition	Imaging Findings	Comments
Yersinia colitis (see Fig GI32-7)	Multiple small colonic ulcerations.	Primarily involves the terminal ileum and cecum (often indistinguishable from Crohn's colitis).
Campylobacter fetus colitis	Ulcerative colitis pattern.	Most common cause of specific infectious colitis. Usually self-limited and probably responsible for most single episodes of alleged ulcerative colitis.
Fungal infections	Mucosal ulcerations are occasionally identified.	Histoplasmosis, mucormycosis, actinomycosis, and candidiasis. More typical appearance is irritable bowel with irregularly thickened mucosal folds.
Lymphogranuloma venereum	Multiple shaggy ulcers primarily involving the rectum.	Venereal disease (especially common in the tropics). A rectal stricture typically develops, and fistulas and sinus tracts often occur.
Herpes zoster	Segmental ulcerating colitis.	Typical clinical history and skin lesions.
Cytomegalovirus	Ulceration primarily involves the cecum.	Major cause of severe lower gastrointestinal bleeding in renal transplant recipients undergoing immunosuppressive therapy.
Strongyloidiasis	Diffuse ulcerating colitis.	Unusual manifestation due to larval invasion of the colon wall.
Pseudomembranous colitis (Fig GI34-5)	Diffuse irregular ulceration associated with multiple flat, raised lesions.	Follows drug administration (tetracycline, penicillin, ampicillin, clindamycin, lincomycin). May reflect infection by a resistant strain of *Clostridium difficile*. The clinical hallmark is a severe debilitating diarrhea.
Radiation injury (see Fig GI35-6)	Fine superficial (occasionally deep) ulceration, primarily involving the rectosigmoid region.	Usually follows pelvic irradiation for carcinoma of the cervix, endometrium, ovary, bladder, or prostate. Strictures and fistulas often develop.
Caustic colitis (see Fig GI35-8)	Severe ulcerating process after an irritating enema (soapsuds, detergents).	Irritant enema tends to produce spasm of the rectosigmoid, resulting in rapid expulsion of the solution from this segment. Because the fluid trapped in the proximal colon is not promptly expelled, corrosive damage is most severe in this region.
Pancreatitis (Fig GI34-6)	Pattern of ulcerating colitis involving the superior margin of the transverse colon and the splenic flexure.	Close anatomic relation between the pancreas and transverse colon provides a pathway for the dissemination of pancreatic inflammatory products.
Adenocarcinoma of colon (Fig GI34-7)	Various patterns of ulceration.	May present as an excavation in a large fungating mass or as mucosal destruction in an annular apple-core tumor.

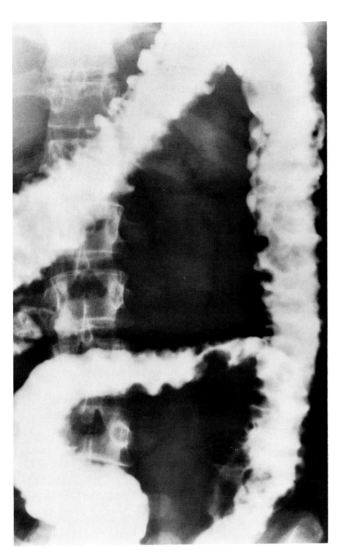

FIG GI34-5. **Pseudomembranous colitis.** The shaggy and irregular margins reflect the pseudomembrane and superficial necrosis with mucosal ulceration.

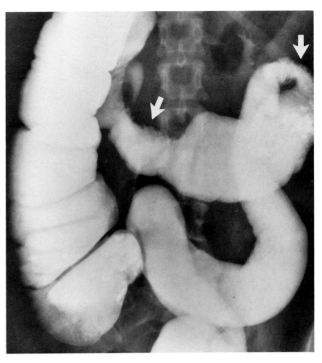

FIG GI34-6. **Pancreatitis.** Spiculation of the proximal transverse colon and splenic flexure (arrows) simulates an ulcerating colitis.

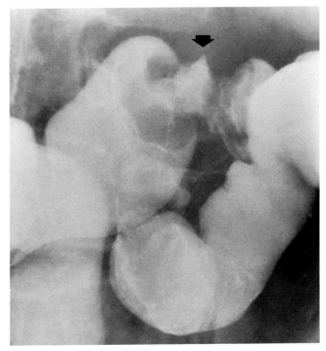

FIG GI34-7. **Ulcerated primary carcinoma** of the sigmoid colon (arrow).

Condition	Imaging Findings	Comments
Metastases (Figs GI34-8 and GI34-9)	Various patterns of ulceration.	May produce marginal and deep ulcerations associated with nodular masses and multiple eccentric strictures.
Behçet's syndrome	Various patterns of ulceration (segmental involvement by multiple discrete ulcers; diffuse ulceration).	Uncommon multiple-system disease characterized by ulceration of the buccal and genital mucosa, ocular inflammation, and a variety of skin lesions. Colitis often leads to perforation or hemorrhage.
Solitary rectal ulcer syndrome	Usually a single ulceration within 15 cm of the anal verge.	Primarily occurs in young patients complaining of rectal bleeding and may lead to stricturing. Often difficult to distinguish from inflammatory bowel disease or malignancy.
Nonspecific benign ulceration of colon (Fig GI34-10)	Usually single (20% are multiple) ulcer primarily involving the cecum and ascending colon in the region of the ileocecal valve.	Associated intense inflammatory reaction produces a masslike effect simulating carcinoma. Suggested causes include peptic ulceration, solitary diverticulitis, drugs, mucosal trauma, infection, and vascular disease.
Amyloidosis	Nonspecific ulcerating colitis.	Histologic material and special amyloid stains (Congo red) required for diagnosis.
Inorganic mercury poisoning	Nonspecific ulcerating colitis.	Clinical history and concomitant renal involvement are usually diagnostic.

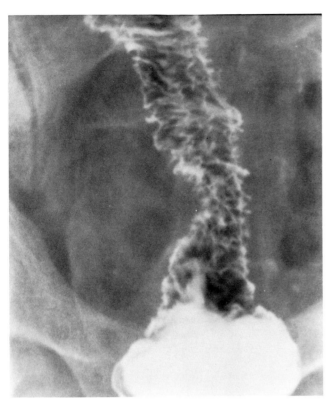

FIG GI34-8. Carcinoma of the prostate metastatic to the rectum and rectosigmoid. The diffuse circumferential ulceration mimics ulcerative colitis.

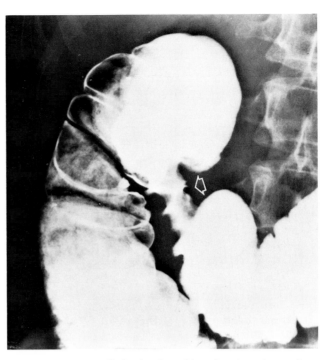

FIG GI34-10. Nonspecific benign ulcer of the colon. Area of narrowing in the proximal transverse colon with ulceration along its inferior aspect and marginal spiculation (arrow).[20]

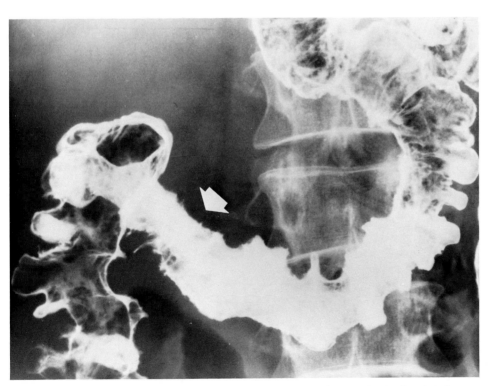

FIG GI34-9. Carcinoma of the stomach metastatic to the transverse colon. Localized right-sided ulceration and narrowing (arrow) simulate Crohn's colitis.

NARROWING OF THE COLON

Condition	Imaging Findings	Comments
Ulcerative colitis (Figs GI35-1 and GI35-2)	Rigidity and narrowing of the bowel lumen ("lead pipe" colon) with foreshortening.	Colonic strictures with smooth contours and pliable, tapering margins occur in up to 10% of patients. Carcinoma in these patients can have an indistinguishable appearance.
Crohn's colitis (Fig GI35-3)	Narrowing and stricture formation.	May appear identical to ulcerative colitis, though there are usually characteristic features of Crohn's disease elsewhere (deep ulcerations, pseudopolyposis, skip lesions, sinus tracts, fistulas).
Infectious colitides **Ischemic colitis** (Fig GI35-4)	Short segment of tubular narrowing.	Rectum is rarely involved because of its excellent collateral blood supply. May produce an annular constricting lesion simulating malignancy.
Amebiasis (Fig GI35-5)	Annular constriction (ameboma) simulating malignancy.	Localized granulomatous mass. Factors favoring ameboma rather than malignancy include multiplicity, longer length and pliability of the lesion, and rapid improvement on antiamebic therapy.
Schistosomiasis	Segmental narrowing, primarily involving the sigmoid colon.	Stenosing granulomatous process simulating Crohn's disease or colonic malignancy.
Bacillary dysentery	Segmental rigidity and tubular narrowing.	Repeated episodes can produce a pattern simulating chronic ulcerative colitis.
Tuberculosis	Segmental narrowing and rigidity.	May produce an annular ulcerating lesion mimicking carcinoma.
Lymphogranuloma venereum (see Fig GI39-2)	Rectal stricture beginning just above the anus.	Varies from a short isolated narrowing to a long stenotic segment with multiple deep ulcers. There are often associated fistulas and sinus tracts.
Other infectious causes	Various patterns of narrowing.	Herpes zoster; cytomegalovirus (in renal transplant patients undergoing immunosuppressive therapy); strongyloidiasis; fungal infestations.
Radiation injury (Fig GI35-6)	Long smooth stricture of the rectum and sigmoid colon.	Develops 6 to 24 months after irradiation. Probably related to chronic ischemia caused by an obliterative arteritis in the bowel wall. A short, irregular, radiation-induced stricture can mimic malignancy.

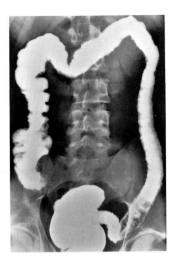

FIG GI35-1. Chronic ulcerative colitis. Fibrosis and muscular spasm cause shortening and rigidity of the colon and a loss of haustral markings.

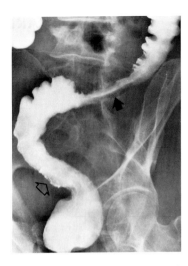

FIG GI35-2. Benign stricture in chronic ulcerative colitis. In addition to the severe narrowing in the sigmoid colon (closed arrow), there are ulcerative changes in the upper rectum and proximal sigmoid colon (open arrow).

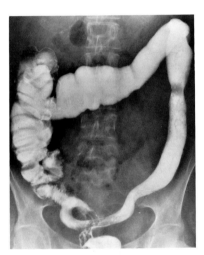

FIG GI35-3. Chronic Crohn's colitis. Foreshortening and loss of haustra involving the colon distal to the hepatic flexure simulate the appearance of chronic ulcerative colitis.

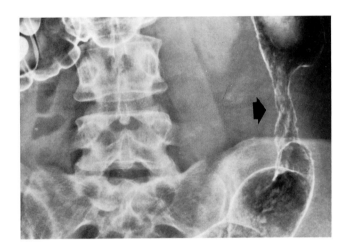

FIG GI35-4. Ischemic colitis. A stricture in the descending colon (arrow) followed healing of the ischemic episode.[21]

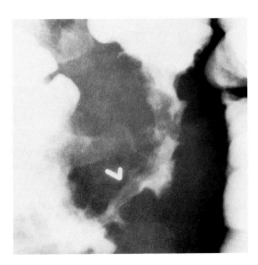

FIG GI35-5. Amebiasis. Irregular constricting lesion in the transverse colon. The relatively long area of involvement tends to favor an inflammatory etiology.

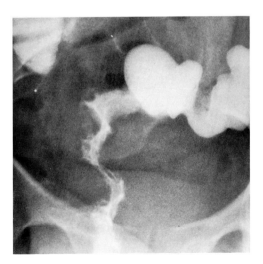

FIG GI35-6. Radiation injury. Smooth stricture of the rectosigmoid (arrow) developed 18 months after irradiation.

Condition	Imaging Findings	Comments
Cathartic colon (Fig GI35-7)	Bizarre contractions and inconstant areas of narrowing, primarily involving the right colon.	Due to the prolonged use of stimulant and irritant cathartics, especially in women of middle age. May mimic "burned-out" chronic ulcerative colitis.
Caustic colitis (Fig GI35-8)	Stricture formation primarily involving the transverse and descending colon.	Fibrosis with luminal narrowing is a late complication.
Solitary rectal ulcer syndrome	Rectal stricture.	Without previous evidence of mucosal nodularity or ulceration, it may be impossible to differentiate this condition from inflammatory bowel disease, lymphogranuloma venereum, or rectal malignancy.
Nonspecific benign ulcer of colon (see Fig GI34-10)	Smooth or irregular area of narrowing, most frequently involving the cecum.	May be radiographically indistinguishable from carcinoma. Perforation and hemorrhage are complications.
Colonic "sphincters"	Transient areas of narrowing, primarily in the transverse, descending, and sigmoid portions.	Areas of spasm that probably reflect localized nerve and muscle imbalance. Unlike annular carcinoma, colonic sphincters change on sequential films, have tapering margins and intact mucosa, and usually can be relieved by intravenous glucagon.
Annular carcinoma of colon (Fig GI35-9)	Short segment of luminal narrowing with an abrupt change from tumor to normal bowel (overhanging margins).	Initially produces a flat plaque of tumor (saddle lesion) involving only a portion of the circumference of the colon wall. In the sigmoid, an apple-core lesion may be difficult to distinguish from diverticulitis (annular carcinoma tends to be shorter with more sharply defined margins and mucosal destruction).
Scirrhous carcinoma of colon (Fig GI35-10)	Long segment (up to 12 cm) of luminal narrowing due to intense desmoplastic reaction infiltrating the bowel wall.	Rare variant of annular carcinoma with a very poor prognosis. Unlike the more common annular form, the mucosa in scirrhous carcinoma is often partially preserved and the margins of the lesion tend to taper.
Metastases (Figs GI35-11 and GI35-12)	Various patterns of narrowing. May be associated with ulceration, extrinsic masses, and a "striped colon" (transverse folds that do not completely traverse the colonic lumen).	Metastases to the colon can arise from direct invasion (prostate, ovary, uterus; stomach and pancreas via mesenteric reflections), intraperitoneal seeding (especially involving the pouch of Douglas, inferomedial border of the cecum, right paracolic gutter, and sigmoid mesocolon), hematogenous spread (especially breast carcinoma; infrequently lung and melanoma), or lymphangitic spread.
Carcinoma complicating other conditions (Fig GI35-13)	Various patterns of narrowing.	Ulcerative colitis (filiform stricture); Crohn's colitis (fungating mass); ureterosigmoidostomy (adjacent to the urine-diverting stoma).

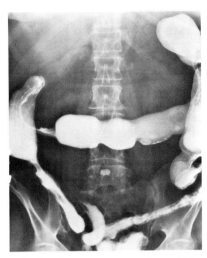

FIG GI35-7. Cathartic colon. Bizarre contractions with irregular areas of narrowing primarily involve the right colon. Although the ileocecal valve is gaping, simulating ulcerative colitis, no ulcerations are identified.

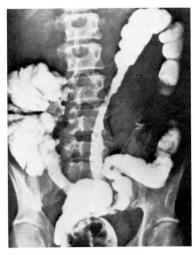

FIG GI35-8. Caustic colitis. Narrowing of the midtransverse colon 2 months after a detergent enema.[22]

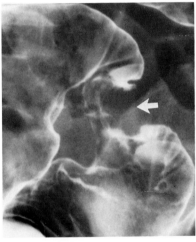

FIG GI35-9. Annular carcinoma of the sigmoid colon. The relatively short lesion (arrow) has sharply defined proximal and distal margins.

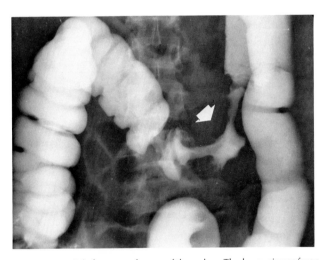

FIG GI35-10. Scirrhous carcinoma of the colon. The long, circumferentially narrowed area (arrow) simulates segmental colonic encasement due to metastatic disease.

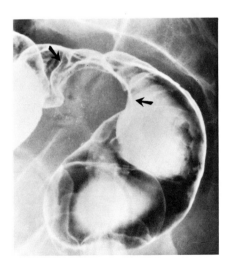

FIG GI35-11. Intraperitoneal metastases from carcinoma of the pancreas. The nodular mass in the region of the pouch of Douglas (arrows) was clinically palpable (Blumer's shelf).

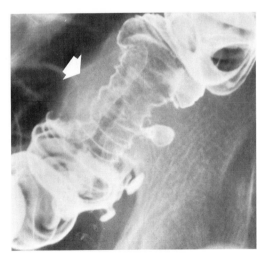

FIG GI35-12. Intraperitoneal seeding of undifferentiated carcinoma involving the sigmoid mesocolon. There is a mass effect and tethering localized to the superior border of the sigmoid colon (arrow).

Condition	Imaging Findings	Comments
Carcinoid tumor	Infiltrating, constricting lesion.	Infrequent presentation (usually produces a polypoid mass).
Lymphoma	Localized annular narrowing.	Rare presentation (more commonly a polypoid mass or diffuse infiltration).
Diverticulitis (Fig GI35-14)	Eccentric narrowing or severe spasm. Definitive diagnosis requires evidence of diverticular perforation (extravasation or a pericolic mass due to a localized abscess).	May be indistinguishable from carcinoma (diverticulitis is usually longer with intact, though often distorted, mucosa and tapering margins).
Pancreatitis	Narrowing primarily involving the distal transverse colon and splenic flexure.	Reflects the spread of liberated digestive enzymes along the mesenteric attachments joining the pancreas and transverse colon. May simulate pancreatic or colon carcinoma.
Amyloidosis	Narrowing and rigidity, primarily in the rectum and sigmoid.	Thickening of the bowel wall due to direct mural deposition of amyloid or secondary to ischemic colitis. May mimic chronic ulcerative colitis.
Endometriosis	Smooth constriction, usually involving the rectosigmoid.	Occurs in women of childbearing age. May simulate malignancy but is usually longer with more tapering margins and an intact mucosa.
Pelvic lipomatosis	Vertical elongation of the sigmoid colon with narrowing of the rectosigmoid. Increased pelvic lucency on plain films.	Benign increased deposition of normal, mature adipose tissue in the pelvis. Almost all cases occur in men. Teardrop bladder. The major complication is urinary tract obstruction.
Retractile mesenteritis (see Fig GI29-5)	Narrowing of the rectosigmoid simulating pelvic carcinomatosis.	Rare condition in which fibroadipose proliferation causes thickening and retraction of the mesentery. Usually involves the small bowel rather than the colon.
Adhesive bands	Short, smooth areas of circumferential narrowing with normal mucosal contours.	Most bands are due to previous abdominal or pelvic surgery, though some are secondary to development of the mesentery or to inflammatory disease of the appendices epiploicae.
Site of surgical anastomosis	Smooth segmental narrowing.	Distensibility of the narrowed area and a history of previous surgery permit distinction from a malignant process.

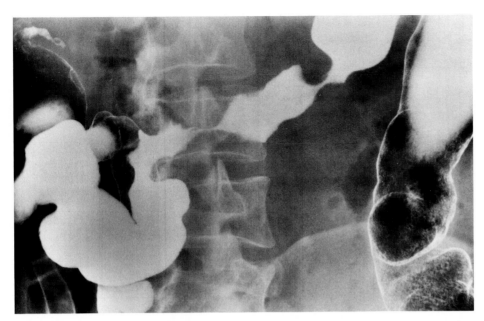

FIG GI35-13. **Carcinoma of the colon** developing in a patient with long-standing chronic ulcerative colitis. There is a long, irregular lesion with a bizarre pattern in the transverse colon. Note the pseudopolyps in the visualized portion of the descending colon.

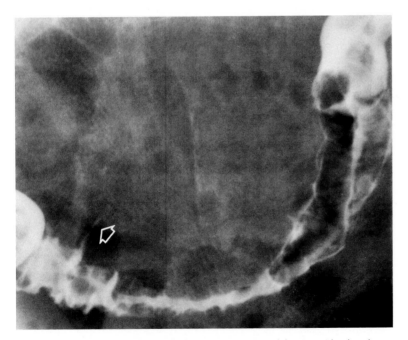

FIG GI35-14. **Acute sigmoid diverticulitis.** Severe spasm of the sigmoid colon due to the intense adjacent inflammation. Note the thin projection of contrast material (arrow) representing extravasation from the colonic lumen.

FILLING DEFECTS IN THE COLON

Condition	Imaging Findings	Comments
Hyperplastic polyp	Smooth, sessile mucosal elevation less than 5 mm in size.	Constitutes more than 90% of all colonic polyps. No malignant potential.
Adenomatous polyp (Fig GI36-1)	Sessile, protuberant, or pedunculated appearance; often multiple. An increasing incidence with advancing age.	Premalignant condition. Adenomas measuring 5 to 9 mm have a 1% probability of containing invasive malignancy. Polyps measuring 1 to 2 cm have a 4% to 10% incidence of malignancy. Polyps more than 2 cm in diameter have a 20% to 40% incidence of malignancy.
Carcinoma (Fig GI36-2)	Various appearances (saddle lesion, discrete intraluminal polyp, annular constriction). Often ulcerated. There is a 1% risk of multiple synchronous colon cancers and a 3% risk of metachronous cancers.	Signs of malignancy include large size; irregular or lobulated surface; retraction (puckering) of the colon wall on profile view; interval growth or change in shape; and short, thick, irregular stalk (if pedunculated).
Villous adenoma (Fig GI36-3)	Bulky mass with barium filling the interstices of the tumor. Usually solitary.	Some 40% have infiltrating carcinoma (usually at the base). There may be mucous diarrhea causing severe fluid, protein, and electrolyte (especially potassium) depletion.
Lipoma (Fig GI36-4)	Smooth submucosal filling defect that is usually single and most often involves the right colon.	Second most common benign colonic tumor. Fatty consistency makes the tumor changeable in size and shape with palpation. Other spindle cell tumors are rare.
Carcinoid tumor (Fig GI36-5)	Small (<1 cm), solitary, polypoid filling defect in the rectum.	Metastases develop in about 10% of patients (primarily when lesions are larger than 2 cm). Most are asymptomatic and found incidentally (rarely cause the carcinoid syndrome).
Metastases (Figs GI36-6 and GI36-7)	Filling defects that are most commonly multiple.	Major primary sites include the breast, lung, stomach, ovary, pancreas, and uterus. Also melanoma.
Lymphoma (Fig GI36-8)	Single (rarely multiple) bulky polypoid mass.	Unlike carcinoma, lymphoma often produces a large mass or extensively infiltrates a longer segment of the colon.

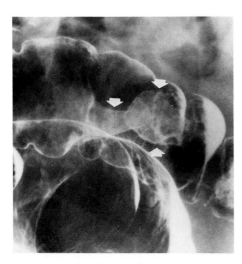

FIG GI36-1. **Pedunculated colonic polyp** (arrows).

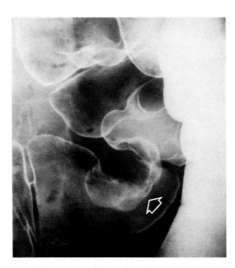

FIG GI36-2. **Saddle cancer of the colon.** The tumor (arrow) appears to sit on the upper margin of the distal transverse colon like a saddle on a horse.

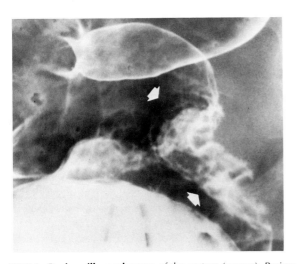

FIG GI36-3. **Benign villous adenoma** of the rectum (arrows). Barium is seen filling the deep clefts between the multiple fronds.

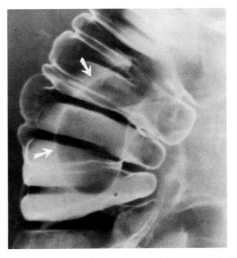

FIG GI36-4. **Lipoma.** Ascending colon mass that is extremely lucent and has smooth margins and a teardrop shape (arrows).

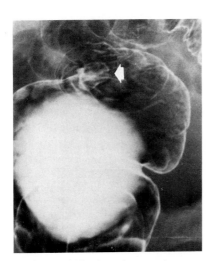

FIG GI36-5. **Rectal carcinoid.** The submucosal mass presents radiographically as a sessile polyp protruding into the lumen (arrow).

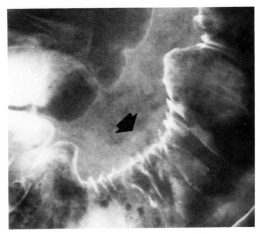

FIG GI36-6. **Carcinoma of the pancreas metastatic to the transverse colon.** Shallow extrinsic pressure defect with multiple spiculations (arrows).

Condition	Imaging Findings	Comments
Polyposis syndromes		
Familial polyposis (Figs GI36-9 and GI36-10)	Multiple adenomatous polyps.	Inherited disorder (autosomal dominant) with a 100% risk of developing colorectal cancer.
Gardner's syndrome (Fig GI36-11)	Multiple adenomatous polyps.	Inherited disorder (autosomal dominant) with a 100% risk of developing colorectal cancer. There are often sinus osteomas and soft-tissue tumors.
Peutz-Jeghers syndrome	Multiple hamartomatous polyps (primarily involving the small bowel).	Inherited disorder (autosomal dominant) with no malignant potential (2% of patients develop gastrointestinal carcinoma elsewhere; 5% of women have ovarian cysts or tumors). Characteristic abnormal mucocutaneous pigmentation (especially affecting the lips and buccal mucosa).
Turcot syndrome	Multiple adenomatous polyps.	Extremely rare. Polyps are associated with brain tumors (usually supratentorial glioblastoma).
Cronkhite-Canada syndrome	Multiple hamartomatous juvenile polyps.	No malignant potential. Presents later in life with malabsorption and severe diarrhea. Associated hyperpigmentation, alopecia, and atrophy of the fingernails and toenails.
Multiple juvenile polyps	Multiple hamartomatous polyps.	Childhood disorder with no malignant potential (polyps tend to autoamputate or regress). Surgery is indicated only if there are significant or repeated episodes of rectal bleeding or intussusception.
Cowden's disease	Multiple hamartomatous polyps.	Rare hereditary disorder associated with multiple malformations and tumors of various organs. Typically there is circumoral papillomatosis and nodular gingival hyperplasia.
Inflammatory pseudopolyposis (Fig GI36-12)	Islands of hyperplastic, inflamed mucosa (between areas of ulceration) mimicking multiple filling defects. Occasionally a large single inflammatory pseudopolyp.	Most commonly a manifestation of ulcerative colitis and Crohn's colitis. Usually there is other radiographic evidence of the inflammatory process (ulceration, absence or irregularity of haustral folds, luminal narrowing) and a history of chronic diarrhea. A similar pattern may develop in infectious colitis (amebiasis, schistosomiasis, strongyloidiasis, trichuriasis).
Ameboma	Single or multiple polypoid filling defects.	Focal hyperplastic granuloma (secondary bacterial infection of an amebic abscess in the bowel wall). Usually produces an annular, nondistensible lesion with irregular mucosa simulating colonic carcinoma.
Fecal material (Fig GI36-13)	Innumerable filling defects or a single large, irregular intraluminal mass (impaction).	Usually freely movable (occasionally tightly adherent and resembling a polyp). Plain radiographs are usually diagnostic of fecal impaction (soft-tissue density in the rectum containing multiple small, irregular lucent areas reflecting pockets of gas in the fecal mass).

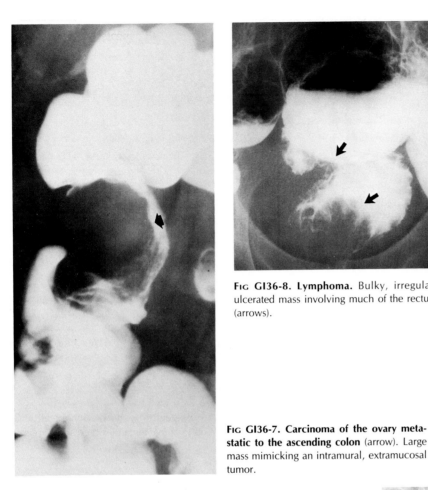

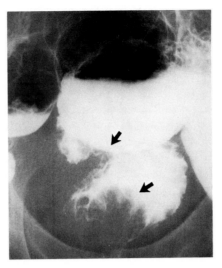

FIG GI36-8. Lymphoma. Bulky, irregular, ulcerated mass involving much of the rectum (arrows).

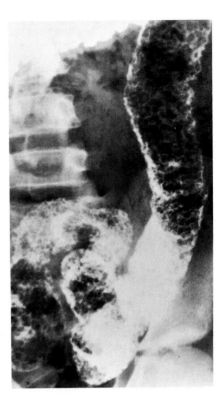

FIG GI36-9. Familial polyposis.

FIG GI36-7. Carcinoma of the ovary metastatic to the ascending colon (arrow). Large mass mimicking an intramural, extramucosal tumor.

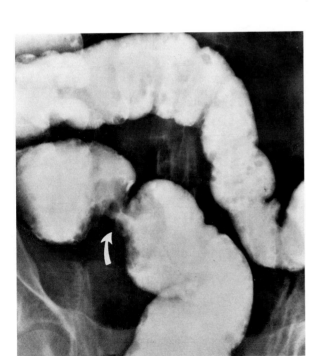

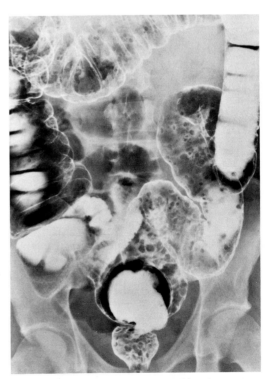

FIG GI36-10. Carcinoma of the sigmoid (arrow) developing in a patient with long-standing familial polyposis.

FIG GI36-11. Gardner's syndrome. Innumerable adenomatous polyps throughout the colon present a radiographic appearance indistinguishable from that of familial polyposis.

Condition	Imaging Findings	Comments
Other artifacts; foreign bodies	Bizarre array of multiple filling defects.	Air bubbles; mucous strands (long and slender); ingested foreign bodies.
Endometriosis (Fig GI36-14)	Single or multiple intramural defects involving the sigmoid colon.	Extrauterine foci of endometrium in women of child-bearing age. May cause pleating of the adjacent mucosa (secondary fibrosis) or present as a constricting lesion simulating annular carcinoma.
Intussusception (Fig GI36-15)	Mass causing obstruction to the retrograde flow of barium. Often the characteristic coiled-spring appearance.	Most occur in children (under age 2) and are ileocolic without a specific leading point. Frequently can be reduced by the increased hydrostatic pressure of a carefully performed barium enema examination.
Gallstone (see Fig GI53-2)	Filling defect in the rectum or distal sigmoid. May contain laminated calcification.	Rare. The gallstone enters the bowel via a cholecystoduodenal fistula (passing through the terminal ileum) or a direct cholecystocolic fistula.
Internal hemorrhoids (Fig GI36-16)	Multiple rectal filling defects simulating polyps.	Usually associated with linear shadows of the veins from which they arise.
Diverticulum	Barium-coated, air-filled diverticulum may mimic a filling defect.	Ring of barium coating a diverticulum has a smooth, well-defined outer border and a blurred, irregular inner border (opposite of a polyp). ''Filling defects'' can be projected clear of the colonic lumen on oblique views.
Pneumatosis intestinalis (see Fig GI37-4)	Intramural collections of gas simulating multiple colonic polyps.	''Filling defects'' are extremely lucent and change shape when the abdomen is palpated.
Colitis cystica profunda	Multiple irregular filling defects in the rectosigmoid. Single rectal mass may mimic a sessile polyp.	Large submucosal, mucous epithelium–lined cysts involving a short segment of the bowel. Benign condition with no malignant potential.
Nodular lymphoid hyperplasia (Fig GI36-17)	Multiple tiny (2 mm), nodular filling defects evenly distributed throughout the involved bowel.	Aggregates of lymphoid tissue that can simulate familial polyposis, pseudopolyposis of inflammatory bowel disease, or nodular lymphoma. Characteristic fleck of barium in the center of each ''polyp'' (umbilication at the apices of the lymphoid nodules).
Lymphoid follicular pattern (Fig GI36-18)	Multiple tiny nodular filling defects evenly distributed throughout the involved bowel.	Normal finding in children. Also occurs in 10% to 15% of adults on double-contrast examination. No flecks of barium in the centers of the ''polyps.''

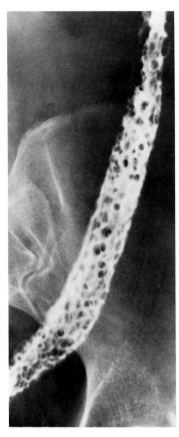

Fɪɢ GI36-12. Inflammatory pseudopolyposis in Crohn's colitis.

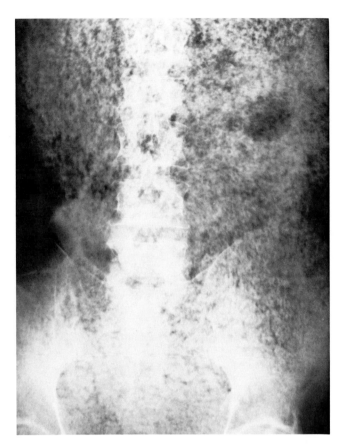

Fɪɢ GI36-13. Fecal impaction.

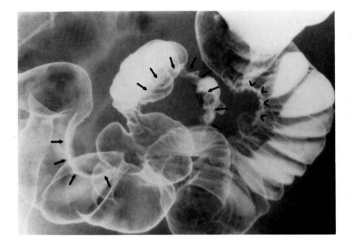

Fɪɢ GI36-14. Endometriosis. Three separate endometrial implants (arrows and arrowheads) in the sigmoid colon. The most distal lesion has a smooth interface with the bowel wall, indicating no intramural invasion. The two more proximal lesions demonstrate crenulations indicating intramural or submucosal invasion.[23]

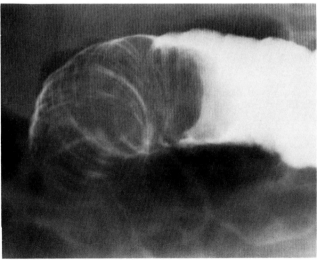

Fɪɢ GI36-15. Intussusception. Obstruction of the colon at the hepatic flexure. Note the characteristic coiled-spring appearance.

Condition	Imaging Findings	Comments
Cystic fibrosis	Multiple poorly defined filling defects simulating polyposis.	Adherent collections of viscid mucus that can rarely be adequately cleansed before a barium enema examination.
Submucosal edema pattern (Fig GI36-19)	Large, round or polygonal, raised plaques in grossly dilated bowel.	Initially described as ''colonic urticaria'' (hypersensitivity reaction predominantly involving the right colon). Can also occur secondary to obstructing carcinoma, cecal volvulus, ischemia, colonic ileus, benign colonic obstruction, and herpes zoster infection.
Ulcerative pseudopolyps proximal to an obstruction	Prominent nodularity with pseudopolyp formation (simulates ulcerating colitis).	Probably caused by ischemia (due to distension of the bowel with decreased bowel flow). Bowel distal to the point of obstruction appears normal.
Amyloidosis	Single or multiple discrete filling defects.	Single collection of amyloid usually involves the rectum and simulates a neoplasm.

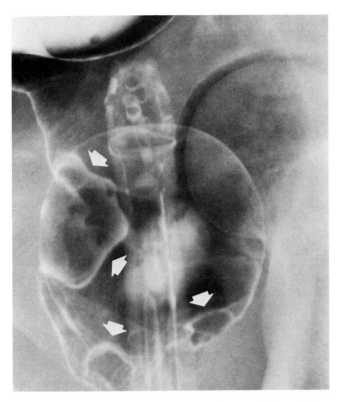

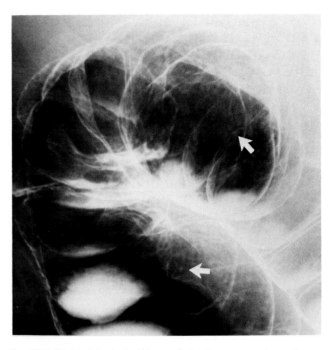

FIG GI36-17. Nodular lyphoid hyperplasia. The arrows point to characteristic flecks of barium in the centers of several of the lymphoid masses.

FIG GI36-16. Internal hemorrhoids. Multiple rectal filling defects (arrows) simulate polyps.

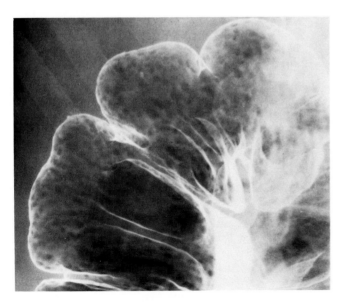

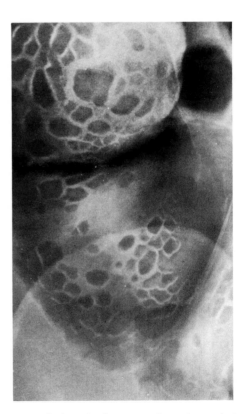

FIG GI36-18. Lymphoid follicular pattern in an adult.[24]

FIG GI36-19. Colonic urticaria. Large polygonal, raised plaques in a dilated cecum and ascending colon.

THUMBPRINTING OF THE COLON*

Condition	Comments
Ischemic colitis (Fig GI37-1)	Segmental involvement resulting from occlusive vascular disease or intramural hemorrhage (anticoagulant overdose, bleeding diathesis). Usually reverts to a normal radiographic appearance if good collateral circulation is established. May heal by stricture formation.
Ulcerative colitis and Crohn's colitis	Multiple symmetric contour defects simulating thumbprinting. Usually involves the rectum in ulcerative colitis (rectal involvement is infrequent in ischemic colitis). Transverse linear ulcers, skip areas, and terminal ileal disease suggest Crohn's colitis.
Infectious colitis	Rare manifestation of amebiasis, schistosomiasis, strongyloidiasis, salmonellosis, and cytomegalovirus.
Pseudomembranous colitis (Fig GI37-2)	Generalized thumbprinting involving the entire colon, unlike the segmental pattern in ischemic disease. Develops after a course of antibiotic therapy, with the thumbprinting reflecting marked thickening of the bowel wall.
Malignant lesion (Fig GI37-3)	Often asymmetric or irregular pattern of thumbprinting that is caused by submucosal cellular infiltrate in lymphoma and hematogenous metastases. Insidious onset, unlike the acute presentation of ischemic colitis.
Endometriosis	Multiple intramural filling defects simulating thumbprinting that develop in women of childbearing age.
Amyloidosis	Deposition of amyloid in the submucosal layer of the colon.
Pneumatosis intestinalis (Fig GI37-4)	The polypoid masses indenting the barium column are composed of air rather than soft-tissue density.
Diverticulosis	Accordionlike effect simulating thumbprinting that reflects accentuated haustral markings due to extensive muscular hypertrophy of the bowel wall. There are usually multiple diverticula and evidence of muscular thickening and spasm.
Hereditary angioneurotic edema	Thumbprinting pattern develops during acute attacks and reverts to a normal radiographic appearance once the acute episode subsides.

*Pattern: Sharply defined, fingerlike marginal indentations along the wall of the colon.

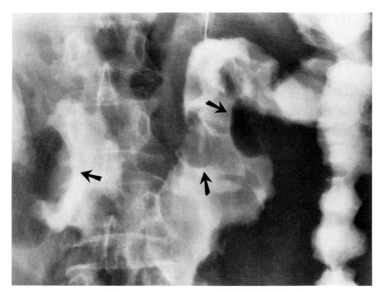

FIG GI37-1. **Ischemic colitis.** Multiple filling defects (arrows) indent the margins of the transverse and descending portions of the colon.

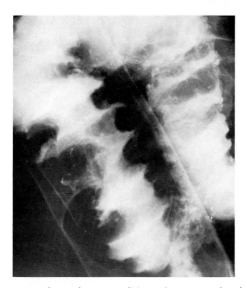

FIG GI37-2. **Pseudomembranous colitis.** Wide transverse bands of mural thickening.[25]

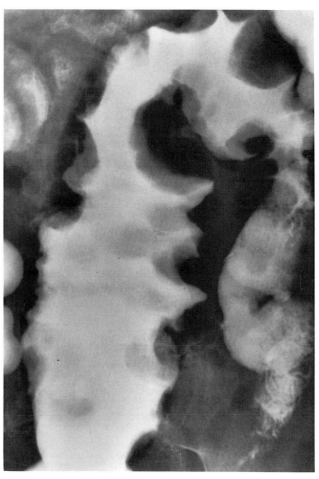

FIG GI37-4. **Pneumatosis intestinalis.** The polypoid masses indenting the barium column are composed of air rather than soft-tissue density.

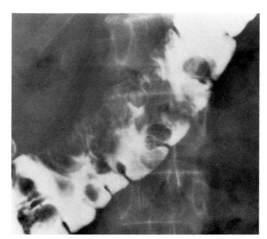

FIG GI37-3. **Lymphoma.** Submucosal cellular infiltrate produces the radiographic pattern of thumbprinting.

DOUBLE TRACKING IN THE COLON

Condition	Comments
Diverticulitis **(Figs GI38-1 and GI38-2)**	Primarily involves the sigmoid region. Represents a dissecting sinus tract that probably resulted from multiple fistulous communications with a paracolic diverticular abscess.
Crohn's disease **(Fig GI38-3)**	Long extraluminal sinus tract that may be indistinguishable from diverticulitis both clinically and radiographically. Ulceration, edematous and distorted folds, and other sites of colon involvement suggest Crohn's disease.
Carcinoma of colon **(Fig GI38-4)**	Primarily involves the sigmoid colon. Caused by transmural ulceration leading to perforation with abscess formation in the pericolic fat. Difficult to distinguish from diverticulitis unless there is clear radiographic evidence of bowel inflammation.

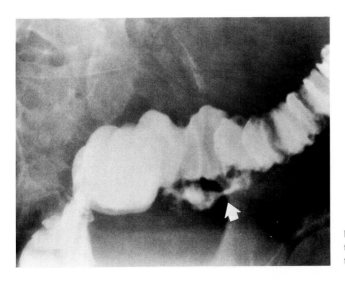

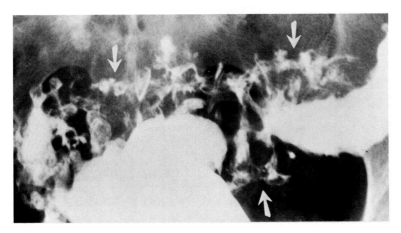

Fig GI38-1. **Dissecting peridiverticulitis.** There is a short extraluminal track (arrow) along the antimesocolic border of the sigmoid colon. Note the apparent absence of other demonstrable diverticula.

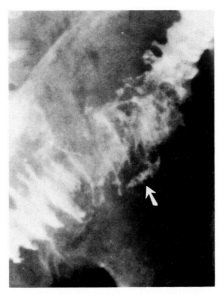

Fig GI38-2. **Dissecting peridiverticulitis.** There is diffuse sigmoid involvement with extraluminal tracks extending along both the mesocolic (upper arrows) and antimesocolic (lower arrow) borders.

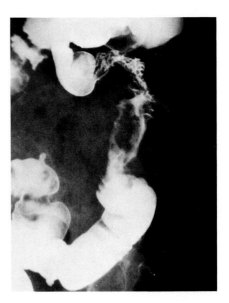

Fig GI38-3. **Crohn's colitis** grafted on diverticulosis. A 1.5-cm track of barium (arrow) is visible along the antimesocolic border of the sigmoid. The mucosal fold pattern appears granular and ulcerated and multiple diverticula are apparent.[26]

Fig GI38-4. **Primary carcinoma** of the distal descending colon producing a double-track appearance due to transmural perforation.[26]

ENLARGEMENT OF THE RETRORECTAL SPACE

Condition	Imaging Findings	Comments
Normal variant (Fig GI39-1)	Widening of the retrorectal space with no evidence of an abnormality of the rectum, sacrum, or presacral soft tissues.	More than one third of individuals have an "enlarged" retrorectal space (>1.5 cm) with no underlying abnormality. Most are large or obese.
Inflammatory bowel disease (Fig GI39-2)	Rectal involvement (ulceration, narrowing).	Most commonly due to ulcerative colitis. Other causes include Crohn's disease and, infrequently, tuberculosis, amebiasis, lymphogranuloma venereum, radiation, or ischemia. Rarely retrorectal abscess from diverticulitis, perforated appendix, malignant perforation, or infected developmental cyst.
Benign retrorectal tumor	Smooth extrinsic impression on the posterior wall. Overlying rectal mucosa remains intact.	Most commonly due to a developmental cyst (especially dermoid cyst). Rare causes include lipomas and hemangioendotheliomas.
Primary or metastatic malignancy (Fig GI39-3)	Irregular narrowing of the rectum. There may be mucosal destruction and shelf formation (even with metastases).	Almost all primary tumors are adenocarcinomas (rare lymphomas, sarcomas, cloacogenic carcinomas). Metastases include carcinomas of the prostate, bladder, cervix, and ovary. It may be difficult to distinguish a widened retrorectal space caused by radiation effects from that due to recurrent tumor.
Neurogenic tumor	Anterior displacement of the rectum without bowel wall invasion.	Chordomas often cause expansion and destruction of the sacrum (50% show amorphous calcifications). A neurofibroma arising in a sacral foramen can enlarge and distort it.
Sacral tumor	Various abnormalities involving the sacrum.	Primary and secondary malignancies cause bone destruction; an anterior sacral meningocele is associated with an anomalous sacrum; and sacrococcygeal teratomas frequently contain calcification.
Pelvic lipomatosis/ Cushing's disease	Narrowed rectum with an excessively lucent retrorectal space.	Massive deposition of fat in the pelvis.
Previous sacral fracture	Evidence of an old sacral fracture.	Bleeding into the presacral soft tissues causes a widened retrorectal space.
Colitis cystica profunda	Multiple intraluminal filling defects in the rectum.	Filling defects represent cystic dilatation of colonic mucus glands.
Partial sigmoid resection (Fig GI39-4)	Shortening of the rectosigmoid colon.	Operative trauma alters the normal anatomic relations in the pelvis.

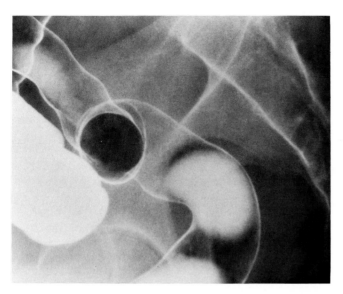

FIG GI39-1. **Normal variant.** Although the retrorectal space measured 2 cm, the patient had no abnormality by clinical history, digital rectal examination, or proctoscopy.

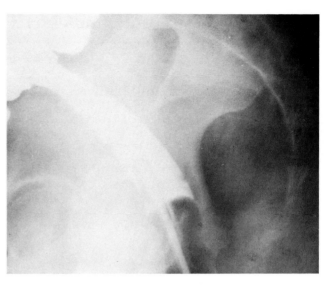

FIG GI39-2. **Lymphogranuloma venereum.** Characteristic smooth narrowing of the rectum with widening of the retrorectal space.

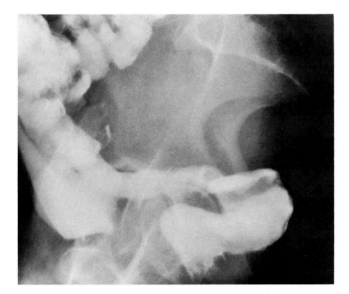

FIG GI39-3. **Lymphoma.** Marked widening of the retrorectal space with narrowing of a long segment of the rectosigmoid.

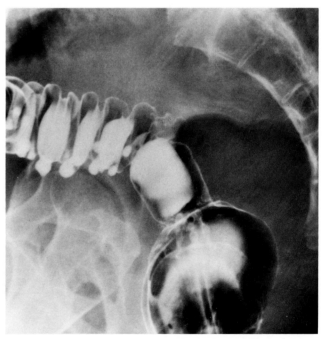

FIG GI39-4. **Sigmoid resection for carcinoma.** Widening of the retrorectal space is due to operative trauma altering the normal anatomic relations in the pelvis.

ALTERATIONS IN GALLBLADDER SIZE

Condition	Imaging Findings	Comments
Courvoisier phenomenon (Fig GI40-1)	Enlarged gallbladder.	Caused by extrahepatic neoplastic disease (arising in the head of the pancreas, duodenal papilla, ampulla of Vater, or lower common bile duct). Usually produces jaundice and a nontender, palpable gallbladder.
Hydrops/empyema	Enlarged gallbladder.	Complications of acute cholecystitis. No jaundice.
Vagotomy	Enlarged gallbladder.	No evidence of biliary tract obstruction. Size of the gallbladder in the resting state is about twice normal after a truncal vagotomy.
Diabetes mellitus	Enlarged gallbladder.	Seen in 20% of patients with diabetes and probably reflects an autonomic neuropathy. Increased incidence of gallstones.
Chronic cholecystitis (Fig GI40-2)	Small, shrunken gallbladder.	Thickening and fibrous contraction of the gallbladder wall.
Cystic fibrosis	Small, contracted gallbladder.	In 30% to 50% of patients with cystic fibrosis, the gallbladder has multiple weblike trabeculations and is filled with thick, tenacious, colorless bile and mucus. Increased incidence of gallstones.
Congenital multiseptate gallbladder	Small gallbladder with honeycomb pattern.	Multiple intercommunicating septa divide the lumen of the gallbladder. Increased incidence of infection and gallstone formation.
Hypoplasia of gallbladder	Very small gallbladder.	Gallbladder is merely a small, rudimentary pouch at the end of the cystic duct.

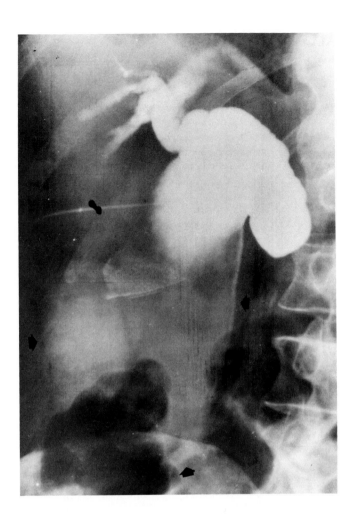

Fig GI40-1. Courvoisier phenomenon. Huge gallbladder (arrows) injected by error at percutaneous hepatic cholangiography. The patient had carcinoma of the pancreas and presented with painless jaundice.

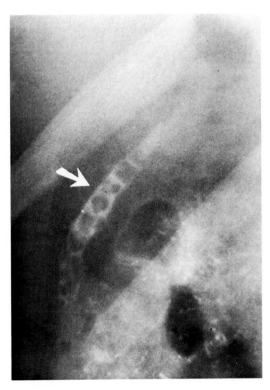

Fig GI40-2. Chronic cholecystitis. Multiple radiolucent stones (arrow) fill the small, shrunken gallbladder.

FILLING DEFECTS IN AN OPACIFIED GALLBLADDER

Condition	Imaging Findings	Comments
Gallstones **(Figs GI41-1 to GI41-3)**	Variable size, shape, number, and degree of calcifications. They are usually freely movable and settle in the dependent portion of the gallbladder (the level depends on the relation of the specific gravity of the stone to that of the surrounding bile).	Approximately 80% are lucent cholesterol stones, while 20% contain sufficient calcium to be radiographically detectable. The incidence of gallstones increases in several disease states (hemolytic anemias, cirrhosis, diabetes, Crohn's disease, hyperparathyroidism, pancreatic disease) and various metabolic disorders. Infrequently, a gallstone coated by tenacious mucus adheres to the gallbladder wall.
Cholesterolosis **(strawberry gallbladder)** **(Fig GI41-4)**	Single or multiple small polypoid filling defects (best seen after a fatty meal).	Abnormal deposits of cholesterol esters in fat-laden macrophages in the lamina propria of the gallbladder wall. No malignant potential.
Adenomyoma **(Figs GI41-5 and GI41-6)**	Single filling defect situated at the tip of the fundus.	In adenomyomatosis, single or multiple oval collections of contrast material (Rokitansky-Aschoff sinuses) are projected just outside the lumen of the gallbladder.
Benign tumor	Fixed filling defect.	Rare. Mainly adenomatous polyps and papillary adenomas (papilloma, villous adenoma).
Carcinoma of gallbladder **(Fig GI41-7)**	Solitary fixed polyp or irregular mural filling defect.	Rare manifestation (the gallbladder is usually not visualized in the presence of a carcinoma). Primarily affects elderly women and is usually associated with cholelithiasis.
Metastases	Single or multiple fixed filling defects.	Most commonly melanoma (occurs in about 15% of patients with the disease but is rarely detectable radiographically).
Parasitic granuloma	Single or multiple fixed nodules.	Eggs of *Ascaris lumbricoides* or *Paragonimus westermani* deposited in the gallbladder wall incite an intense inflammatory cell infiltration.
Metachromatic leukodystrophy	Single or multiple filling defects.	Very rare condition in which there is deposition of metachromatic sulfatides due to an enzyme deficiency.
Pseudopolyp	Fixed filling defect that may simulate a true tumor.	Congenital fold or septum (eg, Phrygian cap); heterotopic gastric or pancreatic tissue; projectional artifacts (folding or coiling of the junction between the neck of the gallbladder and the cystic duct or a lucent cystic duct superimposed on the opaque neck of the gallbladder).

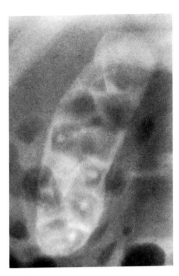

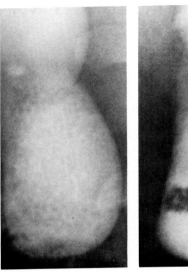

Fig GI41-1. Multiple radiolucent gallstones, many of which contain a central nidus of calcification.

Fig GI41-2. Layering of gallstones. (Left) With the patient supine, the stones are poorly defined and have a gravel-like consistency. (Right) On an erect film taken with a horizontal beam, the innumerable gallstones layer out and are easily seen.

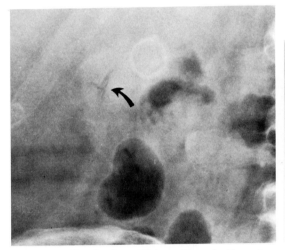

Fig GI41-3. Fissuring in a gallstone. Mercedes-Benz sign (arrow). Note the adjacent gallstone with a radiopaque rim.

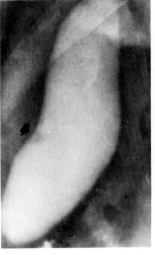

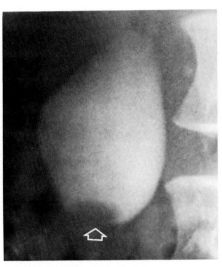

Fig GI41-4. Cholesterol polyp (arrow).

Fig GI41-5. Solitary adenomyoma. A broad mass (arrow) is evident at the tip of the fundus of the gallbladder.

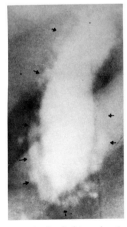

Fig GI41-6. Adenomyomatosis. Rokitansky-Aschoff sinuses are scattered diffusely throughout the gallbladder. The collections of intramural contrast material appear to parallel the opacified gallbladder lumen (arrows), from which they are separated by a lucent space representing the thickness of the mucosa and muscularis.

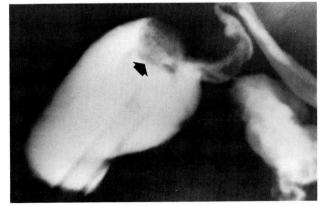

Fig GI41-7. Carcinoma of the gallbladder. Irregular mural mass (arrow) with tumor growth extending into the cystic duct.

FILLING DEFECTS IN THE BILE DUCTS

Condition	Imaging Findings	Comments
Biliary calculi (Figs GI42-1 and GI42-2)	Single or multiple filling defects that move freely and change location with alterations in patient position.	Usually arise in the gallbladder and reach the bile duct either by passage through the cystic duct or by fistulous erosion through the gallbladder wall. May impact in the distal common duct and cause obstruction (smooth, sharply defined meniscus).
Pseudocalculus (Fig GI42-3)	Smooth, arcuate filling defect simulating an impacted gallstone. Serial radiographs show the pseudocalculus disappearing as the sphincter relaxes.	Cyclic contraction of the sphincter of Oddi that occurs after surgical manipulation or instrumentation of the common bile duct. Never completely obstructs the bile duct (some contrast material flows into the duodenum).
Air bubbles	Smooth, round, generally multiple filling defects.	Vexing artifacts on T-tube cholangiography. If the patient is raised toward the upright position, the air bubbles rise (lighter than contrast-laden bile), while true calculi remain in a stationary position or fall with gravity.
Malignant tumors (Fig GI42-4)	Single or multiple filling defects.	Rare manifestation of cholangiocarcinoma, ampullary carcinoma, hepatoma, or villous tumors.
Benign tumors	Small polypoid filling defects.	Very rare. Mostly adenomas and papillomas.
Ascaris lumbricoides	Long, linear filling defects.	Coiling of worms can rarely produce a discrete mass.
Liver flukes (Fig GI42-5)	Smooth filling defects simulating calculi (when viewed en face). Typical linear filling defects when the worms are seen in profile.	*Clonorchis sinensis* (in raw or partially cooked fish) and *Fasciola hepatica* (in pond water or watercress in sheep-growing areas).
Hydatid cyst (*Echinococcus*) (Fig GI42-6)	Round or irregular filling defect in a bile duct or a cyst cavity.	If a liver cyst communicates with the biliary tree, the periodic discharge of cyst membranes, daughter cysts, or scolices causes recurrent episodes of biliary colic.

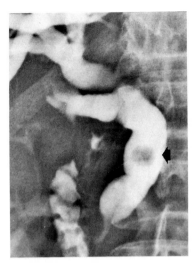

Fig GI42-1. Common bile duct stone (arrow).

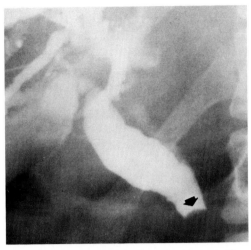

Fig GI42-2. Impacted common bile duct stone (arrow). Characteristic smooth, concave intraluminal filling defect.

A

B

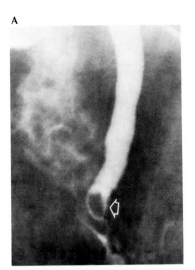

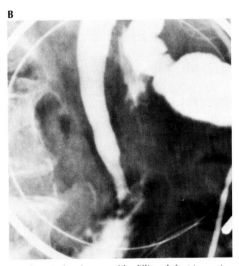

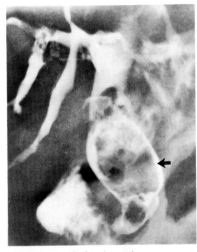

Fig GI42-3. Pseudocalculus. (A) Contrast material encircles the stonelike filling defect (arrow). (B) After relaxation of the sphincter of Oddi, the distal common bile duct appears normal and contrast material flows freely into the duodenum.

Fig GI42-4. Cholangiocarcinoma presenting as a large filling defect (arrow) in the common bile duct.

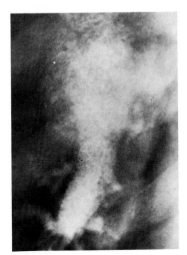

Fig GI42-5. Liver flukes (*Clonorchis sinensis*) causing multiple filling defects in the biliary system. Many of the filling defects represent coexisting calculi, which are often seen in this condition.

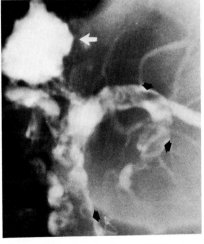

Fig GI42-6. Hydatid disease of the liver and biliary tree. Multiple cysts present as filling defects in the bile ducts (black arrows). Note contrast material filling a large communicating cystic cavity in the liver parenchyma (white arrow).

BILE DUCT NARROWING OR OBSTRUCTION

Condition	Imaging Findings	Comments
Cholangiocarcinoma (Figs GI43-1 and GI43-2)	Short, well-demarcated, segmental narrowing of the bile duct. There may be diffuse ductal narrowing (extensive desmoplastic response). Rarely multicentric (mimicking sclerosing cholangitis).	Most commonly affects the retroduodenal or supraduodenal segments of the common bile duct. Lesions are usually far advanced at the time of diagnosis (extend along the bile duct and spread to regional lymph nodes). Klatskin tumors arising at the junction of the right and left hepatic ducts tend to grow slowly and metastasize late.
Ampullary carcinoma (Fig GI43-3)	Obstruction of the distal end of the bile duct.	Small neoplasm that can appear as a polypoid mass or merely obstruct the bile duct without a demonstrable tumor mass.
Adjacent malignancy (Figs GI43-4 and GI43-5)	Asymmetric narrowing or obstruction of the bile duct.	Primary carcinoma of the pancreas or the duodenum; metastases (usually from a gastrointestinal tract primary); lymphoma (nodes in the porta hepatis).
Benign tumor	Polypoid filling defect with some degree of obstruction.	Extremely rare. Usually occurs in the distal bile duct and simulates a biliary stone.
Cholangitis (Fig GI43-6)	Multiple biliary strictures of various lengths with beading of the duct between narrowed segments. Almost always involves the extrahepatic ducts; there may be progressive involvement of the intrahepatic ducts.	Most commonly an inflammatory disorder secondary to long-standing partial obstruction. Primary sclerosing cholangitis is a rare condition that tends to occur in patients with inflammatory bowel disease.
Cholangiolitic hepatitis (Fig GI43-7)	Diffuse or focal ductal narrowing with diminished branching of the intrahepatic biliary ductal system.	Rare, chronic, slowly progressive intrahepatic disease of unknown etiology. Extrahepatic ducts are not involved (unlike sclerosing cholangitis).
Chronic pancreatitis (Fig GI43-8)	Smooth, concentric inflammatory stricture with gradual tapering.	Involves the intrapancreatic portion of the common bile duct. Often associated with pancreatic calcifications.
Acute pancreatitis	Circumferential narrowing of the common bile duct.	Usually reversible when the acute inflammatory process subsides.

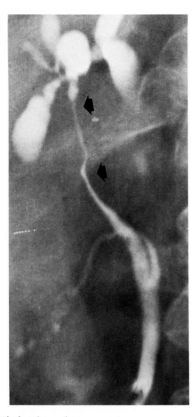

FIG GI43-1. **Cholangiocarcinoma** causing severe narrowing of a long segment of the common hepatic duct (arrows).

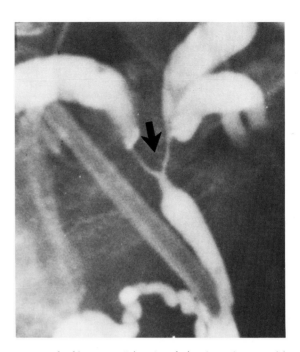

FIG GI43-2. **Klatskin tumor.** Sclerosing cholangiocarcinomas arising at the junction of the right and left hepatic ducts.

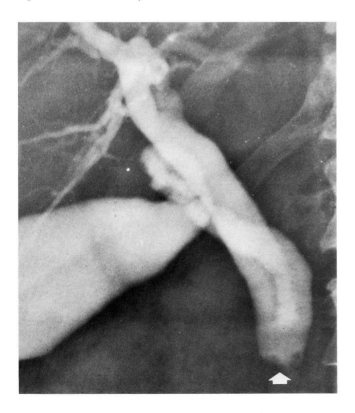

FIG GI43-3. **Ampullary carcinoma.** Abrupt occlusion (arrow) of the distal common bile duct.

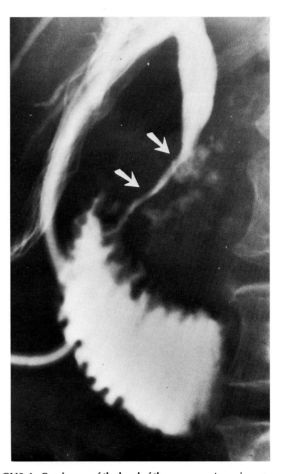

FIG GI43-4. **Carcinoma of the head of the pancreas.** Irregular narrowing of the common bile duct (arrows). The calcifications reflect underlying chronic pancreatitis.

Condition	Imaging Findings	Comments
Papillary stenosis	Smooth narrowing of the terminal portion of the bile duct.	Controversial entity that is associated with chronic inflammatory disease of the biliary tract and pancreas. May be the cause of postcholecystectomy symptoms resembling biliary colic. Successfully treated by surgical relief of the obstruction at the choledocho-duodenal junction.
Parasitic infestation	Relative obstruction usually due to an inflammatory stricture and stone formation.	*Clonorchis sinensis; Fasciola hepatica; Ascaris lumbricoides.* Conglomeration of worms can cause an obstructive mass. In *Echinococcus* infestation, daughter cysts shed into the bile ducts can cause obstruction at the ampullary level.
Granulomatous disease	Compression and narrowing of the bile duct, primarily in the region of the porta hepatis.	Periductal lymph node involvement in tuberculosis, sarcoidosis, and other chronic granulomatous diseases.
Impacted biliary calculus (see Fig GI42-2)	Smooth, concave intraluminal filling defect.	Impacted ampullary stone and papillary edema secondary to a recently passed stone are common causes of bile duct obstruction. Calculi enter the common bile duct via the cystic duct or by erosion.
Surgical or traumatic stricture (Fig GI43-9)	Smooth, concentric narrowing of the bile duct. If the bile duct is obstructed, it appears convex (unlike the concave margin of an obstructing stone).	Most are related to previous biliary tract surgery. Infrequently, blunt abdominal trauma causes torsion injury to the common bile duct. Unlike malignant lesions, benign strictures usually involve long segments and have a gradual transition without complete obstruction.
Biliary atresia	Obliteration of the ductal lumen (often segmental and irregular in distribution).	Most common cause of persistent neonatal jaundice. Rather than a congenital defect, it probably develops postpartum as a complication of a chronic inflammatory process.
Membranous diaphragm (Fig GI43-10)	Luminal web in the common bile duct.	Extremely rare. Chronic partial biliary obstruction results in bile stasis, stone formation, and recurring cholangitis.
Duodenal diverticulum	Distal obstruction of the common bile duct.	Common duct that empties directly into a duodenal diverticulum may be obstructed by anatomic distortion, diverticulitis, or an enterolith in the sac.
Cirrhosis	Irregular tortuous or corkscrew appearance of the intrahepatic bile ducts.	Distortion of the hepatic parenchyma by fatty infiltration and subsequent regenerating nodules and fibrosis.

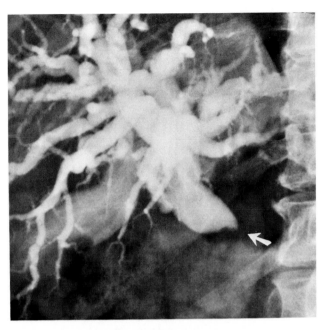

Fig GI43-5. Extrinsic obstruction of the common bile duct (arrow) due to nodal metastases from carcinoma of the colon.

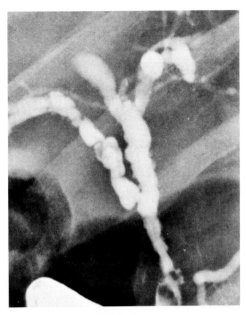

Fig GI43-6. Primary sclerosing cholangitis in a patient with chronic ulcerative colitis.

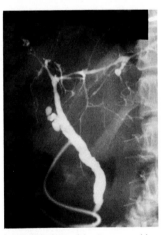

Fig GI43-7. Cholangiolitic hepatitis. Decreased branching of the intrahepatic ducts with associated diffuse and focal narrowing. The extrahepatic bile ducts are normal.[27]

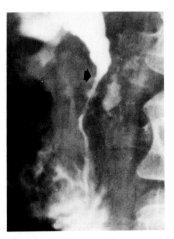

Fig GI43-8. Chronic pancreatitis. Note the abrupt transition between the encased pipe stem segment and the dilated suprapancreatic portion of the common bile duct (arrow). Calcification suggestive of chronic pancreatitis can also be seen.

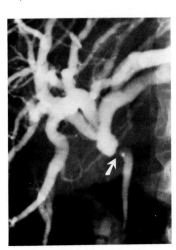

Fig GI43-9. Benign stricture of the common bile duct (arrow) related to previous biliary tract surgery.

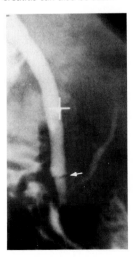

Fig GI43-10. Congenital membranous diaphragm (web) of the common bile duct (arrow).

CYSTIC DILATATION OF THE BILE DUCTS

Condition	Imaging Findings	Comments
Choledochal cyst (Fig GI44-1)	Cystic or fusiform dilatation that primarily affects the common bile duct and adjacent portions of the common hepatic and cystic ducts. There can also be dilatation of intrahepatic bile ducts.	Typically associated with a localized constriction of the distal common bile duct. Classic clinical triad of upper abdominal pain, mass, and jaundice.
Choledochocele (Fig GI44-2)	Cystic dilatation of the intraduodenal portion of the common bile duct.	Well-defined, smooth duodenal filling defect on an upper gastrointestinal series. On cholangiography, it mimics the urographic appearance of a ureterocele.
Caroli's disease (Fig GI44-3)	Segmental saccular dilatation of intrahepatic bile ducts throughout the liver.	Rare condition in which the dilated cystic segments contain bile and communicate freely with the biliary tree and each other. Approximately 80% of patients have associated medullary sponge kidney.
Congenital hepatic fibrosis (Fig GI44-4)	Large or small cystic spaces communicating with intrahepatic bile ducts (lollipop-tree appearance).	Rare condition that radiographically simulates Caroli's disease but is far more serious. Massive periportal fibrosis leads to fatal liver failure and portal hypertension at an early age.
Papillomatosis of intrahepatic biliary ducts	Intrahepatic or extrahepatic bile duct dilatation proximal to multiple filling defects.	Rare condition in which biliary obstruction is caused by thick mucous material produced by the villous tumors, fragmentation of the papillary fronds, or amputation of entire polyps into the biliary tract. High incidence of carcinoma.
Choledocholithiasis (Oriental)	Ductal dilatation proximal to obstructing calculi or masses of worms.	In Oriental countries, intrahepatic lithiasis and cystic dilatation of bile ducts are frequent complications of parasitic infestation (*Ascaris lumbricoides, Clonorchis sinensis*).
Cholangitis (Fig GI44-5)	Areas of cystic dilatation combined with strictures of various lengths.	Caused by diffuse periductal inflammatory fibrosis. Cystic dilatation can also be due to communicating hepatic abscesses.
Cholangiohepatitis (recurrent pyogenic hepatitis) (Fig GI44-6)	Segmental dilatation of bile ducts with areas of rapid peripheral tapering (arrowhead sign).	Major cause of acute abdomen in the Far East. Frequently leads to stone formation, biliary obstruction, and portal septicemia.

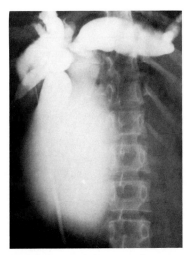

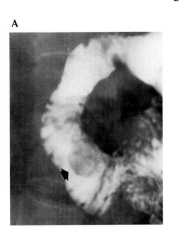

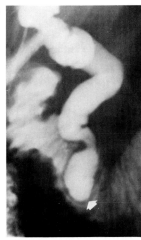

FIG GI44-1. Choledochal cyst. Cholangiographic contrast material fills the huge fusiform dilatation of the common bile duct and the markedly dilated intrahepatic ducts.

FIG GI44-2. Choledochocele. (A) A well-defined, smooth filling defect (arrow) projects into the duodenal lumen on an upper gastrointestinal series. (B) At cholangiography, the bulbous terminal portion of the common bile duct fills with contrast material and projects into the duodenal lumen (arrow). It is separated from contrast material in the duodenum by a radiolucent membrane.

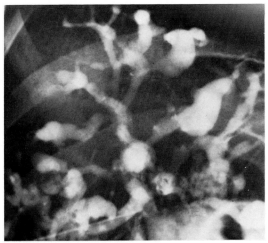

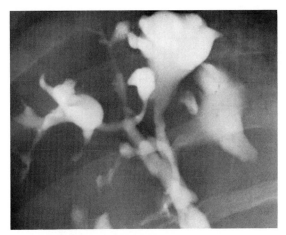

FIG GI44-3. Caroli's disease.

FIG GI44-4. Congenital hepatic fibrosis.[28]

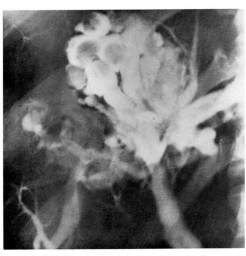

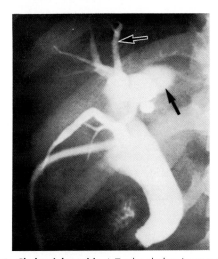

FIG GI44-5. Cholangitis. Communicating hepatic abscess simulating localized cystic dilatation of an intrahepatic bile duct.

FIG GI44-6. Cholangiohepatitis. A T-tube cholangiogram demonstrates that the common bile duct and intrahepatic duct (lower arrow) are dilated. The upper arrow shows a moderately dilated bile duct with short branches arising at right angles to the duct.[29]

PNEUMOPERITONEUM

Condition	Comments
Pneumoperitoneum with peritonitis	
Perforated viscus (Figs GI45-1 and GI45-2)	The most frequent cause is perforated duodenal ulcer (gastric or duodenal). In 30% of perforated peptic ulcers, no free intraperitoneal gas can be detected. The absence of stomach gas with gas present distally suggests gastric perforation, while the absence of colonic gas in the presence of a gastric gas-fluid level and small bowel distension suggests colonic perforation. Colonic perforation can be due to obstructing malignancy, severe ulcerating colitis (toxic megacolon), and, rarely, diverticulitis or appendicitis. A precise diagnosis of the site of perforation often requires a barium study.
Ulcerative bowel disease	Tuberculosis; typhoid fever; ulcerated Meckel's diverticulum; ulcerative colitis (toxic megacolon); lymphogranuloma venereum. There is often evidence of bowel inflammation on the plain abdominal radiograph.
Infection/trauma	Infection of the peritoneal cavity by a gas-forming organism; blunt or penetrating trauma causing rupture of a hollow viscus.
Delayed complication of renal transplantation	Spontaneous perforation of the colon may develop in a patient on long-term immunosuppressive therapy. High mortality rate.
Pneumoperitoneum without peritonitis	
Iatrogenic causes	Abdominal surgery; endoscopy; diagnostic pneumoperitoneum.
Abdominal causes	Pneumatosis intestinalis (rupture of mural gas-filled cysts); forme fruste of perforation; jejunal diverticulosis.
Gynecologic causes	Rubin test for tubal patency; vaginal douching; postpartum exercises or examination; orogenital intercourse (ascent of air through the normal female genital tract into the peritoneal cavity).
Intrathoracic causes	Pneumomediastinum; ruptured emphysematous bullus (dissection of gas downward into the extraperitoneal tissues followed by perforation into the peritoneal cavity).

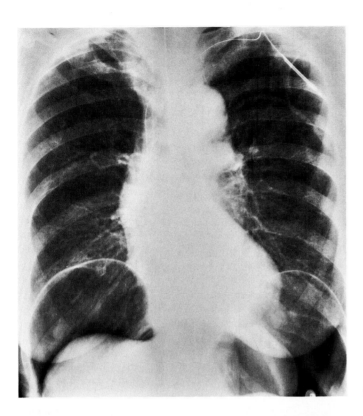

FIG GI45-1. Extensive pneumoperitoneum after colonic perforation.

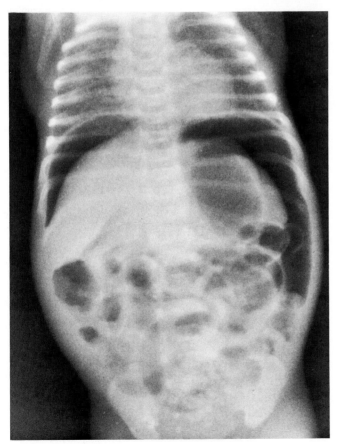

FIG GI45-2. Pneumoperitoneum after perforation of an ulcerated Meckel's diverticulum in a child.

GAS IN THE BOWEL WALL (PNEUMATOSIS INTESTINALIS)

Condition	Imaging Findings	Comments
Primary (idiopathic) pneumatosis intestinalis (Fig GI46-1)	Radiolucent clusters of cysts along the contours of the bowel that are compressible on palpation and can simulate polyps, thumbprinting, or even an annular constriction.	Benign condition with multiple thin-walled, noncommunicating, gas-filled cysts in the bowel wall. Primarily involves the colon (especially the left side). No associated gastrointestinal or respiratory abnormalities, but may cause asymptomatic pneumoperitoneum.
Necrotizing enterocolitis (Fig GI46-2)	Frothy or bubbly appearance of gas in the wall of diseased bowel loops. Often resembles fecal material in the right colon (normal in adults, but abnormal in premature infants).	Primarily occurs in premature or debilitated infants and has a low survival rate. Most commonly affects the ileum and right colon. Pneumoperitoneum and portal vein gas are ominous signs.
Mesenteric vascular disease (Fig GI46-3)	Crescentic linear gas collections in the walls of ischemic bowel loops.	Due to loss of mucosal integrity or increased intraluminal pressure in the bowel (ischemic necrosis; intestinal obstruction, especially if strangulation; corrosive ingestion; primary infection of the bowel wall). Portal vein gas indicates irreversible intestinal necrosis.
Gastrointestinal tract lesion without necrosis of bowel wall (Fig GI46-4)	Short, sharply defined intramural gas collections parallel to the bowel wall.	May develop in conditions resulting in mucosal ulceration or intestinal obstruction (obstructive pyloro-duodenal peptic ulcer disease, inflammatory bowel disease, connective tissue disease, jejunoileal bypass surgery, obstructive colonic lesions in children, steroid therapy, complication of gastrointestinal endoscopy or colonoscopy).
Obstructive pulmonary disease	Segmental intramural gas collections parallel to the bowel wall.	Partial bronchial obstruction and coughing presumably cause alveolar rupture with gas dissecting along peribronchial and perivascular tissue planes into the mediastinum and passing through various diaphragmatic openings to reach the retroperitoneal area. Gas then dissects between the leaves of the mesentery to reach the bowel wall.

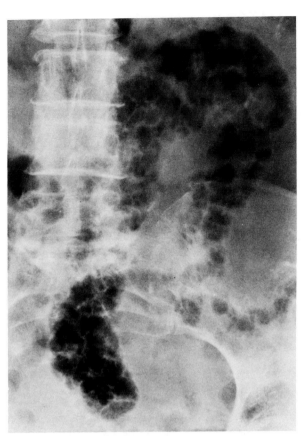

FIG GI46-1. **Primary pneumatosis intestinalis** in an asymptomatic man.

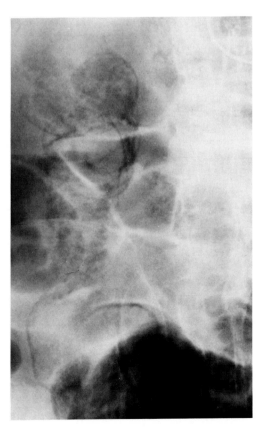

FIG GI46-2. **Pneumatosis intestinalis** in a premature infant with necrotizing enterocolitis. The bubbly appearance of gas in the wall of the diseased colon represents fecal material (arrow).

FIG GI46-3. **Pneumatosis intestinalis** due to mesenteric arterial thrombosis.

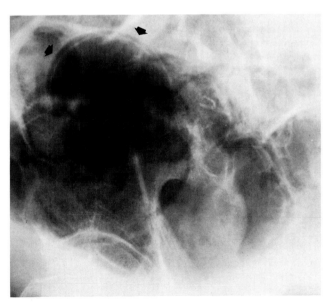

FIG GI46-4. **Pneumatosis intestinalis** involving the colon (arrows) in a patient with severe pyloric stenosis.

EXTRALUMINAL GAS IN THE UPPER QUADRANTS

Condition	Imaging Findings	Comments
Pneumoperitoneum (Fig GI47-1)	Best seen on upright or decubitus views with a horizontal beam. Double-wall, inverted-V, and urachal signs on supine views. Falciform ligament and football signs in children.	Secondary to visceral perforation, surgery, or a variety of nonemergent abdominal, gynecologic, and intrathoracic causes.
Retroperitoneal gas (Fig GI47-2)	Outlines the kidney and, on the right, the undersurface of the liver. Does not move freely when the patient changes position (unlike intraperitoneal gas).	Most common cause is perforation of the duodenum or rectum due to trauma, diverticulitis, or ulcerative disease. Can be a complication of an endoscopic procedure.
Subhepatic gas	Triangular or crescent-shaped gas collection overlying the right kidney inferior to the liver edge. Subhepatic abscess has a round or oval configuration and often contains a gas-fluid level.	Most common cause is perforation of a duodenal ulcer. Less frequently, perforation of the appendix or a sigmoid diverticulum or leakage of a gastroenteric or ileotransverse colon anastomosis. Subhepatic abscess may complicate enteric perforation or pelvic inflammation.
Subphrenic abscess (Fig GI47-3)	Mottled radiolucent appearance, often with a gas-fluid level. Unlike bowel gas, gas in an abscess is constant in multiple projections and on serial films.	Primarily a complication of intra-abdominal surgery and associated with a high mortality rate. Usually there is elevation and restricted motion of the ipsilateral hemidiaphragm and often a nonpurulent (sympathetic) pleural effusion.
Renal or perirenal abscess (Fig GI47-4)	Gas within and surrounding the kidney.	Caused by antecedent urinary tract disease (infection, obstruction, trauma, instrumentation) or direct or hematogenous spread of an extraurinary infection.
Liver abscess	Bubbly gas collection overlying the liver.	Caused by pyogenic organisms (especially *Klebsiella*) or amebic infestation.
Pancreatic abscess (Fig GI47-5)	Mottled lucent pattern in the midabdomen.	Complication of acute pancreatitis that is associated with a high mortality rate.
Lesser sac abscess (Fig GI47-6)	Mottled collection in the left upper abdomen, often with a gas-fluid level.	Displaces the stomach anteriorly and the colon inferiorly. May extend slightly over the midline but does not reach the diaphragm.
Gas in bowel wall (pneumatosis intestinalis) (Fig GI47-7)	Multiple gas-filled mural cysts (primary) or crescentic linear gas collections (secondary).	Benign primary condition or secondary to necrotizing enterocolitis, mesenteric vascular disease, and a variety of gastrointestinal and obstructive pulmonary conditions.

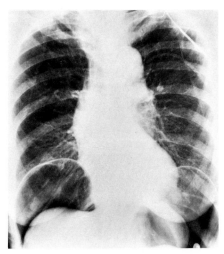

FIG GI47-1. **Pneumoperitoneum.**

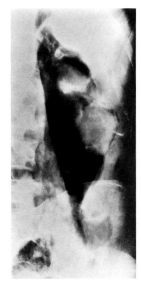

FIG GI47-2. **Retroperitoneal gas** surrounding the left kidney after colonoscopy.

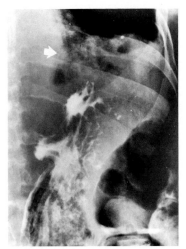

FIG GI47-3. **Left subphrenic abscess.** Characteristic mottled radiolucent appearance of the abscess (arrow), which is located above the fundus of the stomach, is due to gas bubbles intermixed with necrotic material and pus.

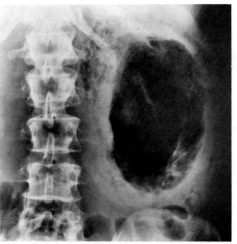

FIG GI47-4. **Renal and perirenal abscess.**

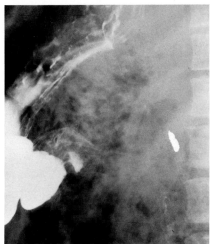

FIG GI47-5. **Pancreatic abscess.**

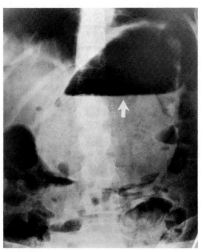

FIG GI47-6. **Lesser sac abscess** with a prominent gas-fluid level (arrow).

Condition	Imaging Findings	Comments
Gas in biliary system (Fig GI47-8)	Gas in larger, more centrally situated bile ducts.	Caused by inflammatory fistulization between the gallbladder or bile duct and the stomach or duodenum, or due to previous surgery (sphincterotomy), cholecystitis, severe peptic ulcer disease, trauma, or a tumor.
Emphysematous cholecystitis (Fig GI47-9)	Gas in the lumen or the wall of the gallbladder or in pericholecystic tissues.	Caused by gas-forming organisms and usually occurs in patients with poorly controlled diabetes mellitus, most of whom have cystic duct obstruction by stones.
Gas in portal venous system (Fig GI47-10)	Radiating tubular lucencies branching from the porta hepatis to the periphery of the liver.	Usually an ominous prognostic sign in children with necrotizing entercolitis or adults with mesenteric ischemia and bowel necrosis. A benign form in children is related to the placement of an umbilical venous catheter.
Chilaiditi's syndrome (Fig GI47-11)	Gas in the hepatic flexture of the colon interposed between the liver and the diaphragm.	No clinical significance. Primarily seen in mentally retarded or psychotic patients with chronic colonic enlargement. Must not be confused with pneumoperitoneum.
Perforation due to foreign body	Offending foreign body seen if opaque.	Most ingested foreign bodies pass through the gastrointestinal tract without incident. Sharp or elongated foreign bodies may cause perforation and localized abscess formation (which may be associated with signs of peritonitis, mechanical bowel obstruction, or pneumoperitoneum).
Abdominal wall gas/abscess (Fig GI47-12)	Gas in the region of the abdominal wall musculature.	May be a normal finding after surgery or reflect postoperative wound infection or localized abscess formation.

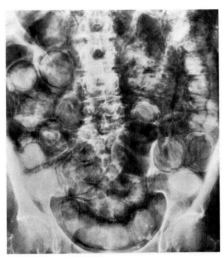

FIG GI47-7. **Pneumatosis intestinalis** secondary to primary amyloidosis of the small bowel.

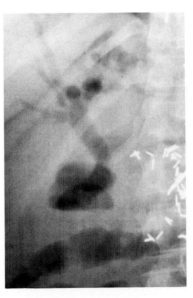

FIG GI47-8. **Gas in the biliary tree** in a patient who had undergone a surgical procedure to relieve biliary obstruction.

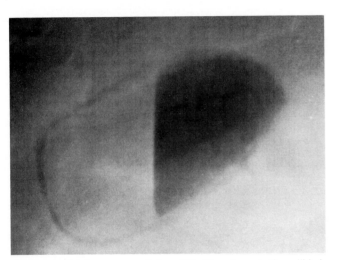

FIG GI47-9. **Emphysematous cholecystitis.** There is gas in the gallbladder lumen and wall.

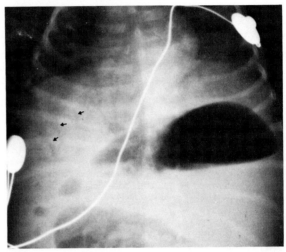

FIG GI47-10. **Portal vein gas** (arrows) in an infant with necrotizing enterocolitis.

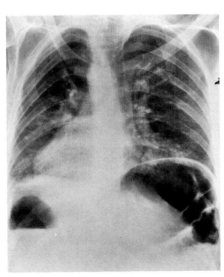

FIG GI47-11. **Chilaiditi's syndrome.**

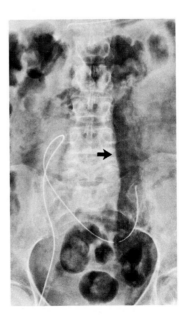

FIG GI47-12. **Gas in a wound infection** in the rectus sheath (arrow) after abdominal surgery.

BULL'S-EYE LESIONS OF THE GASTROINTESTINAL TRACT

Condition	Comments
Melanoma **(Fig GI48-1)**	Multiple ulcerated lesions frequently involve the small bowel and stomach.
Primary neoplasms **(Fig GI48-2)**	Single ulcerated lesion that is most commonly due to a spindle cell tumor (especially leiomyoma). Infrequent manifestation of lymphoma, carcinoma, or carcinoid.
Hematogenous metastases **(Fig GI48-3)**	Multiple ulcerating lesions most commonly due to carcinomas of the breast or lung (especially in the stomach and duodenum).
Kaposi's sarcoma	Multiple ulcerating lesions that primarily involve the small bowel. Associated with characteristic ulcerated hemorrhagic dermatitis in patients with immune deficiency disorders.
Eosinophilic granuloma	Single ulcerated polypoid mass that most frequently involves the stomach, but can occur in the small bowel, colon, or rectum. Unlike eosinophilic gastroenteritis, the inflammatory mass of an eosinophilic granuloma is not associated with specific food intolerance or peripheral blood eosinophilia.
Ectopic pancreas **(Fig GI48-4)**	Single "ulcerated" polypoid mass in the stomach or duodenum. The central barium collection represents umbilication of a rudimentary pancreatic duct rather than necrotic ulceration.

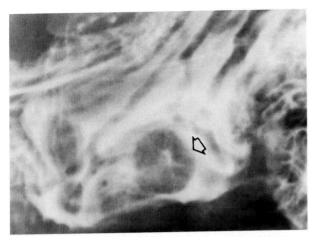

FIG GI48-1. **Metastatic melanoma.** Large, ulcerated filling defect (arrow) in the stomach.

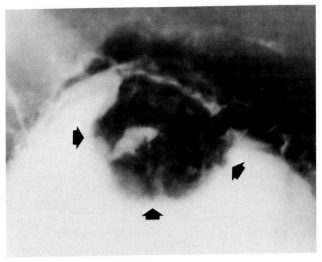

FIG GI48-2. **Ulcerated leiomyoma** of the fundus of the stomach (arrows).

FIG GI48-3. **Carcinoma of the breast metastatic to the stomach**. There is a huge, centrally ulcerated lesion (arrow).

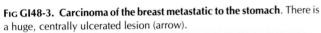

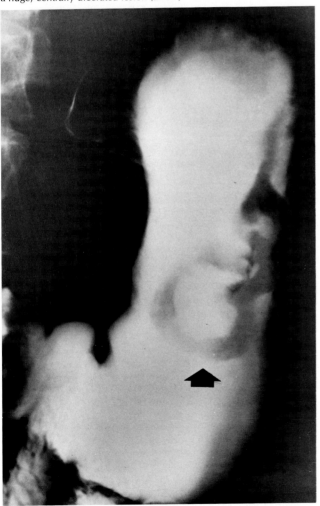

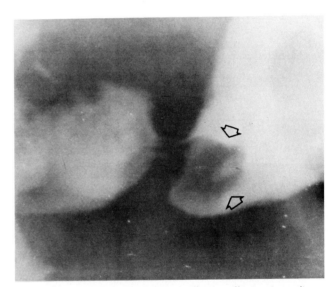

FIG GI48-4. **Ectopic pancreas.** Central collection of barium in a rudimentary duct in a filling defect in the gastric antrum (arrows).

LIVER CALCIFICATION

Condition	Imaging Findings	Comments
Tuberculosis/histoplasmosis	Small (1 to 3 cm), multiple, dense, discrete calcifications scattered throughout the liver.	Healed foci of granulomatous disease are the most common intrahepatic calcifications. Usually there are also calcifications in the lung and spleen.
Echinococcus granulosus **(Fig GI49-1)**	Complete oval or circular calcification at the periphery of a mother cyst. There may be multiple daughter cysts with archlike calcifications.	Hydatid cyst calcification generally develops 5 to 10 years after liver infection. Extensive dense calcifications suggest an inactive cyst, while segmental calcifications suggest cystic activity and are often considered an indication for surgery.
Echinococcus multilocularis **(Fig GI49-2)**	Multiple small lucencies surrounded by rings of calcification which, in turn, lie within large areas of amorphous calcification.	Calcification occurs in about 70% of patients with this rarer and more malignant form (''alveolar type'') of hydatid disease.
Amebic or pyogenic abscess **(Fig GI49-3)**	Dense, mottled calcifications that are usually solitary but are occasionally multiple.	Patient is usually asymptomatic when the hepatic calcification is detected.
Brucellosis **(see Fig GI50-1)**	Snowflake appearance of fluffy calcifications.	Usually there are similar calcifications in the spleen.
Other parasitic infestations **(Fig GI49-4)**	Various patterns of calcification.	*Armillifer armillatus* (tongue worm); guinea worm; filariasis; toxoplasmosis; cysticercosis.
Cavernous hemangioma	Sunburst pattern of spicules of calcification (radiating from the central area toward the periphery of the lesion).	Appearance similar to that of hemangiomas in flat bones (eg, skull and sternum). Most hemangiomas are not calcified. Rarely associated with calcified phleboliths (unlike hemangiomas elsewhere).
Primary carcinoma of liver	Various patterns of calcification (small irregular flecks to discrete spherical calculi).	Tumors most often calcify in children as a result of dystrophic calcification of necrotic tissue.
Metastases to liver **(Fig GI49-5)**	Diffuse, finely granular calcifications.	Calcification most commonly occurs in metastatic colloid carcinoma of the colon or rectum. Less frequently, carcinomas of the breast, stomach, and ovary. Metastases from other primary tumors are usually larger and denser.

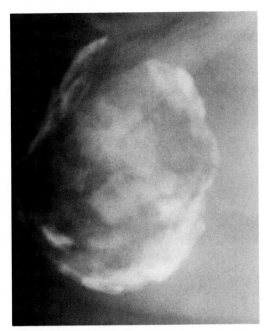

FIG GI49-1. Hydatid liver cyst (*Echinococcus granulosus*). There is complete oval calcification at the periphery of the mother cyst. Within the mother cyst are several small arclike calcifications representing daughter cysts.

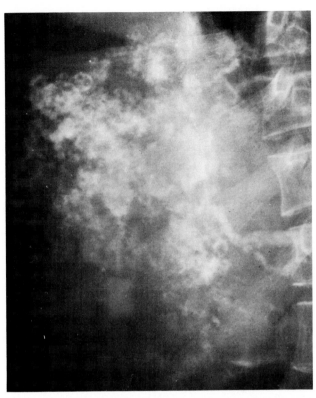

FIG GI49-2. Alveolar hydatic disease (*Echinococcus multilocularis*).[30]

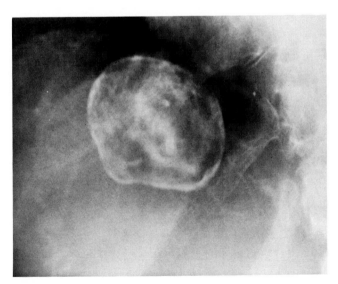

FIG GI49-3. Calcified pyogenic liver abscess.

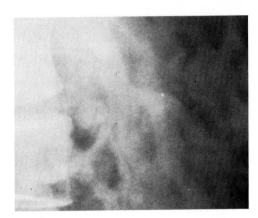

FIG GI49-4. Calcified guinea worm in the right lobe of the liver.[31]

Condition	Imaging Findings	Comments
Portal vein thrombus	Linear opacity crossing the vertebral column.	Usually associated with cirrhosis and portal hypertension.
Hepatic artery aneurysm	Circular, cracked-eggshell pattern.	Most hepatic artery aneurysms do not calcify.
Calcification of liver capsule (Fig GI49-6)	Opaque shell around part or all of the liver.	May reflect alcoholic cirrhosis, pyogenic infection, meconium peritonitis, pseudomyxoma peritonei, or lipoid granulomatosis after the intraperitoneal instillation of mineral oil. A similar pattern can follow the inadvertent introduction of barium into the peritoneal cavity through a colonic perforation.
Generalized increased liver density (without demonstrable calcification) (Figs GI49-7 and GI49-8)	Uniform or patchy increased density.	Causes include hemochromatosis, siderosis, cirrhosis (contracted liver), and a previous injection of Thorotrast.

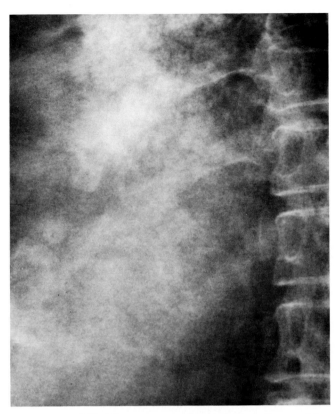

FIG GI49-5. **Calcified liver metastases** from colloid carcinoma of the colon producing a diffuse, finely granular pattern.

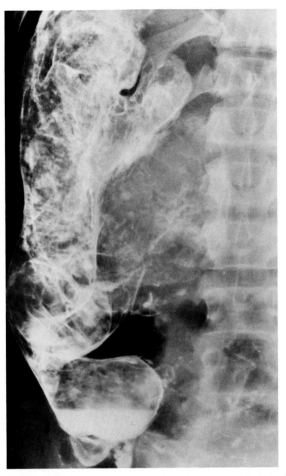

FIG GI49-6. **Appearance simulating intrinsic hepatic calcification** due to inadvertent intraperitoneal extravasation of barium, which produced an opaque shell around the liver.

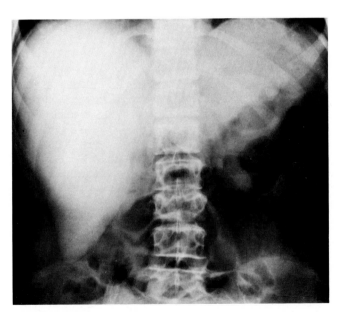

FIG GI49-7. **Hemochromatosis.** Extremely dense liver shadow in the right upper quadrant is caused by parenchymal deposition of iron.[32]

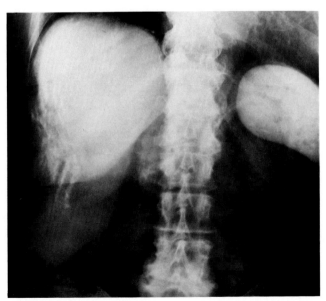

FIG GI49-8. **Calcification of the liver and spleen caused by a prior injection of Thorotrast.**

SPLEEN CALCIFICATION

Condition	Imaging Findings	Comments
Histoplasmosis/tuberculosis (Fig GI50-1)	Multiple small, round or ovoid calcified nodules distributed throughout the spleen.	Healed foci of granulomatous disease are the most common intrasplenic calcifications. There are usually also calcifications in the lung and occasionally in the liver.
Brucellosis (Fig GI50-2)	Snowflake appearance of fluffy calcifications that are generally larger than those in other granulomatous diseases.	The lesions in chronic brucellosis, unlike those in histoplasmosis and tuberculosis, tend to be active and suppurating even in the presence of calcification.
Phleboliths	Small, round or ovoid calcified nodules, often with lucent centers.	Usually diffusely distributed in veins throughout the spleen.
Cyst		
Nonparasitic (Fig GI50-3)	Thin peripheral calcification.	Infrequent manifestation of congenital or post-traumatic cyst.
Echinococcal (hydatid) (Fig GI50-4)	Peripheral calcification that is often multiple and tends to be thicker and coarser than nonparasitic cystic calcification.	Echinococcal calcification can reflect a hydatid cyst in the spleen or extension of cysts arising from neighboring organs.
Calcification of splenic capsule (Fig GI50-5)	Opaque shell around part or all of the spleen.	May be secondary to a pyogenic or tuberculous abscess, infarct, or hematoma. Although they infrequently calcify, splenic infarcts may have a characteristic triangular or wedge-shaped appearance, with the apex of the calcification appearing to point toward the center of the organ.
Splenic artery (Fig GI50-6)	Characteristic tortuous, corkscrew appearance.	Extremely common finding. When viewed end-on, splenic artery calcification appears as a thin-walled ring.
Splenic artery aneurysm (Fig GI50-7)	Circular pattern or bizarre configuration of calcification.	
Generalized increased splenic density (without demonstrable calcification) (Fig GI50-8)	Uniform or patchy increased density.	Causes include sickle cell anemia, hemochromatosis, Fanconi's anemia, multiple transfusions, and a previous injection of Thorotrast.

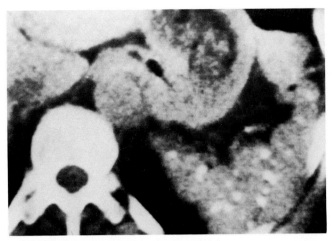

FIG GI50-1. **Histoplasmosis.** CT scan shows multiple small calcifications in the spleen.

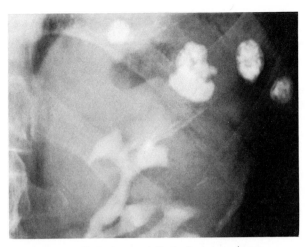

FIG GI50-2. **Brucellosis.** Large calcified splenic granulomas.

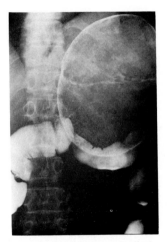

FIG GI50-3. **Huge calcified nonparasitic splenic cyst.**

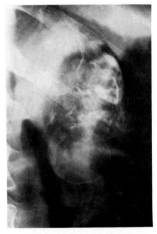

FIG GI50-4. **Calcified hydatid cyst** of the spleen (echinococcal disease).

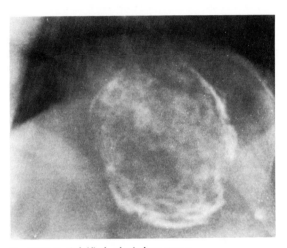

FIG GI50-5. **Calcified splenic hematoma.**

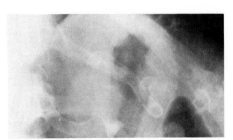

FIG GI50-6. **Calcification of the splenic artery.**

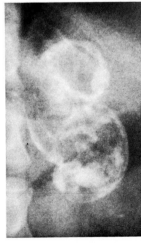

FIG GI50-7. **Splenic artery aneurysm** producing bizarre, lobulated calcification.

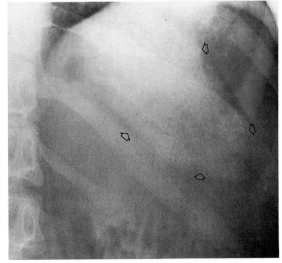

FIG GI50-8. **Sickle cell anemia** causing generalized increase in splenic density.

ALIMENTARY TRACT CALCIFICATION

Condition	Imaging Findings	Comments
Appendicolith (Fig GI51-1)	Round or oval, laminated stones of various sizes.	Found in 10% to 15% of cases of acute appendicitis. Suggests a gangrenous appendix that is likely to perforate and is usually an indication for surgery. May be retrocecal (simulating a gallstone) or pelvic (mimicking a ureteral stone).
Other enterolith (Fig GI51-2)	Faceted, laminated stone in a Meckel's diverticulum, a colonic diverticulum, or the rectum.	Probably results from stasis and is usually found proximal to an area of stricture or within a diverticulum. May cause mucosal ulceration and lower abdominal pain.
Calcified mucocele of appendix	Large crescent-shaped or circular calcification.	Mucocele represents a mucus-containing dilatation of the appendix distal to a fibrotic obstruction of the lumen.
Calcified appendices epiploicae (Fig GI51-3)	Cystlike calcifications adjacent to the gas-filled colon (especially the ascending portion).	May become detached from the colon and appear as small, ring-shaped calcifications lying free in the peritoneal cavity (they change position on serial films).
Ingested foreign bodies (Fig GI51-4)	Various calcific and metallic densities.	Ingested birdshot (metallic) may be trapped in the appendix or colonic diverticula. Trapped seeds and pits may develop ringlike calcium deposits around them.
Mucinous carcinoma of stomach or colon (Fig GI51-5)	Small mottled or punctate deposits of calcium in the tumor.	Calcification may be limited to the tumor mass or involve regional lymph nodes, adjacent omentum, or metastatic foci in the liver.
Leiomyoma of stomach or esophagus (see Fig GI6-1)	Stippled or punctate calcification scattered throughout the mass.	Simulates the pattern of calcification in uterine leiomyomas (fibroids).
Mesenteric calcification (Fig GI51-6)	Various patterns of calcification.	Calcified fat deposits in the omentum; peripheral calcification in mesenteric cysts; rarely, calcified mesenteric lipomas or hydatid cysts in the peritoneal cavity.

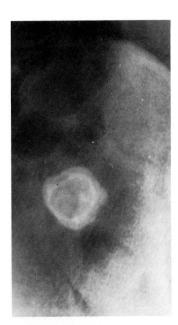

Fig GI51-1. **Appendicolith.**

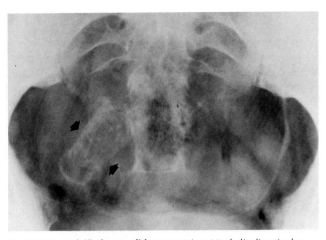

Fig GI51-2. **Calcified enterolith** (arrows) in a Meckel's diverticulum.

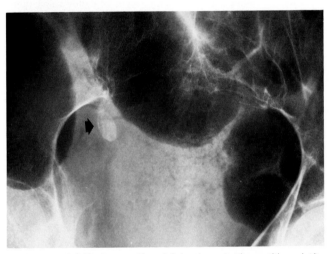

Fig GI51-3. **Calcified appendix epiploica** (arrow). The cystlike calcific density was detached from the colon and changed position on serial films.

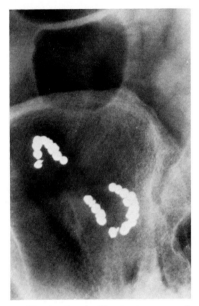

Fig GI51-4. **Metallic foreign bodies** in the appendix representing ingested birdshot.

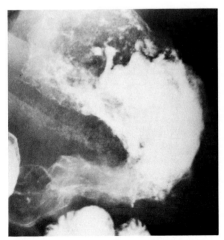

Fig GI51-5. **Calcified mucinous adenocarcinoma** of the stomach causing irregular narrowing of the antrum and body.

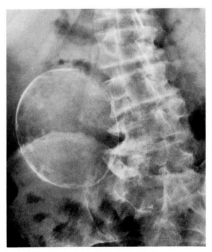

Fig GI51-6. **Calcified mesenteric cyst.**

PANCREATIC CALCIFICATION

Condition	Imaging Findings	Comments
Chronic pancreatitis (Fig GI52-1)	Multiple irregular, small concretions widely scattered throughout the gland (limited to the head or tail in about 25% of cases). Solitary pancreatic calculi are rare.	Primarily alcoholic pancreatitis (calcification in 20% to 40% of patients with chronic alcoholic pancreatitis; 90% of patients with pancreatic calcification have high alcohol intake). Calcification is much less common (2% of cases) in pancreatitis secondary to biliary tract disease.
Pancreatic pseudocyst (Fig GI52-2)	Typical calcifications of chronic pancreatitis, occasionally with a rim of calcification outlining the wall of the pseudocyst.	Calcification can be detected in about 20% of patients who develop a pseudocyst as a complication of chronic pancreatitis.
Hyperparathyroidism	Chronic pancreatitis pattern of calcification.	Pancreatitis occurs in up to 20% of patients with hyperparathyroidism. There is often associated renal calcification (nephrocalcinosis or nephrolithiasis).
Cystadenoma/ cystadenocarcinoma	Sunburst pattern of calcification.	Tumor calcification (often nonspecific) in about 10% of cases. No calcification in adenocarcinoma of the pancreas (though there may be calcification from associated chronic pancreatitis).
Cavernous lymphangioma (Fig GI52-3)	Multiple phleboliths within and adjacent to the pancreas.	Very rare pancreatic tumor.
Hereditary pancreatitis (Fig GI52-4)	Large, rounded calcification (larger than in cystic fibrosis).	More than 50% of children with this inherited (autosomal dominant) condition have pancreatic calcification. Some 20% die from pancreatic cancer.
Cystic fibrosis (Fig GI52-5)	Fine granular calcifications (smaller than in hereditary pancreatitis).	In children and young adults, pancreatic calcification usually implies marked fibrosis with diabetes mellitus.
Kwashiorkor (protein malnutrition)	Various patterns of calcification.	Occurs in underdeveloped countries and is often associated with diabetes and steatorrhea.
Intraparenchymal hemorrhage	Calcified pancreatic mass.	Calcified hematoma due to trauma, infarction, or a bleeding intrapancreatic aneurysm.
Idiopathic pancreatitis	Various patterns of calcification.	No clinical evidence of pancreatic disease. There is usually nonspecific pancreatic ductal stenosis with calculus formation proximal to the site of obstruction.

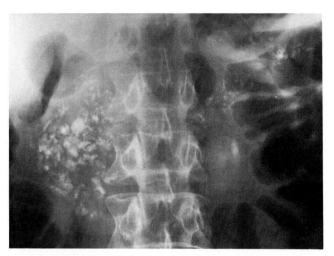

FIG GI52-1. **Chronic alcoholic pancreatitis.**

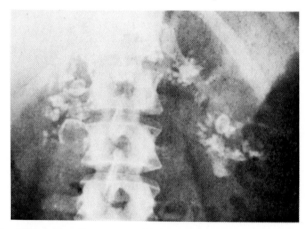

FIG GI52-2. **Pancreatic pseudocyst.** A rim of calcification outlines the wall of the pseudocyst.

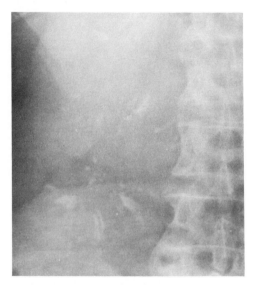

FIG GI52-3. **Cavernous lymphangioma.**

FIG GI52-4. **Hereditary pancreatitis.** The calcifications are rounder and larger than those usually found in other pancreatic diseases.[33]

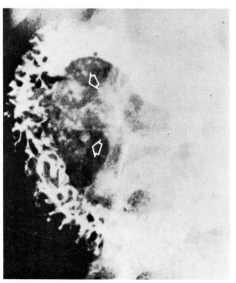

FIG GI52-5. **Cystic fibrosis.** Finely granular calcification primarily found on the head of the pancreas.[33]

GALLBLADDER AND BILE DUCT CALCIFICATION

Condition	Imaging Findings	Comments
Gallstone (Figs GI53-1 and GI53-2)	Single or multiple, smooth or faceted, and often laminated (alternating opaque and lucent rings).	About 20% of gallstones contain sufficient calcium to be radiopaque. If there is a fistula between the biliary and alimentary tracts, a gallstone can be demonstrated at any point in the duodenum, small bowel, or colon.
Porcelain gallbladder (Fig GI53-3)	Extensive mural calcification around the perimeter of the gallbladder.	High incidence of carcinoma (up to 60% of cases). Therefore, a prophylactic cholecystectomy is usually performed even if the patient is asymptomatic.
Milk of calcium bile (Fig GI53-4)	Opacification of the entire gallbladder (simulates a normal gallbladder with contrast material).	Gallbladder is filled with bile that appears opaque because of the high concentration of calcium carbonate. Secondary to chronic cholecystitis with a thickened gallbladder wall and an obstructed cystic duct.
Common duct stone	Single or multiple calcified calculi.	Often difficult to diagnose (the stone is situated close to the spine and often overlies a transverse process).
Mucinous adenocarcinoma of gallbladder	Fine, granular, punctate flecks of calcification.	Rare manifestation. Similar to tumors of the same cell type in the stomach and colon.

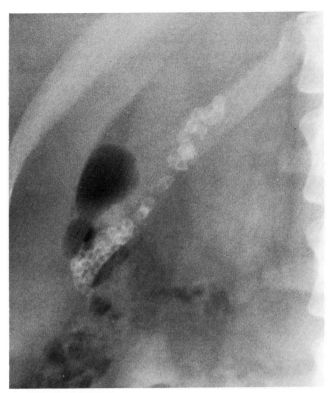

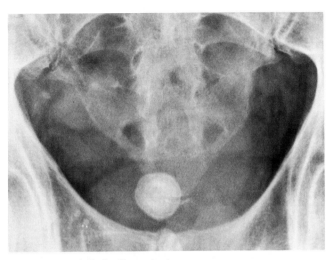

Fig GI53-2. **Calcified gallstone in the rectum.**

Fig GI53-1. **Multiple faceted gallstones.**

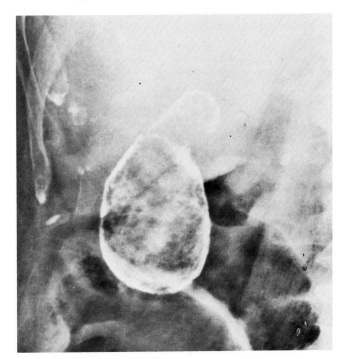

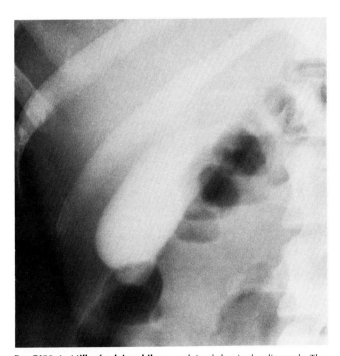

Fig GI53-3. **Porcelain gallbladder.**

Fig GI53-4. **Milk of calcium bile** on a plain abdominal radiograph. The patient had not received any cholecystographic agent.

ADRENAL CALCIFICATION

Condition	Imaging Findings	Comments
Neonatal adrenal hemorrhage (Fig GI54-1)	Triangular or circular calcification about the periphery of the gland.	Most common cause of adrenal calcification. Usually occurs in infants born to diabetic mothers or those with an abnormal obstetric history (prematurity, use of forceps, breech delivery).
Tuberculosis (Fig GI54-2)	Discrete, stippled densities that often outline the entire gland.	Seen in about one fourth of patients with adrenal tuberculosis. Infrequently produces confluent and dense calcific masses.
Neuroblastoma (Fig GI54-3)	Multiple finely stippled, punctate, or flocculent calcifications. May be dense and confluent or extend across the midline.	Calcification with areas of hemorrhage and necrosis occurs in about 50% of cases. There may be calcification in metastatic foci in regional lymph nodes and the liver.
Adrenal cyst	Thin rim of curvilinear calcification outlining the cyst wall.	May represent serous cyst, pseudocyst, (necrosis and resolution of old hemorrhage), parasitic (usually echinococcal) cyst, or cystic adenoma.
Adrenal cortical carcinoma	Scattered calcifications in a mass.	Calcification is fairly common in these tumors.
Pheochromocytoma	Tiny flecks of calcification scattered throughout the tumor.	About 10% are multiple and 10% arise in an extrarenal location (primarily the retroperitoneal ganglia).
Wolman's disease (Fig GI54-4)	Diffuse punctate calcifications throughout both glands.	Rare familial xanthomatosis that causes death in early infancy. Adrenal glands are enlarged but have a normal shape.

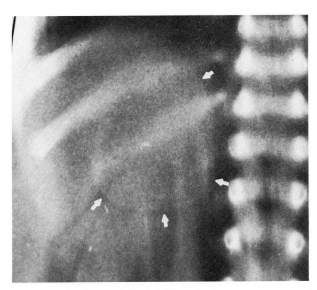

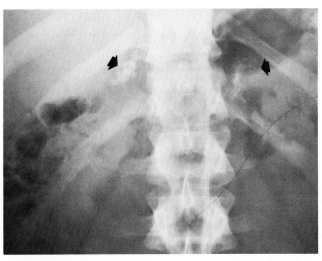

FIG GI54-1. Neonatal adrenal hemorrhage. Circular calcification about the periphery of the gland.[34]

FIG GI54-2. Adrenocortical insufficiency (Addison's disease). There are bilateral adrenal calcifications (arrows) in this patient with tuberculous adrenal disease.

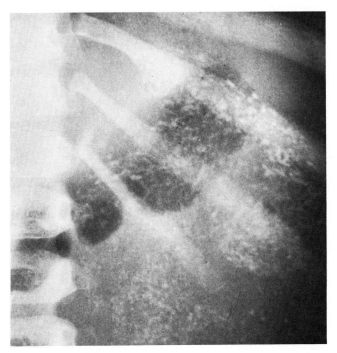

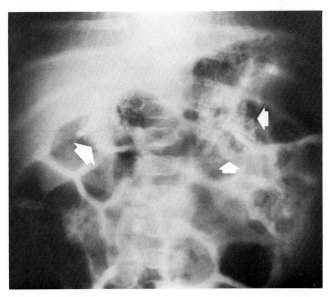

FIG GI54-4. Wolman's disease. Diffuse punctate calcifications in bilaterally enlarged adrenal glands (arrows).

FIG GI54-3. Neuroblastoma. Diffuse granular calcification in the large left upper quadrant mass.

RENAL CALCIFICATION

Condition	Imaging Findings	Comments
Calculus (Fig GI55-1)	Single or multiple stones in the calyces and renal pelvis.	Approximately 80% of renal calculi are opaque. Urinary stasis and infection are important predisposing factors.
Nephrocalcinosis (Fig GI55-2)	Diffuse calcium deposition in the renal parenchyma (especially the medullary pyramids). Varies from a few scattered punctate densities to very dense and extensive calcifications throughout both kidneys.	Causes include skeletal deossification (hyperparathyroidism, primary and secondary bone malignancy, severe osteoporosis, Cushing's syndrome, steroid therapy), increased intestinal absorption of calcium (sarcoidosis, milk-alkali syndrome, hypervitaminosis D), renal tubular acidosis, and hyperoxaluria.
Medullary sponge kidney (Fig GI55-3)	Small, round calculi clustering around the apices of renal pyramids.	Cystic dilatations of the distal collecting ducts.
Papillary necrosis (Fig GI55-4)	Triangular lucency surrounded by a dense opaque band (ring shadow) representing calcification of a sloughed papilla.	Infarction of renal papillae resulting in necrosis with sloughing of involved tissue. Causes include analgesic abuse (phenacetin), diabetes mellitus, sickle cell anemia, pyelonephritis, and urinary tract obstruction.
Tuberculosis	Various patterns of calcification.	Flecks of calcification in multiple tuberculous granulomas. Massive amorphous calcification in nonfunctioning renal parenchyma (autonephrectomy).
Cystic disease (Fig GI55-5)	Thin, curvilinear calcification around the periphery of a renal cyst.	Approximately 3% of simple renal cysts have this pattern (but up to 20% of renal carcinomas have a similar appearance). Peripheral calcification also occurs in polycystic or multicystic disease and in more than half of echinococcal cysts.
Perirenal hematoma/ abscess	Large cystlike calcification.	Calcification tends to be thicker than in a simple renal cyst.
Renal cell carcinoma (Fig GI55-6)	Typically nonperipheral, mottled, or punctate calcification in a mass. There may be cystlike peripheral calcification of the fibrous pseudocapsule.	About 10% contain calcification (primarily in reactive fibrous zones about areas of tissue necrosis). Approximately 90% of masses containing calcium in a nonperipheral location are malignant.
Wilms' tumor	Peripheral cystic calcification in about 10% of cases.	Differs from the fine, granular, or stippled calcification that occurs in 50% of neuroblastomas.
Xanthogranulomatous pyelonephritis (Fig GI55-7)	Diffuse parenchymal calcification, often with an obstructing pelvocalyceal stone.	Chronic inflammatory disease that predominantly occurs in women with a long history of renal infection and is characterized by multiple inflammatory masses that often simulate renal carcinoma.

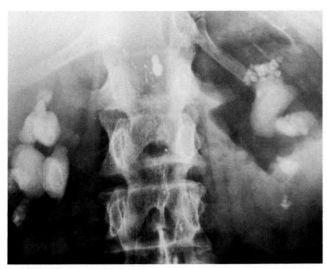

FIG GI55-1. **Bilateral staghorn calculi.**

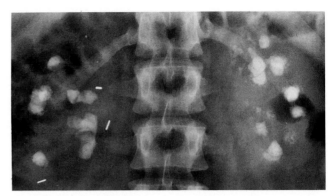

FIG GI55-2. **Milk-alkali syndrome** causing nephrocalcinosis.

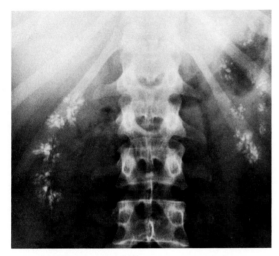

FIG GI55-3. **Medullary sponge kidney.**

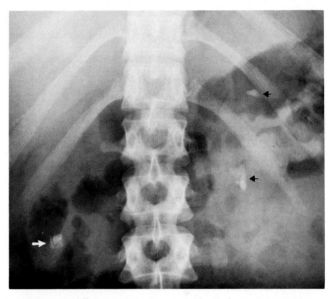

FIG GI55-4. **Papillary necrosis.** Ring-shaped calcifications (arrows) are visible in both kidneys in a young analgesic abuser. This pattern of calcification is associated with sloughing of the entire papillary tip.[35]

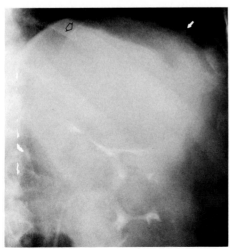

FIG GI55-5. **Simple rental cyst.** Curvilinear, peripheral calcification outlines part of the cyst wall (arrows). Smooth splaying of upper pole calyces is demonstrated on this film from an excretory urogram.[35]

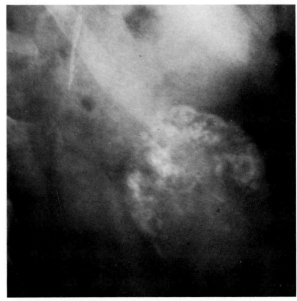

FIG GI55-6. **Calcification in a renal cell carcinoma.** If there is no peripheral calcification, mottled or punctuate calcium that appears to be within a mass is highly indicative of a malignant lesion.[36]

Condition	Imaging Findings	Comments
Cortical calcification	Punctate or linear (tramline) calcification around the renal margin.	Occurs in acute cortical necrosis (rare form of acute renal failure with sparing of the medulla), chronic glomerulonephritis, and hereditary nephritis, and also occurs in dialysis patients.
Renal artery aneurysm (Fig GI55-8)	Circular calcification with a cracked-eggshell appearance.	Calcification develops in one third of these saccular structures situated at the renal hilus.
Arteriovenous malformation	Curvilinear calcification.	Congenital malformation that usually presents with hematuria and frequently an abdominal bruit.
Renal milk of calcium (Fig GI55-9)	Simulates a typical round or oval solid calculus on supine views. Characteristic half-moon contour with the patient in an upright or sitting position (calcific material gravitates to the bottom of the cyst).	Suspension of fine sediment containing calcium that is most commonly found in a cyst or calyceal diverticulum. Usually asymptomatic and an incidental finding. May be related to stasis and infection.
Dysplastic (Fig GI55-10)	Thin curvilinear calcification outlining cyst walls.	Nonhereditary congenital dysplasia, usually unilateral and asymptomatic, in which the kidney is composed almost entirely of large, thin-walled cysts with only a little solid renal tissue. Absent or severely atretic renal artery and an atretic ureter with a blind proximal end.
Residual Pantopaque in renal cyst	Heavy-metal density simulating a swallowed coin.	Pantopaque instilled after renal cyst puncture takes several years to be absorbed (unlike water-soluble contrast material).

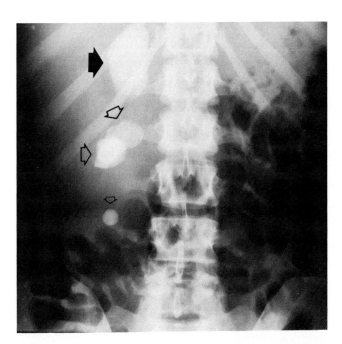

Fig GI55-7. **Xanthogranulomatous pyelonephritis.** Several large radiopaque calculi at the ureteropelvic junction and in the proximal ureter on the right (open arrows). The closed arrow points to an opacified gallbladder. At excretory urography, the right kidney showed no function.

A

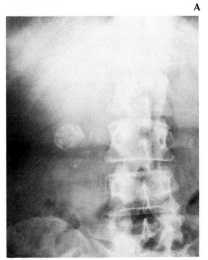

B

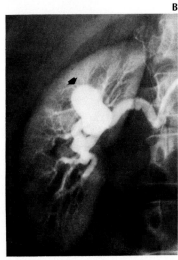

Fig GI55-8. **Calcification in a renal artery aneurysm.** (A) Plain abdominal radiograph demonstrates the circular calcification with a cracked-eggshell appearance at the renal hilus. (B) Selective right arteriogram shows contrast material filling the saccular aneurysm (arrow).

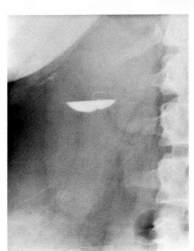

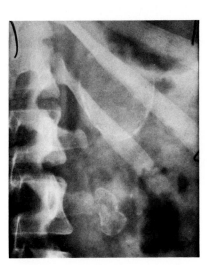

Fig GI55-9. **Renal milk of calcium.** On an upright view, the calcium-containing sediment gravitates to the bottom of the renal cyst, resulting in the characteristic half-moon contour.

Fig GI55-10. **Congenital unilateral multicystic kidney.** There are three peripherally calcified masses, with no excretion of contrast material on excretory urography.[36]

URETERAL CALCIFICATION

Condition	Imaging Findings	Comments
Calculus **(Figs GI56-1 and GI56-2)**	Small, irregular, and poorly calcified. Often oval with its long axis paralleling the course of the ureter.	Most commonly lodges in the lower portion of the ureter (especially at the ureterovesical junction and the pelvic brim). Situated medially above the interspinous line (unlike the far more common phleboliths, which are spherical and located in the lateral portion of the pelvis below a line joining the ischial spines).
Schistosomiasis **(see Fig GI57-1)**	Two roughly parallel, dense lines separated by the caliber of the ureter.	Ureteral calcification occurs in about 15% of patients. It is heaviest in the pelvic portion and gradually decreases proximally. Diffuse bladder calcification is present almost invariably.
Tuberculosis **(Fig GI56-3)**	Linear calcification of the ureteral wall.	Much less frequent than renal calcification in tuberculosis. Calcification of the bladder is relatively rare.

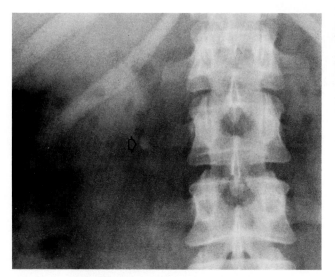

FIG GI56-1. Ureteral calculus (arrow).

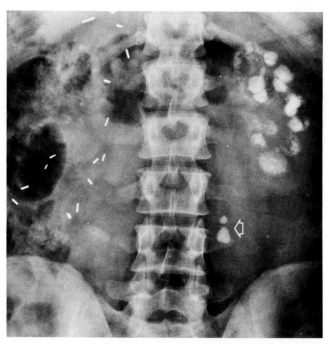

FIG GI56-2. Ureteral calculi. Two stones (one of which is causing obstruction) in the midportion of the left ureter (arrow) in a patient with renal tubular acidosis causing nephrocalcinosis.

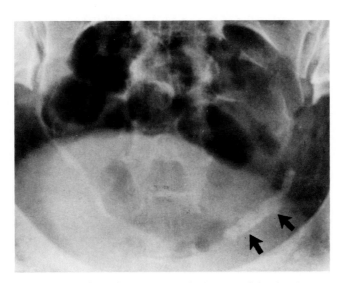

FIG GI56-3. Tuberculosis. Linear calcification of the distal ureter (arrows).

BLADDER CALCIFICATION

Condition	Imaging Findings	Comments
Schistosomiasis (Fig GI57-1)	Linear opaque shadow that initially involves the base of the bladder and eventually encircles the entire bladder.	Worldwide, the most common cause of bladder wall calcification. The bladder often retains relatively normal capacity and distensibility (unlike other inflammatory causes of calcification). Disruption in the continuity of the line of calcification suggests superimposed bladder carcinoma.
Tuberculosis	Faint, irregular rim of calcium outlining the wall of a markedly contracted bladder.	When bladder wall calcification is detectable, extensive tuberculous changes are usually evident in the kidneys and ureters.
Other types of cystitis	Various patterns of amorphous calcification.	Rare manifestation of postirradiation cystitis, bacterial cystitis, and nonspecific infections (encrusted cystitis) with calcium deposited on mucosal erosions.
Bladder calculus (Figs GI57-2 and GI57-3)	Single or multiple and varying in size from tiny concretions to an enormous single calculus occupying the entire bladder lumen.	May represent a migrating stone from the upper urinary tract or a de novo bladder stone (predominantly in elderly men with obstruction or infection of the lower urinary tract). The calcification is usually circular or oval, but may be amorphous, laminated, or spiculated.
Bladder neoplasm (Fig GI57-4)	Punctate, coarse, or linear calcification that is usually encrusted on the tumor surface.	Most common in epithelial lesions (transitional cell and squamous cell carcinomas). Occasionally occurs in mesenchymal tumors (leiomyosarcoma, hemangioma, neuroblastoma, osteogenic sarcoma).

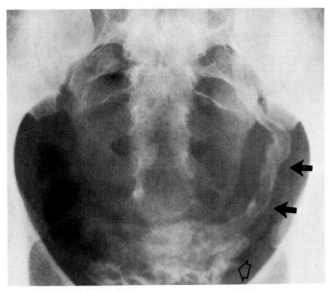

FIG GI57-1. **Schistosomiasis.** Calcification of the bladder (open arrow) and distal ureter (solid arrows).

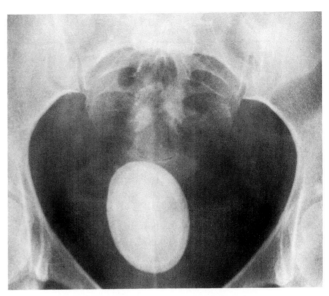

FIG GI57-2. **Bladder calculus.** Single huge, laminated, calcified stone.

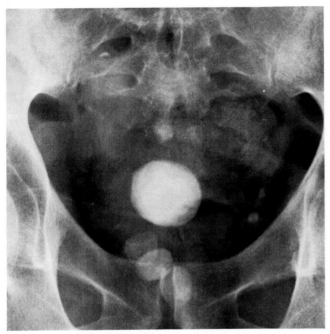

FIG GI57-3. **Multiple bladder stones** of various sizes.

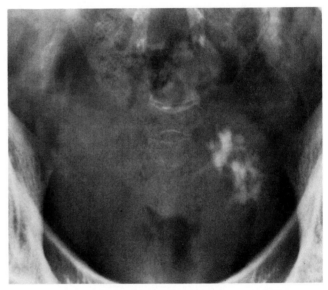

FIG GI57-4. **Calcified transitional cell carcinoma** of the bladder. Coarse tumor calcification was associated with an intravesical mass on excretory urography.

FEMALE GENITAL TRACT CALCIFICATION

Condition	Imaging Findings	Comments
Uterine fibroid (leiomyoma) (Fig GI58-1)	Stippled, mottled, or whorled calcification.	Most common calcified lesion of the female genital tract. A huge fibroid may occupy the entire pelvis or even extend beyond it.
Dermoid cyst (Fig GI58-2)	May contain partially or completely formed teeth. Less frequently, the wall of the cyst is partially calcified.	About half of dermoid cysts contain some calcification. Demonstration of the relatively radiolucent fatty material in the lesion is diagnostic.
Cystadenoma/ cystadenocarcinoma of ovary (Fig GI58-3)	Scattered, fine amorphous shadows (psammomatous bodies), which are barely denser than normal soft tissue.	Calcification is often found in serosal and omental implants throughout the abdomen.
Gonadoblastoma of ovary (Fig GI58-4)	Unilateral or bilateral circumscribed, mottled calcifications.	Rare, potentially malignant gonadal neoplasm that is usually hormonally active and is composed of germ cells, cells of sex cord origin, and mesenchymal elements.
Spontaneous amputation of ovary	Small, coarsely stippled calcified mass that moves on serial films or with changes in patient position.	Probably the result of torsion of the adnexa with subsequent ischemic infarction. Ultrasound or CT shows evidence of a missing ovary on one side.
Pseudomyxoma peritonei (Fig GI58-5)	Curvilinear calcification at the periphery of the jellylike masses.	Complication of spontaneous or surgical rupture of pseudomucinous carcinoma of the ovary or mucocele of the appendix.
Tuberculous salpingitis	Bilateral "string-of-pearls" calcification.	Fallopian tubes have an irregular contour, small lumen, and multiple strictures.
Placental calcification	Fine lacelike pattern outlining the crescentic shape of the placenta.	Physiologic phenomenon associated with involution of the placenta (usually occurs after the 32nd week of fetal life).
Lithopedion (Fig GI58-6)	Calcification or ossification of fetal skeletal parts.	Rare. May be intrauterine (old missed abortion) or extrauterine (previous etopic pregnancy).
Complication of parametrial gold therapy	Bilateral laminated calcification closely approximating the lateral pelvic wall.	Complication of parametrial injections of [198]Au colloid (previous therapy for carcinoma of the cervix). Gold seed implants for pelvic malignancy can appear as multiple short, thin metallic densities.

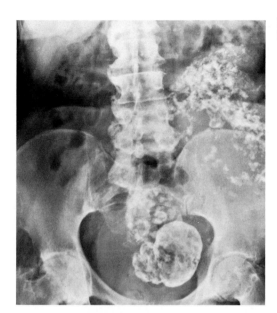

FIG **GI58-1. Calcified uterine fibroid** (leiomyoma). The calcified mass extends well beyond the confines of the pelvis.

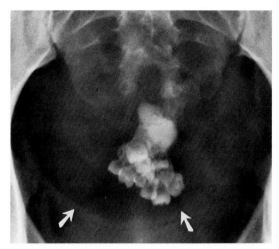

FIG **GI58-2. Dermoid cyst** containing multiple well-formed teeth. Note the relative lucency of the mass (arrows), which is composed largely of fatty tissue.

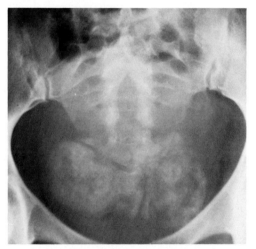

FIG **GI58-3. Calcified cystadenocarcinoma** of the ovary. Diffuse, ill-defined collections of granular amorphous calcification.

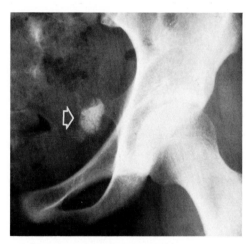

FIG **GI58-4. Calcified gonadoblastoma** of the ovary.[37]

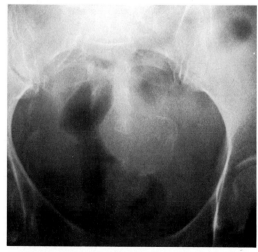

FIG **GI58-5. Pseudomyxoma peritonei**. Complication of spontaneous rupture of pseudomucinous carcinoma of the ovary.

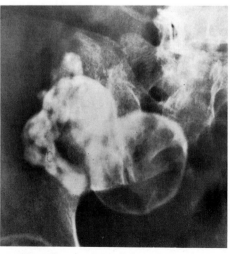

FIG **GI58-6. Lithopedion** in a 78-year-old woman.

WIDESPREAD ABDOMINAL CALCIFICATION

Condition	Imaging Findings	Comments
Psammomatous calcification (cystadenocarcinoma of ovary) (Fig GI59-1)	Scattered granular or sandlike shadows that are often barely denser than normal soft tissue.	May be confined to the primary tumor or diffusely involve metastases throughout the abdomen.
Pseudomyxoma peritonei (see Fig GI58-5)	Widespread abdominal calcifications that are annular and tend to be most numerous in the pelvis.	Caused by rupture of a pseudomucinous cystadenoma of the ovary or a mucocele of the appendix.
Undifferentiated abdominal malignancy (Fig GI59-2)	Bizarre masses of calcification that do not conform to any organ.	Patients with this condition have large soft-tissue masses with multiple linear or nodular calcific densities that can coalesce to form distinctive conglomerate masses.
Tuberculous peritonitis	Widespread mottled abdominal calcifications.	May simulate residual barium in the gastrointestinal tract.
Meconium peritonitis	Multiple small calcific deposits scattered widely throughout the abdomen in a newborn.	Chemical inflammation of the peritoneum caused by the escape of sterile meconium into the peritoneal cavity. Meconium peritonitis usually results from perforation in utero secondary to a congenital stenosis or atresia of the bowel or to meconium ileus.
Oil granulomas (Fig GI59-3)	Widespread annular or plaquelike deposits simulating pseudomyxoma peritonei.	Late effect of the instillation of liquid petrolatum into the peritoneal cavity to prevent adhesions. The calcifications are located in masses of fibrous tissue surrounding the oil droplets. Clinically, oil granulomas can produce hard palpable masses that simulate carcinomatosis or cause intestinal obstruction.

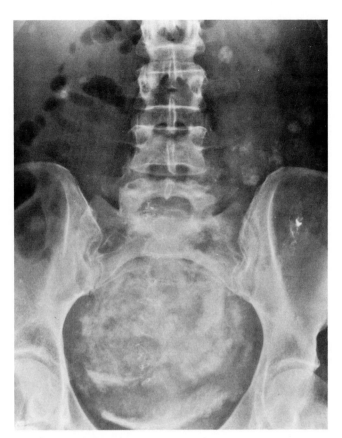

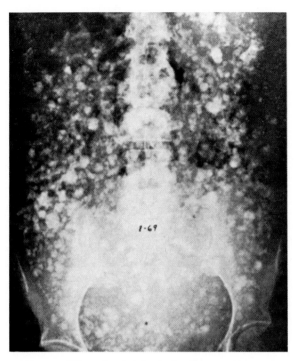

FIG GI59-2. Undifferentiated abdominal malignancy.[38]

FIG GI59-1. Psammomatous calcification of ovarian cystadenocarcinoma. The granular, sandlike calcifications represent metastatic spread throughout the abdomen.

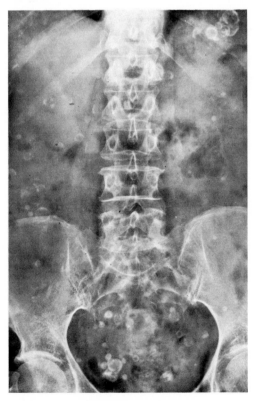

FIG GI59-3. Intraperitoneal granulomatosis.

THICKENED GALLBLADDER WALL (> 2 MILLIMETERS)

Condition	Comments
Cholecystitis (Figs GI60-1 and GI60-2)	Thickening of the gallbladder wall is frequently observed on sonograms of patients with acute cholecystitis, though it is a nonspecific finding that can be seen in several other conditions. Measurements of gallbladder wall thickness should be made on the anterior surface of the gallbladder where it abuts the liver, since the posterior wall is often more difficult to define because of acoustic enhancement and adjacent bowel. Gallbladder wall thickening may occur in patients with chronic cholecystitis (with or without stones) and has also been described in complications of cholecystitis (eg, empyema of the gallbladder, gangrenous necrosis, and pericholecystic abscess).
Hypoalbuminemia (Fig GI60-3)	Thickening of the gallbladder wall may be associated with markedly depressed levels of serum albumin in the absence of any other known etiologic factor. The postulated mechanism for wall thickening in this setting is edema from increased extravascular fluid (due to low plasma oncotic pressure). Hypoalbuminemia may well be the underlying cause for the gallbladder wall thickening seen in patients with ascites, renal disease, and elevated venous pressure secondary to congestive heart disease.
Ascites (Fig GI60-4)	May reflect an underlying hypoalbuminemic state. The apparent gallbladder wall thickening in this condition may result from improper transducer placement or angulation.
Congestive heart failure	Probably reflects edema of the gallbladder wall due to increased systemic and portal venous engorgement.
Hepatitis	A postulated mechanism is that the viruses excreted into the biliary system may produce a mild pericholecystic inflammation that is appreciated as wall thickening on ultrasound.
Incomplete fasting	The most common reason for apparent thickening of the gallbladder wall (not related to any pathologic abnormality). Normal patients who have incompletely fasted will often show a contracted gallbladder with a wall thickness of greater than 2 mm, so an accurate history of dietary intake before the examination is essential. Especially common in infants, in whom prolonged fasting before the examination is not possible.
Extrahepatic portal vein obstruction	Variceal collaterals and edema cause thickening of the gallbladder wall. May be secondary to pancreatitis, carcinoma of the pancreas or stomach, or neonatal omphalitis.

Condition	Comments
Lymphatic obstruction	Nodal enlargement in the porta hepatis causes dilation of lymphatics in the gallbladder wall.
Carcinoma of gallbladder	Diffuse or focal thickening of the gallbladder wall is a relatively unusual manifestation. Metastases may very rarely cause segmental wall thickening.
Adenomyomatosis	Diffuse or focal thickening of the muscular layer of the gallbladder. Characteristic glandlike, barium-filled outpouchings projecting just outside the gallbladder lumen on oral cholecystography.

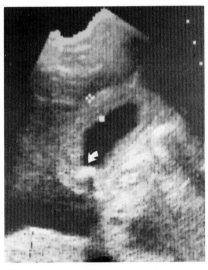

FIG GI60-1. Acute cholecystitis. Marked thickening of the gallbladder neck (1.1 cm between the cursors). There is a densely echogenic stone (arrow) with posterior acoustic shadowing in the neck of the gallbladder.

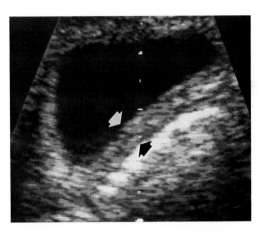

FIG GI60-2. Acalculous cholecystitis. Enlarged gallbladder with a thickened, edematous wall. There is no evidence of gallstones or posterior acoustic shadowing.

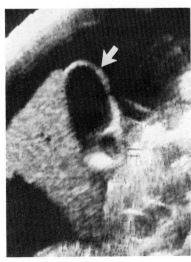

FIG GI60-3. Hypoalbuminemia with marked ascites. Thickening of the gallbladder wall (arrow).

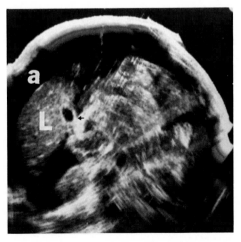

FIG GI60-4. Ascites. A large amount of sonolucent ascitic fluid (a) separates the liver (L) and other soft-tissue structures from the anterior abdominal wall. Note the relative thickness of the gallbladder wall (arrow).

FOCAL ANECHOIC (CYSTIC) LIVER MASSES

Condition	Comments
Congenital cyst (Fig GI61-1)	Most common benign cystic lesion of the liver that develops secondary to an excess of intrahepatic ductules that fail to involute. While generally asymptomatic, hepatic cysts may grow large (even causing obstructive jaundice), become infected, or bleed.
Polycystic disease of liver (Fig GI61-2)	Minimal to virtually complete replacement of the hepatic parenchyma by cystic lesions occurs in about one third of patients with adult-type polycystic kidney disease.
Caroli's disease (Fig GI61-3)	Multiple focal cystic collections throughout the liver representing communicating cavernous ectasia of the biliary tree. Although the appearance superficially is that of polycystic disease, careful scanning usually shows that the collections communicate with the biliary tree (unlike the isolated cysts of polycystic disease).
Acquired cysts	Occasionally develop after an episode of trauma or a localized inflammatory process of the liver. Segmental obstruction of the biliary tree (stricture from previous surgery, infection, or neoplasm) may produce focal anechoic areas that mimic true cysts but generally are not as well defined.
Intrahepatic gallbladder	Most common positional anomaly, which appears as a cystic intrahepatic lesion lying in the main interlobar fissure between the right and left lobes. The diagnosis can usually be made by careful scanning and noting that the gallbladder is not present in its normal location. If unclear on ultrasound, a radionuclide scan can document the biliary origin of the lesion.
Hematoma (Fig GI61-4)	May appear cystic, but generally not as well defined as a simple cyst. Subcapsular hematomas tend to be elliptical and are located peripherally.

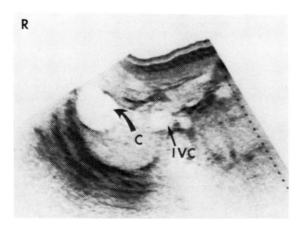

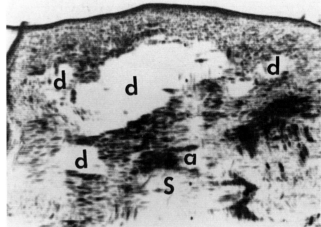

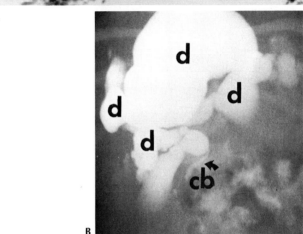

Fig GI61-1. Simple nonparasitic hepatic cyst. Transverse sonogram of the upper abdomen in a patient with suspected metastatic disease and a defect on a radionuclide scan shows a completely sonolucent mass (C) that meets the criteria for a simple uncomplicated cyst. (IVC, inferior vena cava and R, right)[39]

Fig GI61-2. Polycystic liver disease. (A) Multiple anechoic cysts of various sizes throughout the liver in extensive adult-type polycystic kidney disease. (B) Prone longitudinal sonogram on the same patient shows multiple renal cysts.

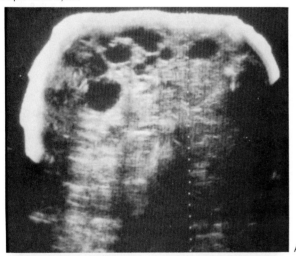

Fig GI61-3. Caroli's disease. (A) Transverse supine sonogram demonstrates multiple dilated bile ducts (d) as sonolucent spaces in the liver. (S, spine and a, aorta). (B) Frontal view of a transhepatic cholangiogram in a projection corresponding to that in (A) shows cystic dilatation of the distal intrahepatic ducts (d) with a normal-sized common bile duct (cb).[40]

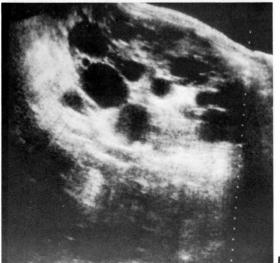

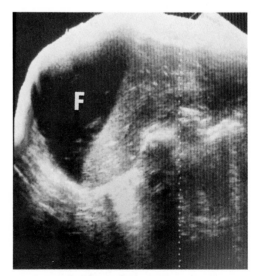

Fig GI61-4. Traumatic subcapsular hematoma. Transverse scan shows an elliptical fluid collection (F) that developed after blunt trauma to the abdomen.

Condition	Comments
Echinococcal cyst **(Fig GI61-5)**	May present as a purely fluid collection in the liver (1 to 20 cm in size) and with localized thickening of the cyst wall. There is often a more complex appearance with multiple septations and daughter cysts or scolices.
Metastases **(Fig GI61-6)**	In one series, 2% of metastases appeared as anechoic masses. Metastatic sarcomas that have undergone necrosis may be difficult to distinguish from simple cysts, though the findings of a thick rim, irregular margins, mural nodules, or a fluid-fluid level should suggest the appropriate diagnosis.

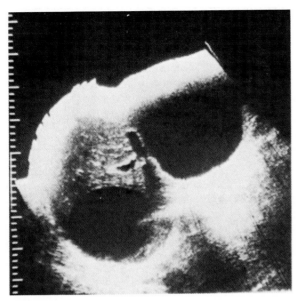

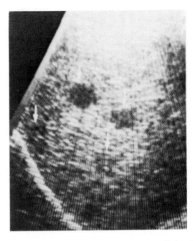

FIG GI61-6. Metastases. Multiple sonolucent nodules.[41]

FIG GI61-5. Echinococcal cysts. Transverse scan shows two large fluid-filled cysts.[41]

COMPLEX OR SOLID HEPATIC MASSES

Condition	Comments
Hepatocellular carcinoma (hepatoma) (Fig GI62-1)	Because primary hepatic carcinoma usually (but not always) arises on a background of underlying liver disease, such as cirrhosis or parasitic infection, the areas of tumor tend to appear hypoechoic when contrasted with the remainder of the liver. When a hepatoma arises in an otherwise normal liver, it may be echogenic. Because the tumor is often multifocal, the demonstration of multiple lesions cannot differentiate between primary and secondary tumors. Unlike metastases, a hepatoma commonly invades the portal venous system and thus should be strongly suspected if tumor thrombus can be visualized in the portal venous radicles.
Metastases (Figs GI62-2 and GI62-3)	Variable pattern (large or small, echogenic or echolucent, partially cystic, focal or diffuse). No correlation between the histology of a metastasis and its sonographic appearance.
Abscess (Figs GI62-4 to GI62-6)	May appear as focal or diffuse areas of increased or decreased parenchymal echoes. In the more chronic stage, an abscess typically appears as a well-defined cavity with various degrees of internal echogenicity and a well-defined, thickened, irregular wall. Microabscesses may appear as "targets" with sonolucent peripheries and echogenic centers. Serial scans may be helpful since echogenic abscesses usually evolve toward a more cystic appearance.
Cavernous hemangioma	Virtually pathognomonic appearance of a small (1 to 3 cm), highly echogenic focus superimposed on a background of normal liver parenchyma. The increased echogenicity is due to the interfaces caused by the walls of the cavernous venous sinuses and the blood in these vessels. A slightly more irregular pattern develops as the hemangioma undergoes degeneration and fibrous replacement.
Echinococcal cyst (Fig GI62-7)	Multiseptate complex cystic lesion that may contain a fluid collection with a split wall or "floating membrane." This condition should be suspected whenever a multicystic mass is seen, especially in areas where echinococcal disease is endemic.

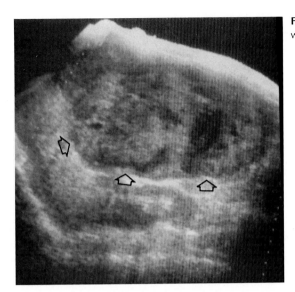

Fig GI62-1. Hepatoma. Complex mass (arrows) with a large echogenic component.

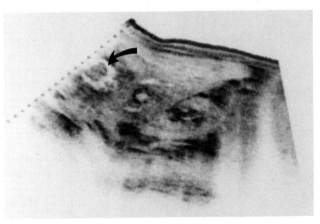

Fig GI62-2. Metastasis from choriocarcinoma. Longitudinal sonogram shows a necrotic metastasis with hemorrhage (arrow) in the liver. The patient died of massive hemoperitoneum from bleeding hepatic metastases.[42]

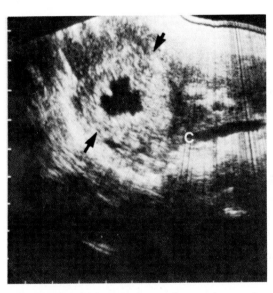

Fig GI62-3. Metastasis. Sagittal scan shows a large echogenic mass (arrows) with central necrosis. (C, inferior vena cava)[41]

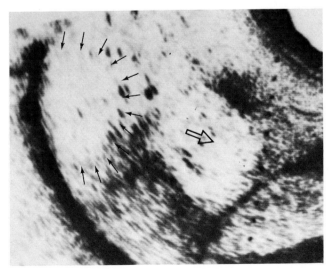

Fig GI62-4. Hepatic amebic abscesses. Sagittal sonogram shows two abscesses in the right lobe, both with low-level, homogeneous fine echoes. One has a small, central, echo-free area (open arrow); the other is homogeneous (small arrows).[43]

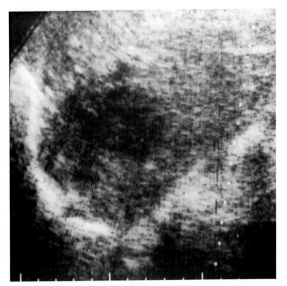

Fig GI62-5. Pyogenic hepatic abscess. Ill-defined complex mass with irregular margins.

Condition	Comments
Focal nodular hyperplasia/ liver cell adenoma (Fig GI62-8)	Sonographically indistinguishable lesions that appear as solid masses of increased or decreased echogenicity. Adenomas may contain sonolucent areas (due to necrosis or hemorrhage) and are frequently seen in women taking oral contraceptives and in patients with type 1 glycogen storage disease (von Gierke's). Unlike hepatic adenoma, which is composed entirely of hepatocytes without Kupffer's cells, focal nodular hyperplasia contains these technetium-avid cells and thus often appears normal on ^{99m}Tc-sulfur colloid scans.
Hemangioendothelioma (Fig GI62-9)	Most common hepatic lesion producing symptoms during infancy (the vast majority of these tumors present before 6 months of age). Although generally considered benign, there have been rare reports of distant metastases. Extensive arteriovenous shunting in the lesion may lead to high-output congestive heart failure. The tumor has a nonspecific sonographic pattern and may appear as a hypoechoic, complex, or hyperechoic lesion.

Fig GI62-6. *Candida albicans* **abscesses** (top and bottom). Numerous rounded, fluid-filled lesions (arrows) with a target appearance.[44]

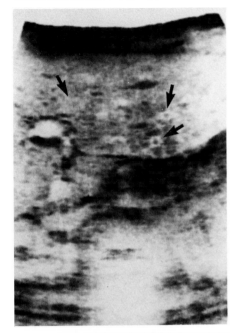

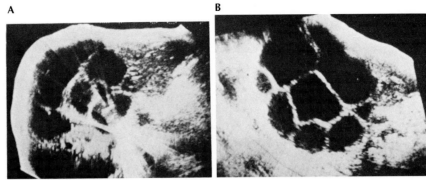

Fig GI62-7. Echinococcal cyst. (A) Transverse scan shows a honeycomb pattern due to the multilocular process. (B) Sagittal scan shows the typical pattern of adjacent daughter vesicles.[41]

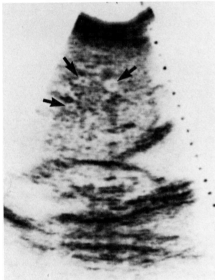

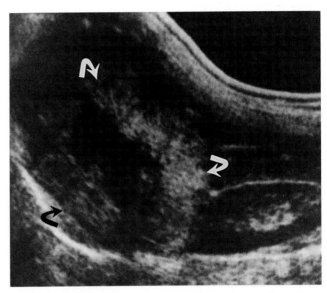

Fig GI62-8. Adenoma. Longitudinal sonogram shows a large dense lesion (arrows) with a central fluid area in the right lobe of the liver.

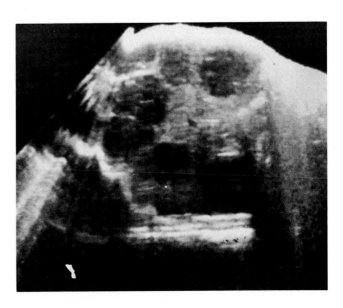

Fig GI62-9. Hemangioendothelioma. Sagittal sonogram shows multiple discrete, hypoechoic solid masses.[45]

FOCAL DECREASED-ATTENUATION MASSES IN THE LIVER

Condition	Imaging Findings	Comments
Cyst		
Nonparasitic cyst (Fig GI63-1)	Sharply delineated, round or oval, near–water attenuation lesion with a very thin wall, no internal septations, and no contrast enhancement.	Most commonly congenital, but may be secondary to inflammation or trauma. Although more frequently single, hepatic cysts may be multiple (innumerable multifocal cysts occur in polycystic liver disease). May occasionally be difficult to differentiate from a cystic neoplasm or an old hematoma (on ultrasound, cystic tumors may have internal septations and irregular inner margins, whereas nonneoplastic hepatic cysts have no internal septations and have completely smooth walls).
Echinococcal cyst (Fig GI63-2)	Sharply defined, rounded, near–water attenuation mass with a thin wall. May appear multilocular with internal septations representing the walls of daughter cysts.	Tissue infection of humans caused by the larval stage of a small tapeworm, for which dogs, sheep, cattle, and camels are the major intermediate hosts. The wall of the cyst may show dense calcification, and gas may form in the cyst because of superimposed infection or communication with the intestinal lumen through the bile duct.
Polycystic disease (Fig GI63-3)	Multiple low-attenuation cysts of various sizes.	About one third of patients with adult polycystic kidney disease have associated cysts of the liver, which do not interfere with hepatic function.
Caroli's disease (Fig GI63-4)	Multiple low-attenuation cystic masses in the liver.	Rare disorder characterized by segmental saccular dilatation of the intrahepatic bile ducts throughout the liver. The dilated cystic segments contain bile and communicate freely with the biliary tree and with each other, in contrast to polycystic liver disease in which the cysts contain a clear serous fluid and do not communicate with the biliary tree or other cysts. About 80% of patients have associated medullary sponge kidney.
Abscess		
Pyogenic abscess (Fig GI63-5)	Sharply defined homogeneous area with an attenuation usually greater than that of a benign cyst but lower than that of a solid neoplasm. No enhancement after intravenous injection of contrast material, though a rim of tissue around the cavity may become more dense than normal liver (also seen with a necrotic neoplasm).	Results from such diverse causes as ascending biliary tract infection (especially secondary to calculi or carcinoma in the extrahepatic biliary ductal system), hematogeneous spread via the portal venous system, generalized septicemia with involvement of the liver by way of the hepatic arterial circulation, direct extension from intraperitoneal infection, and hepatic trauma. May be solitary or multilocular (a single abscess is usually located in the right lobe). The demonstration of gas in a low-density hepatic mass is highly suggestive of an abscess.

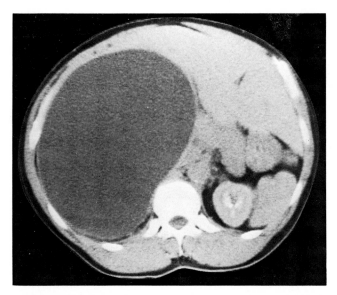

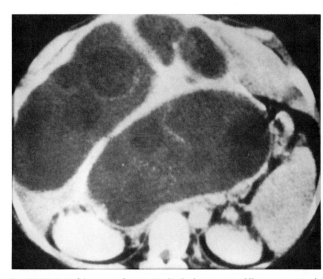

Fɪɢ **GI63-1. Simple hepatic cyst.** A 20-cm fluid-filled mass in the right lobe of the liver displaces the abdominal contents and compresses the inferior vena cava. After aspiration and the instillation of alcohol, there was virtual ablation of the cyst.[46]

Fɪɢ **GI63-2. Echinococcal cyst.** Multiple large cysts filling a massively enlarged liver.

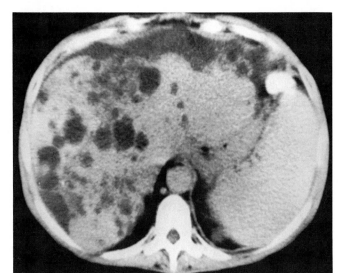

Fɪɢ **GI63-3. Polycystic liver disease.** Innumerable lucent lesions of various sizes in a markedly enlarged liver. The patient also had severe polycystic kidney disease.

A

B

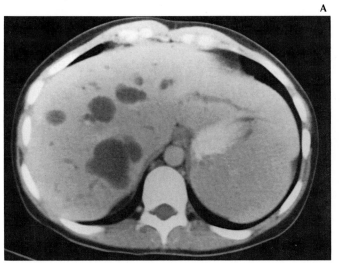

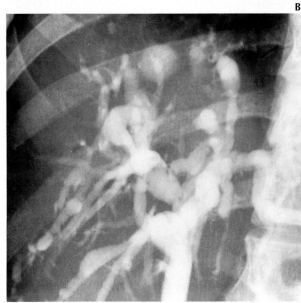

Fɪɢ **GI63-4. Caroli's disease.** (A) CT scan shows fluid-filled cystic masses in the liver. (B) Cholangiogram shows the characteristic dilatation of intrahepatic ducts.

Condition	Imaging Findings	Comments
Amebic abscess	Sharply defined homogeneous area with an attenuation usually greater than that of a benign cyst but lower than that of a solid neoplasm. No enhancement after intravenous injection of contrast material, though a rim of tissue around the cavity may become more dense than normal liver (also seen with a necrotic neoplasm).	Most frequent extracolonic complication of amebiasis, occurring in about one third of patients with amebic dysentery. About two thirds are solitary, with the remainder being multiple and often coalescing into a single large liver abscess. Most often located in the posterior portion of the right lobe of the liver, since this region receives most of the blood draining the right colon (where amebas tend to settle) because of the streaming effect in portal blood flow.
Fungal abscess (Fig GI63-6)	Multiple small, rounded low-attenuation lesions, some of which have a central higher density focus producing a target appearance.	Uncommon condition that usually occurs in patients with compromised immune systems (especially acute myelogeneous and lymphocytic leukemia). The abscesses are usually scattered rather uniformly throughout the liver, spleen, and even the kidneys.
Neoplasm **Cavernous hemangioma** (Fig GI63-7)	Well-circumscribed, low-attenuation area. After the bolus injection of contrast material, the periphery of the lesion becomes hyperdense; serial scans show a centripetally advancing border of enhancement as the central area of low density becomes progressively smaller.	Most common benign tumor of the liver. Usually single, small, and asymptomatic and found incidentally at surgery or autopsy or during an unrelated radiographic procedure. Large symptomatic hemangiomas may present as palpable masses, and spontaneous rupture infrequently causes massive intraperitoneal hemorrhage.
Adenoma (Fig GI63-8)	Low-density or almost isodense mass that demonstrates a variable degree of enhancement. Recent hemorrhage appears as a central area of increased attenuation, while a remote bleeding episode may produce a central area of low attenuation reflecting an evolving hematoma or central cellular necrosis.	Benign lesion that is generally solitary and composed entirely of hepatocytes without Kupffer's cells. The tumor has a strong hormonal association and most often develops in women taking oral contraceptives. When the tumor occurs in men, it may be associated with hormonal therapy of carcinoma of the prostate. Spontaneous hemorrhage, sometimes of life-threatening proportions, is relatively common.
Focal nodular hyperplasia (Fig GI63-9)	Nonspecific low-attenuation mass that often demonstrates substantial enhancement after intravenous injection of contrast material. Central scar may occasionally be large enough to appear as a relatively low-density stellate area in a generally enhancing mass.	Controversial entity that probably represents an uncommon benign liver tumor composed of normal hepatocytes and Kupffer's cells. The characteristic morphologic feature is a central stellate, fibrous scar with peripherally radiating septa that divide the mass into lobules. Often in a subcapsular location or pedunculated along the inferior margin of the liver (infrequently situated deep in the hepatic parenchyma). The normal uptake of ^{99m}Tc-sulfur colloid virtually excludes other hepatic neoplasms that do not contain Kupffer's cells.
Hemangioendothelioma	Multiple well-demarcated masses of decreased attenuation. After a bolus injection of contrast material, there is early enhancement of the lesions, which may be isodense with normal liver on delayed scans.	Most common hepatic lesion producing symptoms during infancy (the vast majority of these tumors present before 6 months of age). Although generally considered benign, there have been rare reports of distant metastases. Extensive arteriovenous shunting in the lesion may lead to high-output congestive heart failure. May rarely occur in adults with long-term exposure to vinyl chloride or who have received Thorotrast.

(continued page 416)

A

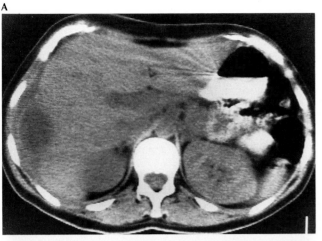

B

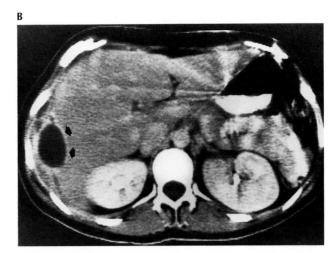

C

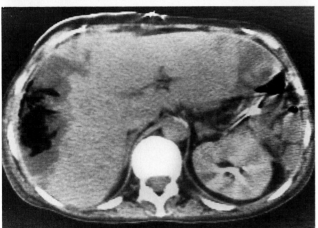

FIG GI63-5. Hepatic abscess. (A) Unenhanced scan shows a single low-density lesion with poorly defined margins at the periphery of the liver. (B) After infusion of contrast material, there is rim enhancement with the margins of the abscess seen as a white line (arrows) of higher density than the surrounding normal liver. (C) CT scan in another patient shows a large collection of gas in a pyogenic abscess in the lateral aspect of the right lobe of the liver.[47]

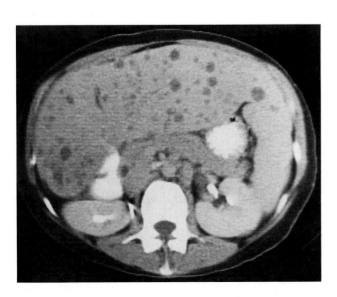

FIG GI63-6. Fungal abscesses. Numerous low-density lesions in a massively enlarged liver representing multiple abscesses containing *Candida albicans*.[44]

Condition	Imaging Findings	Comments
Primary hepatocellular carcinoma (Figs GI63-10 and GI63-11)	Single or multiple solid masses with low attenuation. Dense, diffuse, nonuniform contrast enhancement.	In the United States, primary liver cell carcinoma most commonly occurs in patients with underlying diffuse hepatocellular disease, especially alcoholic or postnecrotic cirrhosis. Extremely common in Africa and Asia, where this tumor may account for up to one third of all types of malignancy. Unlike metastases, primary hepatocellular carcinoma tends to be solitary or to produce a small number of lesions. The demonstration of one or a few large focal lesions in association with a pattern of generalized cirrhosis strongly suggests this diagnosis.
Cholangiocarcinoma	Nonspecific low-attenuation mass that enhances after administration of contrast material.	Most common CT finding of this slow-growing tumor is focal or generalized biliary obstruction.
Lymphoma	Multiple focal masses of diminished attenuation, often associated with lymphadenopathy.	Secondary involvement of the liver is common, though CT is relatively insensitive in detecting the usually small foci. Diffuse lymphomatous infiltration is generally isodense.
Metastases (Figs GI63-12 and GI63-13)	Single or, more commonly, multiple low-density masses adjacent to normally enhancing hepatic parenchyma after contrast material administration. Metastases may rarely have an attenuation value higher than that of liver parenchyma (due to diffuse calcification, recent hemorrhage, or fatty infiltration of surrounding hepatic tissue).	By far the most common malignant tumor involving the hepatic parenchyma. Cystic metastases (sarcoma, melanoma, ovarian and colon carcinoma) may closely simulate benign cysts, though they often have somewhat shaggy and irregular walls. Amorphous punctate deposits of calcification in an area of diminished density may be seen in metastases from mucin-producing tumors (carcinomas of the gastrointestinal tract).
Trauma		
Subcapsular hematoma (Fig GI63-14)	Well-marginated, crescentic or lenticular fluid collection located just beneath the hepatic capsule. Variable attenuation depending on its age and composition.	May be the result of blunt or penetrating abdominal trauma or a complication of surgery, percutaneous cholangiography, biopsy, portography, or biliary drainage procedures. Hematomas generally have high attenuation during the first few days, then diminish gradually over several weeks to become low-density lesions.
Intrahepatic hematoma (Fig GI63-15)	Round or oval mass of variable attenuation depending on its age and composition.	Hematomas generally have high attenuation during the first few days, then diminish gradually over several weeks to become low-density lesions. Dependent layering of cellular debris may produce a fluid-fluid interface in the mass.
Parenchymal laceration (Fig GI63-16)	Irregularly shaped cleft or mass of low attenuation that often extends to the periphery of the liver and may have a branching pattern superficially resembling dilated bile ducts.	Small hyperdense foci, representing clotted blood, are frequently detected in the larger low-density site of a lysed clot and damaged parenchyma. Recent hemorrhage and clot have higher density than older hematomas that have matured.
Biloma (Fig GI63-17)	Low-attenuation mass.	Intrahepatic or extrahepatic collection of bile due to traumatic rupture of the biliary tree.

(continued page 418)

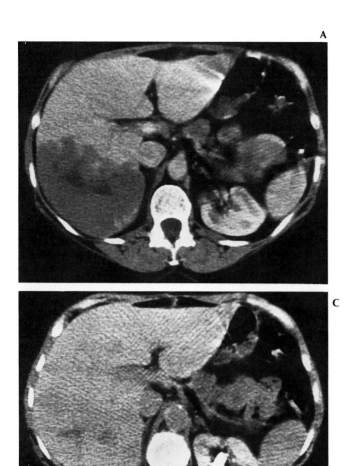

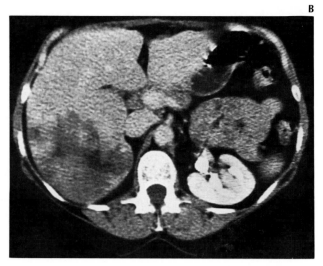

FIG GI63-7. Cavernous hemangioma. (A) Initial scan after a bolus injection of contrast material demonstrates a large low-density lesion in the posterior segment of the right lobe of the liver. (B and C) Delayed scans show progressive enhancement of the lesion until it becomes nearly isodense with normal hepatic parenchyma.

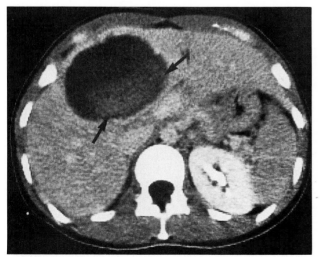

FIG GI63-8. Adenoma. Large low-density mass in the liver. Note the area of higher density (arrows), which represents a blood clot, along the posterior aspect of the lesion.

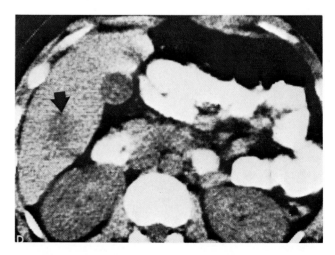

FIG GI63-9. Focal nodular hyperplasia. Noncontrast scan shows an area of low attenuation (arrow) that is indistinguishable from a primary or secondary hepatic neoplasm. The lesion became isodense after the administration of contrast material.[48]

Condition	Imaging Findings	Comments
Radiation injury	Sharply defined band of diminished density in the liver corresponding to the radiation port.	Low attenuation in the irradiated area reflects the histologic combination of panlobar congestion, evolving hemorrhage, and fatty change. May become apparent days to months after radiation therapy (>3,500 rads). Usually a transient phenomenon that is not seen on follow-up scans several months after the initial discovery.
Intrahepatic extension of pancreatic pseudocyst	Low-density, round intrahepatic cystic mass or smaller, circular or tubular lucencies simulating dilated bile ducts (extension of pseudocysts along portal tracts).	The wall of the pseudocyst is initially formed by whatever tissue structures first limit its spread. Gradually, the evoked inflammatory reaction encapsulates the contents of the pseudocyst with granulation tissue and then with a fibrous wall (mature pseudocyst).

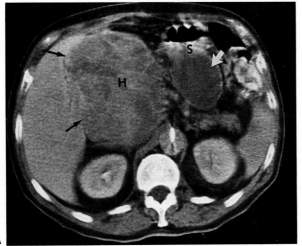
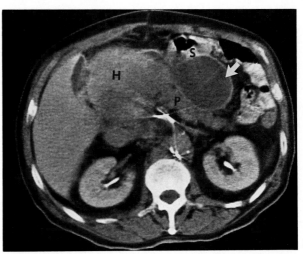

FIG GI63-10. **Primary hepatocellular carcinoma.** (A) Huge mass with an attenuation value slightly less than that of normal liver. The black arrows point to the hepatoma–normal liver interface. Of incidental note is a pancreatic pseudocyst (white arrow) in the lesser sac between the stomach (S) and the pancreas. (B) On a slightly lower scan there is absence of the fat plane surrounding the head of the pancreas (P), indicating invasion of the pancreas by the tumor.

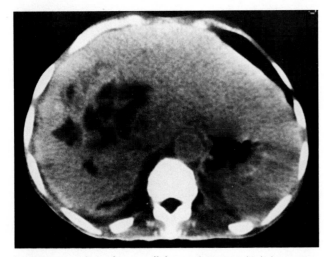
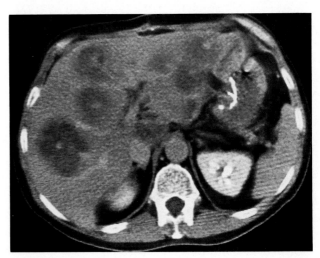

FIG GI63-11. **Primary hepatocellular carcinoma.** Multiple low-attenuation masses in the liver.

FIG GI63-12. **Metastases.** Multiple low-density metastases with high-density centers.

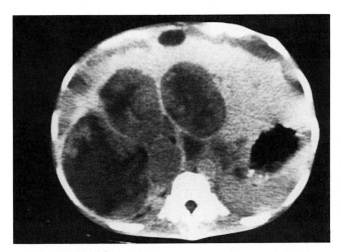

FIG GI63-13. Metastases. Several large, low-density lesions filling much of the liver. Although these lesions simulate benign cysts, their walls are somewhat shaggy and irregular.

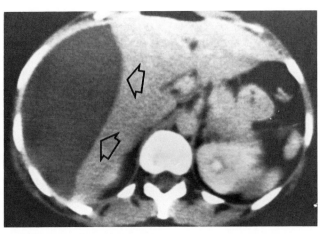

FIG GI63-14. Subcapsular hematoma. Well-circumscribed elliptical area of low-attenuation density (arrowheads) in the periphery of the right lobe of the liver. The patient had sustained blunt trauma to the upper abdomen 2 weeks previously.

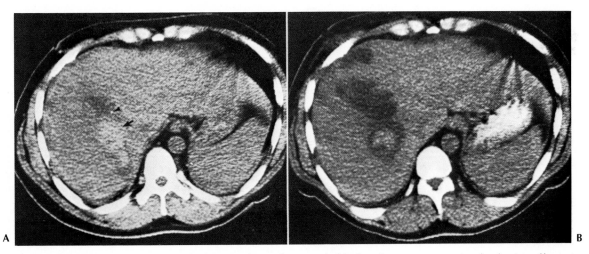

FIG GI63-15. Intrahepatic hematoma. The patient had sustained a gunshot wound of the liver that was not appreciated at the time of laparotomy. (A) CT scan shows the bullet fragment (arrowhead) in a mixed low- and high-density collection. The high-density area (arrow) represents clotted blood. (B) One week later, the hematoma is larger and of lower density.[39]

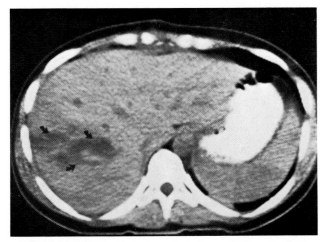

FIG GI63-16. Hepatic laceration. CT scan after blunt trauma shows an irregular low-density plane (arrows) passing through the right lobe of the liver.[39]

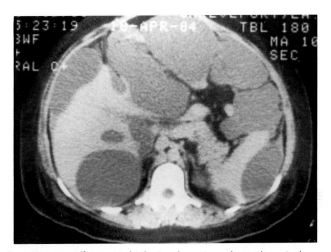

FIG GI63-17. Biloma. Multiple intrahepatic and extrahepatic low-attenuation lesions after traumatic rupture of the biliary tree and bile peritonitis.

GENERALIZED ABNORMALITY OF HEPATIC ATTENUATION

Condition	Imaging Findings	Comments
Fatty infiltration (Figs GI64-1 to GI64-3)	Generalized decrease in the attenuation value of the liver. The portal veins commonly appear as high-density structures surrounded by a background of low density caused by hepatic fat (the opposite of the normal pattern of portal veins as low-density channels on noncontrast scans).	Result of excessive deposition of triglycerides, which occurs in cirrhosis and other hepatic disorders. In normal individuals, the mean liver CT number is never lower than that of the spleen, while in fatty infiltration the hepatic density is much lower. In fatty infiltration of liver due to cirrhosis, there often is prominence of the caudate lobe associated with shrinkage of the right lobe.
Hemochromatosis	Generalized increase in density of the hepatic parenchyma that contrasts sharply with the much lower density of normal intrahepatic blood vessels.	Excessive deposition of iron in body tissues with eventual fibrosis and dysfunction of the severely affected organs. May be a primary inherited disorder (excessive intestinal absorption of iron) or secondary to certain chronic anemias or repeated blood transfusions.
Glycogen storage disease	Generalized increase in hepatic density or, less commonly, a generally low-density liver.	Autosomal genetic disorders of carbohydrate metabolism with various enzymatic defects. The areas of low attenuation in this condition are often nonhomogeneous and result from the fatty infiltration that occurs in long-standing glycogen storage disease.
Thorotrast deposition (Fig GI64-4)	Generalized (often inhomogeneous) increased density of the liver (and spleen and lymph nodes).	Previously used radiographic contrast agent that is retained in endothelial cells of the liver, spleen, and adjacent lymph nodes. The alpha-emitting radionuclide has been associated with the development of hepatobiliary carcinoma, leukemia, and aplastic anemia up to 30 years after the initial injection.

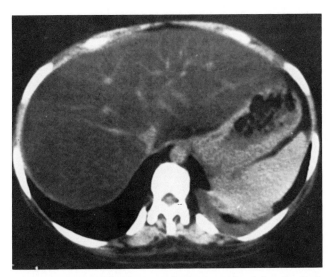

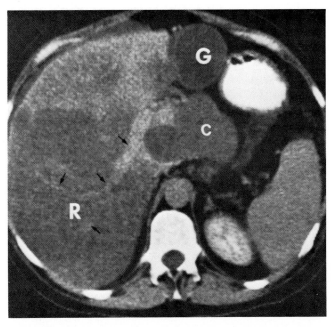

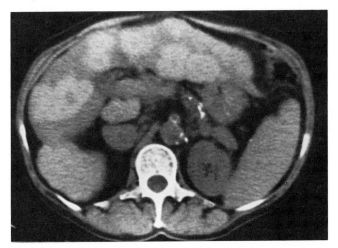

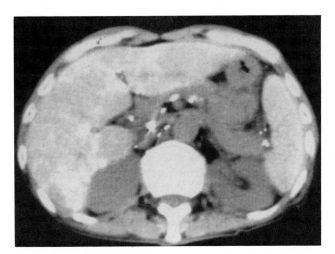

FIG GI64-1. **Fatty infiltration in cirrhosis.** Generalized decrease in the attenuation value of the liver (far less than that of the spleen). The portal veins appear as high-density structures surrounded by a background of low-density hepatic fat.

FIG GI64-2. **Patchy fatty infiltration in cirrhosis.** The right (R) and caudate (c) lobes of the liver are replaced by fat to a degree that makes the density almost equal to that of the gallbladder (G). The medial segment of the left hepatic lobe has a higher CT density but contains foci of low attenuation. The spleen is large and the caudate lobe is prominent. The portal vein (arrow) courses normally through the center of the right hepatic lobe, distinguishing fatty infiltration from a low-density tumor.[48]

FIG GI64-3. **Regenerating nodules in cirrhosis.** Multiple nodules of attenuation equal to that of normal liver are seen superimposed on a background of low-attenuation fatty infiltration. Note the calcifications in the pancreas caused by chronic pancreatitis in this patient, a chronic alcoholic.

FIG GI64-4. **Thorotrast deposition.** Generalized increase in the attenuation of the liver (and spleen).

GENERALIZED INCREASED ECHOGENICITY OF THE LIVER

Condition	Comments
Fatty infiltration	Alcohol abuse is by far the most common cause of fatty liver. Other underlying causes include diabetes, chemotherapy, hyperalimentation, protein malnutrition, intestinal bypass operations, and a variety of toxic substances. At times, fatty infiltration may involve only portions of the liver, producing discrete areas of increased echogenicity alternating with normal parenchyma (may be confused with metastatic disease). Although the ultrasound pattern is indistinguishable from generalized hepatic fibrosis, the two entities can be clearly separated by the different CT attenuation values of fat and fibrous tissue.
Fibrosis **(Fig GI65-1)**	Most commonly the result of cirrhosis. Usually due to alcohol abuse, though it may be secondary to chronic viral hepatitis, schistosomiasis, other parasitic diseases, or glycogen storage disease. Careful sagittal scans of the left lobe should be performed to detect the recanalized umbilical vein, an indicator of portal hypertension.
Technical artifact	Occurs if scanning is performed with too much overall system gain. In most normal patients, the liver and kidney parenchyma are very similar in their gray-scale texture (echogenicity of the liver may be slightly higher). A definite mismatch of the two tissues is strong evidence for parenchymal disease of the organ showing the greater echogenicity.

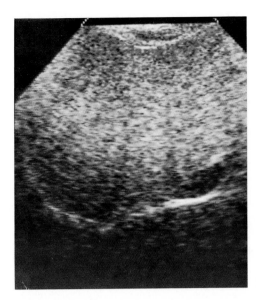

FIG GI65-1. Fibrosis. Diffuse increased echogenicity of the liver secondary to chronic hepatitis.

GENERALIZED DECREASED ECHOGENICITY OF THE LIVER

Condition	Comments
Cellular infiltration	Most commonly due to lymphoma, which may also produce hypoechoic or echogenic focal lesions. Other causes include leukemia and amyloidosis.
Hepatitis	Although the liver parenchyma appears normal in many cases of acute viral hepatitis, swelling of liver cells may produce an overall decreased echogenicity of the liver associated with accentuated brightness of the portal vein walls. In chronic hepatitis, the parenchymal echo pattern is coarsened because of periportal fibrosis and inflammatory cells.

SHADOWING LESIONS IN THE LIVER

Condition	Comments
Calcification **(Figs GI67-1 and GI67-2)**	Usually reflects previous inflammatory disease (granulomatous or parasitic). Also may occur with hepatic metastases (mucinous tumors of the gastrointestinal tract in adults, neuroblastoma in children).
Gas **Biliary tree**	Most commonly due to a surgical connection between the biliary tree and the alimentary tract. If there is no history of previous surgery, the most common causes are gallstone ileus and penetrating duodenal ulcer disease.
Portal vein	Much less common than biliary gas and generally related to necrotizing enterocolitis, mesenteric arterial occlusion and bowel infarction, or an eroding abscess. Shadowing lesions due to portal vein gas appear in the periphery of the liver, unlike the more central location when the shadowing is secondary to gas in the biliary tree.
Normal shadowing	On sagittal scans near the neck of the gallbladder in normal patients, there is often a discrete shadow projected on the posterior aspect of the liver. This may be secondary to a refractive effect caused by tangential incidence of the ultrasound beam to the interface between the liver and gallbladder or to either thick fibrous tissue surrounding the right portal vein or the spiral valves of Heister in the gallbladder. Decubitus scans are required to search for tiny biliary calculi that may be lodged in the cystic duct and produce a similar appearance.

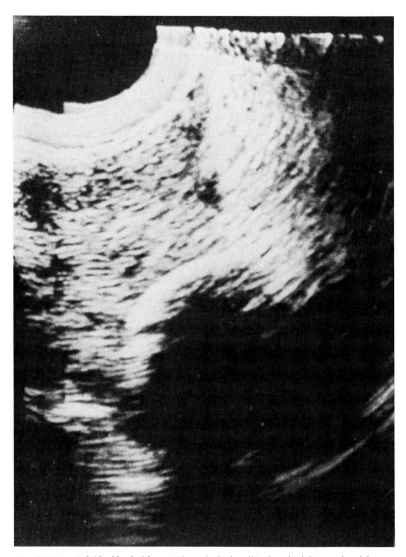

FIG GI67-1. Calcified hydatid cyst. The calcified wall is sharply delineated and there is posterior acoustic shadowing.[41]

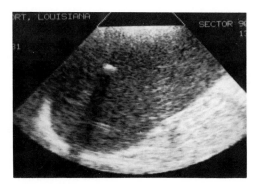

FIG GI67-2. Calcified granuloma in the liver with posterior shadowing.

PANCREATIC MASSES ON ULTRASOUND

Condition	Imaging Findings	Comments
Pancreatic carcinoma	Solid, focally enlarged, lobulated mass with low-level echoes and increased sound absorption. There is often dilatation of the pancreatic duct (and common bile duct) in lesions of the head of the pancreas.	Hypoechoic pancreatic mass may be difficult to separate from a pseudomass produced by overlying bowel gas and its distal reverberation, which creates a false front and back wall. Infrequently, primary pancreatic carcinoma may appear densely hyperechoic. Other sonographic findings suggesting malignancy include liver and nodal metastases, venous compression or obstruction, and ascites.
Islet cell tumor	Well-circumscribed mass that is usually indistinguishable from pancreatic carcinoma but may occasionally contain internal cystic areas.	Rare tumor, usually endocrinologically silent, and most common in the pancreatic body and tail where the greatest concentration of islets of Langerhans is located (unlike carcinoma, which most commonly affects the head of the pancreas).
Metastases	Solid mass with variable echo pattern and increased sound absorption that may be indistinguishable from primary pancreatic carcinoma.	Metastases to the pancreatic bed primarily involve the region of the head and body (where the main lymphatic chains are located). Large masses may compress or displace the pancreas. Compared with primary carcinoma, metastases tend to be lumpier and more diffuse. They frequently are located posterior to and cause anterior displacement of the splenic and portal veins (primary carcinoma tends to be located more anteriorly and to cause posterior displacement of these vessels).
Lymphoma	Solid mass that is relatively anechoic and, when round, may initially appear to be cystic until internal echoes are demonstrated at high power or gain settings.	Primarily involves the region of the head and body (where the main lymphatic chains are located). Large masses may compress or displace the pancreas. Compared with primary carcinoma, lymphoma tends to be lumpier and more diffuse. It frequently is located posterior to and causes anterior displacement of the splenic and portal veins (primary carcinoma tends to be located more anteriorly and causes posterior displacement of these vessels).
Cystadenoma/ cystadenocarcinoma (Fig GI68-1)	Predominantly cystic mass with septations and thick irregular walls. Relatively hypoechoic pattern with decreased sound absorption.	Uncommon tumors, usually occurring in women between ages 30 and 60. Most are located in the pancreatic body and tail, are frequently clinically silent, and can therefore attain sizes greater than 10 cm before becoming palpable. There are no specific criteria to separate benign from malignant tumors.

Condition	Imaging Findings	Comments
Pseudocyst (Figs GI68-2 and GI68-3)	Uncomplicated pseudocysts are usually anechoic with smooth walls and good sound transmission distally. They may infrequently have thick walls, be multiloculated, and contain internal debris and be difficult to differentiate from cystadenoma, cystadenocarcinoma, or abscess.	Frequent complication of acute or chronic pancreatitis. The presence of air or calcification may cause unusually bright echoes. Although most commonly located in the peripancreatic region, pseudocysts may develop apart from the pancreas (the lesser sac, or anywhere from the mediastinum to the groin).
Pancreatic abscess	Complex, predominantly cystic mass, often with irregular walls and internal debris. Bright echoes in the mass (representing gas) confirm the diagnosis of an abscess.	Serious and often fatal complication in severe acute pancreatitis. Although the presence of gas in the pancreatic bed strongly suggests a pancreatic abscess, this appearance may also be demonstrated in patients with a pancreatic pseudocyst that erodes the gastrointestinal tract without forming an abscess.

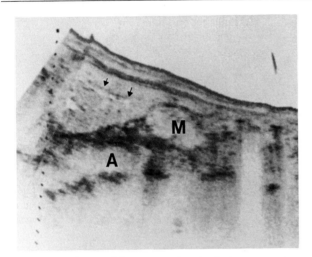

FIG GI68-1. Carcinoma of the pancreas. Longitudinal sonogram demonstrates an irregular mass (M) with a semisolid pattern of intrinsic echoes. There is associated dilatation of the intrahepatic bile ducts (arrows). (A, aorta)[49]

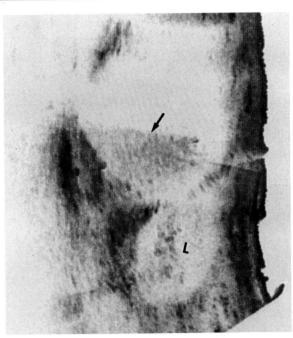

FIG GI68-3. Pancreatic pseudocyst. An erect sonogram demonstrates a fluid-debris level (arrow) in the pseudocyst. (L, left kidney)

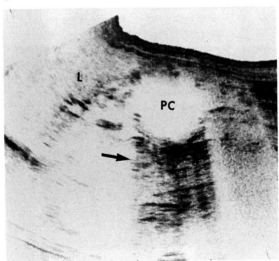

FIG GI68-2. Pancreatic pseudocyst. Longitudinal sonogram of the right upper quadrant demonstrates an irregularly marginated pseudocyst (PC) with acoustic shadowing (arrow). (L, liver)

PANCREATIC MASSES ON COMPUTED TOMOGRAPHY

Condition	Imaging Findings	Comments
Pancreatic carcinoma (Figs GI69-1 and GI69-2)	On noncontrast studies, the tumor usually has an attenuation value similar to that of normal tissue and must alter the contour of the pancreas to be detected. On contrast studies, the relatively avascular tumor appears as an area of decreased attenuation when compared with the normal pancreas.	Some necrotic tumors have well-defined borders and a uniform low density, simulating a pseudocyst. Because a focal mass can also be seen in acute or chronic pancreatitis, a diagnosis of carcinoma requires evidence of secondary signs of malignancy such as obliteration of peripancreatic fat planes (especially posteriorly about vascular structures), lymph node enlargement, and liver metastases.
Islet cell tumor (Fig GI69-3)	Rapid sequential scanning after a bolus injection of contrast material can demonstrate the transient increase in contrast enhancement (tumor blush) that is characteristic of many of these tumors (it is often impossible to differentiate them from surrounding pancreatic tissue on noncontrast scans).	Most tumors are small and isodense with the uninvolved pancreas. Larger tumors may contain low-density areas due to foci of tumor necrosis. Many pancreatic islet cell tumors are malignant, and hepatic metastases may be seen on CT examination.
Cystadenoma/ cystadenocarcinoma	Mass composed of variable numbers of different-sized cysts of fluid attenuation. Multiloculated appearance with septations and sometimes calcification scattered throughout the mass.	Uncommon tumors, usually occurring in women between ages 30 and 60. Most are located in the pancreatic body and tail, are frequently clinically silent, and can therefore attain sizes greater than 10 cm before becoming palpable. There are no specific criteria to separate benign from malignant tumors unless there is evidence of local invasion or metastases.
Metastases **Local invasion**	Obliteration of the fat planes that normally separate the pancreas from adjacent organs.	Hepatomas and carcinoma of the stomach or gallbladder may extend directly into the pancreas. Lesions of the left adrenal and kidney may displace the tail of the pancreas, destroy surrounding fat, and occlude the splenic vein.
Peripancreatic lymph node involvement (Fig GI69-4)	Lobulated mass or masses impinging on the pancreas.	Enlargement of peripancreatic nodes (metastatic tumor, lymphoma, infection) can simulate pancreatic tumor. The boundary of fat between the pancreas and the nodal mass is often preserved (it may be impossible to differentiate primary pancreatic tumor from peripancreatic lymphadenopathy if the fat planes are obliterated).
Lymphoma (Fig GI69-5)	Lobulated mass or masses impinging on the pancreas or diffuse enlargement of the gland due to direct infiltration by lymphomatous tissue.	Lymphomatous involvement of the pancreas or peripancreatic nodes is usually part of a systemic disease in which there is also retroperitoneal and mesenteric lymphadenopathy.

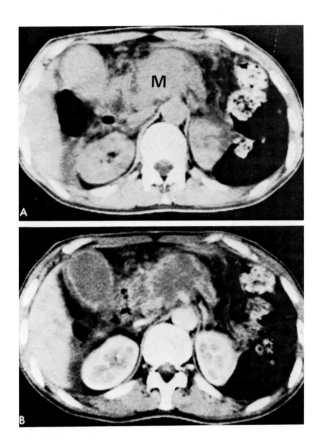

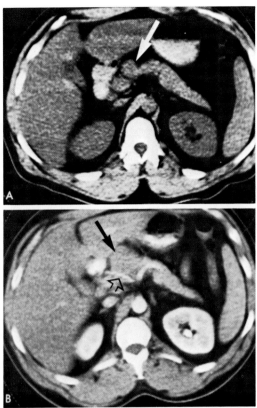

FIG GI69-1. Pancreatic carcinoma. (Top) Noncontrast scan demonstrates a homogeneous mass (M) in the body of the pancreas. (Bottom) Contrast-enhanced scan at the time of maximum aortic contrast shows enhancement of the surrounding vascular structures and normal pancreatic parenchyma while the pancreatic carcinoma remains unchanged and thus appears as a low-density mass.[49]

FIG GI69-2. Pancreatic carcinoma: rapid growth and arterial encasement. (Top) Initial scan demonstrates a focal change in the shape of the ventral contour of the pancreas at the junction of the body and head (arrow). There is no enlargement of the pancreatic tissue. This was initially interpreted as representing an anatomic variant. (Bottom) Three months later, a repeat scan shows a focal tumor mass (closed arrow) in the location of the focal contour abnormality seen in (A). A dynamic CT scan after the intravenous bolus injection of contrast material demonstrates the splenic and hepatic arteries at the base of the tumor. Note that the hepatic artery (open arrow) has an irregular contour. Arteriography showed encasement by this unresectable tumor.[49]

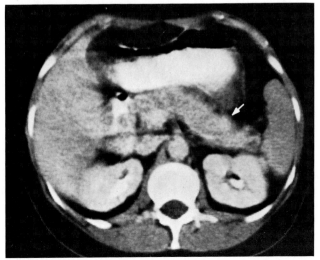

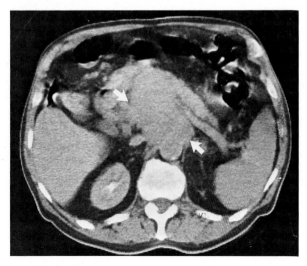

FIG GI69-3. Islet cell tumor. Contrast-enhanced scan shows a small lesion (arrow) in the normal contour of the pancreatic tail. At surgery, there were several small pancreatic gastrinomas in this patient, who had clinical evidence of the Zollinger-Ellison syndrome.[50]

FIG GI69-4. Peripancreatic lymph node metastases. Massive nodal enlargement (arrows) with obliteration of fat planes between the mass and the head of the pancreas.

Condition	Imaging Findings	Comments
Focal pancreatitis (acute or chronic) (Figs GI69-6 to GI69-8)	Focal enlargement of the head of the pancreas that may be indistinguishable from a neoplasm. The presence of evenly distributed calcifications in a focal mass strongly suggests chronic pancreatitis, though a carcinoma can arise in a pancreas that already contains calcifications from chronic inflammatory disease.	In uncomplicated acute pancreatitis, more commonly diffuse enlargement of the gland (often with a decreased attenuation value secondary to edema) or an irregular contour with indistinct margins of the gland and an increased density of the peripancreatic fat planes. In chronic pancreatitis, focal or diffuse pancreatic enlargement often represents edema in association with an acute exacerbation or fibrosis.
Pseudocyst (Figs GI69-9 and GI69-10)	Sharply marginated, unilocular or multilocular, fluid-density mass that is often best delineated after contrast material administration. Older cysts tend to have thicker walls that may contain calcium.	Lobulated fluid collection arising from inflammation, necrosis, or hemorrhage associated with acute pancreatitis or trauma. Because of its ability to image the entire body, CT may demonstrate pseudocysts that have dissected superiorly into the mediastinum or to other ectopic locations, such as the lumbar or inguinal region or within the liver, spleen, or kidney.
Pancreatic abscess (Fig GI69-11 and GI69-12)	Poorly defined, inhomogeneous mass that often displaces adjacent structures and generally has an attenuation value higher than that of a sterile fluid collection or pseudocyst.	The most reliable sign of an abscess is gas in the mass, though this is found in less than 50% of proven abscesses and may also occur in a patient with a pancreatic pseudocyst that erodes into the gastrointestinal tract without abscess formation. Because a pancreatic abscess often has a nonspecific CT appearance, diagnostic needle aspiration is an extremely useful adjunct for early diagnosis.

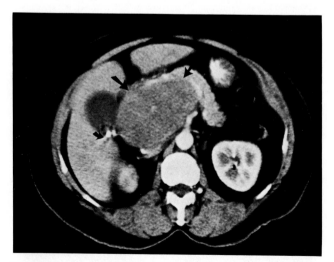

FIG GI69-5. Lymphoma. Huge mass infiltrating the head of the pancreas (straight arrows). The curved arrow points to stones in the gallbladder.

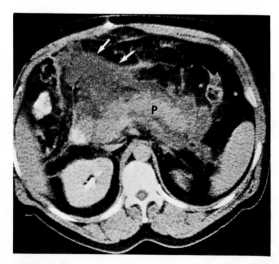

FIG GI69-6. Acute pancreatitis. Diffuse enlargement of the pancreas (P) with obliteration of peripancreatic fat planes by the inflammatory process. Note the extension of the inflammatory reaction into the transverse mesocolon (arrows).[51]

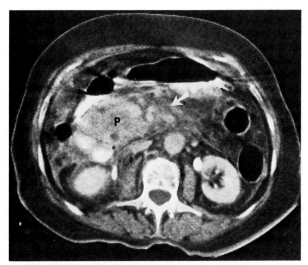
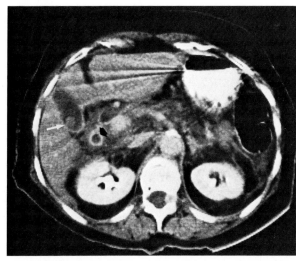

FIG GI69-7. Acute gallstone pancreatitis. (A) There is enlargement of the head of the pancreas (P) with inflammatory reaction surrounding peripancreatic fat planes (arrow). (B) A stone (white arrow) is seen in the gallbladder and the common bile duct is enlarged (black arrow).

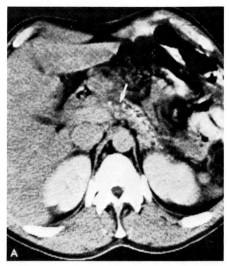

FIG GI69-8. Chronic pancreatitis. There is pancreatic atrophy along with multiple intraductal calculi and dilatation of the pancreatic duct (arrow). The calcifications were not seen on plain abdominal radiographs.[48]

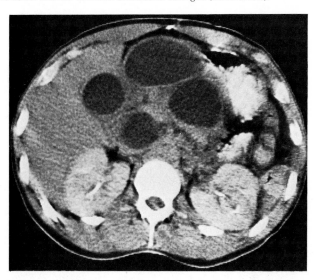

FIG GI69-9. Multiple pancreatic pseudocysts. CT scan after the administration of contrast material demonstrates four sharply marginated, fluid-filled collections.

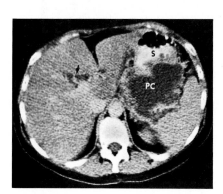

FIG GI69-10. Ectopic pancreatic pseudocyst. The low-attenuation pseudocyst (PC) lies in the superior recess of the lesser sac posterior to the stomach (S). Note the dilated intrahepatic bile ducts (arrow).

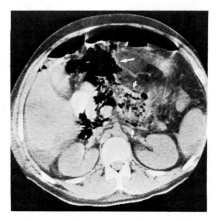

FIG GI69-11. Pancreatic abscess. There is a gas-containing abscess (small arrows) in the pancreatic bed, with marked anterior extension (large arrow) of the inflammatory process.

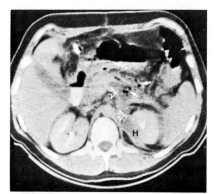

FIG GI69-12. Pancreatic abscess after a gunshot wound. There are multiple intrapancreatic and peripancreatic gas bubbles (closed arrows), bullet fragments (open arrows), a small renal laceration, and an extrarenal hematoma (H).[39]

DILATATION OF THE PANCREATIC DUCT

Condition	Comments
Carcinoma of the pancreas (Fig GI70-1)	Smooth or irregular ductal dilatation. The obstructing ductal lesion can often be demonstrated.
Chronic pancreatitis (Fig GI70-2)	Irregular ductal dilatation with strictures and stenoses. Associated pancreatic calculi produce strong echoes in the duct accompanied by acoustic shadows on ultrasound and high-attenuation areas on CT. Although the diameter of the duct in chronic pancreatitis tends to be smaller than one obstructed by tumor, this is not a reliable differential point. The pancreas is often irregular and lobulated with a variable echo pattern on ultrasound and variable attenuation on CT.
Acute pancreatitis (Fig GI70-3)	Obstruction of the pancreatic duct with proximal dilatation may be due to inflammation, spasm, edema, swelling of the papilla, or an associated pseudocyst. On ultrasound, the pancreas is enlarged and edematous with a uniformly hypoechoic pattern. On CT, there may be diffuse enlargement of the gland (often with decreased attenuation secondary to edema) or an irregular contour with indistinct margins and an increased density of peripancreatic fat planes.

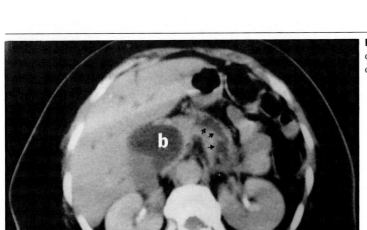

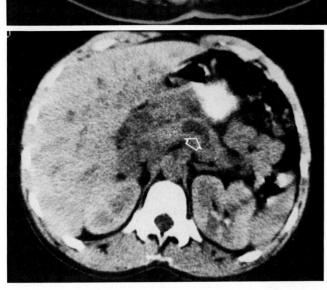

FIG GI70-1. **Carcinoma of the pancreas.** Dilatation of the pancreatic duct (arrows). The tumor (seen on more caudal scans) also causes marked dilatation of the bile duct (b).

FIG GI70-2. **Chronic pancreatitis.** Sonogram performed in the left posterior oblique position (because of gas shadowing) demonstrates dilatation of the pancreatic duct (arrows). The pancreas (P) is displayed between the splenic vein (V) and the liver (L). (G, gallbladder and D, duodenal shadow)[41]

FIG GI70-3. **Acute pancreatitis.** CT scan shows generalized enlargement of the head of the pancreas with dilatation of the pancreatic duct (arrow).

DECREASED-ATTENUATION MASSES IN THE SPLEEN

Condition	Imaging Findings	Comments
Cyst **Nonparasitic** **(Fig GI71-1)**	Unilocular, homogenous, water-density lesion with pencil-thin margins that do not enhance after contrast material administration.	Usually congenital or traumatic in origin. Rarely secondary to pancreatitis, in which dissection of enzymes into the spleen results in an intrasplenic pseudocyst.
Echinococcal **(Fig GI71-2)**	Round or oval mass with sharp margins and near-water density. The noncalcified portions of the cyst wall enhance after contrast material administration.	There may be extensive mural calcification that tends to be thick and irregular, unlike the infrequent calcification of congenital cysts that tends to be thin and smooth. Daughter cysts budding from the outer cyst wall often produce a multiloculated appearance.
Infarction	Wedge-shaped area of decreased attenuation that extends to the capsule of the spleen and does not show contrast enhancement.	Chronic splenic infarction, as in sickle cell anemia, produces a shrunken spleen that often contains areas of calcification.
Hematoma **(Fig GI71-3)**	Initially, a hematoma may appear isodense or even slightly hyperdense on noncontrast scans when compared with normal spleen (may appear to have lower attenuation after contrast material injection as the normal spleen increases in density). As a hematoma ages (1 to 2 weeks), there is a gradual decrease in the attenuation and the nonhomogeneous appearance until the hematoma becomes homogeneous and of low attenuation.	Subcapsular hematomas appear as crescentic collections of fluid that flatten or indent the lateral margin of the spleen. Less common intrasplenic hematomas produce focal masses. The decreasing attenuation of the hematoma as it ages is the result of a decrease in hemoglobin and an increase in the water content of the hematoma.
Abscess **(Fig GI71-4)**	Single or, more commonly, multiple rounded, hypodense or cystic lesions that lack a well-defined wall and do not show contrast enhancement.	Potentially life-threatening condition if appropriate therapy is postponed because of delayed diagnosis. About 75% are associated with the hematogenous spread of infection, 15% with trauma, and 10% with splenic infarction. An abscess may contain gas or show layering of material or different densities in the cavity.
Lymphoma **(Figs GI71-5 and GI71-6)**	Single or multiple low-attenuation masses.	The spleen is involved in about 40% of patients at the time of initial presentation and is often the only site of involvement in patients with Hodgkin's disease. The most common CT appearance is generalized enlargement of a normal-density spleen (homogeneous lymphomatous infiltration).
Metastases **(Fig GI71-7)**	Single or multiple low-attenuation lesions that may appear as ill-defined hypodense areas or as well-delineated cystic masses.	May arise from a variety of neoplasms, most commonly melanoma and carcinomas of the lung and breast. Metastatic nodules with areas of necrosis and liquefaction can contain irregularly shaped regions that approach water density.
Primary angiosarcoma	Nonhomogeneous, complex mass of cystic and solid components.	The spleen is a rare site of primary malignancy. There is a variable degree of tumor enhancement after contrast material administration.

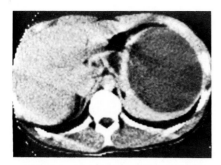

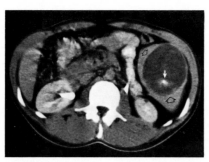

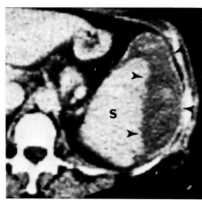

FIG GI71-1. Congenital splenic cyst. Large, low-density mass with pencil-sharp margins filling almost all the spleen.[52]

FIG GI71-2. Echinococcal cyst. Rounded, low-density intrasplenic mass with an area of intracyst calcification (solid arrow). The cyst has pencil-sharp margins and a rim (open arrows) that is enhanced after the injection of contrast material.[52]

FIG GI71-3. Traumatic subcapsular hematoma. Contrast-enhanced scan shows the hematoma as a large zone of decreased attenuation (arrowheads) that surrounds and flattens the lateral and anteromedial borders of the adjacent spleen (S).[53]

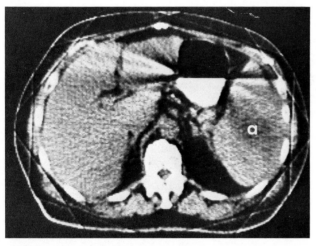

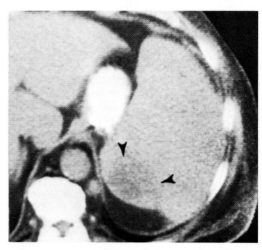

FIG GI71-4. Traumatic subscapsular splenic abscess. The abscess (a) appears as an area of diminished attenuation in the center of spleen.[54]

FIG GI71-5. Lymphoma. Focal low-attenuation lesion (arrowheads) posteriorly in a markedly enlarged spleen.[53]

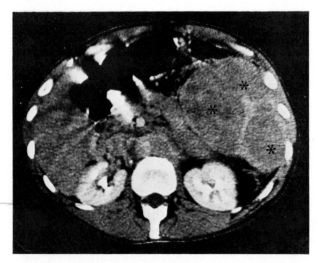

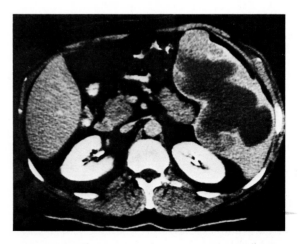

FIG GI71-6. Lymphoma. Multiple low-density lesions (*) involving virtually all of a massively enlarged spleen.

FIG GI71-7. Metastases from melanoma. Multiple confluent lesions, with necrotic central areas showing a cystic appearance. The liver is not involved.[39]

PSEUDOKIDNEY SIGN OR BULL'S EYE APPEARANCE IN THE ABDOMEN

Condition	Comments
Neoplasm **(Figs GI72-1 and GI72-2)**	Thickening of the bowel wall caused by adenocarcinoma, lymphoma, leiomyosarcoma, or serosal metastases.
Intussusception **(Fig GI72-3)**	May present as multiple concentric rings, apparently related to the edematous walls of the intussusceptum and intussuscipiens and the interface between them. The sonolucent mantle correlates with the infiltrated and thickened intestinal walls, while the strong echoes in the center can be explained by the considerable difference in impedance between the bowel wall and the lumen.
Inflammatory or **granulomatous disease** **(Fig GI72-4)**	Thickening of the bowel wall in Crohn's disease, diverticulitis, amyloidosis, and Whipple's disease.
Intramural hematoma	Bowel wall thickening due to trauma or a clotting disorder (anticoagulant therapy or bleeding diathesis).
Hypertrophic pyloric **stenosis** **(Fig GI72-5)**	Sonolucent donut lesion consisting of a prominent anechoic rim of thickened muscle (measuring 3 mm or greater) and an echogenic center of mucosa and submucosa. Classic clinical presentation of projectile, nonbilious vomiting in a 6- to 8-week-old male infant with a characteristic palpable "olive" mass in the epigastrium.

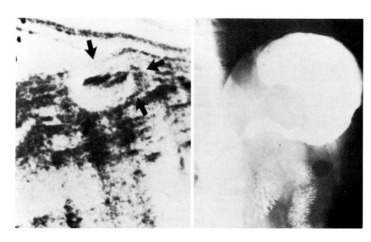

Fig GI72-1. **Carcinoma of the stomach.** The pseudokidney sign (arrows) is located below the left lobe of the liver in this patient, who had narrowing of the antrum characteristic of the linitis plastica pattern.[55]

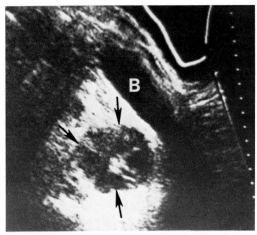

FIG GI72-2. Metastases. Longitudinal sonogram of the pelvis and lower abdomen shows a solid mass with a bull's-eye appearance. The dense central echoes are collapsed mucosa and gut contents, whereas the sonolucent rim represents extrinsic tumor that has infiltrated the bowel serosa circumferentially. At surgery, multiple tumor implants were found in the posterior peritoneum and pelvis, and several extrinsic metastatic lesions were found adhering to the sigmoid colon. Biopsy revealed that the lesions were adenocarcinoma, though the primary site was undetermined. (B, bladder)[56]

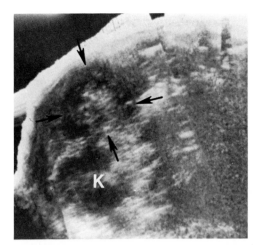

FIG GI72-3. Intussusception. Transverse supine scan in a young boy with abdominal pain, bloody diarrhea, and an anterior right upper quadrant mass demonstrates a bull's-eye lesion (arrows) anterior to the right kidney (K) in the region of the hepatic flexure. The diagnosis of intussusception was confirmed by barium enema examination, and the intussusception was subsequently reduced. The sonolucent rim represents the edematous wall of the intussuscipiens, and the echogenic center represents the intussusceptum.[56]

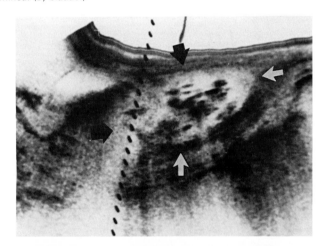

FIG GI72-4. Crohn's disease. Pseudokidney sign below the right lobe of the liver and anterior to the normal position of the right kidney in a patient with the characteristic small bowel changes of Crohn's disease.[55]

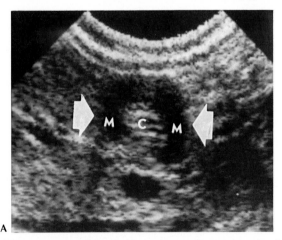

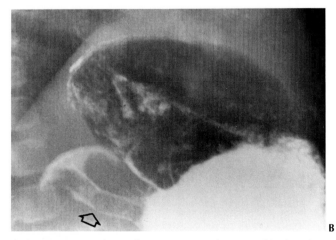

FIG GI72-5. Hypertrophic pyloric stenosis. (A) Characteristic doughnut lesion (arrows) consisting of a prominent anechoic rim of thickened muscle (M) and an echogenic center of mucosa and submucosa (C). (B) Upper gastrointestinal series shows narrowing and elongation of the pyloric canal (arrow) with a typical concave, crescentic indentation at the base of the duodenal bulb.

SOURCES

1. Reprinted with permission from "Functional Disorders of the Pharyngoesophageal Junction" by WB Seaman, *Radiologic Clinics of North America* (1967;7:113–119), Copyright © 1967, WB Saunders Company.

2. Reprinted with permission from "A Roentgen-Anatomic Correlation" by JL Clements et al, *American Journal of Roentgenology* (1974;121:221–231), Copyright © 1974, Williams & Wilkins Company.

3. Reprinted with permission from "Transverse Folds in the Human Esophagus" by VK Gohel et al, *Radiology* (1978;128:303–308), Copyright © 1978, Radiological Society of North America Inc.

4. Reprinted with permission from "*Candida* Esophagitis: Accuracy of Radiographic Diagnosis" by MS Levine, AJ Macones, and I Laufer, *Radiology* (1985;154:581–587), Copyright © 1985, Radiological Society of North America Inc.

5. Reprinted with permission from "Calcified Primary Tumors of the Gastrointestinal Tract" by GG Ghahremani, MA Meyers, and RB Port, *Gastrointestinal Radiology* (1978;2:331–339), Copyright © 1978, Springer-Verlag.

6. Reprinted with permission from "Crohn's Disease of the Stomach: The 'Ram's Horn' Sign" by J Farman et al, *American Journal of Roentgenology* (1975;123:242–251), Copyright © 1975, Williams & Wilkins Company.

7. Reprinted with permission from "Phlegmonous Gastritis" by MA Turner, MC Beachley, and B Stanley, *American Journal of Roentgenology* (1979;133:527–528), Copyright © 1979, Williams & Wilkins Company.

8. Reprinted with permission from "An Evaluation of Nissen Fundoplication" by J Skucas et al, *Radiology* (1976;118:539–543), Copyright © 1976, Radiological Society of North America Inc.

9. Reprinted with permission from "Nonfundic Gastric Varices" by T Sos, MA Meyers, and HA Baltaxe, *Radiology* (1972;105:597–580), Copyright © 1972, Radiological Society of North America Inc.

10. Reprinted with permission from "Suture Granulomas Simulating Tumors: A Preventable Postgastrectomy Complication" by HA Gueller et al, *Digestive Diseases and Sciences* (1976;21:223–228), Copyright © 1976, Plenum Publishing Corporation.

11. Reprinted with permission from "Elevated Lesions in the Duodenal Bulb Caused by Heterotopic Gastric Mucosa" by R Langkamper et al, *Radiology* (1980;137:621–624), Copyright © 1980, Radiological Society of North America Inc.

12. Reprinted with permission from "Chronic Idiopathic Intestinal Pseudo-Obstruction" by JE Maldonado et al, *American Journal of Medicine* (1970;49:203–212), Copyright © 1970, Technical Publishing Company.

13. Reprinted from *Radiology of the Newborn and Young Infant* by LE Swischuk with permission of Williams & Wilkins Company, © 1980.

14. Reprinted with permission from "Tumors of the Small Intestine" by CA Good, *American Journal of Roentgenology* (1963;89:685–705), Copyright © 1963, Williams & Wilkins Company.

15. Reprinted with permission from "The Roentgen Diagnosis of Retractile Mesenteritis" by AR Clemett and DG Tracht, *American Journal of Roentgenology* (1969;107:787), Copyright © 1969, Williams & Wilkins Company.

16. Reprinted with permission from "Giant Duodenal Ulcers" by RL Eisenberg, AR Margulis, and AA Moss, *Gastrointestinal Radiology* (1978;2:347–353), Copyright © 1978, Springer-Verlag.

17. Reprinted with permission from "Intraluminal Duodenal Diverticulum" by JCH Laudan and GI Norton, *American Journal of Roentgenology* (1963;90:756–760), Copyright © 1963, Williams & Wilkins Company.

18. Reprinted with permission from "Cecal Diverticulitis in Young Patients" by JF Norfray et al, *Gastrointestinal Radiology* (1980;5:379–382), Copyright © 1980, Springer-Verlag.

19. Reprinted with permission from "Typhoid Fever" by RS Francis and RN Berk, *Radiology* (1974;112:583–585), Copyright © 1974, Radiological Society of North America Inc.

20. Reprinted with permission from "Nonspecific Ulcers of the Colon Resembling Annular Carcinoma" by GA Gardiner and CR Bird, *Radiology* (1980;137:331–334), Copyright © 1980, Radiological Society of North America Inc.

21. Reprinted with permission from "Colitis in the Elderly: Ischemic Colitis Mimicking Ulcerative and Granulomatous Colitis" by RL Eisenberg, CK Montgomery, and AR Margulis, *American Journal of Roentgenology* (1979;133:1113–1118), Copyright © 1979, Williams & Wilkins Company.

22. Reprinted with permission from "Caustic Colitis Due to Detergent Enema" by SK Kim, C Cho, and EM Levinsohn, *American Journal of Roentgenology* (1980;134:397–398), Copyright © 1980, Williams & Wilkins Company.

23. Reprinted with permission from "Value of the Pre-Operative Barium Enema Examination in the Assessment of Pelvic Masses" by RK Gedgaudas et al, *Radiology* (1983;146:609–616), Copyright © 1983, Radiological Society of North America Inc.

24. Reprinted with permission from "Lymphoid Follicular Pattern of the Colon in Adults" by FM Kelvin et al, *American Journal of Roentgenology* (1979;133:821–825), Copyright © 1979, Williams & Wilkins Company.

25. Reprinted with permission from "Plain Film Findings in Severe Pseudomembranous Colitis" by RJ Stanley et al, *Radiology* (1976;118:7–11), Copyright © 1976, Radiological Society of North America Inc.

26. Reprinted with permission from "Double Tracking in the Sigmoid Colon" by JT Ferrucci et al, *Radiology* (1976;120:307–312), Copyright © 1976, Radiological Society of North America Inc.

27. Reprinted with permission from "Cholangiographic Findings in Cholangiolitic Hepatitis" by DA Legge et al, *American Journal of Roentgenology* (1971;113:16–20), Copyright © 1971, Williams & Wilkins Company.

28. Reprinted with permission from "Congenital Hepatic Fibrosis Associated with Renal Tubular Ectasia" by I Unite et al, *Radiology* (1973;109:565–570), Copyright © 1973, Radiological Society of North America Inc.

29. Reprinted with permission from "Recurrent Pyogenic Cholangitis in Chinese Immigrants" by CS Ho and DE Wesson, *American Journal of Roentgenology* (1974;122:368–374), Copyright © 1974, Williams & Wilkins Company.

30. Reprinted with permission from "Plain Film Roentgenographic Findings in Alveolar Hydatid Disease: *Echinococcus Multilocularis*" by WM Thompson, DP Chisholm, and R Tank, *American Journal of Roentgenology* (1972;116:345–358), Copyright © 1972, Williams & Wilkins Company.

31. Reprinted with permission from "Calcifications in the Liver" by JJ Darlak, M Moskowitz, and KR Kattan, *Radiologic Clinics of North America* (1980;18:209–219), Copyright © 1980, WB Saunders Company.

32. Reprinted with permission from "Radiodense Liver in Transfusion Hemochromatosis" by WL Smith and F Quattromani, *American Journal of Roentgenology* (1977;128:316–317), Copyright © 1977, Williams & Wilkins Company.

33. Reprinted with permission from "Differential Diagnosis of Pancreatic Calcification" by EJ Ring et al, *American Journal of Roentgenology* (1973;117:446–452), Copyright © 1973, Williams & Wilkins Company.

34. Reprinted with permission from "An Early Rim Sign in Neonatal Adrenal Hemorrhage" by PW Brill, IH Krasna, and H Aaron, *American Journal of Roentgenology* (1976;127:289–291), Copyright © 1976, Williams & Wilkins Company.

35. Reprinted from *Radiologic Diagnosis of Renal Parenchymal Disease* by AJ Davidson with permission of WB Saunders Company, © 1977.

36. Reprinted with permission from "Calcified Renal Masses: A Review of Ten Years' Experience at the Mayo Clinic" by WW Daniel et al, *Radiology* (1972;103:503–508), Copyright © 1972, Radiological Society of North America Inc.

37. Reprinted with permission from "Gonadoblastoma: An Ovarian Tumor with Characteristic Pelvic Calcifications" by EQ Seymour et al, *American Journal of Roentgenology* (1976;127:1001–1002), Copyright © 1976, Williams & Wilkins Company.

38. Reprinted with permission from "Calcification in Undifferentiated Abdominal Malignancies" by MK Dalinka et al, *Clinical Radiology* (1975;26:115–119), Copyright © 1975, Royal College of Radiologists.

39. Reprinted from *Alimentary Tract Radiology*, ed 3, by AR Margulis and HJ Burhenne (Eds) with permission of The CV Mosby Company, St Louis, © 1983.

40. Reprinted with permission of "Caroli's Disease: Sonographic Findings" by CA Mittelstaedt et al, *American Journal of Roentgenology* (1980;134:585–587), Copyright © 1980, Williams & Wilkins Company.

41. Reprinted from *Ultrasonography of Digestive Diseases* by FS Weill, The CV Mosby Company, St Louis, with permission of the author, © 1982.

42. Reprinted from *Ultrasonography in Obstetrics and Gynecology* by PW Callen (Ed) with permission of WB Saunders Company, © 1983.

43. Reprinted with permission from "Gray-Scale Ultrasonography of Hepatic Amoebic Abscesses" by PW Ralls et al, *Radiology* (1979;132: 125–132), Copyright © 1979, Radiological Society of North America Inc.

44. Reprinted with permission from "Ultrasonography and Computed Tomography in the Evaluation of Hepatic Microabscesses in the Immunosuppressed Patient" by PW Callen, RA Filly, and FS Marcus, *Radiology* (1980;136:433–434), Copyright © 1980, Radiological Society of North America Inc.

45. Reprinted with permission from "Infantile Hemagioendothelioma of the Liver" by AH Dachman et al, *American Journal of Roentgenology* (1983;140:1091–1096), Copyright © 1983, Williams & Wilkins Company.

46. Reprinted with permission from "Hepatic Cysts: Treatment with Alcohol" by WJ Bean and BA Rodan, *American Journal of Roentgenology* (1985;144:237–241), Copyright © 1985, Williams & Wilkins Company.

47. Reprinted with permission from "Variable CT Appearance of Hepatic Abscesses" by RA Halvorsen et al, *American Journal of Roentgenology* (1984;142:941–947), Copyright © 1984, Williams & Wilkins Company.

48. Reprinted from *Computed Tomography of the Body* by AA Moss, G Gamsu, an HK Genant (Eds) with permission of WB Saunders Company, © 1983.

49. Reprinted from *Diagnostic Imaging in Internal Medicine* by RL Eisenberg with permission of McGraw-Hill Book Company, © 1985. Courtesy of Gretchen AW Gooding, MD.

50. Reprinted with permission from "CT of Pancreatic Islet Cell Tumors" by DD Stark et al, *Radiology* (1983;150:491–494), Copyright © 1983, Radiological Society of North America Inc.

51. Reprinted with permission from "Computed Tomography of Mesenteric Involvement in Fulminant Pancreatitis" by RB Jeffrey, MD Federle, and FC Laing, *Radiology* (1983;147:185–192), Copyright © 1983, Radiological Society of North America Inc.

52. Reprinted with permission from "Computed Tomography of the Spleen" by J Piekarski et al, *Radiology* (1980;135:683–689), Copyright © 1980, Radiological Society of North America Inc.

53. Reprinted from *Computed Body Tomography* by JKT Lee, SS Sagel, and RJ Stanley (Eds) with permission of Raven Press, New York, © 1983.

54. Reprinted with permission from "Sonography of Splenic Abscess" by S Pawar et al, *American Journal of Roentgenology* (1982;138:259–262), Copyright © 1982, Williams & Wilkins Company.

55. Reprinted with permission from "Ultrasonic Evaluation of the Stomach, Small Bowel, and Colon" by EI Bluth, CRB Merritt, and MA Sullivan, *Radiology* (1979;133:677–680), Copyright © 1979, Radiological Society of North America Inc.

56. Reprinted with permission from "Ultrasound Patterns of Disorders Affecting the Gastrointestinal Tract" by CL Morgan, WS Trought, and TA Oddson, *Radiology* (1980;135:129–135), Copyright © 1980, Radiological Society of North America Inc.

Genitourinary Patterns

4

GU1 Misplaced, displaced, or absent kidney **442**

GU2 Unilateral small, smooth kidney **446**

GU3 Unilateral small, scarred kidney **448**

GU4 Unilateral large, smooth kidney **450**

GU5 Unilateral large, multilobulated kidney **452**

GU6 Bilateral small, smooth kidneys **454**

GU7 Bilateral large, smooth kidneys **458**

GU8 Bilateral large, multifocal kidneys **464**

GU9 Focal renal mass **466**

GU10 Cystic diseases of the kidneys **472**

GU11 Depression or scar in the renal margin **478**

GU12 Persistent or increasingly dense nephrogram **480**

GU13 Diminished concentration of contrast material in the pelvocalyceal system **482**

GU14 Solitary or multiple filling defects in the pelvocalyceal system **484**

GU15 Clubbing or destruction of renal calyces **488**

GU16 Effaced pelvocalyceal system **490**

GU17 Filling defects in the ureter **492**

GU18 Obstruction of the ureter **498**

GU19 Ureterectasis **506**

GU20 Small urinary bladder **510**

GU21 Large urinary bladder **512**

GU22 Single or multiple filling defects in the urinary bladder **514**

GU23 Gas in the bladder lumen or wall **520**

GU24 Urinary tract obstruction below the bladder in children **522**

GU25 Calcification of the vas deferens **524**

GU26 Anechoic (cystic) renal masses **526**

GU27 Complex renal masses **528**

GU28 Solid renal masses **530**

GU29 Cystic renal masses on computed tomography **532**

GU30 Focal solid renal masses on computed tomography **534**

GU31 Increased renal cortical echogenicity with preservation of medullary sonolucency (type I lesions) **538**

GU32 Focal or diffuse distortion of normal renal anatomy and elimination of corticomedullary definition (type II lesions) **540**

GU33 Fluid collections around the transplanted kidney **542**

GU34 Adrenal masses on computed tomography **544**

GU35 Cystic-appearing pelvic masses **548**

GU36 Complex pelvic masses **550**

GU37 Solid pelvic masses **554**

GU38 Fluid collection in the scrotum **556**

Sources **558**

MISPLACED, DISPLACED, OR ABSENT KIDNEY

Condition	Imaging Findings	Comments
Unilateral renal agenesis (solitary kidney) (Fig GU1-1)	Filling of the renal fossa with bowel loops (sharply outlined gas or fecal material in the plane of the renal fossa on nephrotomography). The contralateral kidney usually shows compensatory hypertrophy.	Rare anomaly that is associated with a variety of other congenital malformations. It is essential to exclude a nonfunctioning, diseased kidney by ultrasound or CT. After nephrectomy, the renal outline is generally preserved on plain films if the perinephric fat is left in situ.
Renal ectopia (Figs GU1-2 and GU1-3)	Abnormally positioned kidney that can be found in various locations. The ectopic kidney usually functions, though the nephrogram and pelvocalyceal system may be obscured by overlying bone and fecal contents.	Includes pelvic kidney, intrathoracic kidney, and crossed ectopia (the ectopic kidney lies on the same side as the normal kidney and is usually fused with it). Whenever only one kidney is seen on excretory urography, a full view of the abdomen is essential to search for an ectopic kidney.
Nephroptosis	Excessive caudal movement of a mobile kidney (especially the right) when the patient goes from supine to erect position. There may be associated changes in the ureter (angulation at the ureteropelvic junction, loops, kinks, and tortuosity).	Most commonly occurs in thin females. If a ptotic kidney becomes fixed in its dropped state, permanent ureteral kinking causes impaired drainage, increased hydronephrosis, and a greater chance of infection.
Malrotation (Fig GU1-4)	Often bizarre appearance of the renal parenchyma, calyces, and pelvis that may suggest a pathologic condition in an otherwise normal kidney.	Unilateral or bilateral anomaly. When the renal pelvis is situated in an anterior or lateral position, the upper part of the ureter often appears to be displaced laterally, suggesting an extrinsic mass. The elongated pelvis of a malrotated kidney may mimic obstructive dilatation.
Horseshoe kidney (Fig GU1-5)	Characteristic urographic features include vertical or reversed longitudinal axes of the kidneys (upper poles tilted away from the spine), demonstration on the nephrogram phase of a parenchymal isthmus (if present) connecting the lower poles, and projection of the lower calyces medial to the upper calyces on frontal views. The large and flabby pelves may simulate an obstruction.	Most common type of fusion anomaly. Both kidneys are malrotated and their lower poles are joined by a band of normal renal parenchyma (an isthmus) or connective tissue. True ureteropelvic junction obstruction may develop because of the unusual course of the ureter, which arises high in the renal pelvis, passes over the isthmus, and may kink at the ureteropelvic junction.
Hepatomegaly/ splenomegaly (Fig GU1-6)	Downward displacement of a kidney.	Liver enlargement almost always causes downward displacement of the right kidney. Splenomegaly infrequently causes downward and medial displacement of the left kidney.
Intra- or extrarenal mass **Downward displacement (Fig GU1-7)**	Direction of displacement of the kidney depends on the type of underlying mass.	Adrenal tumor or hemorrhage; large upper pole intrarenal mass.
Upward displacement (Fig GU1-8)		Small liver (high right kidney in advanced cirrhosis with a shrunken liver); Bochdalek's hernia (intrathoracic kidney); lower pole intrarenal mass.

(continued page 444)

A

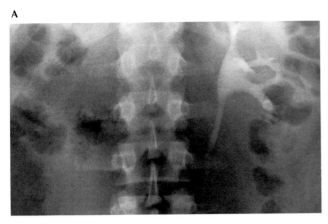

B

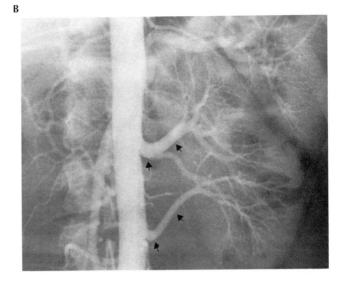

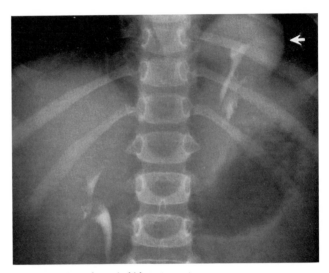

FIG GU1-1. Solitary kidney. (A) Excretory urogram demonstrates a normal left kidney with no evidence of right renal tissue. (B) Aortogram shows two renal arteries to the left kidney (arrows) and no evidence of a right renal artery, thus confirming the diagnosis of unilateral renal agenesis.

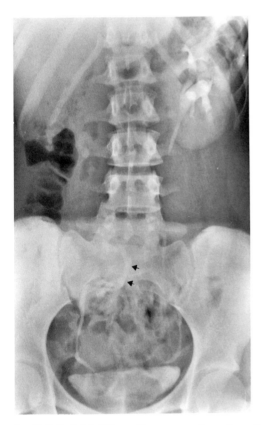

FIG GU1-2. Pelvic kidney. The arrows point to the collecting system.

FIG GU1-3. Intrathoracic kidney (arrow).

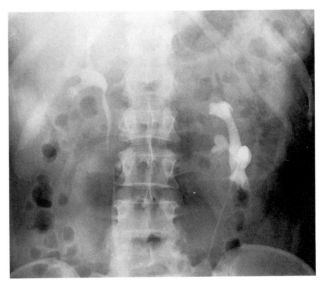

FIG GU1-4. Malrotation of the left kidney. Note the apparent lateral displacement of the upper ureter and the elongation of the pelvis.

Condition	Imaging Findings	Comments
Medial displacement (Fig GU1-9)		Splenomegaly; large extracapsular or subcapsular renal mass (hematoma, lipoma).
Lateral displacement		Lymphoma; lymph node metastases; retroperitoneal sarcoma; expansion of a peripelvic mass (cyst, tumor, abscess, hydronephrosis); aortic aneurysm; adrenal tumor; pancreatic tumor or pseudocyst.
Transplanted kidney (Fig GU1-10)	Kidney overlies the ilium.	Evidence of surgical clips or markers.

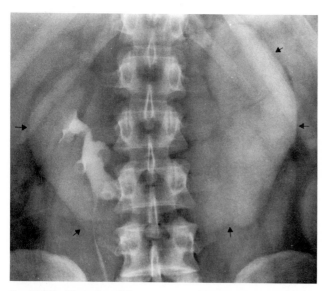

FIG GU1-5. **Horseshoe kidney** (arrows). The prolonged nephrogram and delayed calyceal filling on the left are caused by an obstructing stone at the ureteropelvic junction on that side.

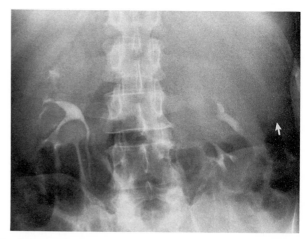

FIG GU1-6. **Splenomegaly.** Downward displacement of the left kidney. The arrow points to the inferior margin of the spleen.

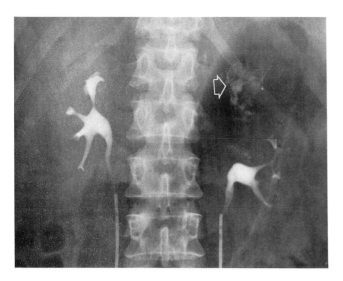

FIG GU1-7. Calcified adrenal teratoma (arrow). Downward displacement of the left kidney.

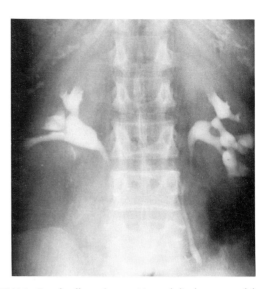

FIG GU1-8. Renal cell carcinoma. Upward displacement of the right kidney and distortion of the collecting system by the large lower pole mass.

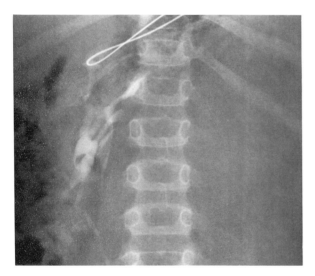

FIG GU1-9. Wilms' tumor. Massive displacement of the left kidney across the midline by a huge mass filling much of the left side of the abdomen.

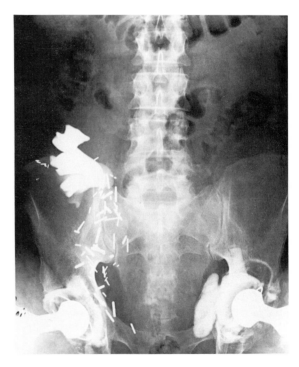

FIG GU1-10. Kidney transplant.

UNILATERAL SMALL, SMOOTH KIDNEY

Condition	Imaging Findings	Comments
Renal ischemia (Fig GU2-1)	Small, smooth kidney. Unilateral delayed appearance and excretion of contrast material with subsequent hyperconcentration. There may be ureteral notching (due to collateral arteries) and vascular calcification.	Chronic ischemia (usually arteriosclerosis or fibromuscular hyperplasia) causes tubular atrophy and shrinkage of glomeruli. Often associated with hypertension, which is likely if the right kidney is at least 2 cm shorter than the left or if the left kidney is at least 1.5 cm shorter than the right. May be bilateral if there is generalized renal arteriosclerosis.
Chronic (total) renal infarction (Fig GU2-2)	Global shrinkage of the kidney with absent opacification. There may be a peripheral rim of opacified cortex during the nephrogram phase (probably reflects viable renal cortex perfused by perforating collateral vessels from the renal capsule).	Renal occlusion is most commonly secondary to an embolism from the heart. A decrease in renal size is detectable within 2 weeks and reaches its maximum extent by 5 weeks. Compensatory enlargement of the contralateral kidney (in individuals young enough to provide this reserve).
Radiation nephritis (Fig GU2-3)	Progressive ischemic atrophy and decreased function produce a unilateral small, smooth kidney with some decrease in renal function.	Diffuse renal ischemia and vasculitis are due to inclusion of the kidney in the radiation field. Tends to become apparent after a latent period of 6 to 12 months. The threshold dose is about 2,300 rads over a 5-week period.
Congenital hypoplasia (Fig GU2-4)	Small, smooth kidney with five or fewer calyces and an enlarged contralateral kidney (compensatory hypertrophy). Generally good function with a normal relation between the amount of parenchyma and the size of the collecting system.	Miniature replica of a normal kidney. Must be differentiated from an acquired atrophic kidney due to vascular or inflammatory disease (may require angiographic demonstration of the aortic orifice of the renal artery, which is small in a hypoplastic kidney but of normal size in an atrophic kidney).
Postobstructive atrophy	Small, smooth kidney with dilated calyces, a thin cortex, and usually effaced papillae. Compensatory hypertrophy of the contralateral kidney depending on the age of the patient, duration of the process, and severity of functional impairment.	Generally appears after surgical correction of urinary tract obstruction. Atrophy probably results from a combination of increased hydrostatic pressure on renal tissue and ischemia from the compression of intrarenal arteries and veins.
Postinflammatory atrophy (acute bacterial nephritis)	Uniform decrease in renal size with smooth or minimally irregular contour.	Unusual form of severe gram-negative bacterial infection in adult patients with altered host resistance (especially diabetes mellitus). The kidney becomes smoothly enlarged with decreased function in the acute phase, then shows a rapid return of function and global loss of tissue over a few weeks after the initiation of appropriate antibiotic therapy.
Reflux atrophy	Small, smooth kidney with dilated calyces, a thin cortex, and effaced papillae.	Structural kidney damage caused by vesicoureteral reflux with resulting increased hydrostatic pressure and tissue ischemia. Unlike reflux nephropathy, there is no infection or focal scarring. The appearance persists after spontaneous or surgical resolution of the vesicoureteral reflux.

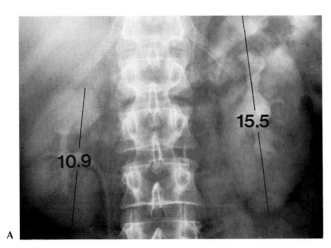

Fig GU2-1. Renal ischemia associated with hypertension. Diminished size of the right kidney (A) due to renal artery stenosis (B).

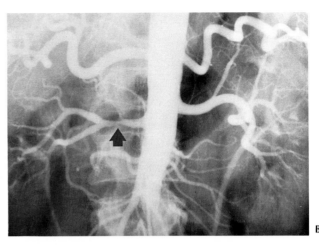

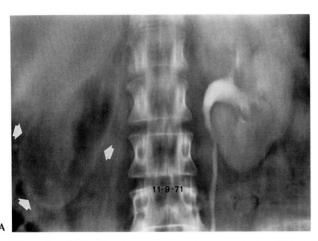

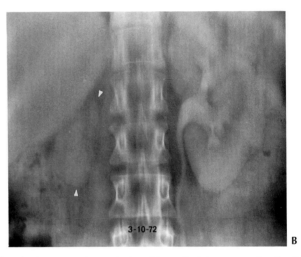

Fig GU2-2. Renal infarction due to acute renal artery occlusion. (A) An initial nephrotomogram demonstrates a thin cortical rim surrounding the right kidney (arrows), reflecting viable renal cortex perfused by perforating collateral vessels from the renal capsule. (B) Four months later a repeat nephrotomogram shows a marked decrease in the size of the atrophic right kidney (arrowheads).[1]

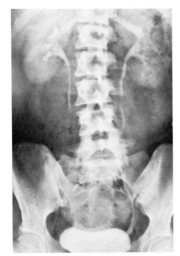

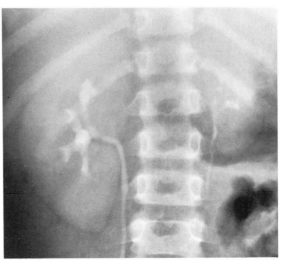

Fig GU2-3. Radiation nephritis. Excretory urogram 5 years after radiation therapy for abdominal lymphoma shows that the left kidney has shrunk markedly. Delayed film showed no contrast material in the collecting system. Although a large left paraspinous mass deviates the axis of the left kidney, ultrasound revealed no obstruction; the intensity of the nephrogram excludes long-standing obstructive atrophy.[2]

Fig GU2-4. Congenital hypoplasia. The small left kidney, a miniature replica of a normal kidney, has good function and a normal relation between the amount of parenchyma and the size of the collecting system. Note the compensatory hypertrophy of the right kidney.

UNILATERAL SMALL, SCARRED KIDNEY

Condition	Imaging Findings	Comments
Reflux nephropathy (chronic atrophic pyelonephritis) (Fig GU3-1)	Unifocal or multifocal reduction in parenchymal thickness (most frequently in the upper pole). Cortical depression overlying retracted papilla whose calyx is secondarily smoothly dilated. May be bilateral (but usually asymmetric).	Related to chronic pyelonephritis and vesicoureteral reflux. By the teenage years, the lesions are fully developed and are no longer progressive unless there are complicating factors (stone formation, obstruction, neurogenic bladder). Cortical depressions must be differentiated from fetal lobulation (which occurs between calyces rather than directly over them). In children, reflux nephropathy may inhibit growth of all or a portion of the affected kidney.
Lobar infarction (Fig GU3-2)	Initially, local failure of calyceal filling with a triangular nephrographic defect whose base is in the subcapsular region. After about 4 weeks, a wide-based cortical depression develops with a normal underlying papilla and calyx. May be multifocal or bilateral.	Usually caused by cardiac embolism (mitral stenosis and atrial fibrillation, infective endocarditis, or mural thrombus overlying a myocardial infarct). In the less common total infarction (occlusion of a main renal artery), the kidney does not function, often has a peripheral rim of opacified cortex, and progressively shrinks after 2 to 3 weeks.
Renal tuberculosis (Fig GU3-3)	Scarring with retraction of the underlying papilla (indistinguishable from reflux nephropathy) or a small, calcified nonfunctioning kidney (autonephrectomy).	Bizarre array of calyceal deformities with papillary destruction, stricture formation (pelvocalyceal system and ureter), and often calcified masses. Bilateral in about 25% of cases.

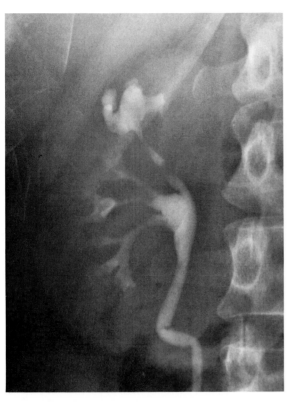

FIG GU3-1. **Chronic atrophic pyelonephritis.** Focal reduction in parenchymal thickness involving the upper pole of the right kidney.

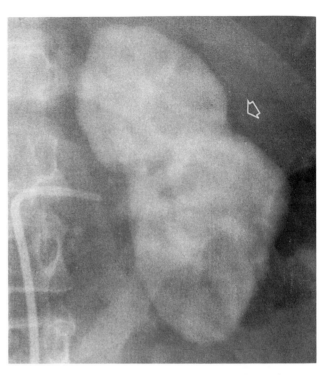

FIG GU3-2. **Segmental renal infarction.** Film from the nephrogram phase of a selective arteriogram demonstrates a typical peripheral triangular defect with its base in the subcapsular region (arrow).

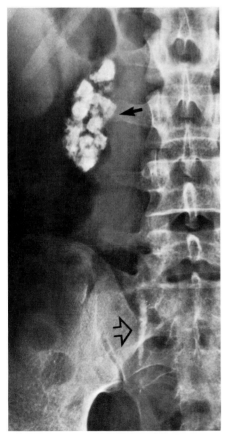

FIG GU3-3. **Tuberculous autonephrectomy.** Plain film shows coarse irregular calcification that retains a reniform shape (black arrow). Note also the tuberculous calcification of the distal right ureter (open arrow).[3]

UNILATERAL LARGE, SMOOTH KIDNEY

Condition	Imaging Findings	Comments
Obstructive uropathy (Fig GU4-1)	Unilateral (or bilateral) large, smooth kidney with a dilated pelvocalyceal system and delayed contrast material excretion. Prolonged hydronephrosis causes diffuse narrowing of the renal parenchyma.	Acute urinary obstruction is most commonly associated with the passage of a calculus or blood clot. Causes of chronic obstruction include benign and malignant tumors of the ureter and adjacent organs, inflammatory strictures and masses, and retroperitoneal tumor or fibrosis.
Renal vein thrombosis (see Fig GU12-4)	Unilateral large, smooth kidney. Little or no opacification in acute thrombosis. Some contrast material excretion if venous occlusion is partial or is accompanied by adequate collateral formation. The collecting system is attenuated by surrounding interstitial edema.	May be a primary event in severely dehydrated infants and children. In adults, most often a complication of another renal disease (amyloidosis, membranous glomerulonephritis, pyelonephritis), trauma, or extension of thrombus or tumor from the inferior vena cava. If unresolved, may produce renal infarction and a small, smooth, nonfunctioning kidney. Enlargement of collateral pathways for renal venous flow causes extrinsic indentations on the pelvis and ureter.
Acute arterial infarction	Unilateral large, smooth, nonopacified kidney. A retrograde pyelogram shows a normal pelvocalyceal system that is effaced by surrounding interstitial edema. Characteristic cortical rim of contrast (peripheral cortex that continues to be perfused by capsular collateral arteries).	Follows embolic, thrombotic, or traumatic occlusion of a renal artery. After 2 to 3 weeks, the kidney begins to shrink and eventually becomes small in the late stage.
Acute pyelonephritis (Fig GU4-2)	Unilateral global enlargement of the kidney with decreased and delayed contrast material excretion and mild dilatation of the collecting system. There is often focal polar swelling and calyceal compression. Characteristic wedge-shaped zones of diminished enhancement radiating from the collecting system to the renal surface on CT.	Primarily affects women 15 to 40 years of age and is most commonly due to *Escherichia coli*. The most severe form (acute bacterial nephritis) occurs in patients with altered host resistance (diabetes mellitus, immunosuppressant therapy). In uncomplicated acute pyelonephritis, the radiographic abnormalities revert to normal after appropriate therapy. In severe disease, there may be marked parenchymal wasting and a small smooth kidney.
Compensatory hypertrophy (Fig GU4-3)	Unilateral smooth, large kidney that is normal in all respects except for its size and the thickness of the renal parenchyma. The pelvocalyceal system and ureter may appear distended (high urinary flow rate).	Response to congenital absence, surgical removal, or disease of the contralateral kidney. The ability of the kidney to undergo compensatory hypertrophy diminishes with age (some state that it does not occur after age 30). After surgical removal of the opposite kidney, the contralateral kidney reaches its maximum size in about 6 months.
Duplicated pelvocalyceal system (Fig GU4-4)	Unilateral (or bilateral) large, smooth kidney. Normal function and appearance of the duplex pelvocalyceal system.	Represents earlier than normal dichotomous branching of the ureteral bud. The two branches encounter a greater mass of metanephric blastema than otherwise would have occurred (causing a larger than normal amount of renal parenchyma associated with the duplex collecting system).

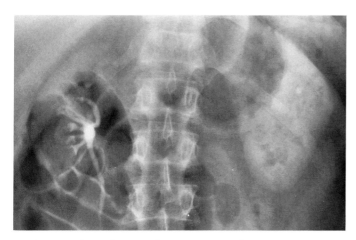

Fɪɢ GU4-1. Obstructive uropathy. Acute urinary obstruction causes a large smooth left kidney with delayed contrast excretion and prolonged nephrogram.

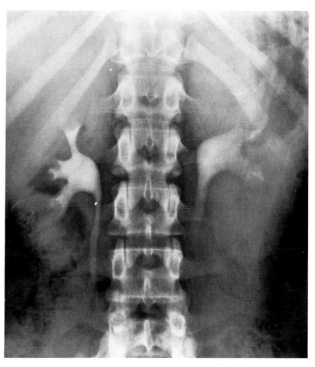

Fɪɢ GU4-2. Acute pyelonephritis. Generalized enlargement of the left kidney with decreased density of contrast material in the collecting system.

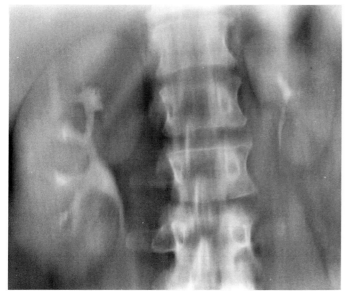

Fɪɢ GU4-3. Compensatory hypertrophy. Markedly enlarged right kidney in a patient with a hypoplastic left kidney.

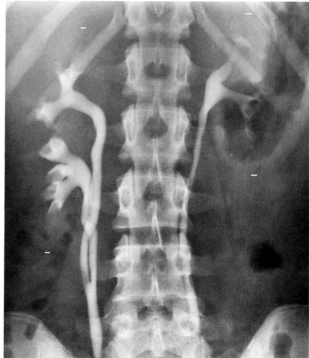

Fɪɢ GU4-4. Duplicated right pelvocalyceal system.

UNILATERAL LARGE, MULTILOBULATED KIDNEY

Condition	Imaging Findings	Comments
Xanthogranulomatous pyelonephritis (Fig GU5-1)	Unilateral nonfunctioning kidney with multifocal enlargement and an obstructing radiopaque calculus at the ureteropelvic junction. There is obstructive dilatation of the collecting system on retrograde pyelography. In the tumefactive form, single or multiple irregular inflammatory masses distort the opacified collecting system or renal margins (simulates renal abscess or neoplasm).	Nodular replacement of renal parenchyma by large lipid-filled macrophages (foam cells) that develop in chronically infected kidneys. May cause multiple small nodules coalescing to form several large masses, a single granulomatous mass, or diffuse replacement of the renal parenchyma. CT shows the characteristic fatty consistency of the xanthogranulomatous mass.
Multicystic dysplastic kidney	Unilateral, multilobulated, nonfunctioning mass in the area normally occupied by the kidney. Thin curvilinear calcification may outline cyst walls. The vascularized walls of individual cysts may become slightly opaque during urography (cluster-of-grapes sign). Usually there is compensatory hypertrophy of the contralateral kidney.	Nonhereditary congenital dysplasia, usually asymptomatic, in which the kidney is composed almost entirely of large thin-walled cysts with only little solid renal tissue. Most common cause of an abdominal mass in the newborn. Other manifestations include an atretic ureter with a blind proximal end (on retrograde pyelography) and an absent or severely atretic renal artery. Ultrasound can differentiate the disorganized pattern of cysts and the lack of renal parenchyma and reniform contour in multicystic kidney disease from the precise organization of symmetrically positioned fluid-filled spaces in hydronephrosis.
Malacoplakia	Unilateral multifocal kidney enlargement with diminished or absent contrast material excretion. Multiple granulomas produce a mass effect on the pelvocalyceal system. No calcification.	Rare inflammation of renal parenchyma characterized by cortical and medullary granulomatous masses containing large mononuclear cells with abundant cytoplasm. Usually associated with *Escherichia coli* infection. About 75% of cases are multifocal and 50% are bilateral. Malacoplakia of the urinary tract most commonly affects the bladder.

A   B

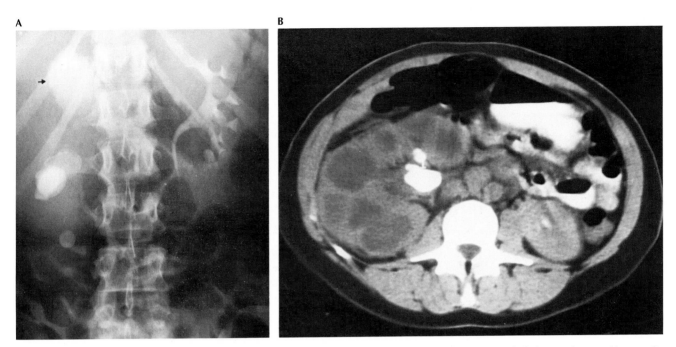

Fɪɢ GU5-1. Xanthogranulomatous pyelonephritis. (A) Excretory urogram shows a unilateral nonfunctioning right kidney with several large radiopaque calculi at the ureteropelvic junction and in the proximal ureter. The arrow points to an opacified gallbladder. (B) CT scan shows the characteristic fatty consistency of the multiple xanthogranulomatous masses. Note the dense zone at the ureteropelvic junction.

BILATERAL SMALL, SMOOTH KIDNEYS

Condition	Imaging Findings	Comments
Generalized arteriosclerosis (Fig GU6-1)	Bilaterally small kidneys that may be smooth or show focal depressions (scars) representing infarctions. Uniform loss of cortical thickness but normal nephrogram, papillae, and pelvocalyceal system. Increased radiolucency in the renal pelvis is due to proliferation of renal sinus fat.	Generalized arteriosclerosis involving most of the interlobar and arcuate arteries causes uniform shrinkage of both kidneys. A similar appearance may develop in scleroderma, chronic tophaceous gout, and polyarteritis (due to the accelerated atherosclerotic or necrotic arterial lesions associated with these diseases). Usually not detected before age 50.
Nephrosclerosis (benign and malignant) (Fig GU6-2; see Fig GU13-2)	Radiographic appearance of benign nephrosclerosis is similar to that of arteriosclerotic kidney disease. In malignant nephrosclerosis, there is invariably diminished opacification of the kidneys. Occasionally there may be subcapsular bleeding (concave, inward displacement of the parenchyma).	Benign nephrosclerosis consists of thickening and subendothelial hyalinization of afferent arterioles associated with hypertension. In malignant nephrosclerosis, there is accelerated or malignant hypertension with proliferative endarteritis. It is controversial whether the elevated blood pressure is the cause or the result of the afferent arteriolar lesion.
Atheroembolic renal disease	Radiographic appearance similar to that of malignant nephrosclerosis.	Caused by the dislodgement from the aorta of multiple atheromatous emboli that occlude intrarenal arteries. May be spontaneous or result from external trauma or from a direct insult to the aorta during surgery or catheter manipulation.
Chronic glomerulonephritis (Figs GU6-3 and GU6-4)	Globally small kidneys with smooth contours, normal calyces and papillae, and occasional peripelvic fat proliferation. The density of the nephrogram and pelvocalyceal system varies with the severity of the disease. There may be cortical calcification (best seen on CT).	Develops weeks or months after an episode of acute glomerulonephritis (not always poststreptococcal). Associated with progressive hypertension and renal failure. About 50% of patients eventually develop the nephrotic syndrome.
Papillary necrosis (see Figs GU15-1 and GU15-2)	Bilateral globally shrunken kidneys with impaired function sometimes occur in severe disease (most patients have normal-sized kidneys). Earlier signs include papillary enlargement followed by disruption (tract formation, cavitation, papillary slough). Sloughed, eventually calcified, papillae may cause urinary tract obstruction and predispose to infection.	Bilateral small, smooth kidneys primarily occur in papillary necrosis associated with analgesic abuse. Small kidneys are not reported in papillary necrosis due to diabetes mellitus or sickle cell disease. Usually unilateral if papillary necrosis is secondary to noninfected urinary tract obstruction, renal vein thrombosis, or trauma.
Hereditary nephropathy **Hereditary chronic nephritis (Alport's syndrome)**	Small, smooth kidneys with impaired excretion of contrast material.	Distinctive histologic feature of fat-filled macrophages (foam cells), especially in the corticomedullary junction. Males are affected by a more severe form of renal disease and usually die before age 50. No hypertension. Most patients also have nerve deafness and ocular abnormalities.

(continued page 456)

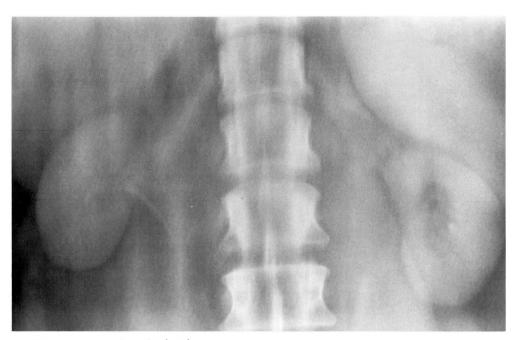

Fɪɢ **GU6-1.** **Generalized arteriosclerosis.**

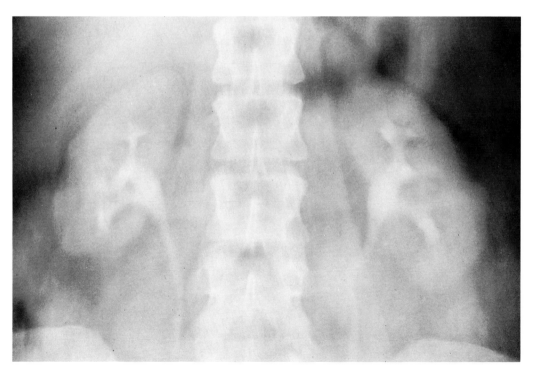

Fɪɢ **GU6-2.** **Benign nephrosclerosis.** Bilaterally small kidneys with several shallow infarct scars. The pelvocalyceal systems and renal opacitication are normal.[4]

Condition	Imaging Findings	Comments
Medullary cystic disease (see Fig GU10-5)	Normal or small kidneys with smooth contour and impaired excretion of contrast material. Large medullary cysts may produce sharply defined radiolucent defects on nephrotomography (best seen on CT). The cysts are usually too small to cause pelvocalyceal displacement or lobulation of the renal contour.	Variable number of often very small cysts in the corticomedullary junction and medulla. More often involves females. Clinical findings include anemia, polyuria, hyposthenuria, and salt wasting. No hypertension.
Amyloidosis (late)	Typically causes smooth enlargement of both kidneys. In long-standing disease, amyloid kidneys become small with preservation of their normal contours and pelvocalyceal relations.	Shrinkage of the kidneys presumably occurs as a result of ischemic atrophy of nephrons induced by the involvement of renal blood vessels by amyloid deposits.
Arterial hypotension	Bilateral small, smooth kidneys with their nephrograms becoming progressively denser over time or remaining unchanged.	May be secondary to shock or a reaction to contrast material. Once the hypotension is reversed, the urogram usually reverts to normal.

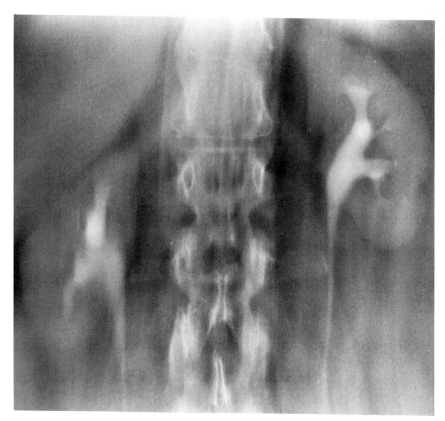

FIG **GU6-3. Chronic glomerulonephritis.** Nephrotomogram shows bilateral small smooth kidneys. The uniform reduction in parenchymal thickness is particularly apparent in the right kidney. Note that the pelvocalyceal system is well opacified and without the irregular contours and blunted calyces seen in chronic pyelonephritis.

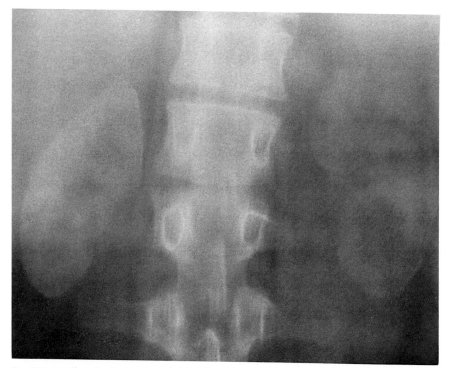

FIG **GU6-4. Chronic glomerulonephritis.** Plain film tomogram shows bilateral small smooth kidneys with diffuse fine calcification in the renal parenchyma.

BILATERAL LARGE, SMOOTH KIDNEYS

Condition	Imaging Findings	Comments
Proliferative or necrotizing disorders		
Acute glomerulonephritides (Fig GU7-1)	Bilateral large kidneys (may be of normal size) with global parenchymal thickening and smooth contours. The nephrogram is homogeneously faint or normal. The pelvocalyceal system is normal, though opacification is often faint (ultrasound is the most efficacious test to show that the calyces are not dilated and thus not obstructed).	Kidneys may remain enlarged or normal throughout the course of illness. If the disease progresses to a chronic stage (especially in the poststreptococcal type), the kidneys become bilaterally small with smooth contours. (*Note:* A patient with renal failure must be well hydrated before excretory urography is performed.)
Glomerular abnormality in multisystem diseases	Nonspecific findings of acute glomerular disease (large, smooth, nonobstructed kidneys with or without impaired excretion of contrast material).	Specific extrarenal findings vary depending on the underlying disease (see below).
Polyarteritis nodosa (Fig GU7-2)	Multiple small aneurysms that most often arise at arterial bifurcations and predominantly involve small arteries of the kidneys, mesentery, liver, pancreas, heart, muscles, and nerves.	Necrotizing inflammation involving all layers of the walls of arterioles and small arteries. Hypertension and hematuria are common. Rupture of an intrarenal aneurysm may cause renal infarction or perinephric or parenchymal hematoma.
Systemic lupus erythematosus (see Figs C28-4 and C29-11)	Subluxation and malalignment of joints without erosions (eg, boutonnière and swan neck deformities). Pleural and pericardial effusions. Patchy infiltrates at lung bases.	Connective tissue disorder primarily involving young or middle-aged women. Probably an immune complex disease. Characteristic butterfly rash.
Wegener's granulomatosus (see Fig C8-12)	Granulomatous lesions in the kidneys, upper respiratory tract (especially the paranasal sinuses), and lungs (multiple pulmonary nodules that often cavitate).	Necrotizing vasculitis and granulomatous inflammation. Renal involvement in more than 90% of patients (primarily focal or acute glomerulonephritis).
Allergic angiitis	Fleeting, patchy pulmonary consolidations with nonsegmental distribution. Confluent densities may cavitate.	Necrotizing vasculitis separated from polyarteritis nodosa because of prominent eosinophilia, the presence of perivascular granulomas, lung involvement, and clinical association with bronchial asthma (except for pulmonary manifestations, organ involvement is similar to that of polyarteritis nodosa).
Goodpasture's syndrome (see Fig C2-11)	Pulmonary hemorrhage causing patchy air-space consolidation (especially in the perihilar region, simulating pulmonary edema) followed by a reticular pattern that initially clears. Repeated attacks cause interstitial deposition of hemosiderin and progressive interstitial fibrosis.	Most likely an autoimmune disease with circulating antibodies to the glomerular and alveolar basement membranes. Usually occurs in young adult men.
Henoch-Schönlein purpura (Fig GU7-3)	Bleeding into joints and the gastrointestinal tract (regular thickening of small bowel folds with separation of loops).	Acute vasculitis characterized by purpura, nephritis, abdominal pain, and joint pain. Most commonly occurs in the first two decades and frequently develops several weeks after a streptococcal infection. Usually self-limited.
Thrombotic thrombocytopenic purpura	Bilateral large, smooth kidneys.	Hemolytic anemia, hemorrhage, and oliguric or anuric renal failure occur as a result of arterial thrombosis and proliferative lesions of the glomerular epithelium.

(continued page 460)

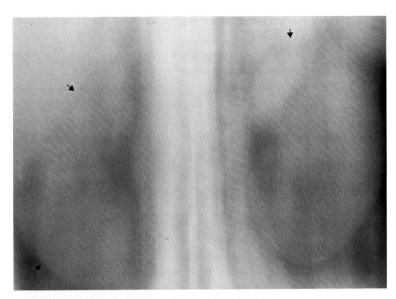

Fig GU7-1. Acute glomerulonephritis. Nephrotomogram demonstrates bilateral large kidneys with smooth contours (arrows). The nephrographic density, although faint, was maximal at this time. The calyces were never visualized.[4]

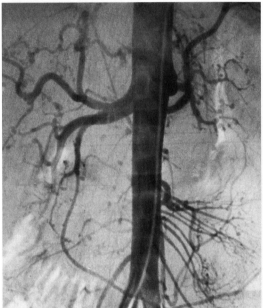

Fig GU7-2. Polyarteritis nodosa. An aortogram demonstrates innumerable small aneurysms arising from vessels throughout the abdomen. The aorta and its major branches are spared.

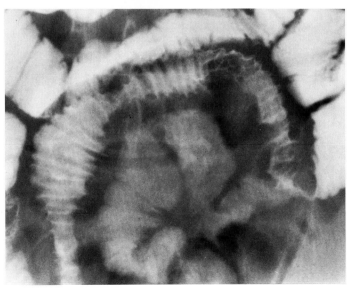

Fig GU7-3. Henoch-Schönlein purpura. Hemorrhage and edema in the intestinal wall causes regular thickening of small bowel folds.

Condition	Imaging Findings	Comments
Diabetic glomerulosclerosis (Fig GU7-4)	Wide spectrum of radiographic changes in diabetes mellitus.	Nodular sclerosis of renal glomeruli and arterioles (Kimmelstiel-Wilson syndrome) may occur in chronic diabetics and lead to the development of the nephrotic syndrome or chronic renal failure.
Subacute infective endocarditis	Focal or diffuse glomerulonephritis.	Diffuse glomerulonephritis that is indistinguishable from other types of immune complex disease. Small emboli may produce a focal glomerulitis, while large emboli to the kidneys may cause infarction. The spleen is frequently involved and petechial skin lesions are common.
Abnormal protein deposition **Amyloidosis** (Fig GU7-5)	Bilateral large, smooth kidneys with normal or impaired opacification and normal pelvocalyceal systems. With time, the kidneys decrease in size and eventually become small.	Kidneys affected in over 80% of patients with amyloidosis secondary to chronic suppurative or inflammatory disease. Renal involvement in about 35% of patients with primary amyloidosis. May be complicated by renal vein thrombosis (produces decreased kidney opacification).
Multiple myeloma	Bilateral large, smooth kidneys with reduced opacification. The pelvocalyceal system is normal but often diffusely attenuated in patients with severe renal involvement. In late stages, the kidneys may eventually shrink.	Abnormal proteins precipitated in the tubules cause renal insufficiency in up to 50% of cases. Diffuse renal infiltration of plasma cells is rare. Renal function may also be compromised by impaired renal blood flow (increased blood viscosity) and nephrocalcinosis due to hypercalcemia. (*Note:* A patient with renal failure must be well hydrated before excretory urography is performed.)
Abnormal fluid accumulation **Acute tubular necrosis**	Bilateral large, smooth kidneys with characteristic immediate and prolonged increased nephrogram (increasingly dense nephrogram in 25% of cases) that may persist for more than 1 day. The pelvocalyceal system is faintly or not opacified and is usually globally attenuated because of increased parenchymal thickness.	Reversible renal failure with or without oliguria that follows exposure of the kidney to certain toxic agents (mercury, ethylene glycol, carbon tetrachloride, bismuth, arsenic, urographic contrast material) or to a period of prolonged severe ischemia (shock, crush injury, burns, transfusion reaction, severe dehydration, renal transplantation, aortic resection). Usually reversible, but may require temporary dialysis. The proximal convoluted tubules may rarely calcify after recovery.
Acute cortical necrosis (Fig GU7-6)	Bilateral large, smooth kidneys with poor opacification. Normal pelvocalyceal systems on retrograde studies. Classic appearance of punctate or linear (tramline) calcification confined to the renal cortex develops within about 1 month.	Very uncommon form of acute renal failure in which there is patchy or universal necrosis of the renal cortex with sparing of the medulla. May be associated with severe burns, multiple fractures, internal hemorrhage, transfusions of incompatible blood, and especially complications of pregnancy (abruptio placentae, septic abortion, or placenta previa).

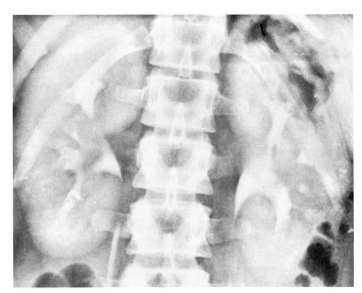

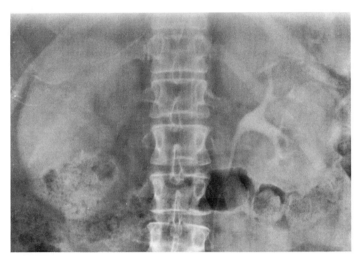

Fig GU7-4. Diabetic glomerulosclerosis with nephrotic syndrome and chronic renal failure. An excretory urogram demonstrates bilateral large smooth kidneys with normal calyces.[2]

Fig GU7-5. Amyloidosis. Bilateral large smooth kidneys. Decreased opacification and prolonged nephrogram on the right are secondary to superimposed ureteral obstruction.

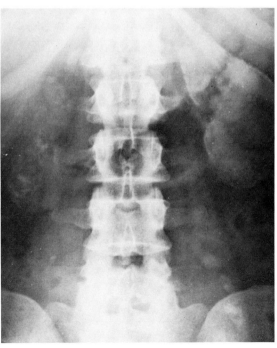

Fig GU7-6. Bilateral acute renal cortical necrosis. There is punctate calcification in the right kidney and a peripheral rim of calcification surrounding the left kidney.

Condition	Imaging Findings	Comments
Other conditions **Leukemia** **(Fig GU7-7)**	Bilateral large, smooth kidneys with nephrographic and pelvocalyceal density varying from normal to markedly depressed. The collecting systems may be attenuated by neoplastic cell infiltration.	Most common malignant cause of bilateral global renal enlargement. More frequent in children with acute leukemia, especially of the lymphocytic type. Superimposed hemorrhage may produce a focal parenchymal mass, a subcapsular collection of blood, or obstructive or nonobstructive clots in the renal pelvis or ureters.
Acute interstitial nephritis	Bilateral large, smooth kidneys with normal to diminished opacification. There is a return to normal apearance after withdrawal of the offending drug.	Inflammatory cell infiltration representing a complication of exposure to certain drugs (most commonly methicillin; also phenindione, diphenylhydantoin, sulfonamides, ampicillin, cephalothin). Probably represents an allergic or idiosyncratic reaction rather than direct drug nephrotoxicity.
Acute urate nephropathy	Bilateral large, smooth kidneys with unopacified pelvocalyceal systems and increasing nephrographic density.	Flooding of nephrons with large amounts of uric acid crystals (which deposit in the collecting tubules and interstitium). Most commonly a complication of therapy of leukemia, lymphoma, myeloproliferative disorders, or polycythemia vera (cytotoxic agents release large amounts of nucleoprotein that is metabolized to uric acid). (*Note:* Contrast material may be dangerous in these patients because of its uricosuric effect.)
Acromegaly **(Fig GU7-8)**	Bilateral large, smooth kidneys with normal structure and function.	Manifestation of the generalized organomegaly.
Nephromegaly associated with other diseases	Bilateral large, smooth kidneys with normal structure and function.	Hepatic cirrhosis (especially in patients with marked fatty changes in the liver); hyperalimentation (increase in the fluid compartments of the kidney related to the hyperosmolality of administered solutions); diabetes mellitus (even in the absence of diabetic glomerulosclerosis); hemophilia; Fabry's disease (lipid deposition in the renal parenchyma).
Sickle cell disease (homozygous)	Bilateral large, smooth kidneys. Eventually there is impaired concentration of contrast material and dilated pelvocalyceal systems and ureters.	Reflects vascular dilatation, engorgement of vessels, glomerular enlargement, interstitial edema, and increased renal blood flow. Lobar infarction may develop. Papillary necrosis is more common in patients with heterozygous disease.
Bilateral duplication	Bilateral long, smooth kidneys (normal width). Two pelvocalyceal systems on both sides.	May mimic a neoplasm if one of the collecting systems is obstructed and nonfunctioning.
Physiologic response to contrast material and diuretics	Bilateral large, smooth kidneys with normal structure and function.	Vasodilatation or diuresis may increase renal size, presumably because of volume expansion of the vascular tree, tubular lumens, or interstitial fluid space. Renal area may increase up to 35% (mean increase, only 5%).
Bilateral hydronephrosis	Bilateral large, smooth kidneys with dilated pelvocalyceal systems and delayed excretion. Prolonged hydronephrosis causes diffuse parenchymal narrowing and small, smooth kidneys.	May be congenital or acquired (bladder outlet obstruction or an inflammatory mass obstructing both ureters).

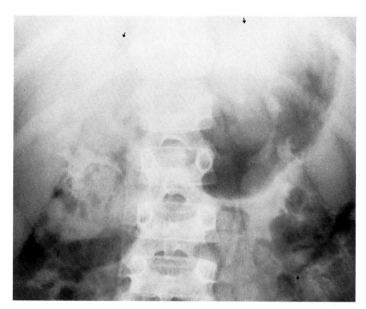

FIG GU7-7. Chronic leukemia. Diffuse infiltration of leukemic cells has caused bilateral enlargement of the kidneys (arrows).

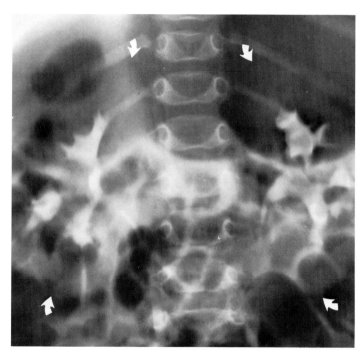

FIG GU7-8. Acromegaly. Bilateral enlargement of well-functioning kidneys. The arrows point to the superior and inferior margins of the kidneys, both of which are about five vertebral bodies in length.

BILATERAL LARGE, MULTIFOCAL KIDNEYS

Condition	Imaging Findings	Comments
Adult polycystic kidney disease (Figs GU8-1 and GU8-2)	Bilateral large kidneys with multilobulated contours. The pelvic and infundibular structures are elongated, effaced, and often displaced around larger cysts to produce a crescentic outline. Characteristic mottled nephrogram (Swiss cheese pattern) due to the presence of innumerable lucent cysts of various sizes throughout the kidneys. Plaques of calcification occasionally occur in the cyst walls.	Inherited disorder in which many progressively growing cysts cause lobulated enlargement of the kidneys and progressive renal impairment (presumably due to cystic compression of nephrons that causes localized intrarenal obstruction). About 35% of patients have associated cysts of the liver (they do not interfere with hepatic function). About 10% have one or more saccular (berry) aneurysms of cerebral arteries (may rupture and produce fatal subarachnoid hemorrhage). Hypertension is common. Patients tend to be asymptomatic during the first three decades of life (early diagnosis is made by chance or as the result of a specific search prompted by a positive family history).
Acquired cystic kidney disease	Bilateral large kidneys with multilobulated contours and no renal function. Requires ultrasound or CT for detection.	Multiple cyst formation occurs in chronically failed kidneys of patients undergoing long-term hemodialysis. The degree of enlargement may approach that of adult polycystic kidney disease. The process may reverse after successful renal transplantation.
Lymphoma	Bilaterally enlarged kidneys with multifocal bulges of renal contours and displacement of the pelvocalyceal systems. There may be a single mass in one kidney or a normal urogram (lymphomatous nodules too small to displace the collecting structures or distort the renal contour). Opacification of the kidneys progressively diminishes as the lymphomatous masses grow, coalesce, and replace nephrons.	Renal involvement occurs much more frequently in non-Hodgkin's lymphoma than in Hodgkin's disease. Usually asymptomatic unless there is a palpable mass, hypertension (mass impressing renal artery or causing renal vein occlusion), or obstructive uropathy (ureteral encasement by lymphomatous tissue in the retroperitoneum. Radiation or chemotherapy may produce uric acid nephropathy or radiation nephritis.

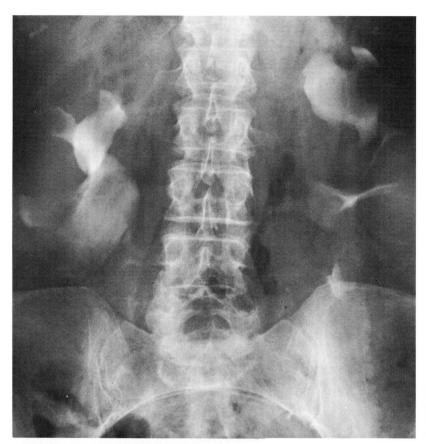

FIG GU8-1. Adult polycystic kidney disease. Excretory urogram shows marked multifocal enlargement of both kidneys, focal displacement of the collecting structures, and normal opacification.[4]

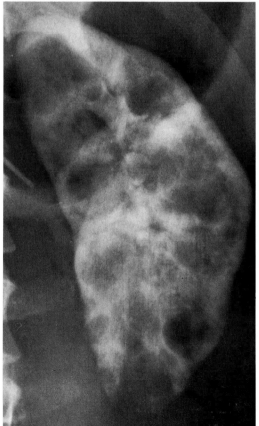

FIG GU8-2. Adult polycystic kidney disease. Nephrogram phase from selective arteriography of the left kidney demonstrates innumerable cysts ranging from pinhead size to 2 cm. The opposite kidney had an identical appearance.[5]

FOCAL RENAL MASS

Condition	Imaging Findings	Comments
Normal variant	Focal ''mass'' on the surface of a kidney that may be confused with a neoplasm.	Fetal lobulation (prominence of the centrilobar cortex where two adjacent lobes abut); dromedary hump; hilar bulge (prominence of the suprahilar region of the left kidney that may cause focal displacement of the upper pole collecting system).
Congenital renal pseudotumor (column of Bertin) (Fig GU9-1)	Focal ''mass'' apparently arising from the surface of the kidney with compression and splaying of the pelvocalyceal system. May simulate a true neoplasm.	Mass of normal cortical tissue in the renal parenchyma. Most commonly develops at the junction of the middle and upper thirds of a duplex kidney. The correct diagnosis can be made by radionuclide scanning, which reveals normal or even increased uptake of isotope in the pseudotumor in contrast to decreased uptake in other renal masses.
Simple renal cyst (Figs GU9-2 and GU9-3)	Focal contour expansion of the kidney outline on the nephrogram. The cortical margin appears as a very thin, smooth radiopaque rim about the bulging lucent cyst (beak sign). A thickened wall suggests bleeding into a cyst, cyst infection, or a malignant lesion. When a simple cyst is completely embedded in the kidney parenchyma, the thin rim and beak are absent and the renal size and contour are normal. A renal cyst causes focal displacement of adjacent portions of the pelvocalyceal system with the collecting structures remaining smooth and attenuated rather than shaggy and obliterated as with a malignant neoplasm.	Unifocal fluid-filled mass that is usually unilocular, though septa sometimes divide the cyst into chambers that may or may not communicate with each other. Cysts vary in size and may occur at single or multiple sites in one or both kidneys. Thin curvilinear calcification occurs in about 3% of simple cysts (not pathognomonic of a benign process since 20% of masses with this appearance are malignant). Ultrasound or CT can unequivocally demonstrate a simple renal cyst. Cyst puncture is necessary if there is an atypical appearance or a strong clinical suspicion of abscess or if the patient has hematuria or hypertension.
Malignant neoplasm (Figs GU9-4 to GU9-6)	Focal mass with indistinct outlines and a density similar to that of normal parenchyma (unlike the classic radiolucent mass with sharp margins and a thin wall representing a benign cyst). Necrotic neoplasms may appear cystic, though they are usually surrounded by thick, irregular walls. Initially, there is elongation of adjacent calyces, followed by distortion, narrowing, or obliteration of part or all of the collecting system due to progressive tumor enlargement and infiltration. Large tumors may partially obstruct the pelvis or upper ureter and cause proximal dilatation or even a nonfunctioning kidney.	Renal cell carcinoma (hypernephroma) is the most common malignant renal neoplasm, predominantly occurring in patients over age 40. About 10% of hypernephromas contain calcification (usually located in reactive fibrous zones about areas of tumor necrosis). Of all masses containing calcium in a nonperipheral location, almost 90% are malignant (peripheral curvilinear calcification is more suggestive of a benign cyst, but a hypernephroma can have a calcified fibrous pseudocapsule and present an identical radiographic appearance). Bilateral carcinomas occur in about 2% of cases (especially in von Hippel–Lindau disease). Nephroblastoma (Wilms' tumor) is common in children. Sarcomas, metastases, and invasive transitional cell carcinoma are rare.

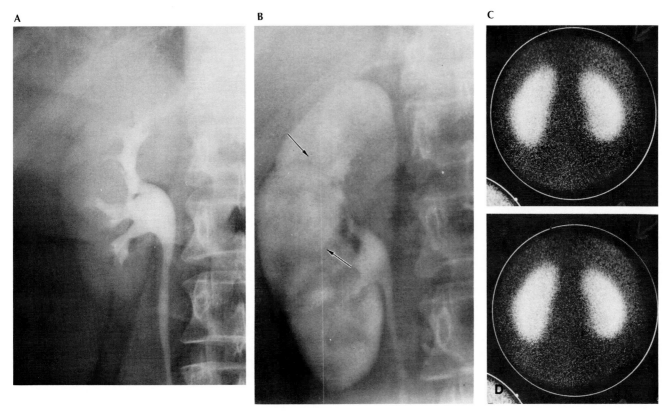

FIG GU9-1. Congenital renal pseudotumor. (A) Excretory urogram shows displacement of the upper calyceal system of the right kidney. (B) Film from the nephrotomogram phase of a selective right renal arteriogram shows the large cortical column (arrows), which appears denser than the medullary substance. (C) Renal scan shows normal functioning parenchyma.[6]

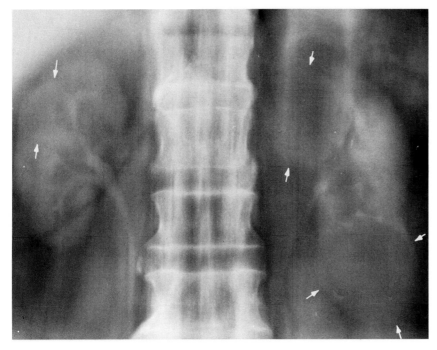

FIG GU9-2. Renal cysts. Nephrotomogram demonstrates bilateral renal cysts (arrows).

Condition	Imaging Findings	Comments
Benign neoplasm (Figs GU9-7 to GU9-9)	Unifocal renal mass enlarging the kidney and causing distortion and displacement of the adjacent portion of the pelvocalyceal system. No tumor calcification or irregular obliteration of the pelvocalyceal system as in malignant disease. Fat in an angiomyolipoma may produce a well-defined area of mottled radiolucency on plain films.	Most common benign tumor of the kidney is hamartoma (angiomyolipoma), which develops in a large percentage of patients with tuberous sclerosis in whom involvement is usually multifocal and bilateral. Angiomyolipomas typically appear as intensely echogenic masses on ultrasound and have a high fat content on CT. Other benign tumors include adenoma (usually small, asymptomatic, and discovered incidentally), reninoma (uncommon benign tumor of juxtaglomerular cells associated with increased renin secretion and hypertension), and mesenchymal tumors (fibroma, lipoma, leiomyoma, angioma).
Renal/perirenal abscess (Fig GU9-10)	Focal, usually polar, renal mass that may displace or efface adjacent portions of the pelvocalyceal system. In a chronic abscess, a nephrographic radiolucent defect in the well-defined mass corresponds to a central collection of necrotic tissue (thick-walled cavity with an irregular inner margin). Perirenal infection causes partial or complete obscuration of the renal outline, loss of the psoas margin, immobility of the kidney with respiration, and lumbar scoliosis concave to the side of involvement. The demonstration of extraluminal gas around or inside the kidney is virtually pathognomonic of renal or perirenal abscess.	Most renal and perirenal abscesses occur by direct extension from renal pelvic infection, especially if there is a calculus obstructing the ureter or pelvis. Since the introduction of antibiotics, renal abscess is infrequently due to direct or hematogenous spread of an extraurinary infection. A renal abscess usually does not spread to the contralateral side because the medial fascia surrounding the kidney is closed and the spine and great vessels act as natural deterrents. An inflammatory process can extend around the entire kidney, though it usually is most pronounced on the dorsal and superior aspects where the renal fascia is open and the surrounding tissues offer little resistance. The radiographic appearance may be indistinguishable from that of a renal neoplasm.
Focal hydronephrosis	Increased renal length and a localized bulge in contour. Sharply marginated lucency corresponds to the dilated calyces filled with nonopacified urine seen during the nephrogram phase. The obstructed area slowly opacifies as contrast material passes into the dilated, urine-filled system (may require films as late as 24 to 36 hours after injection). Nonobstructed calyces draining the remainder of the kidney opacify normally, though they may be displaced by the mass effect of the hydronephrotic segment.	Caused by obstruction to drainage of one portion of the kidney (most often the upper pole of a kidney with partial or complete duplication of the collecting system). May reflect a congenital ureteropelvic duplication with an ectopic ureterocele or be the result of infection (especially tuberculosis). Retrograde or antegrade pyelography may be of value to visualize precisely the point of obstruction (if not determined on delayed films).
Multilocular cyst	Unifocal mass, usually in a polar location, that produces a sharply defined lucent nephrographic defect and often displaces the pelvocalyceal system. Calcification and faint septa may be detected.	Uncommon unilateral mass composed of multiple cysts of various sizes and adjoining primitive cellular elements. May be detected as a palpable mass in infants. May represent a form of congenital cystic dysplasia or a benign renal neoplasm. Differs from multicystic (dysgenetic) kidney in that it is unilateral, involves only a segment of an otherwise normal kidney, and has no associated abnormalities of the ureter or renal artery.

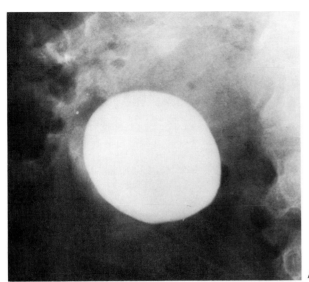

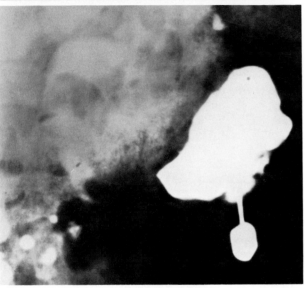

FIG GU9-3. Renal cyst puncture. (A) The instillation of contrast material shows the smooth inner wall characteristic of a benign cyst. (B) In another patient, the introduction of contrast material reveals the markedly irregular inner border of a necrotic renal cell carcinoma.

FIG GU9-5. Renal cell carcinoma. Left renal arteriogram demonstrates a large hypervascular mass with striking enlargement of capsular vessels.

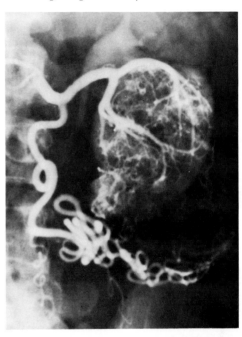

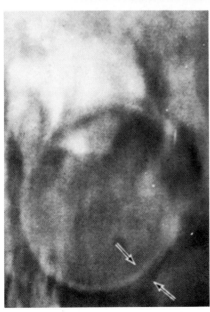

FIG GU9-4. Renal cell carcinoma. Nephrotomogram demonstrates a lucent, well-demarcated renal mass with a thick wall (arrows).[7]

FIG GU9-6. Wilms' tumor. Huge mass in the right kidney distorts and displaces the pelvocalyceal system.[2]

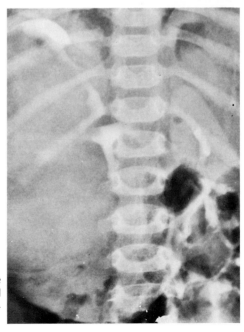

Condition	Imaging Findings	Comments
Congenital arteriovenous malformation	Unifocal mass, most commonly in a parapelvic or medullary location, which impresses the pelvocalyceal system. Cirsoid vascular channels occasionally produce multinodular impressions on the pelvocalyceal system. Curvilinear calcification may form in the walls of the mass.	Most commonly cirsoid (multiple coiled vascular channels grouped in a cluster). The much rarer cavernous form is composed of a single well-defined artery feeding into a single vein. Usually presents with hematuria and may produce an abdominal bruit.
Xanthogranulomatous pyelonephritis (see Fig GU5-1)	Unifocal or multifocal masses with displacement of nondilated calyces and normal or diminished opacification. Calcification is common.	Nodular replacement of renal parenchyma by large lipid-filled macrophages (foam cells) that develops in chronically infected kidneys. Most commonly appears as a unilateral nonfunctioning kidney with multifocal enlargement and an obstructing radiopaque calculus at the ureteropelvic junction. May simulate a renal neoplasm (CT shows the characteristic fatty consistency of the xanthogranulomatous mass).
Subcapsular hematoma	Nonopacifying mass between opacified renal parenchyma and the renal capsule that flattens and compresses the underlying renal parenchyma. May extrinsically compress the pelvocalyceal system and even result in a nonfunctioning kidney.	Posttraumatic or spontaneous (often associated with neoplasm, arteriosclerosis, or polyarteritis nodosa). A large subcapsular hematoma may produce hypertension (Page kidney).

A

B

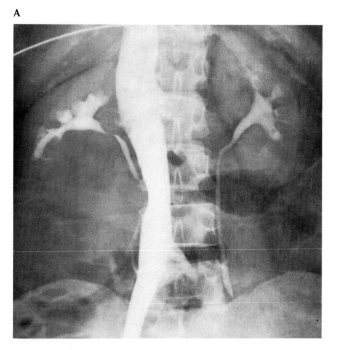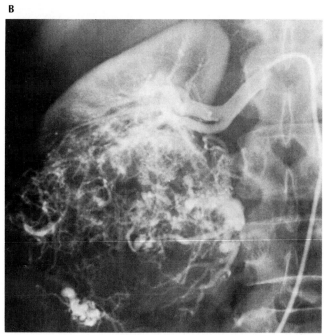

FIG GU9-7. Renal hamartoma. (A) A combined excretory urogram and inferior vena cavagram shows a large mass in the lower pole of the right kidney with displacement but no invasion of the pelvocalyceal system and inferior vena cava. (B) Arteriography shows the mass to be hypervascular. The overall radiographic appearance is indistinguishable from that of renal cell carcinoma.

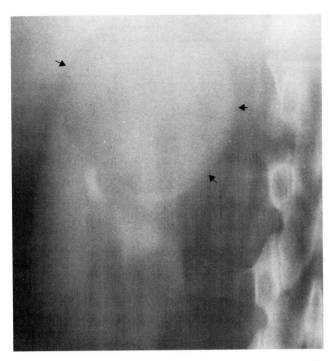

FIG GU9-8. Renal adenoma. Nephrotomogram shows the tumor to be a smooth, relatively lucent mass (arrows) that is indistinguishable from a cyst.

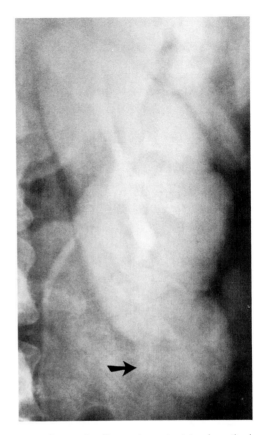

FIG GU9-9. Reninoma. Small mass (arrow) arising from the lower pole of the left kidney.[8]

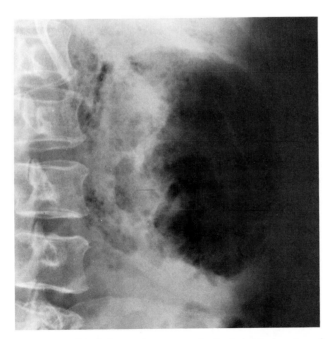

FIG GU9-10. Renal abscess. Large amounts of extraluminal gas in and around the left kidney.

CYSTIC DISEASES OF THE KIDNEYS

Condition	Imaging Findings	Comments
Simple renal cyst **(Fig GU10-1)**	Focal contour expansion of the renal outline on the nephrogram phase. The cortical margin appears as a very thin, smooth radiopaque rim about the bulging lucent cyst (beak sign). A thickened wall suggests bleeding into the cyst, cyst infection, or a malignant lesion. Thin curvilinear calcification is seen in about 3% of cases (not pathognomonic of a benign process, since 20% of masses with this appearance are malignant).	Unifocal, fluid-filled mass. Usually unilocular, though septa sometimes divide the cyst into chambers that may or may not communicate with each other. Cysts vary in size and may occur at single or multiple sites in one or both kidneys. Ultrasound or CT scans unequivocally demonstrate simple renal cysts. Cyst puncture is necessary if there is an atypical appearance or a strong clinical suspicion of an abscess or if the patient has hematura or hypertension.
Parapelvic cyst	Hilar mass displacing the kidney laterally and rotating it on its anteroposterior axis. Occasionally compresses hilar fat to produce a thin, lucent fat line separating the cyst from the adjacent renal parenchyma.	Extraparenchymal cyst occurring in the region of the renal hilum. Most parapelvic cysts lie lateral to the renal pelvis and can spread, elongate, and compress adjacent calyces (may even cause obstruction).
Adult polycystic kidney disease	Bilateral large kidneys with a multilobulated contour. The pelvic and infundibular structures are elongated, effaced, and often displaced around larger cysts to produce a crescentic outline. The characteristic mottled, "Swiss cheese" nephrogram is due to the presence of innumerable lucent cysts of various sizes throughout the kidneys. Plaques of calcification occasionally occur in cyst walls.	Inherited disorder in which many progressively growing cysts cause lobulated enlargement of the kidneys and progressive renal impairment. About 35% of patients have associated cysts of the liver (they do not interfere with hepatic functions). About 10% have one or more saccular (berry) aneurysms of the cerebral arteries (may rupture and produce fatal subarachnoid hemorrhage). Hypertension is common.
Infantile polycystic kidney disease **(Fig GU10-2)**	Kidneys appear as large soft-tissue masses occupying much of the abdomen and displacing the stomach and bowel. Smooth cortical margins (unlike the adult form). If there is sufficient renal function, urography results in a nephrogram with a streaky pattern of alternating dense and lucent bands reflecting contrast material puddling in elongated cystic spaces that radiate perpendicular to the cortical surface.	Rare, usually fatal, autosomal recessive disorder that manifests itself at birth by diffusely enlarged kidneys, renal failure, and maldevelopment of intrahepatic bile ducts. In the childhood form, renal abnormality is usually milder but is associated with severe congenital hepatic fibrosis and portal hypertension.
Medullary sponge kidney (renal tubular ectasia) **(Fig GU10-3)**	Ectatic tubules appear either as fine linear striations of contrast producing a brush border pattern or as more cystic dilatation simulating a cluster of grapes. Plain radiographs often demonstrate small, smoothly rounded calculi occurring in clusters or in a fanlike arrangement in the papillary tip of one or more renal pyramids.	Cystic dilatation of distal collecting tubules in the renal pyramids. The ectatic changes may be limited to a single pyramid, but are usually more extensive and bilateral (often asymmetric). Renal function is preserved, though tubular stasis predisposes to calculus formation and pyelonephritis. Generally asymptomatic, except when medullary calculi become dislodged and produce renal colic or hematuria.

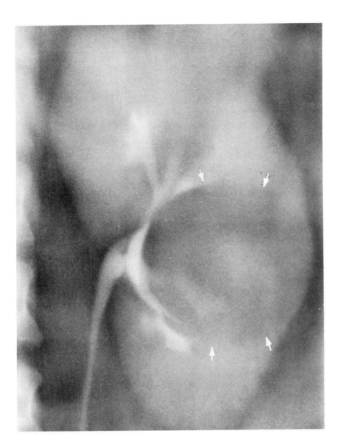

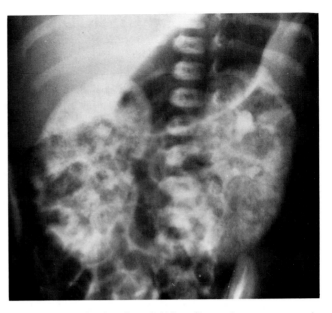

Fig GU10-2. Infantile polycystic kidney disease. Excretory urogram in a young boy with large, palpable abdominal masses demonstrates renal enlargement with characteristic streaky densities leading to the calyceal tips. There is only minimal distortion of the calyces.

Fig GU10-1. Simple renal cyst. Nephrotomogram shows the smooth-walled, fluid-filled mass (arrows).

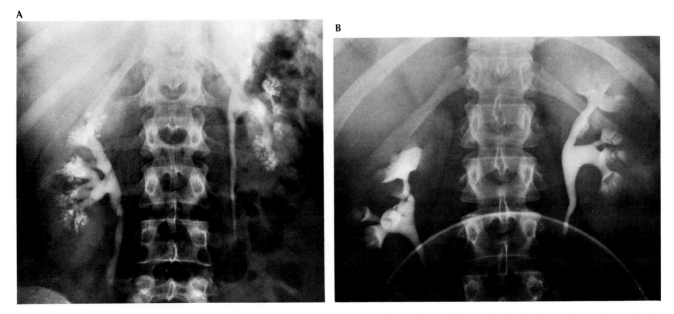

Fig GU10-3. Medullary sponge kidney. (A) Excretory urogram demonstrates multiple small, smoothly rounded calculi occurring in clusters in the papillary tips of multiple renal pyramids. (B) In another patient, the ectatic tubules appear as fine linear striations of contrast producing the characteristic brush border pattern.

Condition	Imaging Findings	Comments
Multicystic dysplastic kidney (Fig GU10-4)	Unilateral, multilobulated, nonfunctioning mass in the area normally occupied by the kidney. There may be thin curvilinear calcification outlining cyst walls. The vascularized walls of individual cysts may become slightly opaque during urography to produce the cluster-of-grapes sign (round lucent cysts separated from each other by slightly opacified septa). Usually there is compensatory hypertrophy of the contralateral kidney.	Nonhereditary congenital dysplasia (usually asymptomatic) in which the kidney is composed almost entirely of large thin-walled cysts with little solid renal tissue. Most common cause of an abdominal mass in the newborn. Other manifestations include an atretic ureter with a blind proximal end (on retrograde pyelography) and an absent or severely atretic renal artery. Ultrasound can differentiate the disorganized pattern of cysts and lack of renal parenchyma and reniform contour in multicystic kidney disease from the precise organization of symmetrically positioned fluid-filled spaces in hydronephrosis.
Calyceal cyst or diverticulum (pyelogenic cyst)	Sharply defined, often spherical cystic space. Delayed urographic opacification occurs by retrograde filling through a narrow channel that typically arises from a calyceal fornix.	Possible causes include a parenchymal cyst draining into a calyx, a ruptured cortical abscess, and dilatation of a renal tubule or the blind end of a branching wolffian duct.
Medullary cystic disease (Fig GU10-5)	Normal or small kidneys with smooth contours and impaired excretion of contrast material. A large medullary cyst may produce a sharply defined radiolucent defect on a nephrotomogram (best seen on CT). The cysts are usually too small to cause pelvocalyceal displacement or lobulation of the renal contours.	Hereditary nephropathy consisting of a variable number of cysts (often very small) in the corticomedullary junction and medulla. More often involves females. Clinical findings include anemia, polyuria, hyposthenuria, and salt wasting. No hypertension.
Multilocular cyst	Unifocal mass that is usually in a polar location. Sharply defined lucent nephrographic defect. Calcification and faint septa may be detected. Often displacement of the pelvocalyceal system.	Uncommon unilateral mass composed of multiple cysts of various sizes and adjoining primitive cellular elements. May be detected as a palpable mass in infants. Represents either a form of congenital cystic dysplasia or a benign renal neoplasm. Differs from multicystic (dysgenetic) kidney in that a multilocular cyst is unilateral, involves only a segment of an otherwise normal kidney, and has no associated abnormality of the ureter or renal artery.
Perinephric cyst (pararenal pseudocyst, urinoma)	Elliptical soft-tissue mass in the flank with upward and lateral displacement of the lower pole of the kidney, medial displacement of the ureter, and often obstructive hydronephrosis. Usually reduced or absent excretion of contrast material. Infrequently, evidence of extravasation into the mass.	Most cases result from accidents, operative trauma, or renal transplantation. In infants and children, congenital obstruction of the urinary tract may be a factor. Most common clinical finding is a palpable flank mass (usually a normal urinalysis and no fever).
Acquired cystic kidney disease	Bilateral large kidneys with multilobulated contours and no renal function. Requires ultrasound or CT for detection.	The development of multiple cysts occurs in the chronically failed kidneys of patients undergoing long-term hemodialysis. The degree of enlargement may approach that of adult polycystic kidney disease. The process may reverse after successful renal transplantation.

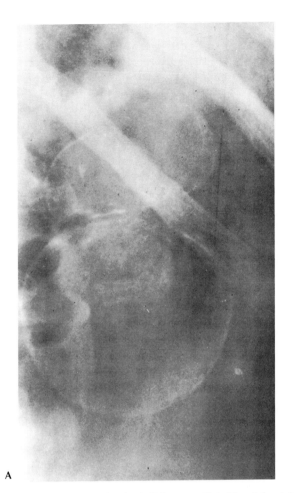

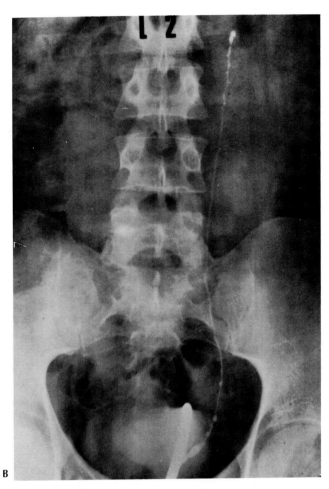

A

B

FIG GU10-4. Multicystic dysplastic kidney. (A) Plain film of the abdomen demonstrates multiple thin, curvilinear calcifications outlining the cysts. (B) Retrograde pyelogram shows atresia of the proximal ureter.[9]

Condition	Imaging Findings	Comments
Echinococcal cyst	Thick-walled cyst with nonhomogeneous lucency. Often produces narrowing or even obstruction of an adjacent calyx. There may be a permanent or intermittent communication between the cyst and the calyceal system.	Usually a solitary cyst, predominantly in the polar region, that may have a calcified wall. Communication with the collecting system almost always occurs through the calyx rather than directly to the pelvis.
Congenital cortical cystic disease	Kidneys usually appear normal. A large cortical cyst may cause a focal contour bulge or calyceal distortion.	In young infants with congenital heart disease and the trisomy syndromes, numerous small cysts may occur along the capsular surface and outline fetal fissures (no functional or clinical abnormality). In tuberous sclerosis the cysts are of tubular origin and severe involvement may lead to hypertension and renal failure.
Cystic dysplasia (associated with lower urinary tract obstruction)	Rarely detected on excretory urography (accompanying hydronephrosis obscures evidence of the multiple cortical cysts).	Rarely recognized as a clinical entity but relatively common on pathologic examination of the kidneys in children with lower urinary tract obstruction in fetal life (especially boys with congenital urethral valves). The increased pressure presumably results in malformation of the renal parenchyma and the development of numerous cortical cysts, especially beneath the capsule. Mild involvement is apparently compatible with a normal life span.

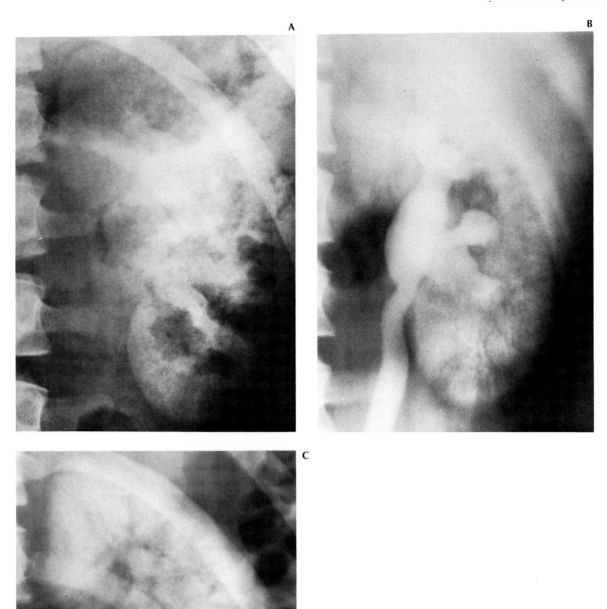

FIG GU10-5. Medullary cystic disease. (A) A 4-minute radiograph from an excretory urogram shows a normal-sized kidney with a smooth margin, delayed contrast excretion, and a poor but homogeneous nephrogram over the entire kidney. (B) Tomogram taken at 10 minutes shows opacification of the collecting system with mild blunting of the calyces. The nephrogram is composed of many streaky collections of contrast material radiating from the calyces to the periphery. (C) Radiograph taken at 120 minutes shows a high-density nephrogram confined to the medulla. This is probably caused by accumulation of contrast material in dilated tubules. The cortex and the columns of Bertin are recognizable as radiolucent areas.[10]

DEPRESSION OR SCAR IN THE RENAL MARGIN

Condition	Imaging Findings	Comments
Fetal lobulation	Slight notching of the renal contour that is located between normal calyces. May be multifocal or bilateral.	Common normal variant. The notches represent points at which the centrilobar cortex of one lobe abuts that of an adjacent lobe.
Splenic impression	Flattening of the upper lateral margin of the left kidney.	The impression on the renal contour is probably made by the spleen during development of the left kidney. There is often an associated bulge lower on the lateral margin of the kidney (dromedary hump).
Renal infarction (Fig GU11-1; see Fig GU3-2)	Wide-based cortical depression with normal underlying papilla and calyx. May be multifocal or bilateral.	Usually caused by cardiac embolism (mitral stenosis and atrial fibrillation, infective endocarditis, or mural thrombus overlying a myocardial infarct).
Chronic atrophic pyelonephritis (Fig GU11-2; see Fig GU3-1)	Cortical depression overlying a retracted papilla whose calyx is secondarily smoothly dilated. May be bilateral (but usually is asymmetric).	Related to chronic pyelonephritis and vesicoureteral reflux. Cortical depressions must be differentiated from fetal lobulation (which occurs between calyces rather than directly overlying them).
Tuberculosis (see Fig GU3-3)	Single or multiple cortical depressions that may give the renal surface an irregular appearance.	May produce a pattern indistinguishable from that of chronic atrophic pyelonephritis.

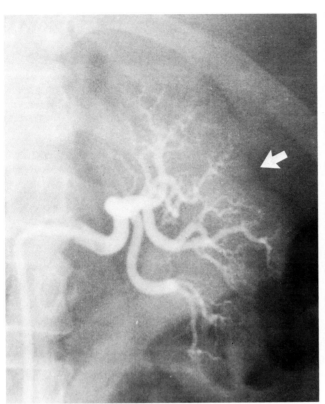

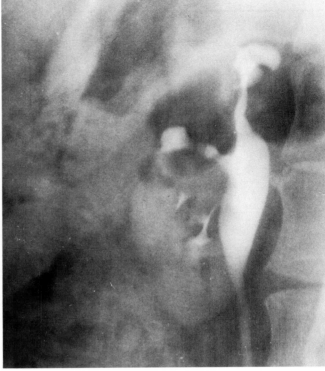

FIG GU11-1. Renal infarction. Selective left renal arteriogram shows a wide-based cortical depression (arrow) reflecting an infarct scar. Note the tortuosity and rapid tapering of interlobar arteries and their branches that is characteristic of arteriolar nephrosclerosis.

FIG GU11-2. Chronic pyelonephritis. Focal areas of parenchymal loss and calyceal clubbing in the upper pole of the right kidney.[11]

PERSISTENT OR INCREASINGLY DENSE NEPHROGRAM

Condition	Imaging Findings	Comments
Acute extrarenal obstruction (Fig GU12-1)	Unilateral (rarely bilateral) increasingly dense nephrogram that may have striations. Delayed and decreased excretion of contrast material into a dilated (hydronephrotic) collecting system.	Most common cause of an increasingly dense nephrogram. Usually due to a ureteral calculus or blood clot and associated with symptoms of ureteral colic.
Renal ischemia (see Fig GU13-3)	Unilateral increasingly dense nephrogram. Delayed and decreased excretion of contrast material, decreased kidney size, and often notching of the ipsilateral proximal ureter.	Severe stenosis of the main renal artery causes diminished renal perfusion pressure and the development of arterial collaterals.
Hypotension/shock	Bilateral increasingly dense nephrograms. Decreased or absent excretion of contrast material.	Diminished perfusion pressure of both kidneys. Once normal blood pressure is restored, there is rapid pelvocalyceal opacification and a return to normal nephrographic density. Most commonly an adverse reaction to contrast material during urography (kidney size decreased compared to scout film).
Acute tubular necrosis	Bilateral immediate and persistent dense nephrograms (may be increasingly dense). Decreased or absent excretion of contrast material.	Causes include severe ischemia (shock, crush injuries, burns, transfusion reactions) and exposure to toxic agents (carbon tetrachloride, ethylene glycol, mercury, bismuth, arsenic). An uncommon cause is contrast material nephrotoxicity (dose-related and potentiated by pre-existing dehydration, low-flow states, and chronic renal disease, especially diabetic nephropathy).
Acute tubular blockage	Bilateral increasingly dense or persistent dense nephrograms. Decreased excretion of contrast material into nondilated collecting systems.	Causes include multiple myeloma, urate nephropathy, amyloidosis, hemo- or myoglobulinuria, sulfonamide therapy, and massive precipitation of Tamm-Horsfall protein (may be a complication of contrast material given to severely dehydrated infants and children).
Acute bacterial nephritis (severe pyelonephritis) (Fig GU12-2)	Unilateral immediate and persistent dense nephrogram. Minimal or absent excretion of contrast material.	Most often seen with acute suppurative pyelonephritis, especially in patients with diabetes mellitus.
Acute glomerulonephritis (Fig GU12-3)	Bilateral increasingly dense nephrograms.	Probably reflects reduced glomerular perfusion due to obliterative changes in the renal microvasculature.
Acute renal vein thrombosis (Fig GU12-4)	Unilateral increasingly dense nephrogram. Decreased or absent excretion of contrast material.	Most frequently occurs in children who are severely dehydrated. In adults, generally a complication of another renal disease (chronic glomerulonephritis, amyloidosis, pyelonephritis), trauma, extension of thrombus from the inferior vena cava, and direct invasion or extrinsic pressure secondary to a renal tumor.
Acute papillary necrosis (see Fig GU15-1)	Increasingly dense nephrogram. Characteristic central or eccentric cavitation of papillae or complete sloughing of papillary tips (may calcify).	Unusual presentation due to tubular obstruction by necrotic papillary tips. Underlying causes include analgesic abuse (especially phenacetin), sickle cell anemia, diabetes, and pyelonephritis.

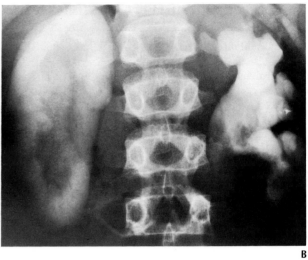

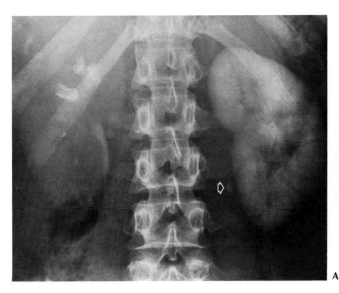

FIG GU12-1. **Acute urinary tract obstruction.** (A) Excretory urogram demonstrates a prolonged nephrogram on the left with fine cortical striations (alternating radiolucent and radiopaque lines) and no calyceal filling. An arrow points to the obstructing stone in the proximal left ureter. (B) In another patient, there is a prolonged and intensified obstructive nephrogram of the right kidney. On the left, there is marked dilatation of the pelvocalyceal system but no persistent nephrogram, reflecting an intermittent chronic obstruction on this side.

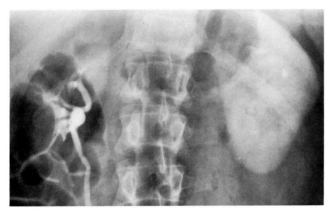

FIG GU12-2. **Acute bacterial nephritis.** Persistent dense nephrogram on the left with minimal opacification of the collecting system.

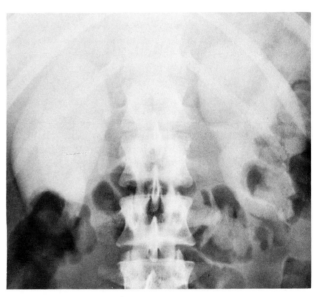

FIG GU12-3. **Acute renal failure.** Film from an excretory urogram 20 minutes after the injection of contrast material shows bilateral persistent nephrograms with no calyceal filling.

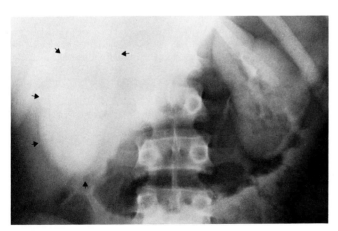

FIG GU12-4. **Acute renal vein thrombosis.** Film of the right kidney taken 5 minutes after the injection of contrast material shows a dense nephrogram and the absence of calyceal filling.

DIMINISHED CONCENTRATION OF CONTRAST MATERIAL
IN THE PELVOCALYCEAL SYSTEM

Condition	Comments
Bilateral	
Overhydration/ inadequate dehydration	Causes dilution of the contrast material (the kidneys may be entirely normal).
Polyuria	Excretion of large volumes of hypotonic urine due to diuretic therapy, diabetes insipidus (lack of anti-diuretic hormone secreted by the posterior lobe of the pituitary gland), diabetes mellitus, and intrinsic renal diseases.
Renal failure (uremia) (Fig GU13-1)	Severely decreased renal function due to a variety of underlying causes.
Nephrosclerosis (Fig GU13-2)	Long-standing hypertension causes narrowing of extra- and intrarenal arteries with prolonged intrarenal circulation time and decreased excretion of contrast material.
Technical	Injection of an inadequate dose of contrast material.
Unilateral	
Urinary tract obstruction	Elevated pressure in the dilated collecting system causes diminished filtration of contrast material. Delayed parenchymal opacification compared with the nonobstructed kidney, with the nephrogram eventually becoming more dense than normal because of a decreased rate of flow through the tubules (enhanced water resorption by the nephrons and greater concentration of the contrast material).
Renal parenchymal infection	Most commonly due to tuberculosis (obstruction of the pelvocalyceal system or ureter, autonephrectomy, or severe narrowing of the renal artery).
Trauma	Spasm of the pelvocalyceal system. Decreased renal function may result in failure to detect extravasation of poorly opacified urine.
Renal artery stenosis involving opposite kidney (Fig GU13-3)	On rapid-sequence studies, the affected kidney demonstrates delayed appearance and excretion of contrast material. Eventually, increased water reabsorption produces an increased concentration of contrast material on the affected side, making the normal side appear to have diminished concentration.

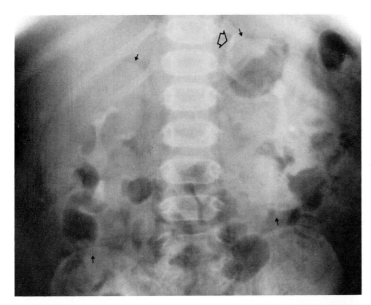

FIG GU13-1. Nephrotic syndrome causing renal failure. Excretory urogram demonstrates striking enlargement of both kidneys. (Arrows point to the tips of the upper and lower poles of the kidneys.) There is decreased opacification of both collecting systems. Of incidental note is calcification in the left adrenal gland (open arrow).

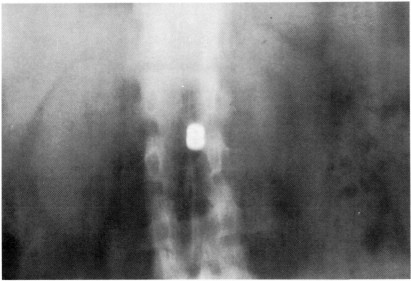

FIG GU13-2. Malignant nephrosclerosis. Nephrotomogram obtained 5 minutes after the injection of contrast material shows minimum opacification of small smooth kidneys.[4]

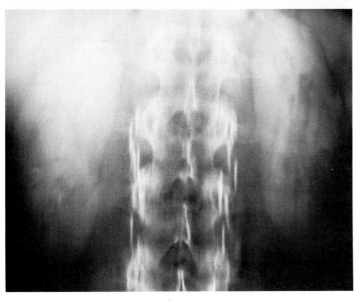

FIG GU13-3. Renovascular hypertension. A film from a rapid-sequence urogram obtained 3 minutes after the injection of contrast material shows no calyceal opacification on the left in a patient with left renal artery stenosis.

SOLITARY OR MULTIPLE FILLING DEFECTS IN THE PELVOCALYCEAL SYSTEM

Condition	Imaging Findings	Comments
Calculus (Figs GU14-1 and GU14-2)	Round or oval, frequently mobile filling defect. Often multiple and bilateral. A large calculus may form a cast of the pelvocalyceal system (staghorn calculus). If the obstruction is acute, the increased intrapelvic pressure may permit little or no glomerular filtration and produce the radiographic appearance of a delayed but prolonged nephrogram and the lack of calyceal filling on the affected side.	More than 80% of renal calculi are radiopaque and detectable on plain abdominal radiographs. These typically develop secondary to hyperparathyroidism, renal tubular acidosis, hyperoxaluria, or any cause of increased calcium excretion in the urine (20% are idiopathic). Radiodense calcium stones are often invisible in the midst of opaque urine. Completely lucent calculi are composed of uric acid or urates, xanthine, or matrix concentrations. Struvite (magnesium ammonium phosphate) stones are moderately radiopaque with variable internal density (found mainly in women with chronic urinary tract infection). Cystine calculi are mildly opaque.
Blood clot (Fig GU14-3)	Single or multiple nonopaque filling defects. Asymptomatic unless it causes pelvocalyceal obstruction. Usually becomes significantly smaller or disappears within 2 weeks (though rarely a residual fibrin mass that may eventually calcify).	Causes of urinary tract bleeding include trauma, tumor, instrumentation, nephritis and vasculitis, rupture of arterial aneurysm, vascular malformation, bleeding disorder, and anticoagulant therapy.
Air	Single or multiple, round, freely movable filling defects that are not associated with any signs of obstruction. Must be differentiated from superimposed intestinal gas that projects at least partially outside the urinary tract in different positions or on subsequent films.	Causes include instrumentation (retrograde pyelogram), trauma, surgery, ureterointestinal anastomosis, and vesicovaginal fistula. Rarely a manifestation of emphysematous pyelonephritis in diabetics (also gas in the renal parenchyma and perirenal soft tissues).
Transitional cell carcinoma (Figs GU14-4 and GU14-5)	Single or multiple, smooth or irregular filling defect. Characteristic stippled pattern reflects trapping of small amounts of contrast material in the interstices of papillary tumor fronds. May develop stippled calcific deposits visible on CT. A wide area of superficial spreading occasionally causes an irregular mucosal pattern and thickening of the pelvocalyceal wall.	Usually occurs in patients 50 to 70 years of age and presents with hematuria and pain. The tumor is infrequently palpable (unless it causes chronic obstruction and pronounced hydronephrosis). Primary squamous cell carcinoma and sarcomas rarely cause pelvocalyceal filling defects.
Benign tumor	Single or multiple filling defects.	Mesenchymal tumor; papilloma; hemangioma; fibrous ureteral polyp.
Sloughed papilla (Fig GU14-6)	Triangular lucent filling defect with the remaining calyx having a round, saccular, or club-shaped configuration. A sloughed papilla may stay in place and become calcified (typically ring-shaped with a lucent center) or pass down the ureter (simulating a stone and even causing obstruction).	Usually develops in a patient with renal papillary necrosis due to analgesic abuse (less frequently secondary to severe urinary tract infection, obstruction, or acute bacterial nephritis).

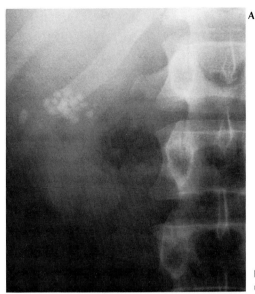

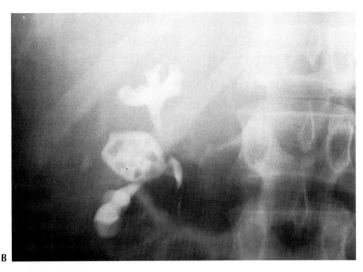

FIG GU14-1. Cystine stones. (A) Plain film shows multiple radiopaque calculi. (B) Excretory urogram demonstrates the stones as lucent filling defects in the opacified renal pelvis.

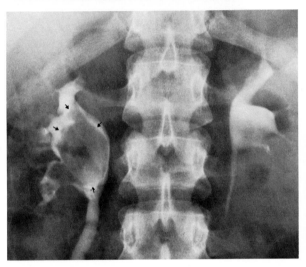

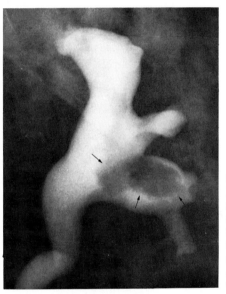

FIG GU14-2. Xanthinuria. A large lucent stone (arrows) almost fills the right pelvocalyceal system.

FIG GU14-3. Blood clot. Large filling defect with a smooth contour (arrows). A CT scan showed the attenuation value of the blood clot to be 62 H, a density higher than that of transitional cell carcinoma but lower than that of a nonopaque stone.[12]

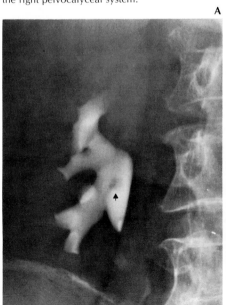

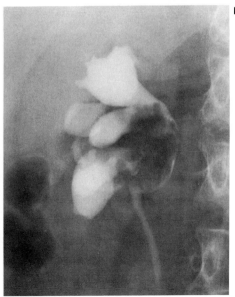

FIG GU14-4. Transitional cell carcinoma of the renal pelvis in two patients. (A) A small filling defect (arrow) in the renal pelvis simulates a blood clot, stone, fungus ball, or sloughed papilla. (B) A huge mass fills virtually all the renal pelvis.

Condition	Imaging Findings	Comments
Fungus ball (mycetoma) (Fig GU14-7)	Single or multiple, large, nonopaque mass that often fills the renal pelvis and may cause obstruction. Contrast material may fill the interstices to produce a lacelike radiodense pattern.	Most mycetomas are caused by *Candida albicans*. *Aspergillus* is the second most common organism. Usually there is involvement of the renal parenchyma (hematogenous dissemination) with the fungus ball forming from mycelia shed into the pelvis.
Cholesteatoma	Single round mass or multiple stringy filling defects with indistinct margins. Contrast material extends into concentric laminations to produce an onion skin pattern of alternating density and lucency.	Unusual form of tissue slough resulting from keratinizing squamous metaplasia of the uroepithelium. Generally associated with chronic infection and impaired urinary drainage. About half the patients have calculi.
Aberrant papilla	Oval or round filling defect in a major infundibulum without any signs of obstruction.	Papilla without a calyx. Must be differentiated from a normal calyx seen end-on (which appears normal when viewed in profile on other projections).
Inspissated pus/ necrotic debris	Irregular filling defect.	Pyelonephritis of suppurative, xanthogranulomatous, or tuberculous origin. There may also be mucosal ulceration, irregularity, and scarring from the infectious process.
Pyelitis cystica (see Fig GU17-6)	Multiple small, sharply defined, unchanging filling defects in the pelvocalyceal system.	Multiple small cysts in the pelvic wall that typically develop in older women with chronic urinary tract infection.
Acute pyelonephritis (Fig GU14-8)	Linear striations in the renal pelvis (and proximal ureter).	Probably reflects acute mucosal edema.
Leukoplakia	Localized or generalized irregularity of the pelvocalyceal wall.	Squamous metaplasia of transitional cells that develops in patients with a history of chronic infection. Unlike cholesteatoma, leukoplakia is smaller and is frequently associated with carcinoma. Coexisting calculi occur in about 50% of patients.
Blood vessels/vascular malformation	Varying pattern of single or multiple, intraluminal or extrinsic filling defects.	Normal renal artery or major branch (solitary, extrinsic defect); arterial collaterals (multiple small marginal defects, especially in the proximal ureter); aneurysm or arteriovenous fistula; renal vein thrombosis; venous collaterals.
Extrinsic compression (see GU16)	Generalized narrowing of part or all of the pelvocalyceal system.	Peripelvic or parenchymal cyst impinging on the renal pelvis; renal sinus lipomatosis.

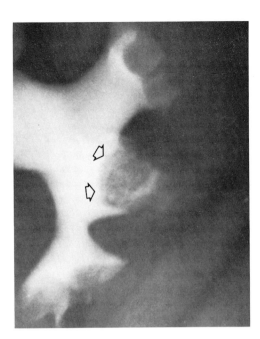

Fig GU14-5. Transitional cell carcinoma of the renal pelvis. A small filling defect occupies an interpolar calyx (arrows). Although the defect might at first be mistaken for a large but otherwise normal papilla, the many small contrast stipples and the suggestively irregular border make its neoplastic nature evident.[13]

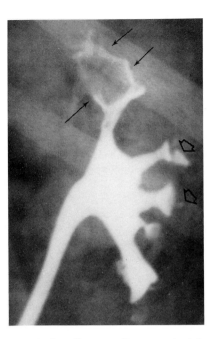

Fig GU14-6. Sloughed papillae in papillary necrosis. A ring of contrast material (long arrows) surrounds a triangular lucent filling defect, which represents an almost complete papilla that has been separated from the rest of the renal parenchyma. The short arrows point to less severe extension of contrast material from the calyces into the papillae.[6]

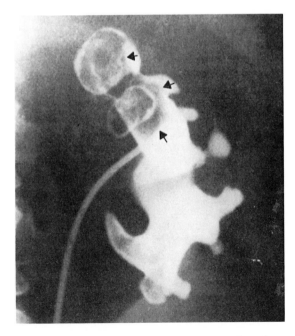

Fig GU14-7. Fungus ball in renal candidiasis. Retrograde pyelogram demonstrates a large filling defect (arrows) in the left renal pelvis.[14]

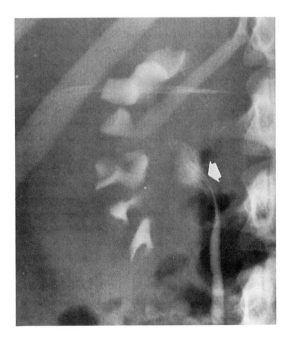

Fig GU14-8. Acute pyelonephritis. Linear striations (arrow) in the right renal pelvis.

CLUBBING OR DESTRUCTION OF RENAL CALYCES

Condition	Imaging Findings	Comments
Papillary necrosis **(Figs GU15-1 and GU15-2)**	Cavitation of the central portion of the papilla or complete sloughing of the papillary tip. The cavitation may be central or eccentric with its long axis paralleling that of the papilla. The cavity varies from long and thin to short and bulbous and the margins may be sharp or irregular. With sloughing, the remaining calyx has a round, saccular, or club-shaped configuration and there is a ring of contrast material surrounding the triangular lucent filling defect that represents the sloughed necrotic tissue (which may calcify or pass down the ureter).	Ischemic coagulative necrosis involving various amounts of the medullary papillae and pyramids. Most often occurs in patients with diabetes, pyelonephritis, urinary tract infection or obstruction, sickle cell disease, or phenacetin abuse. The earliest radiographic sign (often overlooked on excretory urography) is a cleavage plane that develops in a zone of ischemia and communicates with the calyx, producing a faint streak of contrast material oriented parallel to the long axis of the papilla and usually extending from the fornix (also can arise in the papillary tip).
Tuberculosis **(Fig GU15-3)**	Initially, irregularity of one or several papillae or calyces (indistinguishable from papillary necrosis from other causes). Progressive destruction produces large irregular cavities. Fibrosis and stricture formation in the pelvocalyceal system cause narrowing or obstruction of the infundibulum to the affected calyx.	Other characteristic radiographic manifestations in the advanced stage of hematogenously spread tuberculosis include cortical scarring and parenchymal atrophy (simulating chronic bacterial pyelonephritis); focal intrarenal masses mimicking neoplasms (tuberculous granulomas that do not communicate with the collecting system); a densely calcified, nonfunctioning shrunken kidney (autonephrectomy); and ureteral changes (corkscrew and pipe stem ureter).
Chronic pyelonephritis **(Fig GU15-4)**	Clubbed, dilated calyces are caused by retraction of papillae and most frequently involve the poles. Depressed cortical scars typically develop over involved calyces.	May be unifocal or multifocal, unilateral or bilateral (but usually asymmetric). End stage of vesicoureteral reflux and recurrent urinary tract infection in childhood.
Hydronephrosis **(Fig GU15-5)**	Dilatation of the entire pelvocalyceal system. The kidneys may be small and smooth (postobstructive renal atrophy).	Most commonly the result of one prolonged or several intermittent episodes of obstruction. Nonobstructive hydronephrosis may be due to reflux, bacterial endotoxins, pregnancy, or nephrogenic diabetes insipidus.
Localized caliectasis **(Fig GU15-6)**	Calyceal dilatation due to the obstruction of an infundibulum.	Causes include neoplasm (renal cell or transitional cell carcinoma), tuberculosis, inflammatory stricture, calculus, and anomalous vessel.
Congenital megacalyces	Dilated calyces that often have a polygonal or faceted appearance. The renal cortex and kidney size are normal. Bilateral in about 20% of cases.	Congenital nonobstructive enlargement of calyces due to malformations of the renal papillae that are probably secondary to temporary intrauterine obstruction.
Medullary sponge kidney **(tubular ectasia)** **(Fig GU15-7)**	Broadening, increased cupping, and distortion of calyces. The ectatic tubules appear as fine linear striations of contrast producing a brush border pattern. With increasing dilatation, the tubules become more cystic and simulate a cluster of grapes. Plain films often demonstrate multiple small, smoothly rounded calculi occurring in clusters or in a fanlike arrangement in the papillary tip of one or more renal pyramids.	Cystic dilatation of distal collecting tubules in the renal pyramids. The ectatic changes may be limited to a single pyramid, but are usually more extensive and bilateral (though often asymmetric). Although renal function is preserved, tubular stasis predisposes to calculus formation and pyelonephritis. Generally asymptomatic, except when medullary calculi become dislodged and produce renal colic or hematuria.

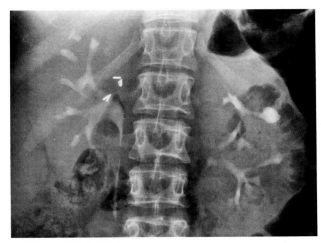

Fig GU15-1. **Papillary necrosis.** Generalized saccular or club-shaped configuration of both calyces bilaterally in a patient with sickle cell disease.

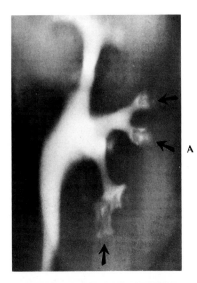

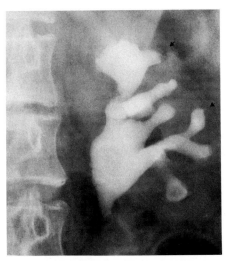

Fig GU15-3. **Chronic pyelonephritis.** Diffuse rounded clubbing of multiple calyces with atrophy and thinning of the overlying renal parenchyma. The arrows indicate the outer margin of the kidney.

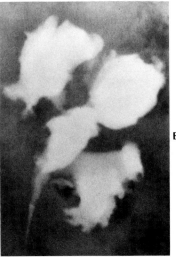

Fig GU15-2. **Stages of papillary destruction** by active tuberculosis. (A) Early. (B) Advanced.[3]

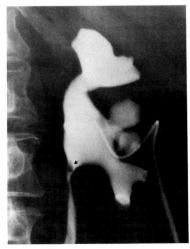

Fig GU15-4. **Hydronephrosis.** Dilatation of the entire pelvocalyceal system proximal to an obstructing cryptococcus fungus ball (arrow) at the ureteropelvic junction.

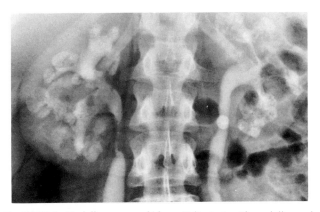

Fig GU15-5. **Medullary sponge kidney.** Caliectasis with medullary calculi throughout both kidneys.

EFFACED PELVOCALYCEAL SYSTEM

Condition	Imaging Findings	Comments
Extrinsic compression **Global enlargement of renal parenchyma**	Bilateral large smooth kidneys with effaced pelvocalyceal systems (see GU7).	Excessive renal bulk occurs with cellular infiltration or proliferation, deposition of abnormal proteins, or accumulation of interstitial edema or blood.
	Unilateral large smooth kidney with effaced pelvocalyceal system (see GU4).	Renal vein occlusion; acute arterial infarction; acute bacterial nephritis.
Renal sinus mass or masslike abnormality **Renal sinus lipomatosis** **(Fig GU16-1)**	Elongation and attenuation of the pelvocalyceal system caused by the accumulation of an excessive amount of fat-density material in the renal sinus (diagnosis easily confirmed on CT).	Often a normal variant in an obese person or a reflection of the loss of kidney parenchyma due to ischemia, infarction, or infection. May mimic single or multiple peripelvic masses.
Parapelvic cysts **(Fig GU16-2)**	Elongation and attenuation of the pelvocalyceal system by multiple or multiloculated water-density cysts.	Can be differentiated from renal sinus lipomatosis by ultrasound or CT. A single parapelvic cyst causes focal displacement and smooth effacement of the adjacent portion of the pelvocalyceal system.
Hemorrhage into renal sinus	Attenuation of the pelvocalyceal system with impaired excretion of contrast material.	Spontaneous hemorrhage into the renal sinus may be a self-limited complication of anticoagulant therapy.
Spasm/inflammation **Infection**	Generalized effacement of the pelvocalyceal system.	Acute pyelonephritis and acute bacterial nephritis (may result from spasm of smooth muscles of the collecting system wall, swelling of the kidney, or paralysis of smooth muscle due to bacterial endotoxins). Uroepithelial tuberculosis produces submucosal granulomas and mucosal ulcerations that render the collecting system nondistensible.
Hematuria	Generalized effacement of the pelvocalyceal system. The appearance reverts to normal as the bleeding ceases.	Upper urinary tract bleeding (from the kidney or directly from uroepithelial structures) irritates pelvocalyceal smooth muscles.
Infiltrating malignant uroepithelial tumor **(Figs GU16-3 and GU16-4)**	Generalized effacement of the pelvocalyceal system associated with a nodular mucosal pattern.	Most commonly a transitional cell carcinoma that grows superficially or infiltrates deeply over a large portion of the pelvocalyceal system.
Oliguria	Unilateral or bilateral collapse of the pelvocalyceal system.	Low-flow states such as water deprivation, renal ischemia, and oliguric renal failure.

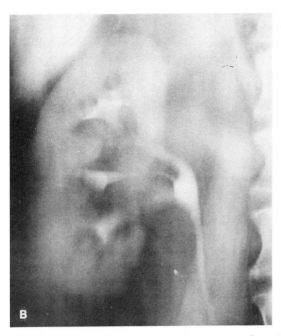

FIG GU16-1. Renal sinus lipomatosis. Nephrotomogram shows increased radiolucency (fat) around the renal sinuses and calyces causing stretching and elongation of the pelvocalyceal system.[6]

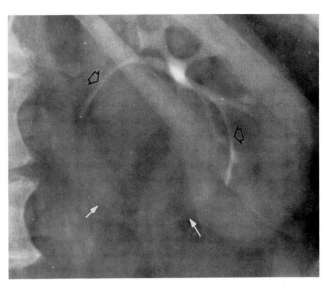

FIG GU16-2. Renal cyst. Smooth displacement of the attenuated lower pole calyces (open arrows). The solid arrows indicate the inferior extent of the cyst.

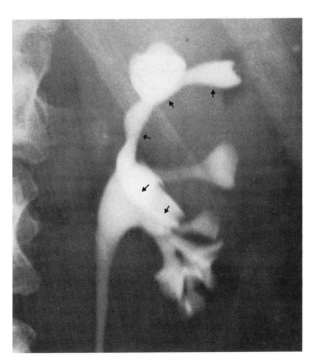

FIG GU16-3. Renal hamartoma. Large mass distorting and displacing the pelvocalyceal system (arrows).

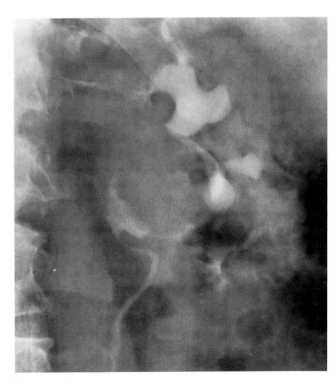

FIG GU16-4. Transitional cell carcinoma of the renal pelvis. A large mass distorts the pelvocalyceal system and causes deviation of the ureter.

FILLING DEFECTS IN THE URETER

Condition	Imaging Findings	Comments
Calculus (Fig GU17-1)	Round or oval filling defect that tends to become impacted in areas of normal anatomic narrowing (ureteropelvic and urtererovesical junctions and the site where the ureter crosses the sacrum and the iliac vessels).	Extremely common and clinically associated with hematuria and ureteral colic. About 80% of ureteral calculi are radiopaque.
Blood clot (Fig GU17-2)	Single or multiple nonopaque filling defects of various sizes and shapes that may cause temporary ureteral obstruction. They typically become much smaller or disappear within several weeks.	Causes of urinary tract bleeding include trauma, tumor, instrumentation, nephritis and vasculitis, rupture of an arterial aneurysm, vascular malformation, bleeding disorder, and anticoagulant therapy.
Air bubble	Single or multiple, round, freely movable filling defects that are not associated with any signs of obstruction.	Air bubbles are most commonly introduced into the ureter (and pelvocalyceal system) during a retrograde study. Other causes include trauma, surgery, infection, and fistula. Must be distinguished from superimposed intestinal gas, which projects at least partially outside the ureter in different positions or on subsequent films.
Blood vessels and vascular malformations (Fig GU17-3)	Various patterns of single or multiple extrinsic defects.	Normal renal artery or major branch (solitary); arterial or venous collaterals (multiple small marginal defects, especially in the proximal ureter, related to renal artery stenosis or renal vein thrombosis); ovarian vein syndrome (solitary compression of the right ureter at the S1 level after several pregnancies).
Transitional cell carcinoma (Figs GU17-4 and GU17-5)	Smooth or irregular shaggy filling defect. Characteristic stippled pattern represents the trapping of small amounts of contrast material in the interstices of papillary tumor fronds. Lesions that are predominantly infiltrating may produce short or long strictures.	Usually occurs in patients 50 to 70 years of age and presents with hematuria and pain. May reflect metastatic seeding from a more proximal lesion of the urogenital tract. There is often localized dilatation of the ureter below the level of the expanding intraluminal tumor, in contrast to ureteral collapse distal to an obstructing stone.
Ureteral polyp	Elongated, smoothly marginated filling defect that is generally located in the proximal ureter.	Usually occurs in patients 20 to 40 years of age. Intermittent pain is common, while hematuria and ureteral obstruction are rare.
Papilloma	Round, irregular, often multiple filling defects most commonly located in the lower ureter. Frequently causes ureteral obstruction.	Although histologically benign, papillomas often recur and therefore may be considered as low-grade malignancies. Associated tumors may occur in the bladder.
Mesenchymal tumor	Single small, smooth filling defect.	Fibroma; lipoma; hamartoma; hemangioma (bleeding tendency); fibroepithelial polyp (often multiple).

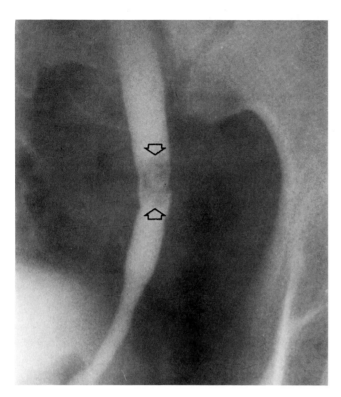

Fɪɢ GU17-1. **Nonopaque ureteral calculus** (arrows).

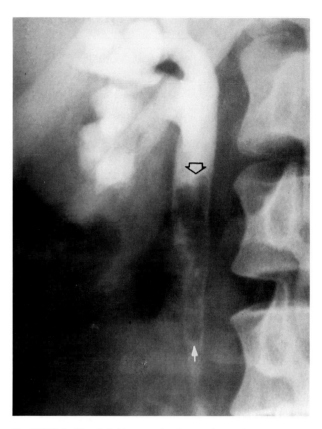

Fɪɢ GU17-2. **Blood clot** in a proximal ureter (arrows).

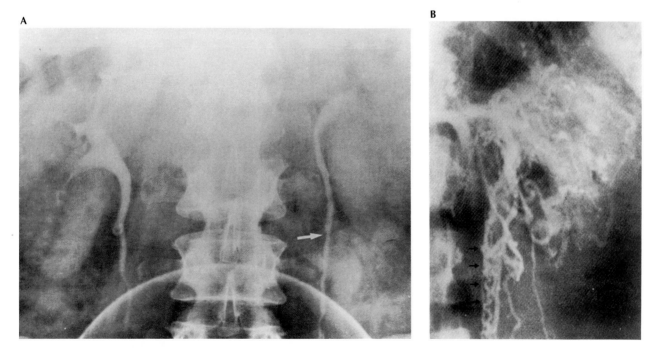

Fɪɢ GU17-3. **Renal vein thrombosis.** (A) Excretory urogram shows characteristic notching (arrow) of the upper ureter. There is enlargement of the left kidney with poor calyceal function due to compression from parenchymal engorgement. (B) In another patient with renal vein thrombosis and ureteral notching, a venogram demonstrates exuberant periureteral collaterals (arrows).[15]

Condition	Imaging Findings	Comments
Metastases	Irregular narrowing of the ureteral lumen. Extension of the lesion may produce an intraluminal mass.	Metastases to the ureter from distant sources are rare and generally a late event (other evidence of distant metastases is usually present). They may arise from almost any organ in the body but have been reported with slightly greater frequency from tumors of the prostate, stomach, breast, lung, and colon. Metastases may occur at any site along the ureter and frequently are seen in both ureters. Many malignant lesions, particularly the lymphomas, cause displacement of the ureters (due to retroperitoneal nodal metastases) without actual invasion.
Ureteritis cystica (Fig GU17-6)	Multiple small, smooth, rounded lucent filling defects that primarily involve one or both proximal ureters. There may also be involvement of the pelvocalyceal system and bladder.	Multiple inflammatory cysts that typically develop in older women, usually in association with chronic urinary tract infection. A single cyst may simulate a transitional cell tumor (but persists unchanged over many years).
Tuberculosis (Fig GU17-7)	Diffuse irregularity of the ureteral wall simulating multiple filling defects. As the disease heals there are usually multiple areas in which ureteral strictures alternate with dilated segments (beaded, or corkscrew, appearance).	Almost always tuberculous involvement of the kidney. In advanced disease, the ureter becomes thickened, fixed, and aperistaltic (pipe stem ureter). Often there is irregular calcification of the vas deferens and seminal vesicles.
Schistosomiasis (see Fig GI57-1)	Multiple filling defects in the distal ureter, almost always associated with a similar process in the bladder.	Usually caused by *Schistosoma hematobium*. Characteristic calcification of the bladder wall.
Malacoplakia (Fig GU17-8)	Smooth, single or multiple, round or oval filling defects that predominantly occur in the distal ureter. May produce a scalloped appearance and occasionally a stricture.	Uncommon chronic inflammatory disease that primarily affects women, most of whom have a history of recurrent or chronic urinary tract infection. Malacoplakia more frequently involves the bladder.
Sloughed papilla/ inspissated pus/ tissue debris	Irregular filling defect that may cause ureteral obstruction.	Papillary necrosis; necrotizing tumor; necrotizing pyelonephritis (especially in diabetics); pyonephrosis.
Endometriosis	Single or multiple filling defects in the distal ureter below the pelvic brim. May cause ureteral stricture or extrinsic ureteral compression.	Uncommon condition presenting with pain or cyclic urinary symptoms including hematuria in a woman in the childbearing years. Often a history of previous gynecologic or abdominal surgery.
Benign ureteral stricture	Usually a smooth, conical narrowing. If short and eccentric, may occasionally simulate an extrinsic defect.	May be congenital or secondary to trauma, surgery, instrumentation, stone passage, inflammation, or radiation therapy.

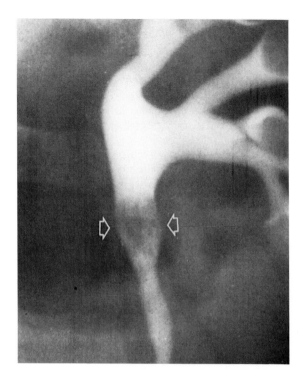

FIG GU17-4. Transitional cell carcinoma of the ureter. The presence of stippling throughout this proximal ureteral filling defect (arrows) and the suggestive papillary contour of its proximal and distal margins allow the correct diagnosis to be made preoperatively.[13]

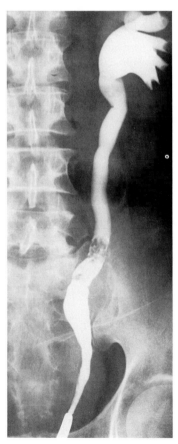

FIG GU17-5. Transitional cell carcinoma of the midureter. Irregular stricture (arrow) with proximal ureteral and pelvocalyceal dilatation.

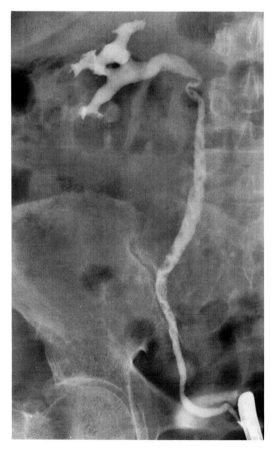

FIG GU17-6. Ureteritis cystica. Multiple small, smooth lucent filling defects in the contrast-filled ureter and pelvis in a patient with chronic urinary tract infection.

Condition	Imaging Findings	Comments
Compression or invasion from adjacent malignancy or nodes	Extrinsic defect that may be smooth or irregular.	Direct extension of retroperitoneal or pelvic malignancy or extrinsic compression by enlarged lymph nodes.
Ureteral diverticulum	Localized extrinsic compression by a cystic lesion that causes slightly delayed opacification.	Very rare solitary (occasionally multiple) outpouching along the course of the ureter. An enlarged diverticulum due to infection, stone formation, or obstruction may make an extrinsic impression on the adjacent ureter.
Ureteral spasm and peristalsis	May simulate a localized filling defect or vascular notching.	Transitory appearance, unlike a true ureteral filling defect.

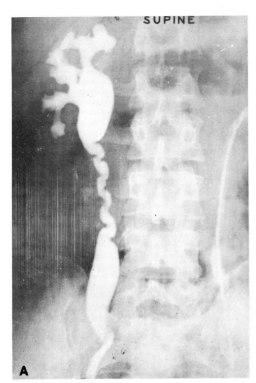

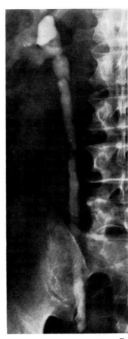

A

Fig GU17-7. Ureteral tuberculosis. (A) Segmental areas of dilatation and constriction produce a corkscrew, or beaded, pattern.[6] (B) Thickening and fixation of the ureter (pipe stem ureter).[16]

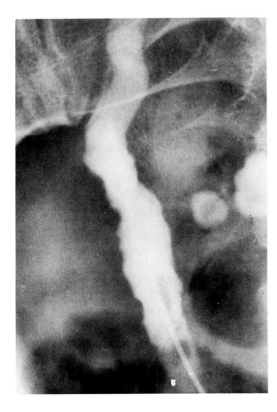

Fig GU17-8. Malacoplakia of the ureter. Magnified view of the distal right ureter shows multiple filling defects simulating ureteritis cystica.[17]

OBSTRUCTION OF THE URETER

Condition	Imaging Findings	Comments
Calculus **(Fig GU18-1)**	About 80% are radiopaque enough to be seen on plain films. Often oval with its long axis paralleling the course of the ureter. A calculus most commonly lodges in the lower portion of the ureter, especially at the ureterovesical junction and the pelvic brim. A nonopaque ureteral calculus appears as a lucent filling defect on excretory urography (retrograde pyelography may be necessary to demonstrate a ureteral calculus if renal function is insufficient).	Ureteral calculi are extremely common and their detection is clinically important. An obstructing distal calculus must be differentiated from far more common phleboliths, which are spherical and located in the lateral portion of the pelvis below a line joining the ischial spines (ureteral calculi are situated medially above the interspinous line). Calculi produce characteristic posterior shadowing on ultrasound and high attenuation values on CT.

Stricture
  Congenital ureteropelvic
  junction (UPJ)
  obstruction
  (Fig GU18-2)
	Sharply defined UPJ narrowing with dilatation of the pelvocalyceal system that persists even when the patient is placed in a position favoring gravity drainage of the pelvis. Late manifestations of long-standing UPJ obstruction include wasting of kidney substance, diminished parenchymal and pelvocalyceal opacification, and the "rim" sign (nephrogram of remaining renal parenchyma rimming the dilated calyces).	May be caused by an intrinsic stenosis of the ureter or by extrinsic compression of the UPJ by a crossing blood vessel or fibrous band. Most patients have no demonstrable anatomic abnormality and the decreased urine flow through the UPJ is secondary to abnormal muscle development, inadequate distensibility, or a deficiency of transmitter substance at nerve endings. UPJ obstruction is especially common in patients with horseshoe and incompletely rotated kidneys. Characteristic kinks, angulations, and "high insertions" of the ureter are most likely the result rather than the cause of pelvic distension.

Tuberculosis	Healing produces multiple areas of ureteral stricture alternating with dilated segments to produce a beaded, or corkscrew, appearance. In advanced disease, the wall of the ureter becomes thickened and fixed with no peristalsis (pipe stem ureter) and a straight course to the bladder.	Ureteral obstruction is a late manifestation, which is almost always associated with renal tuberculosis. There is often a contracted bladder with a thickened wall. Calcification of the ureter and bladder is infrequent.
Schistosomiasis **(see Fig GI57-1)**	Stricture, aperistalsis, and calcification (usually linear) of the distal ureter.	Almost always associated with dense calcification of the bladder wall.
Postsurgery/ **instrumentation** **(Fig GU18-3)**	Localized narrowing of the ureter.	Causes include accidental ligation of the ureter, edema of the ureteral wall, and instrumental perforation (most heal rapidly and without sequelae if less than 50% of the ureteral circumference is involved and there is no distal obstruction). Postsurgical abscess, hematoma, or urinoma may cause diffuse narrowing and displacement of the ureter by extrinsic compression.
Radiation therapy	Ureteral narrowing that gradually develops several months to years after treatment. Most commonly occurs just above the ureterovesical junction after pelvic irradiation (eg, for uterine carcinoma).	Most commonly occurs if the ureter was originally involved with malignancy. A radiation-induced stricture may be impossible to differentiate from tumor recurrence.

(continued page 500)

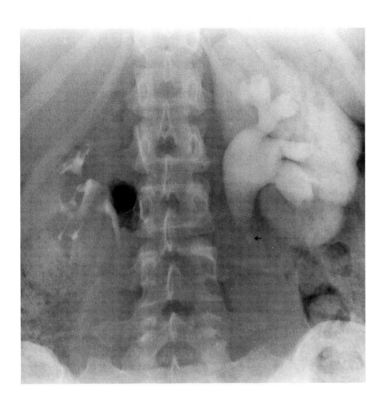

FIG GU18-1. **Obstructing ureteral calculus.** Excretory urogram demonstrates a prolonged nephrogram and marked dilatation of the collecting system and pelvis proximal to the obstructing stone (arrow).

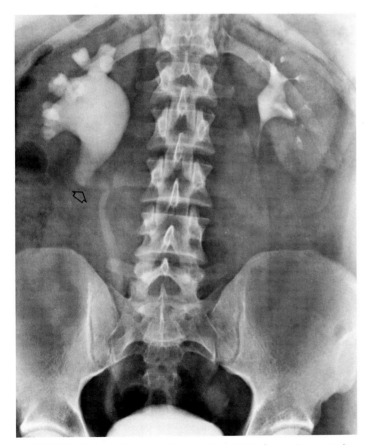

FIG GU18-2. **Congenital ureteropelvic junction (UPJ) obstruction.** Note the characteristic kink or angulation at the UPJ (arrow).

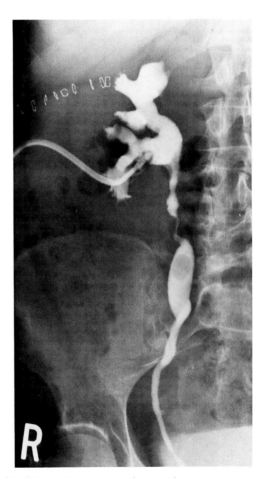

FIG GU18-3. **Postsurgery stricture.** Fibrotic narrowing of the proximal ureter secondary to stone removal.

Condition	Imaging Findings	Comments
Posttraumatic	During surgery, one or both ureters may be sectioned, causing nonfunction of the involved kidney or formation of a local abscess.	Cutting or ligating the ureters usually produces prompt symptoms, and the presence of anuria for 8 to 10 hours after major pelvic surgery should suggest the possibility of bilateral ureteral injury. Kinking, crushing, or clamping of the vascular supply to the ureters may not produce evidence of injury until several weeks after surgery, when necrosis of the ureteral wall may occur leading to fistulization. Unilateral injury that does not produce anuria may not be recognized. External trauma rarely injures the ureters, since they lie deep in the retroperitoneal area adjacent to the lumbar spine and are well protected throughout their course.
Adjacent inflammatory disease	Extrinsic narrowing and displacement of one or both ureters (most often the pelvic portion).	Causes include diverticulitis, Crohn's disease, appendiceal abscess, and postoperative abscess.
Invasion or compression by extrinsic malignancy **Retroperitoneal tumor**	Extrinsic compression, encasement, or invasion causing often irregular narrowing of the proximal ureter. The affected ureter is usually displaced laterally (rarely medially).	Most frequently lymphoma or metastases (pancreas, melanoma, colon). Primary retroperitoneal tumors (eg, liposarcoma) are much less common.
Pelvic tumor **(Fig GU18-4)**	Extrinsic narrowing and often irregularity of the distal ureter. The ureter is typically straightened or displaced medially.	Causes include carcinoma of the cervix or other pelvic organ (direct extension or lymph node metastases) and pelvic lymphoma.
Bladder carcinoma	Unilateral or bilateral obstruction of the distal ureters.	Most common with infiltrating tumors, especially those arising in the trigone. The distal ureters may also be obstructed by lymph node metastases.
Cystitis	Unilateral or bilateral obstruction of the distal ureters.	In acute cystitis, there is compression of the intramural portion of the ureters by edema and inflammation. In chronic cystitis, the ureterovesical junction is obstructed by fibrosis or an inflammatory mass.
Ureterocele **Simple** **(Fig GU18-5)**	Unilateral or bilateral, round or oval density of opacified urine (in the dilated distal segment of the ureter) separated from opacified urine in the bladder by a thin (2- to 3-mm) radiolucent halo representing the wall of the prolapsed ureter and the bladder mucosa (cobra head sign).	Cystic dilatation of the distal intravesical segment of the ureter with protrusion into the bladder lumen. Probably caused by congenital or acquired stenosis of the ureteral orifice that predisposes to infection and stone formation, both of which may aggravate the degree of obstruction.
Ectopic **(Fig GU18-6)**	Ureteral obstruction with hydronephrosis or nonvisualization of the upper segment of a duplicated collecting system.	If the ectopic ureteral orifice is stenotic, proximal distension of the ureter under the submucosa of the bladder produces a characteristic eccentric filling defect at the base of the bladder.

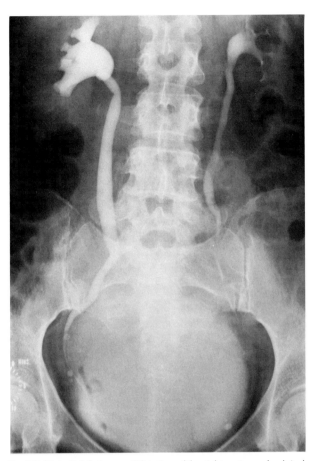

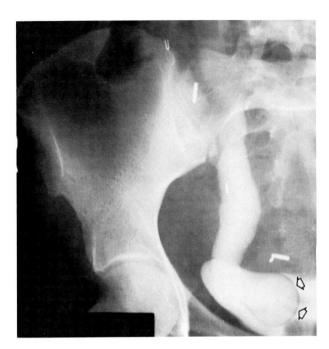

Fɪɢ **GU18-5. Simple ureterocele** (arrows).

Fɪɢ **GU18-4. Pelvic tumor.** Dilatation of the right ureter and pelvis due to partial obstruction by a large ovarian mass.

A

B

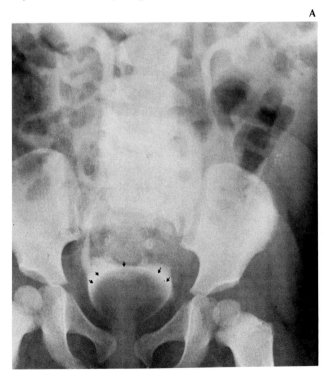

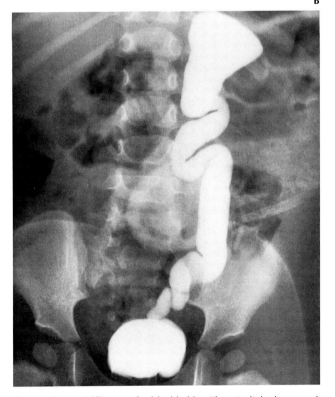

Fɪɢ **GU18-6. Ectopic ureterocele.** (A) Excretory urogram demonstrates a large lucency (arrows) filling much of the bladder. There is slight downward and lateral displacement of the visualized collecting system on the left. (B) Cystogram shows contrast material refluxing to fill the markedly dilated collecting system draining the upper pole of the left kidney. Note the severe dilatation and tortuosity of the ureter.

Condition	Imaging Findings	Comments
Blood clots	Irregular radiolucent filling defects that may produce temporary (usually incomplete) obstruction.	Causes of bleeding include trauma, tumor, instrumentation, vascular malformation, hemorrhagic inflammation, bleeding disorder, and anticoagulant therapy.
Vascular compression **Renal artery**	Extrinsic tubular impression, usually with mild dilatation of the more proximal ureter but rarely significant obstruction.	Normal and aberrant renal arteries in the proximal ureter; iliac vessels in the lower ureter (L5-S1 level).
Ovarian vein syndrome	Extrinsic compression of the right ureter at the S1 level producing mild to moderate obstruction.	Caused by a markedly dilated ovarian vein or possibly by locally induced periureteral fibrosis that develops after several pregnancies.
Aneurysm of abdominal aorta or iliac artery	Extrinsic compression with localized or diffuse lateral displacement of the ureter above the pelvic brim.	The aneurysm is most commonly of arteriosclerotic origin and is often calcified. Ureteral obstruction may also be due to dissecting or mycotic aneurysms.
Retrocaval ureter **(Fig GU18-7)**	Abrupt medial swing of the right ureter, which usually lies over or medial to the vertebral pedicles at the L4-L5 level.	Developmental defect of the inferior vena cava. Compression of the ureter between the inferior vena cava and the posterior abdominal wall often causes narrowing or obstruction of the ureter with progressive hydronephrosis.
Transitional cell carcinoma of the ureter **(Fig GU18-8)**	Smooth or irregular filling defect. Infiltrating carcinoma usually appears as an irregular stricture with overhanging margins (occasionally concentric smooth narrowing with tapering edges that may be difficult to differentiate from ureteral narrowing due to an inflammatory process, calculus, or extrinsic compression).	Rare manifestation. There may be characteristic localized dilatation of the distal ureter, in contrast to the ureteral collapse distal to an obstructing stone. Retrograde pyelography may demonstrate the typical meniscus appearance of the superior border of the contrast column (wine glass sign outlining the lower margin of the tumor).
Benign ureteral tumor	Smooth or irregular filling defect in the ureter. Obstruction is rare, except with papilloma.	Papillomas occur in older patients (50 to 70 years of age), often involve the lower third of the ureter, and tend to produce short filling defects with shaggy and irregular margins and no pedicle. Polyps generally affect young adults, primarily involve the upper third of the ureter, and appear as long, narrow filling defects that have smooth margins and are frequently pedunculated. Submucosal mesenchymal tumors also occur.
Benign pelvic mass **(Fig GU18-9)**	Extrinsic narrowing and lateral deviation of one or both pelvic ureters.	Causes include uterine fibroid, ovarian cyst, enlarged uterus (pregnancy or postpartum), and occasionally a markedly distended rectosigmoid colon.
Pelvic lipomatosis **(see Fig GU20-4)**	Bilateral, symmetric medial displacement and compression of the ureters. Increased radiolucency in the pelvis is caused by the excessive deposition of fat (easily confirmed on CT).	Benign condition with increased deposition of normal, mature adipose tissue in the extraperitoneal pelvic soft tissues around the urinary bladder, rectum, and prostate. Almost all reported cases have been in men. Elevation, elongation, and compression of the rectosigmoid colon and the pear-shaped bladder along with widening of the retrorectal space.

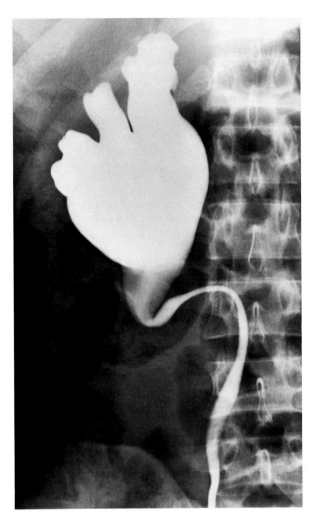

FIG **GU18-7. Retrocaval ureter.** Note the medial swing of the right ureter just distal to the ureteropelvic junction.

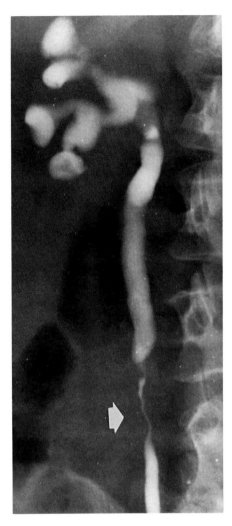

FIG **GU18-8. Transitional cell carcinoma** of the ureter. Irregular stricture (arrow) causing proximal ureteral and pelvocalyceal dilatation.

Condition	Imaging Findings	Comments
Retroperitoneal fibrosis (Fig GU18-10)	Smooth and conical narrowing and frequently medial deviation of both ureters between L4 and S2 with proximal ureteral dilatation.	Fibrosing inflammatory process enveloping but not invading retroperitoneal structures. Although the etiology is unknown, many cases are associated with drug ingestion (eg, methysergide, ergot derivatives, phenacetin, and methyldopa). May coexist with similar fibrotic processes in other sites (fibrosing mediastinitis, sclerosing cholangitis, retro-orbital pseudotumor, retractile mesenteritis, Riedel's thyroiditis).
Retroperitoneal abscess/ hematoma	Extrinsic compression and lateral displacement of the ureter (and kidney). A retroperitoneal gas collection is diagnostic of an abscess. Calcification suggests a tuberculous psoas abscess.	An abscess may originate from spondylitis (especially tuberculous), perinephric abscess, urinary tract infection, pancreatitis, or a perforated duodenum or be a complication of retroperitoneal surgery. A hematoma may be caused by trauma, ruptured aortic aneurysm, bleeding disorder, or anticoagulant therapy or be a complication of surgery.
Papillary necrosis with sloughed papilla	Irregular filling defect simulating an obstructing ureteral stone.	Evidence of papillary necrosis involving other papillae and calyces.
Inspissated pus	Irregular filling defect simulating an obstructing ureteral stone.	Ureteral obstruction is due to a mass of pus from a proximal infectious process. A similar appearance may be caused by tissue debris from a necrotic tumor.
Bladder diverticulum	Single (if congenital) or multiple outpouchings from the bladder that occasionally are large enough to obstruct the distal ureter by extrinsic compression.	Congenital diverticula are usually located near the ureteral orifice and more commonly cause urinary infection and vesicoureteral reflux. Acquired diverticula are usually multiple and result from obstruction of the bladder outlet or urethra. A ''Hutch'' diverticulum in a paraplegic occurs above and lateral to the ureteral orifice and often produces an obstructed ureter just above the bladder (''notch'' sign).
Herniation of ureter	Abnormal course of a redundant ureter that may lead to obstruction.	May be congenital (in femoral, inguinal, sciatic, or internal hernia) or secondary to pelvic surgery.
Endometriosis	Extrinsic obstruction of the distal ureter, usually below the pelvic brim. May produce an intraluminal mass or a stricture and mimic a ureteral tumor.	Uncommon condition in which heterotopic foci of endometrium occur in extrauterine locations. Cyclical urinary symptoms (including hematuria) in women of childbearing age.
Amyloidosis	Narrowing, rigidity, and partial obstruction of the ureter.	Caused by a localized accumulation of amyloid in primary or secondary disease.
Ureteral valve	Sharp horizontal obstruction that usually involves the distal ureter.	Transverse folds or redundant ureteral mucosa that may be either congenital or secondary to chronic inflammation.

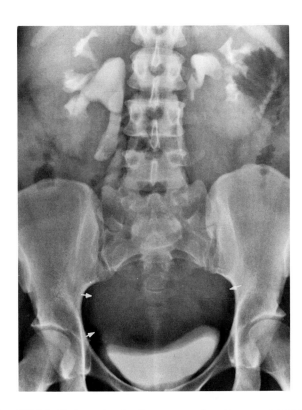

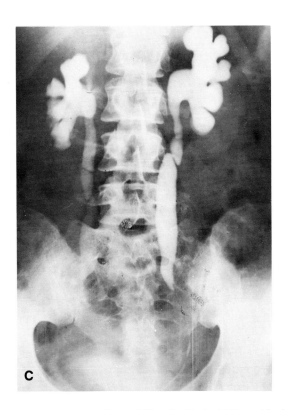

FIG GU18-9. Hydronephrosis of pregnancy. Excretory urogram performed 3 days postpartum demonstrates bilateral large kidneys with dilatation of the ureters and pelvocalyceal systems, especially on the right. The large pelvic mass (arrows) indenting the superior surface of the bladder represents the uterus, which is still causing extrinsic pressure on the ureters.

FIG GU18-10. Retroperitoneal fibrosis. Marked bilateral hydronephrosis with bilateral ureterectasis above the level of the sacral promontory. Below this point both ureters, where visualized, appear to be normal in caliber. No definite ureteral deviation is seen. An excretory urogram performed 1 year previously was entirely normal.[6]

URETERECTASIS

Condition	Imaging Findings	Comments
Ureteral obstruction (Figs GU19-1 and GU19-2; see GU18)	Ureteral dilatation proximal to the point of obstruction. Most often unilateral, but may be bilateral due to an extrinsic lesion.	Causes include calculus, tumor, stricture (congenital, traumatic, surgical, radiation, inflammatory), ureterocele, and extrinsic compression (malignancy, inflammation, pelvic lipomatosis, retroperitoneal fibrosis, pregnancy).
Vesicoureteral reflux (Fig GU19-3)	Generalized dilatation of one or both ureters (and pelvocalyceal systems) occurring with severe reflux.	Most common in children. The relation between reflux and urinary tract infection is controversial, though the combination of the two can produce severe renal scarring as well as dilated and tortuous ureters that may require reimplantation.
Obstruction of urethra or bladder outlet (see Figs GU18-6 and GU24-1)	Bilateral dilatation of the ureters and pelvocalyceal systems. If the obstruction is chronic, the bladder is usually dilated and has trabeculation and diverticula.	Causes include posterior urethral valves, ectopic ureterocele, prostatic hypertrophy or carcinoma, stricture, and diverticulum.
Postobstructive hydronephrosis and hydroureter	Unilateral or bilateral dilatation of the pelvocalyceal system and ureter without evidence of obstruction.	Results from one prolonged or several intermittent episodes of obstruction.
Congenital ureterectasis	Diffuse or segmental dilatation of the ureter (most commonly the lower third) with a normal pelvocalyceal system and no demonstrable ureteral abnormality.	Congenital, nonprogressive malformation of the ureteral wall.
Congenital megaloureter	Functional, smoothly tapered narrowing of the juxtavesical segment with minimal to extensive dilatation (up to 5 cm in diameter) of the pelvic ureter. Vigorous, nonpropulsive peristaltic waves in the dilated segment are similar to those in esophageal achalasia. Bilateral in 20% to 40% of cases.	Represents failure of the juxtavesical segment of the ureter to transmit peristaltic waves (no demonstrable ureteral obstruction and a relaxed, opened, nonrefluxing ureteral orifice). Usually diagnosed in adults, either as an incidental finding or in a patient with vague lower quadrant pain. May remain unchanged for years, but if infection or decompensation occurs the condition may progress to produce massive dilatation of the entire ureter and collecting system.
Infection	Dilatation of the lower third of the ureter is a relatively common result of urinary tract infection (especially recurring cystitis).	Probably related to smooth muscle paralysis in the urinary tract due to bacterial endotoxins. Mild to moderate dilatation of the ureter and pelvocalyceal system may occur in acute pyelonephritis.
Neurogenic bladder (see Figs GU20-2 and GU21-1)	Unilateral or bilateral dilatation of the ureter and pelvocalyceal system. The bladder may be large and flaccid or contracted with mural trabeculation and diverticula formation.	Disease or injury involving the spinal cord or peripheral nerves supplying the bladder. Causes include congenital anomalies (spina bifida, myelomeningocele, sacral agenesis), spinal cord trauma or tumor, syphilis, and diabetes mellitus.

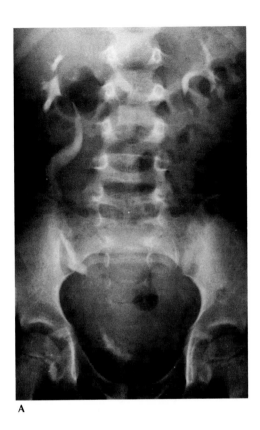

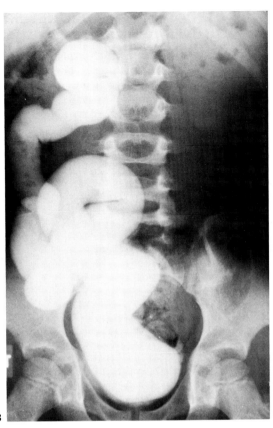

Fig GU19-1. Complete duplication with ureteral obstruction. (A) Excretory urogram demonstrates dilatation and lateral displacement of the right ureter. Ureteral duplication was not suspected. (B) A delayed film following a voiding cystogram demonstrates contrast material filling a dilated and tortuous ureter to the upper segment. This ureter, which was not seen on the excretory urogram, has laterally displaced the ureter to the lower segment.[18]

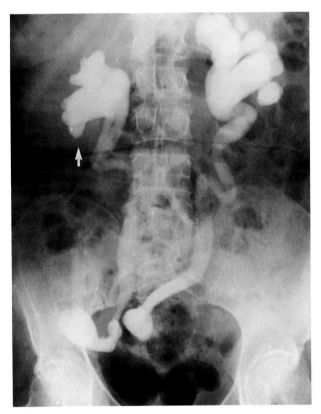

Fig GU19-2. Ileal conduit stenosis. (A) Drainage film from an ileal loopogram shows bilateral hydronephrosis, right lower pole parenchymal scarring (arrow), and failure of the conduit to empty.[19]

Condition	Imaging Findings	Comments
Chagas' disease	Bilateral ureteral dilatation, usually with dilatation of the bladder.	Destruction of myenteric plexuses due to infection by the protozoan *Trypanosoma cruzi* (endemic to South America and Central America).
Diabetes insipidus	Bilateral dilatation of the ureters and pelvocalyceal systems. Often an overdistended bladder.	Continual overloading of the urinary tract in nephrogenic diabetes insipidus (no tubular response to endogenous or exogenous antidiuretic hormone). Rare in pituitary diabetes insipidus.
Absent abdominal musculature (Eagle-Barrett, or prune belly, syndrome) (Fig GU19-4)	Diffuse dilatation of the ureters, pelvocalyceal systems, and bladder.	Rare congenital condition, occurring almost exclusively in males. Bulging of the flanks (due to a lack of support by abdominal muscles) is a characteristic finding on plain films.

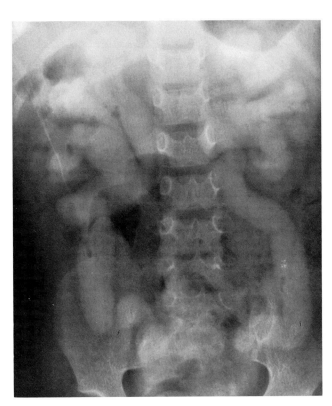

FIG GU19-3. Vesicoureteral reflux. Voiding cystogram in a young girl shows bilateral reflux with gross dilatation of the upper tracts.

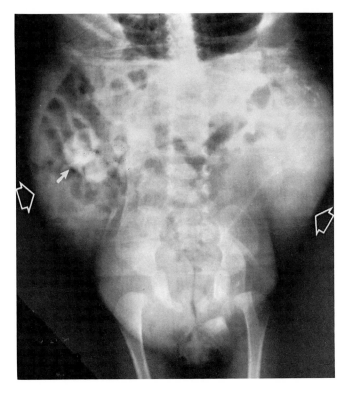

FIG GU19-4. Prune belly syndrome. Pronounced bulging of the flanks (open arrows). The patient had multiple genitourinary anomalies including hydronephrosis of the right collecting system (small arrow).

SMALL URINARY BLADDER

Condition	Imaging Findings	Comments
Transitional cell carcinoma (infiltrating)	Asymmetric bladder contraction with an irregular, thickened wall and mural filling defects. Localized tumor infiltration causes marked bladder deformity. There is often unilateral or bilateral ureteral obstruction.	The wall of the urinary bladder is the most common site of transitional cell cancer. Plain radiographs may demonstrate punctate, coarse, or linear calcifications that are usually encrusted on the surface of the tumor but occasionally lie within it (see Fig GI57-4).
Cystitis (Fig GU20-1)	Small bladder with trabeculation and mural irregularities in chronic disease or severe acute cystitis. There may be associated filling defects (fungus balls, blood clots). Characteristic mural and luminal gas in emphysematous cystitis.	Acute inflammation of the urinary bladder generally does not produce any radiographically detectable abnormality (the wall may be thickened and irregular because of severe mucosal and intramural edema with spasm).
Neurogenic bladder (Fig GU20-2)	Small, spastic, heavily trabeculated bladder with an irregular thickened wall and diverticula formation. May have a pointed dome (pine tree bladder).	Disease or injury involving the spinal cord or peripheral nerves supplying the bladder. Causes include spinal neoplasm or trauma, syphilis, diabetes mellitus, and congenital anomalies (spina bifida, myelomeningocele, sacral agenesis). A neurogenic bladder can also be large and atonic with little trabeculation.
Extrinsic bladder compression (Figs GU20-3 and GU20-4)	Bilaterally symmetric narrowing, elevation, and elongation of the bladder, often resulting in a teardrop or pear-shaped configuration.	Causes include pelvic hematoma (associated with pelvic fractures), pelvic lipomatosis (fat density compressing the bladder), pelvic edema (inferior vena caval occlusion), and pelvic neoplastic or inflammatory disease.
After surgery or radiation therapy	Small bladder with a smooth or irregular surface.	Radiation cystitis develops several months to several years after irradiation (especially intracavitary).
Schistosomiasis (see Fig GI57-1)	Small, fibrotic bladder with characteristic mural calcification. The calcification is initially most apparent and extensive at the base of the bladder, but may surround the bladder completely. There may be ureteral calcification (parallel dense lines, especially in the pelvic portion of the ureter).	Blood fluke with a snail host. The irritative effect of ova passing through or lodging in the wall of the bladder stimulates an inflammatory response (granuloma formation, obliterative vasculitis, progressive fibrosis). The development of squamous cell carcinoma of the bladder is a frequent complication (especially in Egypt).
Tuberculosis	Initially, thickening and trabeculation of the bladder wall. Later there is a progressive decrease in bladder capacity and a smoother wall. Eventually, the bladder virtually disappears and the ureters seem to enter directly into the urethra. Calcification is infrequent in the bladder but common in the vas deferens.	Almost invariably associated with renal and ureteral involvement. There may be reflux and, occasionally, dilatation of one or both ureters and pelvocalyceal systems secondary to bladder muscular hypertrophy that produces ureteral constriction.

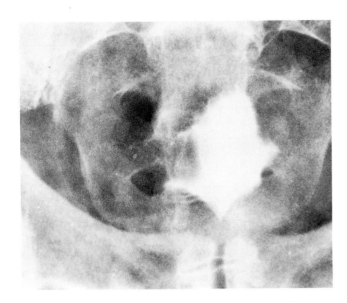

FIG GU20-1. Cyclophosphamide (Cytoxan) cystitis. Six months after repeated cycles of cyclophosphamide therapy, the bladder volume is greatly reduced and the bladder wall appears ulcerated and edematous.[2]

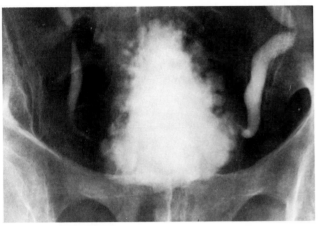

FIG GU20-2. Neurogenic bladder. Small, spastic, trabeculated bladder with a pointed dome.[20]

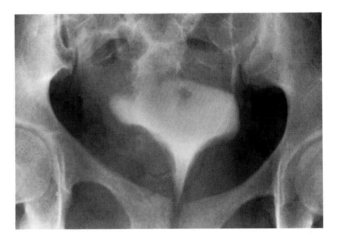

FIG GU20-3. Pelvic hematoma. Symmetric narrowing of the base of the bladder.

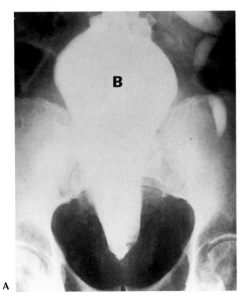

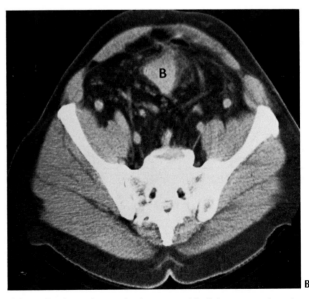

FIG GU20-4. Pelvic lipomatosis. (A) Excretory urogram demonstrates bilateral hydronephrosis, displacement of the left ureter, and an abnormal pear-shaped urinary bladder (B). (B) A CT scan reveals that the compressed bladder (B) is surrounded by low-density fat, confirming the diagnosis of pelvic lipomatosis.

LARGE URINARY BLADDER

Condition	Imaging Findings	Comments
Obstruction of bladder outlet or urethra (see Figs GU18-6 and GU24-1)	Dilated bladder with trabeculation and diverticula formation. With prolonged obstruction, the bladder may become thin-walled and atonic.	Causes include prostatic hypertrophy or carcinoma, stricture, diverticulum, posterior urethral valve, and ectopic ureterocele. Congenital bladder neck obstruction is a controversial entity.
Neurogenic bladder (Figs GU21-1 and GU21-2)	Dilatation of a smooth, thin-walled, atonic bladder with little or no trabeculation.	Suggests underlying diabetes, tabes dorsalis, or syringomyelia. Differs from a spastic neurogenic bladder, which is small and heavily trabeculated.
Bladder prolapse (Fig GU21-3)	Bladder dilatation caused by outlet obstruction. The base of the bladder projects below the inferior margin of the symphysis pubis (may be evident only in the upright position).	After childbirth, the bladder and anterior vaginal wall may prolapse into the vaginal cavity (cystocele). May be associated with incontinence.
Chagas' disease	Dilatation of the bladder and both ureters.	Destruction of myenteric plexuses due to infection by the protozoan *Trypanosoma cruzi* (endemic to South America and Central America).
Megacystis syndrome	Large, smooth-walled bladder with bilateral or unilateral ureteral reflux occurring either at low pressure or only during voiding. The bladder neck and proximal urethra commonly fail to funnel and distend normally during voiding.	Most commonly occurs in childhood, especially in girls. The bladder trigone is twice or triple normal size and the ureteral orifices are gaping. Postvoiding films show no significant bladder residual.
Diabetes insipidus	Dilatation of the bladder and both ureters.	Continual overloading of the urinary tract in nephrogenic diabetes insipidus (no tubular response to endogenous or exogenous antidiuretic hormone). Rare in pituitary diabetes insipidus.
Absent abdominal musculature (Eagle-Barrett, or prune belly, syndrome) (see Fig GU19-4)	Diffuse dilatation of the bladder, ureters, and pelvocalyceal systems.	Rare congenital condition that occurs almost exclusively in males. Bulging of the flanks (due to a lack of support by the abdominal muscles) is a characteristic finding on plain films.
Psychogenic/drug-induced	Smooth-walled, markedly distended bladder with normal function.	No underlying neurologic disease. May be associated with the use of tranquilizers and muscle relaxants.

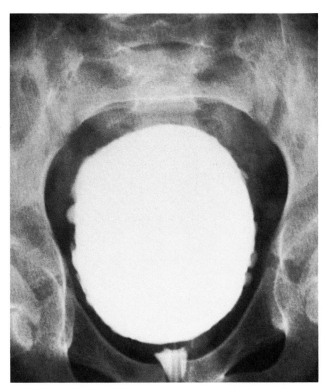

FIG GU21-1. Neurogenic bladder. Large, atonic bladder in a child with traumatic paralysis of the lower extremities.

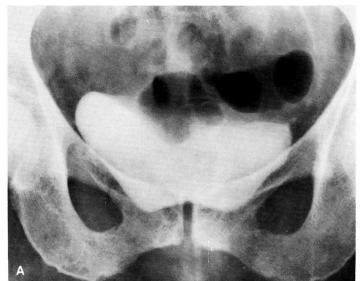

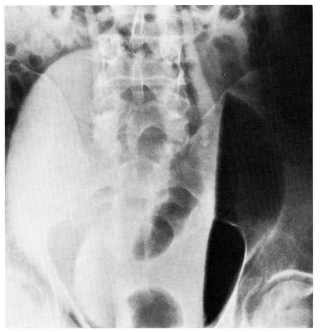

FIG GU21-2. Neurogenic bladder in diabetes. Lateral decubitus view shows the massively enlarged, atonic bladder containing an air-urine level secondary to severe vesical infection by a gas-forming organism.

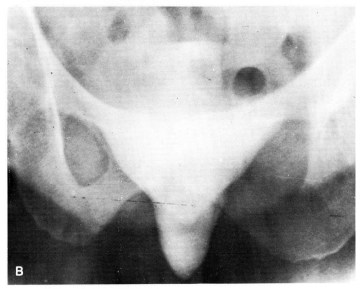

FIG GU21-3. Cystocele. (A) Supine view. The lowermost portion of the bladder is visualized slightly below the upper edge of the symphysis pubis, a finding that is consistent with that in a cystocele. (B) Upright position. Contrast material is well below the symphysis pubis, indicating a marked cystocele. Note the superimposed urethrocele.

SINGLE OR MULTIPLE FILLING DEFECTS IN THE URINARY BLADDER

Condition	Imaging Findings	Comments
Calculus (Fig GU22-1)	Single or multiple filling defects that vary in size from tiny concretions, each the size of a grain of sand, to an enormous single calculus occupying the entire bladder lumen. Most are circular or oval, but they can be amorphous, laminated, or even spiculated. Calculi frequently occur in bladder diverticula, lying in an unusual position close to the lateral pelvic wall or having a dumbbell shape with one end lodged in the diverticulum and the other projecting into the bladder.	Stone formation in the bladder is primarily a disorder of elderly men who have obstruction or infection of the lower urinary tract. Frequently associated lesions include bladder outlet obstruction, urethral stricture, neurogenic bladder, bladder diverticulum, and cystocele. Upper urinary tract stones that migrate down the ureter are occasionally retained in the bladder.
Blood clot	Irregular intraluminal filling defects of various sizes. Large clots may occupy almost the entire bladder lumen but are still completely surrounded by contrast material (unlike tumors). Blood clots often change in size and shape or disappear over several days.	Common causes of bleeding (originating from the kidneys or the bladder itself) include tumor, trauma, instrumentation, vascular malformation, hemorrhagic inflammation, bleeding disorder, and anticoagulant therapy.
Air bubble	Smooth, round, freely movable intraluminal defect. A large amount can produce an air-fluid level on a film obtained with a horizontal beam. There may be associated intramural gas (linear streaks or small round lucencies) in emphysematous cystitis.	Causes of air in the bladder include instrumentation, surgery, penetrating trauma, fistulas to gas-containing hollow organs, and emphysematous cystitis (usually in diabetic patients). Both intraluminal and intramural gas must be differentiated from superimposed bowel gas.
Instrument	Opaque or nonopaque intraluminal filling defect.	Most commonly the inflated balloon of a Foley catheter.
Neoplasm Transitional cell carcinoma (Fig GU22-2)	Single or multiple polypoid defects that arise from the bladder wall and are fixed in position (unlike a calculus, blood clot, or air). May produce only focal bladder wall thickening and rigidity. Punctate, coarse, or linear calcification is occasionally encrusted on the surface of the tumor (rarely lying within it).	Predominantly involves men over age 50. Hematuria, frequency, and dysuria are the most common presenting symptoms. Tumors originating near the ureteral orifices may cause early ureteral obstruction. May be associated with other transitional tumors of the pelvocalyceal system or ureter. Because urography can detect only about 60% of symptomatic bladder carcinomas, all patients with lower urinary tract hematuria should undergo cystoscopy.
Polyp	Single or multiple filling defects that may be pedunculated and movable.	Common tumor consisting of a fibrous stalk with a covering of normal transitional epithelium.
Papilloma	Solitary or multiple polypoid defects with smooth or irregular margins. May be pedunculated. No evidence of bladder wall invasion.	Benign, frondlike tumor that usually arises on the trigone. Often recurs and therefore may be considered as a low-grade malignancy.
Metastases	Direct extension of tumor causes an extrinsic defect with irregular margins. Hematogenous metastases produce solitary or multiple filling defects with smooth or irregular margins. Noninvading pelvic lymph node metastases cause a smooth extrinsic impression on the bladder wall.	Direct extension from primary carcinomas of the prostate, uterus, rectosigmoid, cervix, or ovary. Hematogenous metastases (rare) from lung, breast, and stomach tumors and melanoma. Bladder tumors may also be secondary to papillary tumors of the kidney or ureter and clear cell adenoma of the kidney.

(continued page 516)

A   B

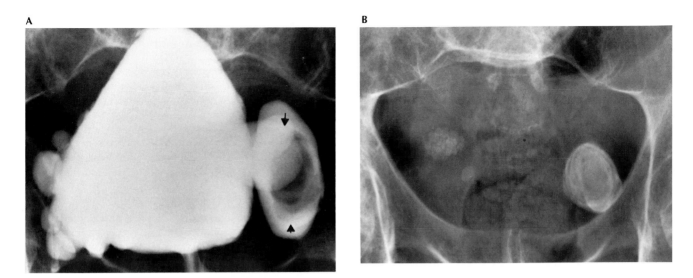

FIG GU22-1. **Bladder calculi.** (A) Excretory urogram demonstrates a large stone (arrows) in a left-sided bladder diverticulum. (B) Plain radiograph of the pelvis shows the laminated stone and multiple smaller calculi that were obscured by contrast material in the right-sided bladder diverticula on the contrast-filled view.

A   B

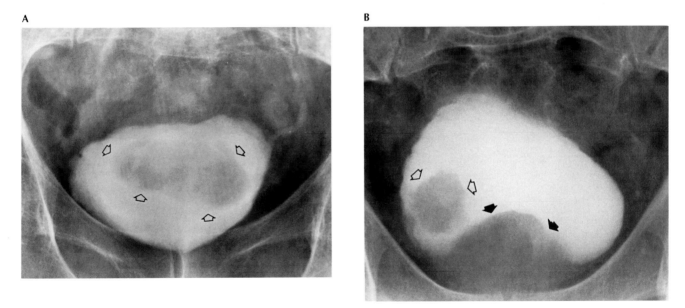

FIG GU22-2. **Transitional cell carcinoma.** (A) Large, irregular filling defect (arrows) in the bladder. (B) In another patient, the irregular tumor (open arrows) is associated with a large filling defect (closed arrow), representing benign prostatic hypertrophy, at the base of the bladder.

Condition	Imaging Findings	Comments
Lymphoma	Direct invasion from perivesical lymphoma causes an irregular defect. Lymph node enlargement without invasion (more common) causes an extrinsic impression. There may be single or multiple well-circumscribed foci limited to the bladder wall.	Primary lymphoma of the bladder is extremely rare. Secondary involvement is not uncommon with advanced lymphoma. Diffuse infiltration or localized bladder masses occasionally occur in leukemia.
Mesenchymal tumor	Various patterns (small polypoid filling defect to large, often fungating, mass). May be pedunculated.	Impossible to differentiate benign from malignant varieties unless there is evidence of wall invasion. Histologic types include leiomyoma, neurofibroma, hemangioma, fibroma, pheochromocytoma, and rhabdomyosarcoma (most common bladder tumor in children and often termed sarcoma botryoides).
Prostatic enlargement (Figs GU22-3 and GU22-4)	Smooth or irregular extrinsic filling defect of varying size at the base of the bladder. If a chronic process, there is trabeculation of the bladder wall and diverticula formation. Bladder outlet obstruction causes dilatation of the pelvocalyceal systems and the ureters. The distal ureters often have a fishhook deformity (due to elevation of the trigone).	Most common causes are benign prostatic hypertrophy and carcinoma of the prostate. Although the contour of the filling defect is usually more irregular in carcinoma, benign hypertrophy and carcinoma usually cannot be differentiated unless there is evidence of tumor invasion into neighboring structures or distal metastases.
Simple ureterocele (Fig GU22-5)	Round or oval density of opacified urine (in the dilated distal segment of the ureter) separated from opacified urine in the bladder by a thin (2- to 3-mm) radiolucent halo representing the wall of the prolapsed ureter and the bladder mucosa (cobra head sign).	Cystic dilatation of the distal intravesical segment of the ureter with protrusion into the bladder lumen. Often an incidental finding, but may predispose to obstruction, infection, and stone formation. May be unilateral or bilateral.
Ectopic ureterocele (see Fig GU18-6)	Smooth or lobulated, usually eccentric filling defect at the base of the bladder. Associated with a duplicated collecting system (ureterocele arises from the ureter draining the upper segment, which is nonfunctioning or hydronephrotic).	Congenital lesion generally found in children (especially females). The ectopic ureter enters the bladder wall near its normal site of insertion. Instead of communicating with the lumen, the ectopic ureter continues for a variable distance before opening into the bladder neck or posterior urethra. If the orifice is stenotic, proximal distension of the ureter under the submucosa of the bladder produces the eccentric filling defect.
Endometriosis	Smooth, round or lobulated, extrinsic or intrinsic filling defect (usually located on the posterior wall).	Uncommon condition that presents with pain or cyclic urinary symptoms, including hematuria. Often a history of previous gynecologic or abdominal surgery.
Amyloidosis	Irregular, lobulated filling defect.	Very rare manifestation of primary or secondary disease.
Schistosomiasis (see Fig GI57-1)	Single or multiple discrete filling defects (may produce a honeycomb appearance).	Usually caused by *Schistosoma hematobium*. Characteristic calcification of the bladder wall.

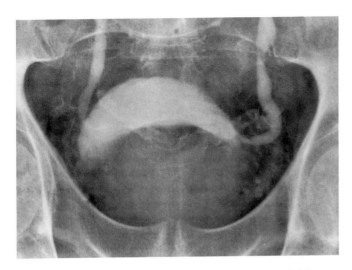

FIG GU22-3. **Benign prostatic hypertrophy.** Large, smooth filling defect at the base of the bladder. Note the fish-hook appearance of the distal ureters and the calcification in the vas deferens.

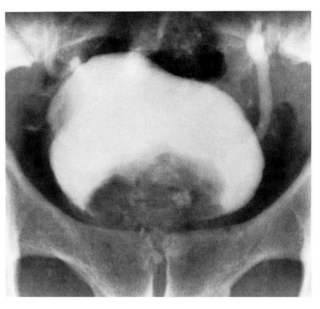

FIG GU22-4. **Carcinoma of the prostate.** Elevation of and markedly irregular impression on the floor of the contrast-filled bladder.

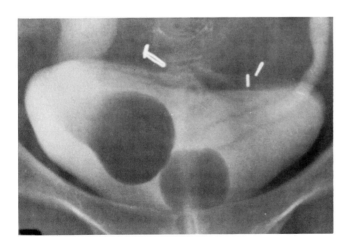

FIG GU22-5. **Bilateral simple ureteroceles.**

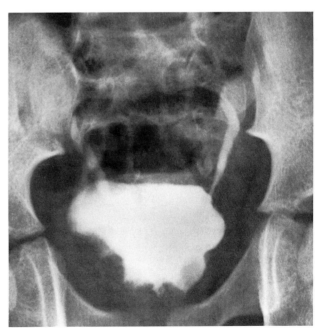

FIG GU22-6. **Cystitis.** Irregular, lobulated filling defects (representing intense mucosal edema) at the base of the bladder.

Condition	Imaging Findings	Comments
Fungus ball	Single large or multiple small filling defects that often contain gas that produces a mottled appearance. Contrast material occasionally enters the fungus ball and accentuates its laminated appearance.	Most often caused by *Candida albicans* in patients with debilitating diseases, diabetes mellitus, or prolonged antibiotic or steroid therapy.
Cystitis (Figs GU22-6 and GU22-7)	Various patterns of irregular wall thickening and mural or mucosal filling defects. Intraluminal or intramural gas in emphysematous cystitis. Multiple cysts project into the lumen in cystitis cystica. There may be amorphous calcification.	Multiple conditions including hemorrhagic cystitis (''honeymoon cystitis''), interstitial cystitis (chronic inflammation in women), granulomatous cystitis (complication of chronic granulomatous disease of childhood or secondary to extension of Crohn's disease or granulomatous prostatitis), radiation cystitis, tuberculous cystitis, and cyclophosphamide (Cytoxan) cystitis.
Malacoplakia (Fig GU22-8)	Smooth, single or multiple, round or oval filling defects that are most commonly located on the bladder floor. The radiographic pattern may suggest a neoplastic process or severe cystitis.	Uncommon chronic inflammatory disease that predominantly affects women, most of whom have a history of recurrent or chronic urinary tract infection. There may also be ureteral involvement (general dilatation with multiple filling defects or a scalloped appearance and occasionally a stricture).
Intramural hematoma	Smooth or irregular mural defect. There may be associated intraluminal filling defects (blood clots).	Follows surgery, trauma, or instrumentation.
Foreign body	Opaque or nonopaque filling defect.	Foreign material may become the nidus for calculus formation.

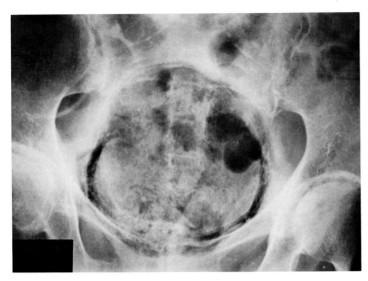

Fig GU22-7. Emphysematous cystitis. Plain film of the pelvis shows radiolucent gas in the wall of the bladder.[6]

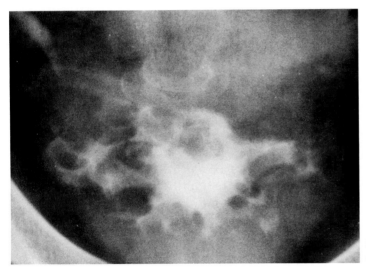

Fig GU22-8. Malacoplakia. Postvoiding excretory urogram shows multiple smooth, nodular filling defects.[17]

GAS IN THE BLADDER LUMEN OR WALL

Condition	Imaging Findings	Comments
Emphysematous cystitis (Fig GU23-1)	Intraluminal gas associated with a ring of lucent gas outlining all or part of the bladder wall.	Inflammatory cystitis that most often occurs in diabetic patients and is caused by gas-forming bacteria.
Iatrogenic	Intraluminal gas.	Follows cystoscopy, surgery, or trauma.
Bladder fistula (Fig GU23-2)	Intraluminal gas.	Fistula formation between the intestinal or genital tract (or both) and the urinary tract. Major underlying causes include diverticulitis (about 50%); carcinomas of the colon, rectum, bladder, cervix, and uterus; and Crohn's disease. Less frequent causes include trauma, radiation therapy, foreign bodies, and abscesses.
Fungus ball in bladder	Soft-tissue mass containing gas (contrast material may enter the fungus ball and further accentuate its laminated appearance).	Composed of layers of mycelia separated by air and proteinaceous material. Usually due to infection by *Candida albicans*, especially in severely debilitated patients undergoing prolonged antibiotic or steroid therapy. Gas results from the chemical action of fungi on glucose in the urine (producing CO_2 and butyric and lactic acid).

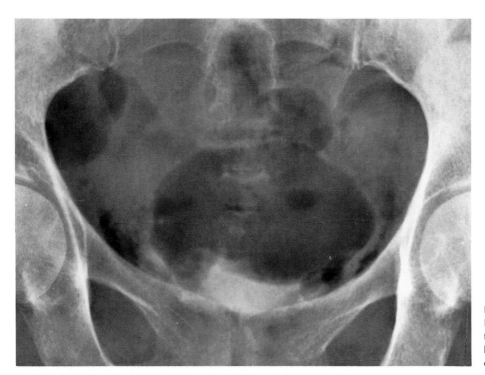

Fig GU23-1. Emphysematous cystitis.
Large amount of air in the bladder. Note the small clusters of air in the wall of the bladder in this patient with severe infection complicating diabetes.

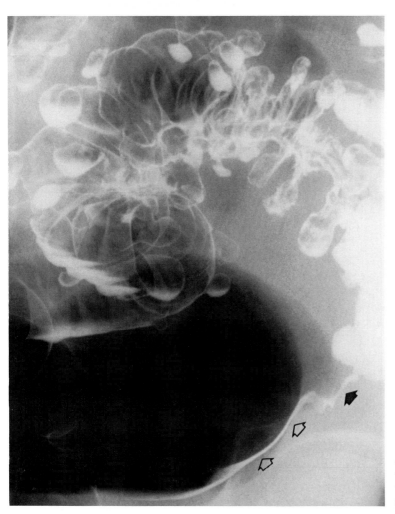

Fig GU23-2. Colovesical fistula in diverticulitis. Barium enema examination demonstrates contrast material in the fistulous tract (solid arrow) between the sigmoid colon and the bladder. Barium can also be seen lining the base of the gas-filled bladder (open arrows).

URINARY TRACT OBSTRUCTION BELOW THE BLADDER
IN CHILDREN

Condition	Imaging Findings	Comments
Meatal stenosis	Distal urethral narrowing, often with severe proximal dilatation.	Much more common in males. May be congenital or secondary to infection or trauma. Often associated with hypospadiac openings.
Urethral stricture	Smooth narrowing of the urethral lumen of varying length (multiple in about 10% of cases).	Almost all congenital strictures occur in boys and are located in the bulbomembranous portion. Most commonly iatrogenic (instrumentation or repair of hypospadias) or due to trauma (straddle injury or kick).
Posterior urethral valve (Fig GU24-1)	Elongation and dilatation of the posterior urethra with a characteristic thin, sail-like lucent defect representing the bulging valve.	Thin transverse membrane, found almost exclusively in males, that causes outlet obstruction and may lead to severe hydronephrosis and renal damage. The bladder neck often appears narrow (although it is usually normal in width) because of the disparity in size between it and the urethra bulging posteriorly beneath it. Anterior urethral valves are extremely rare.
Ectopic ureterocele (see Fig GU18-6)	Smooth or lobulated, usually eccentric filling defect at the base of the bladder associated with a duplicated collecting system (the ureterocele arises from the ureter draining the upper segment, which is nonfunctioning or hydronephrotic).	Congenital lesion in which the ectopic ureter enters the bladder wall near its normal site of insertion. Instead of communicating with the lumen, the ureter continues for a variable distance before opening into the bladder neck or posterior urethra. If the orifice is stenotic, proximal distension of the ureter under the submucosa of the bladder produces the eccentric filling defect.
Foreign body	Single or, less frequently, multiple filling defects that are usually radiopaque.	In addition to causing urinary tract obstruction, a foreign body may be the nidus for calculus formation.
Congenital bladder neck obstruction	Small, narrowed bladder neck. There may occasionally be an anterior or posterior indentation, diaphragm, or collar at the bladder neck opening and failure of funneling during voiding.	Controversial entity with such postulated causes as muscular hypertrophy, fibrous ring, and bladder neck dyskinesia.
Urethral diverticulum	Tubular, round or oval, smooth outpouching that is separate from the urethra but communicates with it.	Diverticulum of the urethra distal to the external sphincter is an uncommon but important cause of urinary obstruction in male children.
Congenital urethral duplication	Accessory urethra may be completely duplicated, join the main urethra distally, or end blindly.	Extremely rare anomaly that almost always occurs in males.

Condition	Imaging Findings	Comments
Hypertrophy of verumontanum	Round or oval filling defect in the prostatic urethra.	Rare cause of obstruction that is probably transient and may be the result of maternal estrogen stimulation near term. May be secondary to inflammatory lesions of the urethra and bladder in older boys and men.
Hydrometrocolpos	Extrinsic pressure narrowing of the urethra with proximal dilatation of the bladder and ureters.	Rare congenital anomaly associated with obstruction of the vaginal outlet and secondary dilatation of the vagina and uterus by retained nonsanguinous secretions.

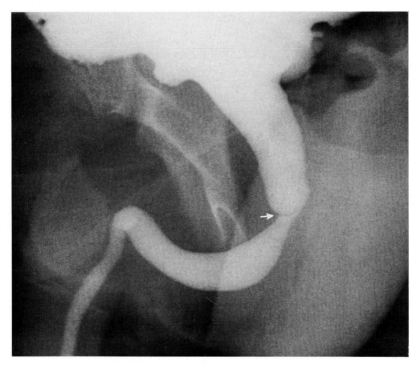

Fɪɢ GU24-1. Posterior urethral valve. Voiding cystourethrogram shows the spinnaker-sail shape of the valve (arrow). Distally, the caliber of the bulbous urethra is normal.[21]

CALCIFICATION OF THE VAS DEFERENS

Condition	Comments
Diabetes mellitus **(Fig GU25-1)**	Most common cause. There is generally bilaterally symmetric calcification in the muscular elements of the vasa with the lumens remaining widely patent.
Degenerative change **(aging)** **(Fig GU25-2)**	Appearance identical to that of vas deferens calcification in a diabetic patient, but develops in individuals with no evidence of diabetes or other predisposing factor. Calcification presumably occurs with greater frequency and at a younger age in diabetic men because this disease accelerates the degenerative process.
Tuberculosis	Inflammation causes partial or complete thrombosis of the lumen of the vas deferens, resulting in intraluminal calcification. The calcification is more frequently unilateral and irregular than in the noninflammatory form (diabetes, degenerative change).
Other infections	Inflammatory intraluminal calcification, often unilateral and irregular like tuberculosis, can develop in gonorrhea, syphilis, schistosomiasis, and chronic nonspecific urinary tract infection.

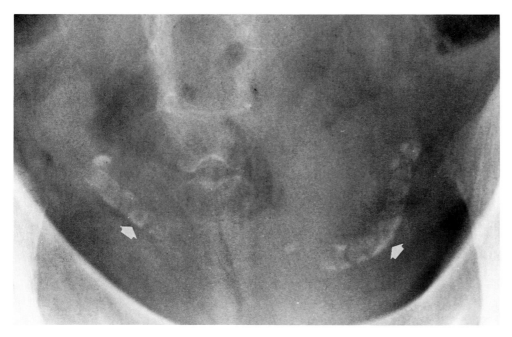

FIG GU25-1. Diabetes mellitus.

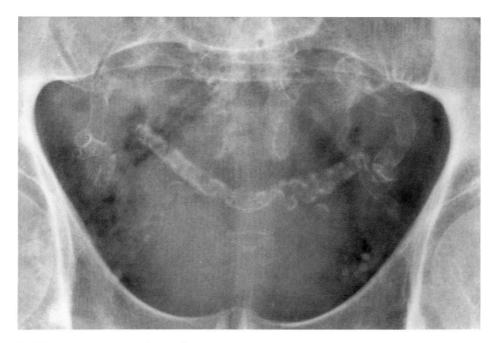

FIG GU25-2. Degenerative change of aging.

ANECHOIC (CYSTIC) RENAL MASSES

Condition	Comments
Simple renal cyst (Fig GU26-1)	Thin-walled, fluid-filled anechoic mass with strongly enhancing posterior wall.
Adult polycystic kidney disease (Fig GU26-2)	Enlarged kidneys containing many anechoic areas of variable size representing multiple cysts. Often associated hepatic and pancreatic cysts.
Parapelvic cyst (Fig GU26-3)	Medially placed, fluid-filled anechoic mass with an echogenic wall. The cyst displaces the pelvocalyceal echo complex, but does not separate it as would be expected in hydronephrosis. Unlike hydronephrosis, the calyces are not dilated nor do they communicate with the mass.
Medullary cystic disease	Multiple anechoic cystic structures (often very small) in the corticomedullary junction and the medulla. Clinical findings include anemia, polyuria, hyposthenuria, salt wasting, and renal failure.
Lesions that may mimic renal cyst (Fig GU26-4)	An anechoic cystic pattern can be produced not only by liquids but by any tissues or substances that acoustically behave like a liquid. For example, uniform gelatin like clots, abscesses consisting only of leukocytes without debris, and unclotted blood (as in hematomas and intrarenal vascular malformations and aneurysms) all show cystic patterns. A few solid lesions also occasionally produce a pattern that so closely simulates a cyst that only the most scrupulous and meticulous technique can differentiate them. In addition to vascular anomalies, hematomas, and abscesses, other lesions that may mimic renal cysts on ultrasound include urine collections (localized hydronephrosis, urinoma), cysts containing small mural tumors, and necrotic and hemorrhagic tumors.

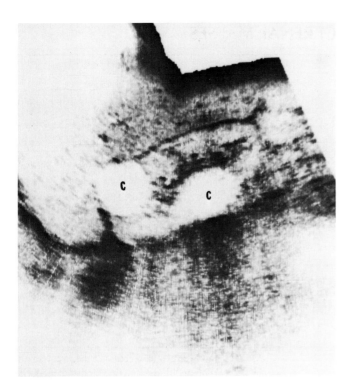

FIG GU26-1. **Simple renal cysts.** Anechoic fluid-filled masses (C) with strongly enhanced posterior walls.

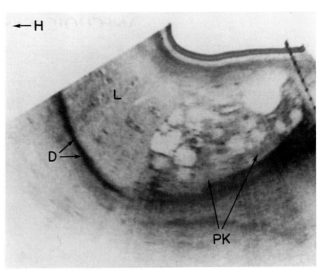

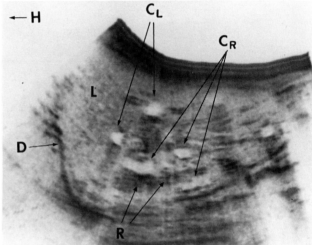

FIG GU26-2. **Adult polycystic kidney disease.** (Top) Parasagittal sonogram of the right kidney (PK) shows a random distribution of multiple cysts that vary dramatically in size. The normal reniform contour is maintained. (Bottom) Parasagittal sonogram in a young, asymptomatic member of the family shows multiple cysts (C_R, C_L) in the right kidney (R) and liver (L). (D, diaphragm and H, head)[2]

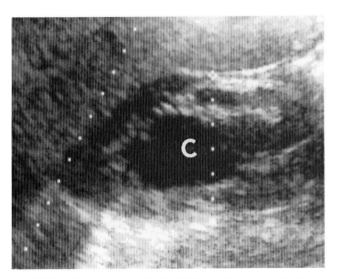

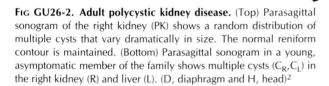

FIG GU26-3. **Parapelvic cyst (C).** Fluid-filled collection that displaces but does not separate the pelvocalyceal echo complex.

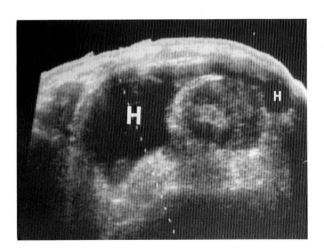

FIG GU26-4. **Hematoma.** Extensive anechoic collection (H) about a renal transplant.

COMPLEX RENAL MASSES

Condition	Comments
Renal neoplasm	Although they usually produce a solid pattern, renal cell carcinomas that are partly cystic or those associated with a large amount of hemorrhage assume fluid-like characteristics that acoustically may overshadow their basically solid nature. A similar appearance is seen with a neoplasm that has become necrotic and contains debris that is jellylike and acts as a homogeneous sound-transmitting medium. With meticulous technique, low-level internal echoes are almost always detectable. In questionable cases, needle aspiration of the mass may be necessary to confirm the correct diagnosis.
Cyst	Multilocular or multiple cysts placed very close together (eg, polycystic disease) may produce an overall complex mass, although each clear space actually represents an individual cyst. Cysts containing debris (infected cysts) or clot (hemorrhagic cysts) are also complex. Dysplastic kidney (the most common cause of an abdominal mass in the newborn) produces a disorganized cystic pattern with lack of renal parenchyma and reniform contour (unlike the precise organization of symmetrically positioned fluid-filled spaces in hydronephrosis due to congenital ureteropelvic junction obstruction).
Abscess (see Fig GU33-3)	Variable pattern that may be primarily solid or cystic with a well-defined or poorly defined wall that is generally not as smooth as an uncomplicated cyst. Characteristically contains low-level echoes representing inflammatory debris. A fluid-debris level may sometimes be noted.
Hematoma/hemorrhagic infarct (see Fig GU33-4)	Hematomas may demonstrate fragments of clot, and, although predominantly cystic, their walls tend to be less smooth than those of uncomplicated renal cysts. Hemorrhagic infarcts (as in renal vein thrombosis) produce a complex pattern (expecially during the acute phase) that is due to areas of hemorrhage and necrosis. A thrombus may occasionally be seen in the renal vein. In contrast, ischemic infarcts secondary to renal artery stenosis tend to appear normal on ultrasound.
Hydronephrosis/ pyonephrosis (Figs GU27-1 and GU27-2)	Internal echoes may occur from the edges of dilated calyceal rims and fornices, converting the fluid pattern of hydronephrosis to an apparently complex one. If the urine in an obstructed kidney is heavily infected (pyonephrosis), the degree of echogenicity is increased.

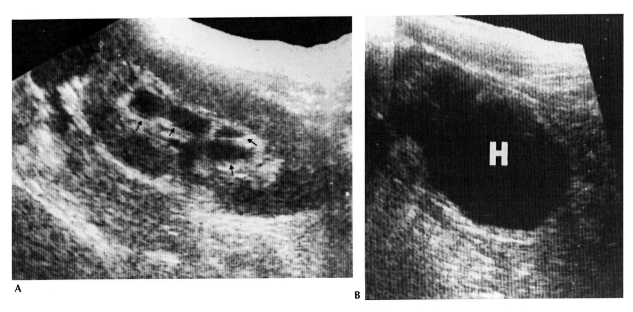

FIG GU27-1. Hydronephrosis. (A) In a patient with moderate disease, the dilated calyces and pelvis appear as echo-free sacs (arrows) separated by septa of compressed tissue and vessels. (B) In a patient with severe hydronephrosis, the intervening septa have disappeared, leaving a large fluid-filled sac (H) with no evidence of internal structure and no normal parenchyma apparent at its margins.

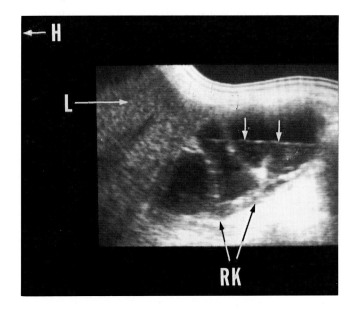

FIG GU27-2. Pyonephrosis. Parasagittal sonogram of the right kidney (RK) demonstrates marked hydronephrosis and a characteristic fluid level (arrows). The fluid level indicates sediment in the renal collecting system and is a typical finding of pyonephrosis. (L, liver and H, head)[2]

SOLID RENAL MASSES

Condition	Comments
Renal cell carcinoma (Fig GU28-1)	Solid mass with numerous internal echoes and no evidence of acoustic enhancement. There is often an irregular or poorly defined interface with the remaining normal parenchyma. May contain sonolucent areas representing hemorrhage, necrosis, or cystic degeneration. Bright echoes around or within the mass may represent circumferential or intratumoral calcification. Extension of tumor into the renal vein or inferior vena cava can be easily detected.
Angiomyolipoma (Fig GU28-2)	Single or multiple renal masses that are extremely echogenic (probably because of the numerous fatty-fibrous interfaces with the lesion). Although most occur as isolated, unilateral kidney lesions in otherwise normal persons, these benign tumors also develop in a large percentage of patients with tuberous sclerosis, in whom the involvement is usually multifocal and bilateral. The characteristic high fat content of an angiomyolipoma can be well demonstrated by CT.
Wilms' tumor (Fig GU28-3)	Mass of generally homogeneous increased echogenicity that may contain relatively sonolucent areas due to cystic necrosis.
Leukemia	Diffusely enlarged kidneys with increased echogenicity. Loss of the corticomedullary demarcation but preservation of the renal sinus echo pattern.
Lymphoma	Characteristically produces a mass effect with one or several areas of decreased echogenicity because it is composed of tissue of fairly uniform type so that there is little difference in specific acoustic impedance between adjacent internal structures.
Infantile polycystic kidney disease	Innumerable ectatic renal tubules (''cysts'') in the large kidneys are so small that their lumens are not resolved by ultrasound. Instead, the interfaces produced by the walls of these tubules cause increased echogenicity throughout the parenchyma of the kidney. Increased echoes from ectatic tubules in the cortex as well as in the medulla cause a loss of the normal sharp distinction between the medullary and cortical areas and its replacement by a homogeneous parenchyma of increased echoes.
Calcified renal mass	Mural calcification, usually in the wall of a cyst but occasionally in the wall of a hematoma or abscess, can cause marked reflection of sound that prevents the through-transmission of enough sound to define the far wall. Correlation with plain radiographs is essential to document the presence of calcification causing this appearance.

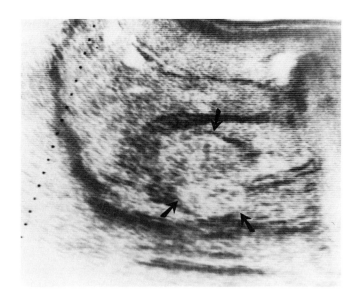

FIG GU28-1. **Renal cell carcinoma.** Echo-filled solid mass (arrows) with no posterior enhancement.

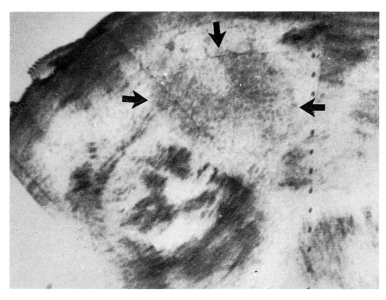

FIG GU28-2. **Angiomyolipoma.** Transverse supine sonogram demonstrates a generally echogenic mass (arrows) arising from the kidney. Less echogenic foci in the mass represent hemorrhage in the fatty tumor.[22]

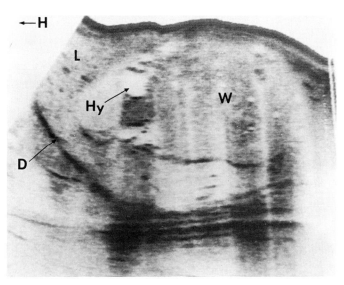

FIG GU28-3. **Wilms' tumor.** Parasagittal supine sonogram demonstrates a huge mass (W) involving the lower pole of the right kidney and resulting in hydronephrosis of the upper collecting system (Hy). Wilms' tumors tend to have a moderately low internal echogenicity and, as in this patient, often contain multiple tiny cystic spaces. The large mass dramatically displaces the liver.[2]

CYSTIC RENAL MASSES ON COMPUTED TOMOGRAPHY

Condition	Imaging Findings	Comments
Benign renal cyst (Figs GU29-1 and GU29-2)	Sharply delineated, near-water attenuation lesion with a very thin wall, no internal septations, and no contrast enhancement.	Most common unifocal mass of the kidney. A renal cyst may have a high attenuation due to hemorrhage into the cyst, calcification of the cyst wall, infection, leakage of contrast material into the cyst by a communication with the collecting system or by diffusion, or image degradation by high-density streak artifacts.
Parapelvic cyst (Fig GU29-3)	Appearance identical to that of a simple benign renal parenchymal cyst though it is located adjacent to the renal sinus.	May be difficult to distinguish from a dilated or an extrarenal pelvis on nonenhanced scans. After administration of contrast material, the unenhanced parapelvic cyst is easily detected adjacent to contrast-filled hilar collecting structures.
Polycystic kidney disease (Fig GU29-4)	Multiple cysts in lobulated and enlarged kidneys.	Splaying and distortion of the renal collecting system. Hepatic or pancreatic cystic disease can be demonstrated in about one third of patients.
Dysplastic kidney	Entire kidney consists of numerous cystic masses that vary in size.	No functioning renal parenchyma is detectable after administration of contrast material (unlike multilocular cystic nephromas or unilateral polycystic disease).
Multilocular renal cyst	Multiple fluid-filled cysts separated by thick septa and sharply demarcated from normal renal parenchyma.	Rare condition. May contain peripheral or central calcification with a circular, stellate, flocculent, or granular pattern.
Lesions that may mimic renal cyst (Fig GU29-5)	Low-attenuation masses that often have somewhat more irregular margins than a simple cyst.	Necrotic tumor; hematoma; vascular anomaly; urine collections (localized hydronephrosis, urinoma).

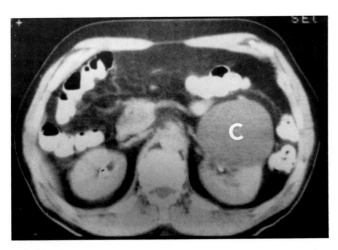

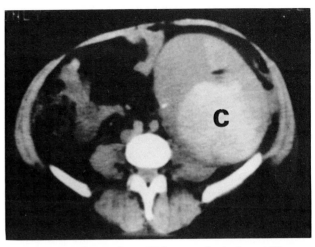

Fig GU29-1. Benign renal cyst. Nonenhancing left renal mass (C) with a sharply marginated border and a thin wall.

Fig GU29-2. Benign renal cyst. High attenuation in the cyst (C) represents hemorrhage.

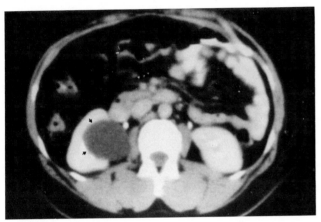

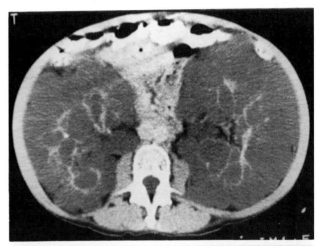

Fig GU29-3. Parapelvic cyst. Well-marginated water-density mass (arrows).

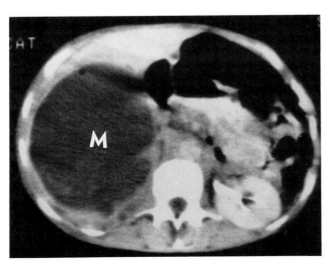

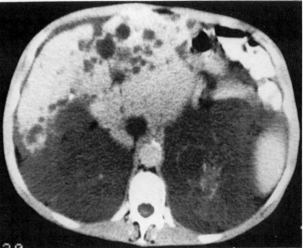

Fig GU29-5. Necrotic renal cell carcinoma. The huge nonenhancing, cystlike mass (M) has irregular margins (especially on its medial and posterior aspects).

Fig GU29-4. Polycystic disease. (Top) Rim of contrast enhancement in the severely thinned renal parenchyma about the innumerable large renal cysts. (Bottom) Scan at a higher level also shows diffuse cystic involvement of the liver.

FOCAL SOLID RENAL MASSES ON COMPUTED TOMOGRAPHY

Condition	Imaging Findings	Comments
Renal cell carcinoma (hypernephroma) (Fig GU30-1)	Renal contour abnormality that is frequently irregularly shaped, poorly demarcated from normal parenchyma, and has an attenuation value near that of normal renal tissue (unlike a simple cyst that is smooth, sharply demarcated, and has a uniform attenuation value near that of water).	After the injection of contrast material, a solid renal neoplasm demonstrates a small but definite increase in density that is probably due primarily to vascular perfusion (unlike a simple cyst, which shows no change in attenuation value). However, this increased density is much less than that of the surrounding normal parenchyma, which also tends to concentrate the contrast material, and thus the renal neoplasm becomes more apparent on contrast-enhanced scans.
Angiomyolipoma (hamartoma) (Figs GU30-2 and GU30-3)	Single or multiple renal masses having zones of different density ranging from -150 H (fat) to $+150$ H (calcification). After contrast injection, portions of the tumor may be enhanced, though fatty tissue in areas of necrosis does not increase in density.	Although the CT diagnosis of angiomyolipoma is highly specific, renal lipoma, liposarcoma, or retroperitoneal liposarcoma invading the kidney cannot be absolutely excluded. If the diagnosis is in doubt, ultrasound can demonstrate the highly echogenic foci characteristic of fat rather than fluid or nonfatty solid tissue.
Renal oncocytoma	Homogeneous mass that is only slightly less dense than renal parenchyma after injection of contrast material. The tumor is sharply separated from the normal cortex and does not invade the calyceal system or adjacent structures.	Rare benign renal tumor thought to originate from proximal tubular epithelial cells. May be impossible to differentiate from a renal adenoma or renal cell carcinoma without additional diagnostic studies (angiography, radionuclide scanning).
Lymphoma (Fig GU30-4)	Various patterns including bilaterally enlarged kidneys without demonstrable masses; multiple focal, nodular, solid masses that have decreased density on postcontrast scans; focal, irregular, solitary, solid intrarenal masses; dilatation of intrarenal collecting structures produced by diffuse interstitial infiltration of the kidneys; and perirenal disease extending into the renal pelvis.	Renal involvement by lymphoma is commonly found at postmortem examination (30% to 50%), but is seldom detected by conventional urographic studies. Multiple parenchymal nodules are by far the most common manifestation of renal lymphoma. Bilateral involvement occurs in about 75% of cases.
Metastases	Solid mass indistinguishable from a primary renal malignancy.	Most commonly from primary tumors of the lung, breast, stomach, colon, cervix, or pancreas. Leukemic infiltration may produce bilateral renal enlargement and intrarenal masses.
Transitional cell carcinoma (Fig GU30-5)	After intravenous injection of contrast material, the tumor appears as a pelvic filling defect with a smooth, lobulated, or irregular margin.	Small pelvic tumors that do not produce hydronephrosis or invade the peripelvic fat are usually not detected on precontrast CT scans.
Wilms' tumor (Figs GU30-6 and GU30-7)	Large, at least partially intrarenal mass that usually has a central density lower than that of normal renal parenchyma while the periphery of the tumor is virtually isodense.	Most common primary malignant renal tumor of childhood. Renal vein thrombosis or tumor extension, which occurs in up to 10% of cases, may be demonstrated as a low-density intraluminal defect after injection of contrast material.

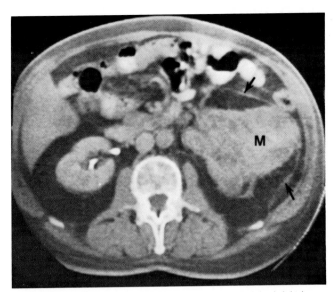

FIG GU30-1. Renal cell carcinoma. Large mass (M) of the left kidney with thickening of Gerota's fascia (arrows).[23]

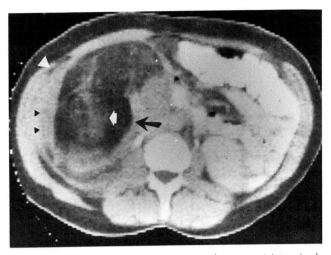

FIG GU30-2. Angiomyolipoma. Fatty mass (long arrow) intermixed with (short arrow) and surrounded by (arrowheads) areas of tissue density, representing intratumoral and perinephric hemorrhage, respectively.[22]

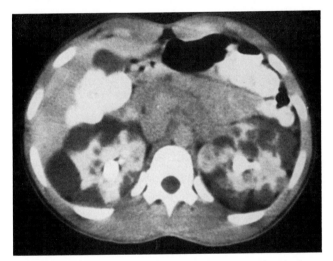

FIG GU30-3. Multiple renal hamartomas in tuberous sclerosis. Innumerable low-attenuation masses in both kidneys.

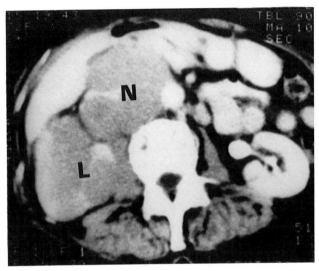

FIG GU30-4. Lymphoma. The right kidney is completely replaced by a lymphomatous mass (L). Note the extensive nodal involvement (N).

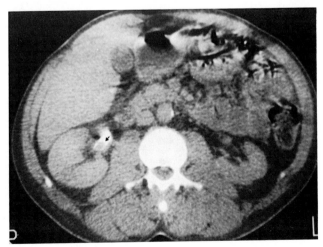

FIG GU30-5. Transitional cell carcinoma. Filling defect (arrow) in the opacified renal pelvis.

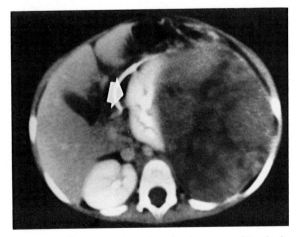

FIG GU30-6. Wilms' tumor. Large low-density mass pushing the functioning portion of the left kidney (arrow) across the midline.

Condition	Imaging Findings	Comments
Infection		
Acute pyelonephritis (focal bacterial nephritis) (Fig GU30-8)	Single or multiple, poorly marginated masses of decreased density.	After injection of contrast material, there may be a characteristic striated appearance of regularly oriented zones of increased density in the affected kidney.
Renal abscess (Fig GU30-9)	Often well-defined mass of decreased density that typically has a thick, irregular wall.	After injection of contrast material, there is a variable pattern of wall enhancement. May be difficult to distinguish from a centrally necrotic renal cell carcinoma.
Xanthogranulomatous pyelonephritis (Fig GU30-10)	Multiple nonenhancing, round areas of decreased attenuation that may be of a characteristic fatty consistency.	Unusual nodular replacement of renal parenchyma by large lipid-filled macrophages (foam cells) that may develop in chronically infected kidneys. Typically a large calculus in the renal pelvis or collecting system and absence of contrast material excretion in the kidney or an area of focal involvement.
Infarction (Fig GU30-11)	Low-attenuation, often wedge-shaped mass.	Frequently a higher attenuation subcapsular rim on contrast-enhanced scans.
Hematoma		
Subcapsular (Fig GU30-12)	Lenticular low-density fluid collection with flattening of the renal parenchyma.	Shortly after injury, a subcapsular hematoma has a higher density than the surrounding kidney because of the fresh extravasation of blood. Follow-up scans show that the hematoma diminishes in intensity as it liquefies.
Intrarenal (Fig GU30-13)	Focal area of decreased attenuation in the kidney.	After injection of contrast material, there is decreased enhancement of the hematoma compared with the normal renal parenchyma.

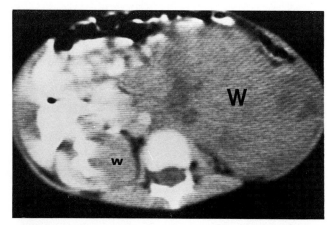

FIG GU30-7. Bilateral Wilms' tumor. Huge left renal mass (W) that crosses the midline. There is also a small separate mass (w) in the right kidney.[2]

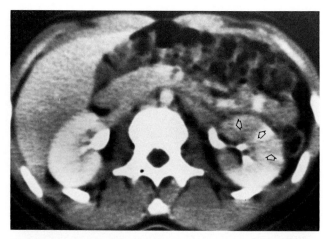

FIG GU30-8. Acute pyelonephritis. Postcontrast scan shows characteristic low-density striations (arrows) in the left kidney.

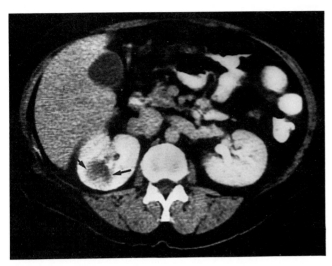

FIG GU30-9. Renal abscess. Contrast-enhanced CT scan through both kidneys demonstrates a discrete low-density area (arrows), which proved to be an abscess on diagnostic needle aspiration.

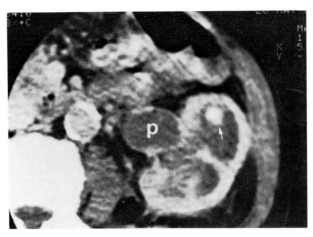

FIG GU30-10. Xanthogranulomatous pyelonephritis. The renal pelvis (p) and intrarenal collecting structures are filled with low-density pus. Note the prolonged opacification of the left renal cortex and the high-density focus (arrow) representing a renal calculus.[24]

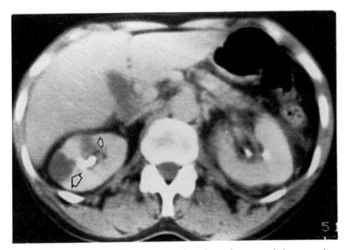

FIG GU30-11. Infarction. Two wedge-shaped areas of decreased attenuation (arrows) in the right kidney.

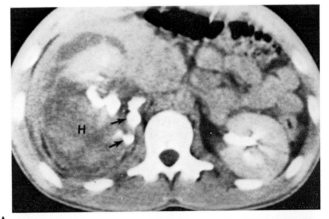

A

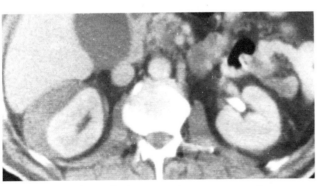

FIG GU30-12. Subcapsular hematoma. Postcontrast scan shows a crescent-shaped extrarenal fluid collection partially encircling and compressing the right kidney. Note that, while the right kidney still remains in the nephrogram phase, contrast material has been excreted into the pelvocalyceal system in the left kidney. The abnormally prolonged nephrogram is due to compression of the right kidney by the subcapsular hematoma.[23]

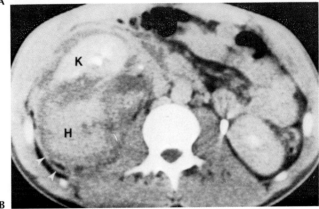

B

FIG GU30-13. Renal trauma. (A) Postcontrast CT scan demonstrates a large hematourinoma (H) from a fracture through the midpole of the right kidney. Extravasation of contrast material (arrows) is seen. (B) On a scan 2 cm more caudal, there is a large hematoma (H) with thickening of the renal fascia (arrowheads). The remaining normal right kidney (K) is displaced anteriorly by the hematoma.[23]

INCREASED RENAL CORTICAL ECHOGENICITY WITH PRESERVATION OF MEDULLARY SONOLUCENCY (TYPE I LESIONS)*

Condition	Comments
Renal parenchymal disease (Figs GU31-1 and GU31-2)	Acute and chronic glomerulonephritis; systemic lupus erythematosus; nephrosclerosis; diabetic nephropathy; acute tubular necrosis; renal cortical necrosis; Alport's syndrome; renal transplant rejection.
Deposition disorders	Amyloidosis; leukemic infiltration.
Diffuse nephrocalcinosis	Deposition of calcium salts, primarily in the renal cortex, causes diffuse high echogenicity of this region. If the calcification is predominantly medullary, there is a reversed pattern with the medulla appearing extremely echogenic.
Normal variant	Corticomedullary differentiation is exaggerated in normal kidneys when there is enhanced amplification of echoes due to passage of the sound beam through a medium of low attenuation between the kidney and the transducer (eg, fluid-filled gallbladder, ascites, or cystic mass anterior to the liver).

*Pattern: Exaggeration of the normal separation between cortex and medulla. Increased renal parenchymal echogenicity correlates with the degree of interstitial (not glomerular) change and the deposition of collagen or calcium.

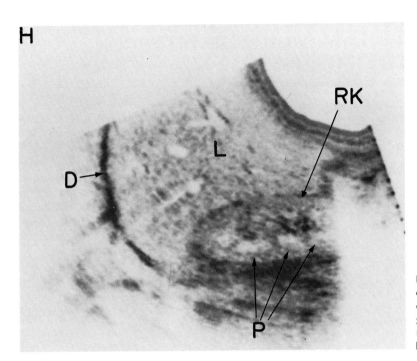

Fɪɢ GU31-1. Chronic renal failure. Parasagittal sonogram of the right kidney (RK) shows that the echogenicity of renal cortical tissue has increased to such an extent that it is now greater than that of the hepatic parenchyma (L). The renal medullary pyramids (P) are clearly visible in the right kidney. (H, head and D, diaphragm)[2]

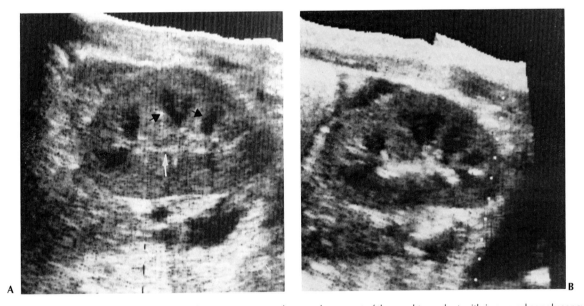

Fɪɢ GU31-2. Renal transplant rejection. (A) Sagittal supine sonogram shows enlargement of the renal transplant with increased sonolucency of the medullary pyramids (black arrows) and thinning of the central echogenic hilar structures (white arrow). (B) Another patient with markedly dilated medullary pyramids of an enlarged renal allograft.[25]

FOCAL OR DIFFUSE DISTORTION OF NORMAL RENAL ANATOMY AND ELIMINATION OF CORTICOMEDULLARY DEFINITION (TYPE II LESIONS)

Condition	Comments
Focal acute bacterial nephritis (lobar nephronia) (Fig GU32-1)	Inflammatory infiltrate appears as a renal mass displacing adjacent calyces. It is more lucent than renal cortical tissue and may be difficult to differentiate from an abscess. Unlike an abscess, focal acute bacterial nephritis does not have accentuation of the far wall, does not contain shifting debris, and lacks a sharp or rounded contour. After appropriate antibiotic therapy there is rapid resolution of the process (an abscess cavity tends to persist).
Chronic atrophic pyelonephritis (Fig GU32-2)	Focal increase in echoes (representing parenchymal scarring) in the involved area of the cortex and medulla.
Healing renal infarct	Focal increase in echoes (representing parenchymal scarring) in the involved area of the cortex and medulla.
Infantile polycystic kidney disease	Generalized increase in parenchymal echoes with loss of corticomedullary definition (can even be diagnosed in utero by means of these criteria).
Congenital hepatic fibrosis with tubular ectasia	Nephromegaly with generalized increase in parenchymal echoes and loss of corticomedullary definition. Usually associated with high-level echoes in the liver representing hepatic fibrosis.
End-stage renal disease (Figs GU32-3 and GU32-4)	Some renal parenchymal disorders originally classified as type I can occur as type II abnormalities late in the course of the disease when the kidney is small and demonstrates high-intensity echoes throughout its substance (making differentiation between cortex and medulla no longer possible).

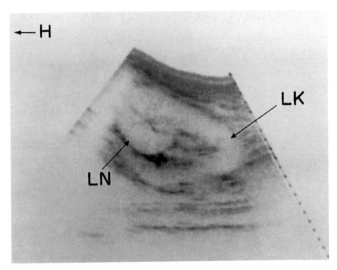

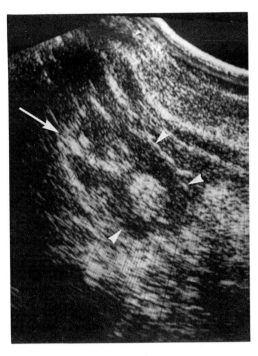

FIG GU32-1. Focal acute bacterial nephritis. Prone parasagittal sonogram of the left kidney (LK) demonstrates acute focal bacterial nephritis (LN) as focal prominence of the renal parenchyma with poor definition of medullary pyramids in the upper pole.[2]

FIG GU32-2. Chronic atrophic pyelonephritis. Prone sonogram of the kidney (arrowheads) shows a focal loss of renal parenchyma and extension of the calyces peripherally from the renal sinus to the renal margin. Note the associated focal area of increased echogenicity due to fibrosis (arrow) in the upper pole.[11]

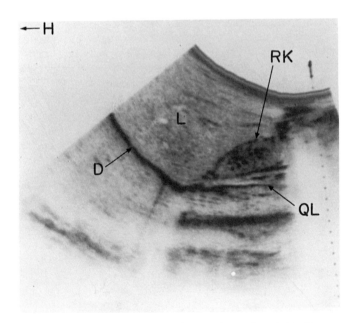

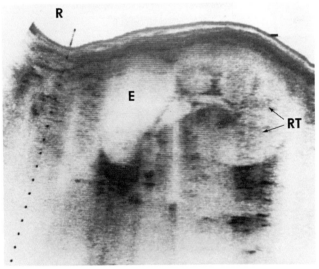

FIG GU32-3. Renal failure due to chronic glomerulonephritis. Parasagittal sonogram demonstrates a tiny right kidney (RK) with marked thinning of the renal parenchyma. The echogenicity of the renal tissue greatly exceeds that of the adjacent liver (L). The medullary pyramids are no longer distinguishable. Scans of the left kidney showed similar findings. (H, head; D, diaphragm; QL, quadratus lumborum muscle)[2]

FIG GU32-4. Renal transplant rejection. Transverse sonogram shows that the renal transplant (RT) has become huge and has lost its corticomedullary definition. The renal vascular pedicle is compressed as it enters the renal hilum. An effusion (E), sometimes seen with acute transplant rejection, is noted medial to the kidney.[2]

FLUID COLLECTIONS AROUND THE TRANSPLANTED KIDNEY

Condition	Imaging Findings	Comments
Lymphocele **(Fig GU33-1)**	Well-defined cystic area that often contains numerous internal septations.	Localized accumulation of lymph in the extraperitoneal space that occurs either as a result of interruption of the recipient's lymphatics or secondary to leakage of lymph from the surface of the transplanted kidney. Lymphocele is the most common type of extraurinary fluid collection, seen in 1% to 15% of renal transplant patients. Generally a late complication in patients who have had a prior episode of graft rejection.
Urinoma **(Fig GU33-2)**	Purely cystic extraurinary fluid collection. Often accompanied by hydronephrosis secondary to compression of the ureter. Rarely contains internal septations.	Early posttransplant complication that develops because of extravasation from the collecting system. The urinary leak may result from poor surgical technique at the ureteroneocystostomy site or ureteral necrosis due to a compromised blood supply, or it may be a manifestation of ureteral graft rejection. Radionuclide demonstration of a urinary leak confirms the diagnosis.
Abscess **(Fig GU33-3)**	Complex mass that typically contains numerous internal echoes (caused by septa and debris) and has relatively poorly defined borders (inflammation and edema around the lesion). Debris in an abscess may shift with changes in patient position.	Early complication that produces unexplained postoperative fever. Increased isotope uptake on ^{67}Ga scintigraphy confirms the presence of an abscess, though a false-positive scan may be produced by wound healing or rejection.
Hematoma **(Fig GU33-4)**	Acute hematoma produces a well-defined, hypoechoic or anechoic extraurinary fluid collection. An old hematoma appears as a complex mass containing echogenic and cystic components (may be difficult to distinguish from an abscess).	Small, clinically insignificant hematomas are frequently seen in the immediate postoperative period. A large hematoma may develop because of graft rupture or injury to the vascular pedicle of the transplanted kidney.

R

RT

Ly

Ca

Ca

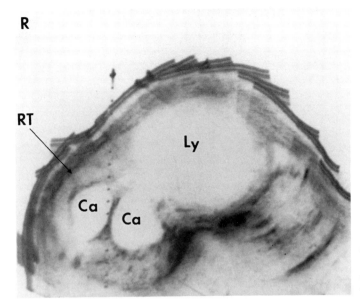

FIG GU33-1. Lymphocele. Transverse sonogram of the right iliac fossa shows a large lymphocele (Ly) obstructing the transplanted kidney (RT) and causing gross dilatation of the calyces (Ca) and slight thinning of the overlying renal parenchyma. A small amount of ascites is seen adjacent to the lymphocele.[2]

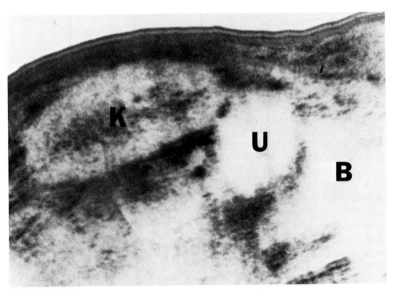

K

U

B

FIG GU33-2. Urinoma. Longitudinal sonogram shows the cystic fluid collection (U) separate from the kidney (K) and bladder (B).[26]

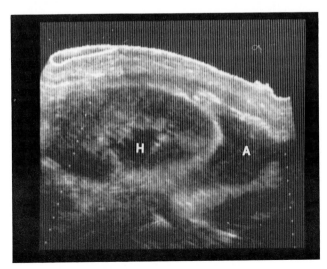

FIG GU33-3. Abscess. Complex mass with internal echoes (A) adjacent to the transplanted kidney. Note the hydronephrosis (H).

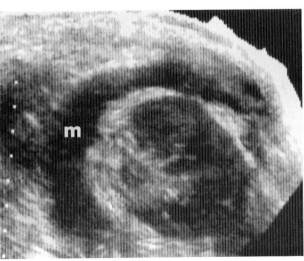

FIG GU33-4. Hematoma. Hypoechoic fluid collection (m) about the transplanted kidney.

ADRENAL MASSES ON COMPUTED TOMOGRAPHY

Condition	Imaging Findings	Comments
Cushing's syndrome **Functioning cortical adenoma** **(Fig GU34-1)**	Solid mass that may have a low attenuation value due to a high lipid content.	Found in 10% to 15% of patients with Cushing's syndrome. May be impossible to differentiate from adrenal carcinoma (found in about 5% of patients with Cushing's syndrome).
Adrenal hyperplasia **(Fig GU34-2)**	Diffuse, bilateral adrenal enlargement with preservation of shape (may have a nodular component).	Associated CT findings in patients with Cushing's syndrome are an abnormally low attenuation value of the liver resulting from hepatic fat deposition and an increase in retroperitoneal and subcutaneous fat.
Aldosteronoma **(Fig GU34-3)**	Contour abnormality (often small). Often contains a large amount of fat that produces a low attenuation value.	Aldosteronomas tend to be much smaller than the large cortical adenomas in patients with Cushing's syndrome. Low-attenuation tumors may be difficult to distinguish from retroperitoneal fat.
Carcinoma **(Figs GU34-4 and GU34-5)**	Often bilateral solid masses that frequently contain low-density areas resulting from necrosis or prior hemorrhage.	Usually grows slowly and can become extremely large before producing symptoms. Because lymphatic and hepatic metastases are common at the time of initial presentation, CT scans at multiple abdominal levels should be performed before a resection is attempted.
Metastases **(Fig GU34-6)**	Masses of soft-tissue density that vary considerably in size and are frequently bilateral.	Common site of metastatic disease (especially from primary tumors of the lung, breast, thyroid, colon, and melanoma). May appear nonhomogeneous or even cystic if tumor necrosis has occurred.
Nonfunctioning adenoma **(Fig GU34-7)**	Unilateral mass that may be large.	Usually cannot be distinguished from carcinoma or metastases unless there is evidence of direct tumor extension into adjacent organs.
Myelolipoma/adenolipoma	Well-circumscribed mass that has an attenuation value in the range of fat and frequently contains areas of calcification.	Rare tumors that may be indistinguishable from cortical adenomas and aldosteronomas, which also can have low attenuation values as a result of their high fat content.
Pheochromocytoma **(Figs GU34-8 to GU34-10)**	Usually a unilateral (10% are bilateral) adrenal mass of soft-tissue density. May have an attenuation value less than that of liver or renal parenchyma and simulate a thick-walled cystic lesion.	If the adrenal glands are normal despite strong clinical suspicion of a pheochromocytoma, the rest of the abdomen and pelvis should be examined to detect the approximately 10% of tumors that are ectopic. The examination may be expanded to the neck and chest if the abdomen and pelvis are normal.

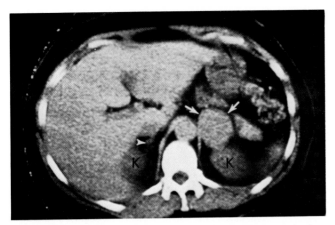

FIG GU34-1. **Cushing's syndrome** due to functioning cortical adenoma. A 4-cm mass in the left adrenal gland (arrows) is seen posterior to the tail of the pancreas and anterior to the kidney (K). The arrowhead points to the normal right adrenal gland.[23]

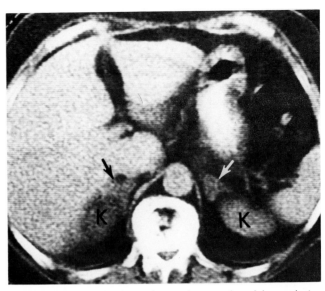

FIG GU34-2. **Cushing's syndrome** due to adrenal hyperplasia. Although the adrenal glands are enlarged (arrows), their normal configuration is maintained. (K, kidneys)[23]

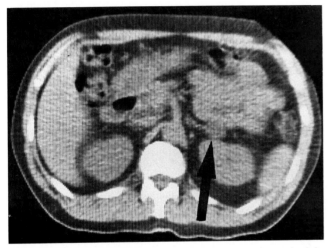

FIG GU34-3. **Aldosteronoma.** Small mass (arrow) anterior to the left kidney.

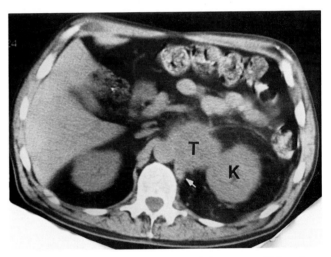

FIG GU34-4. **Adrenal carcinoma.** Large soft-tissue tumor (T) invading the anteromedial aspect of the left kidney (K) and left crus of the diaphragm (arrow).[27]

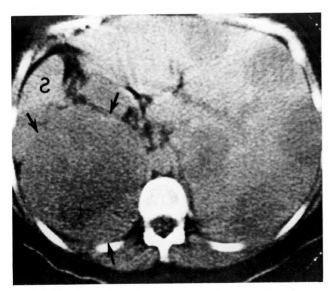

FIG GU34-5. **Adrenal carcinoma** causing adrenogenital syndrome. Large mass in the left upper quadrant (arrows) displacing the spleen (S) anteriorly. Multiple round metastases are present in the liver.[28]

Condition	Imaging Findings	Comments
Neuroblastoma	Soft-tissue or fatty mass that often contains calcification and may have cystic components.	Computed tomography can detect calcification that is not readily apparent on conventional radiography. It also can easily demonstrate hepatic, skeletal, and pulmonary metastases for accurate staging as well as assess the response to treatment and detect recurrent disease.
Adrenal cyst	Rounded, low-density mass. Rim of calcification occurs in about 15% of cases.	Most commonly a pseudocyst, which results from degenerative necrosis and hemorrhage into an adrenal mass. Other types of cysts include parasitic, epithelial, and endothelial (lymphangiectatic, angiomatous, and hamartomatous).

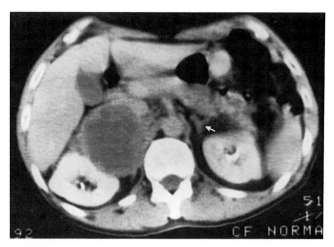

FIG GU34-6. Metastases. Huge irregular low-attenuation mass representing an adrenal metastasis from oat cell carcinoma of the lung. The left adrenal gland (arrow) is normal.

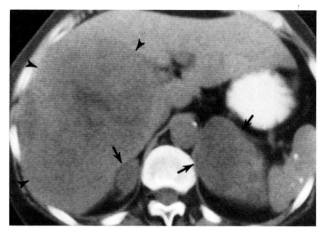

FIG GU34-7. Metastases. Bilateral adrenal metastases (arrows) in a patient with colonic carcinoma. A large liver metastasis (arrowheads) is also present.[23]

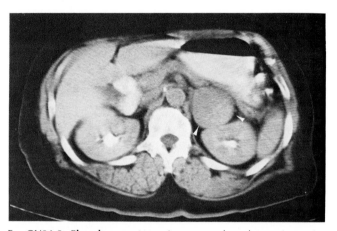

FIG GU34-8. Pheochromocytoma. Large pear-shaped mass (arrows) anterior to the left kidney.

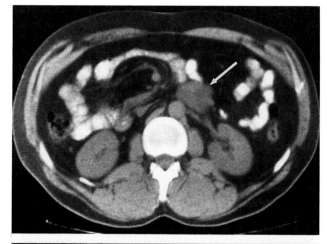

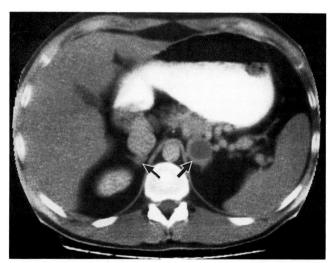

FIG GU34-9. Bilateral pheochromocytomas (arrows). The left adrenal lesion shows peripheral contrast enhancement and a low-density center, producing an appearance simulating that of a thick-walled cystic mass. The patient also had medullary thyroid carcinoma (multiple endocrine neoplasia type II).[29]

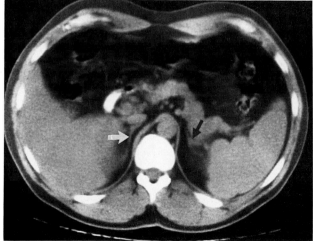

FIG GU34-10. Ectopic pheochromocytoma. (Top) Soft-tissue mass (arrow) adjacent to the aorta and in front of the left renal vein. (Bottom) Scan taken at a higher level demonstrates that both the right and the left adrenal glands are normal (arrows).[29]

CYSTIC-APPEARING PELVIC MASS

Condition	Comments
Physiologic ovarian cyst (**Fig GU35-1**)	Follicular cysts (unruptured, enlarged graafian follicles) and corpus luteum cysts (occur after continued hemorrhage or lack of resolution of the corpus luteum). Most common in the female infant and in women of childbearing age.
Paraovarian cyst	Arises from remnants of the wolffian duct system, which courses within the mesovarium. Like ovarian epithelial tumors and endometriomas, paraovarian cysts do not demonstrate the cyclical regression and growth associated with physiologic ovarian cysts.
Hydrosalpinx (**Fig GU35-2**)	Unilateral or bilateral dilatation of the fallopian tubes that develops as a consequence of tubal adhesions secondary to pelvic inflammatory disease. Massive tubal distension may produce an appearance indistinguishable from that of other large cystic adnexal masses.
Serous cystadenoma (**Fig GU35-3**)	Benign ovarian tumor. May contain an occasional septum.
Endometrioma (**Fig GU35-4**)	Endometriosis can produce a broad spectrum of ultrasound appearances, one of which is an almost completely sonolucent mass.
Hydrocolpos (**Figs GU35-5 and GU35-6**)	Large, tubular, midline retrovesical mass in a newborn girl with an imperforate hymen. Retained secretions and cellular debris may produce internal echoes. If not discovered in the newborn period, the genital tract obstruction tends to go unnoticed until menarche, when it becomes a hematometrocolpos.

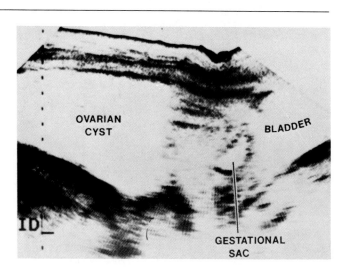

FIG GU35-1. **Physiologic ovarian cyst.** Longitudinal midline section shows a large ovarian cyst superior to the uterus, which contains a gestational sac.[6]

A B

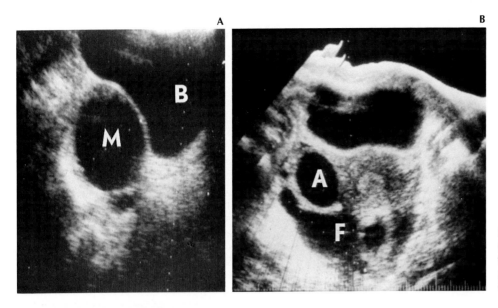

FIG GU35-2. **Tubo-ovarian abscess.** (A) Large sonolucent mass (M) posterior to the bladder (B). (B) In another patient, there is fluid in the cul-de-sac (F) posterior to the cystic abscess (A).

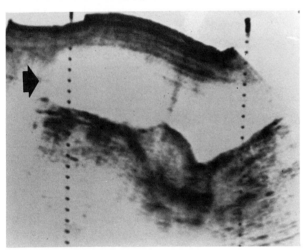

FIG GU35-3. **Serous cystadenoma.** Longitudinal sonogram in an asymptomatic girl demonstrates a large, sonolucent, completely cystic mass.[30]

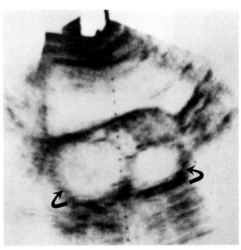

FIG GU35-4. **Endometrioma.** Several sonolucent masses (arrows), simulating multiple follicular cysts, arising from the ovary.[30]

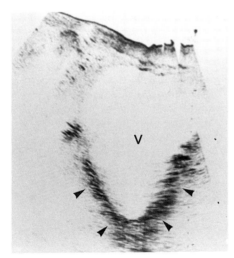

FIG GU35-5. **Hydrocolpos.** Postvoiding midsagittal sonogram of a newborn girl shows a large cystic area (V) with good through-transmission of sound (arrowheads).[31]

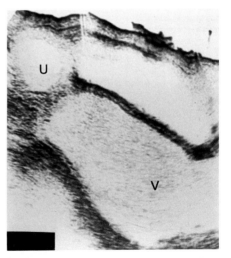

FIG GU35-6. **Hematometrocolpos.** Longitudinal pelvic sonogram in a 15-year-old girl with primary amenorrhea and pain demonstrates marked distension of the vagina (V) and uterus (U).[31]

COMPLEX PELVIC MASSES

Condition	Comments
Cystadenocarcinoma/ mucinous cystadenoma (Fig GU36-1)	Typically appears as a large cystic mass with well-defined internal septa. The number and arrangement of the internal septa do not appear to correlate with whether the mass is benign or malignant. In general, however, the more solid and irregular the areas in the mass, the more likely that it represents a malignant tumor. Other findings suggesting underlying malignancy include ascites, hepatic metastases (usually relatively hypoechoic masses in the liver), and peritoneal implants.
Dermoid cyst (Fig GU36-2)	Complex, predominantly solid mass containing high-level echoes arising from hair or calcification in the mass. This highly echogenic nature may make it difficult to delineate the mass completely or to distinguish it from surrounding gas-containing loops of bowel. As with other ovarian tumors, the more irregular and solid the internal components of the mass, the more likely that it is malignant.
Endometrioma	May appear as a predominantly cystic mass with some thickness or irregularity of the wall and a variable amount of solid internal components related to clot formation and retraction, fibrosis, and liquefaction.
Tubo-ovarian abscess (Fig GU36-3)	Complex adnexal mass that often has a thick and irregular wall or contains echoes or fluid levels representing the layering of purulent debris. Free pelvic fluid suggests superimposed peritonitis. The free fluid may become loculated into a peritoneal abscess, especially in the cul de sac (the most dependent portion of the peritoneal space in the supine patient). Some abscesses have a very echogenic appearance due to small gas bubbles produced by gas-forming organisms.
Ectopic pregnancy (Figs GU36-4 to GU36-6)	Extrauterine, extraovarian adnexal mass. More than 95% of ectopic pregnancies occur in the fallopian tubes, especially the isthmic and ampullary portions. More than half the patients with this complication of pregnancy have a history or pathologic evidence of pelvic inflammatory disease, which appears to provide an environment receptive to tubal implantation. Often associated with urine or plasma levels of human chorionic gonadotropin (HCG) that are substantially lower for the expected date of gestation than those in patients with normal intrauterine pregnancies. The classic ultrasound appearance consists of an enlarged uterus that does not contain a gestational sac and is associated with an irregular adnexal mass, an "ectopic fetal head," or fluid in the cul-de-sac. The incidence of coexisting ectopic and intrauterine pregnancies is only 1 in 30,000.

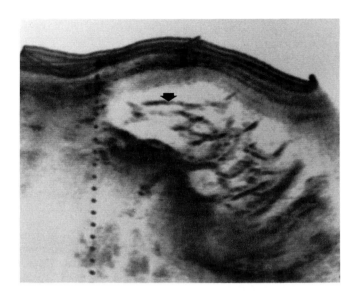

Fig GU36-1. Cystadenoma. Longitudinal sonogram demonstrates a complex, predominantly cystic mass containing several thin and well-defined septations (arrow), an appearance characteristic of mucinous cystadenoma.[30]

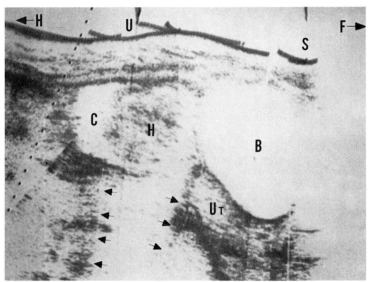

Fig GU36-2. Dermoid cyst. Longitudinal sonogram demonstrates a mass containing fluid and hair (H). Note the characteristic acoustic shadow (between arrows) cast by the hair. (C, cyst; B, bladder; Ut, uterus; S, symphysis pubis; U, umbilicus; H, head; F, feet)

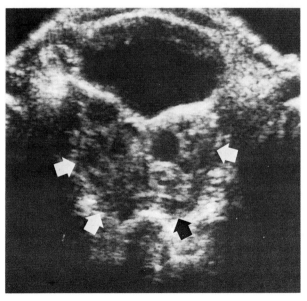

Fig GU36-3. Chronic pelvic inflammatory disease. Transverse sonogram demonstrates large, complex cystic and echogenic masses (arrows).[30]

Condition	Comments
Hemorrhagic corpus luteum cyst	Complex adnexal mass that may be associated with intraperitoneal blood if rupture has occurred. May be extremely difficult to distinguish from ectopic pregnancy, though in most cases the complex mass can be shown to be located within the ovary rather than separate from both the uterus and the ovary, as in an ectopic pregnancy. Corpus luteum cysts may be associated with early intrauterine pregnancies and elevated levels of human chorionic gonadotropin.

A

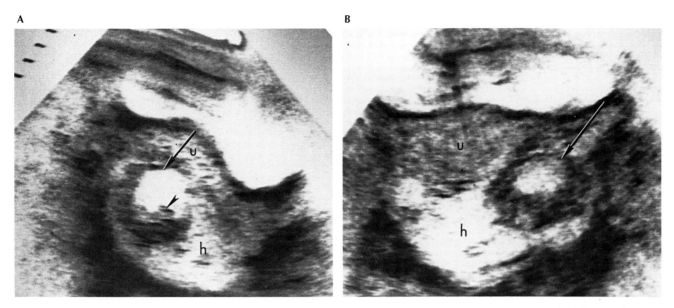

B

FIG GU36-4. Ectopic pregnancy. (A) Sagittal and (B) transverse sonograms show an extrauterine gestational sac (arrow) on the left with a fetus in it (arrowhead). Note the complex cystic mass (h), which represents a hematoma, in the cul de sac. No fetal heart activity was noted. (U, uterus).[32]

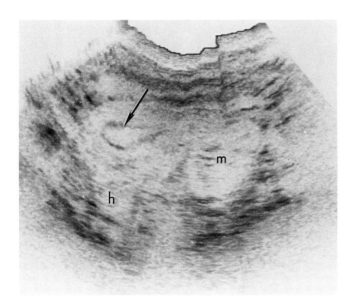

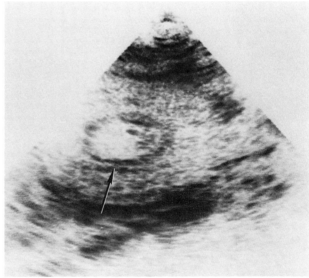

FIG GU36-5. Pseudogestational sac in ectopic pregnancy. Transverse sonogram shows a saclike structure with no fetal pole (arrow) in the uterus. There is also a solid collection in the cul de sac (h) and a left adnexal mass (m).[32]

FIG GU36-6. Double decidual sac in ectopic pregnancy. Transverse sonogram shows a second line (arrow) parallel to a portion of the decidual sac.[32]

SOLID PELVIC MASSES

Condition	Comments
Leiomyoma (fibroid) of the uterus (Figs GU37-1 and GU37-2)	Hypoechoic, solid, contour-deforming mass in an enlarged, inhomogeneous uterus. Fatty degeneration and calcification cause focal increased echogenicity (calcification may result in acoustic shadowing). Degeneration or necrosis may result in decreased echogenicity and increased through-transmission of sound, sometimes simulating a cystlike mass. A subserosal leiomyoma attached to the uterus by a large stalk may occasionally simulate an adnexal mass or ovarian tumor.
Leiomyosarcoma of the uterus	May arise from a pre-existing leiomyoma or from muscle or connective tissue in the myometrium or blood vessels. Although less than 0.2% of all leiomyomas undergo sarcomatous change, leiomyosarcoma is a not uncommon uterine tumor because of the frequency of leiomyomas. The tumor may be too small to be seen on ultrasound or may be indistinguishable from a benign leiomyoma.
Endometrial carcinoma (Fig GU37-3)	Enlarged uterus with irregular areas of low-level echoes and bizarre clusters of high-intensity echoes. Unless evidence of local invasion can be demonstrated, the ultrasound findings are indistinguishable from those of fibroid tumors (which often occur in patients with endometrial carcinoma).
Cervical carcinoma (Fig GU37-4)	Solid retrovesical mass that usually appears indistinguishable from a benign cervical myoma. Ultrasound is of value in staging cervical carcinoma since it may detect thickening of parametrial or paracervical soft tissues, involvement of the pelvic side walls, extension into the bladder, and pelvic adenopathy.
Ovarian tumors (Fig GU37-5)	Carcinoma and dysgerminoma appear as solid pelvic masses of various sizes.
Trophoblastic disease (Fig GU37-6)	Spectrum of pregnancy-related disorders ranging from a benign hydatidiform mole to the more malignant and frequently metastatic choriocarcinoma. Typically appears as a large, soft-tissue solid mass of placental (trophoblastic) tissue filling the uterine cavity and containing echoes of low to moderate amplitude. Numerous small cystic fluid-containing spaces are scattered throughout the lesion. Multiple larger sonolucent areas represent degeneration or internal hemorrhage in the molar tissue.

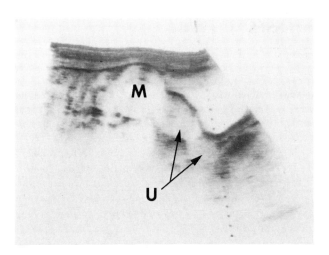

FIG GU37-1. **Uterine fibroid.** Longitudinal sonogram demonstrates a pedunculated leiomyoma as a hypoechoic mass (M) projecting from the fundus of the uterus (U). Decreased sound transmission through the mass indicates its solid nature.[30]

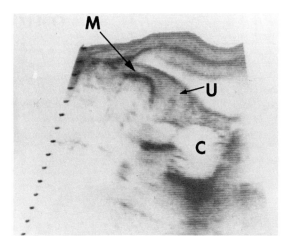

FIG GU37-2. **Calcified uterine fibroid.** Longitudinal sonogram shows the calcification as a high-amplitude echo (M) in the uterus (U), with resultant acoustic shadowing. Incidentally noted is a cystic adnexal mass (C).[30]

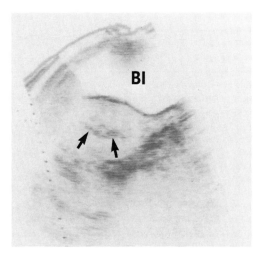

FIG GU37-3. **Endometrial carcinoma.** Longitudinal sonogram shows the uterus to be enlarged and bulbous. There are clusters of high-amplitude echoes (arrows) in the region of the central cavity echo. (BI, bladder)[30]

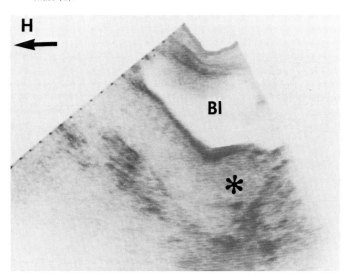

FIG GU37-4. **Carcinoma of the cervix.** Solid, echogenic retrovesical mass (*) that is indistinguishable from a cervical myoma. (BI, bladder)[30]

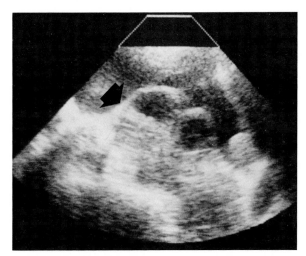

FIG GU37-5. **Mucinous cystadenocarcinoma of the ovary.** Predominantly solid mass with some cystic components and associated ascites.[30]

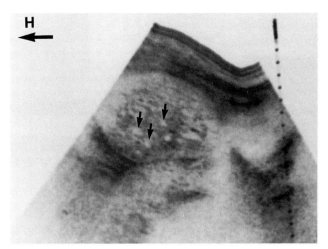

FIG GU37-6. **Hydatidiform mole.** Longitudinal sonogram in a patient in the second trimester demonstrates a large, moderately echogenic mass filling the central uterine cavity. Note the numerous small cystic spaces (arrows) that represent the markedly hydropic chorionic villi.[30]

FLUID COLLECTION IN THE SCROTUM

Condition	Imaging Findings	Comments
Hydrocele (Fig GU38-1)	Echo-free zone with strong posterior sound transmission. The wall shows various degrees of thickness and may contain calcific deposits. The underlying testis is well visualized and is smoothly surrounded by fluid, except on its posterior surface where the testis is attached to the epididymis.	Abnormal accumulation of serous fluid between the tunica vaginalis and its contents. May be congenital (because of a direct communication with the abdominal cavity as a result of failure of the processus vaginalis to close) or secondary to an adjacent disease process (epididymitis, tuberculosis, trauma, mumps). Septations in a hydrocele suggest hemorrhage or infection. Internal echoes represent fibrous bodies that originate from a detached villous projection or from the tunica vaginalis.
Varicocele (Fig GU38-2)	Tubular, serpiginous, anechoic fluid collection in the region of the epididymis just proximal to the upper pole of the testicle. The multicystic pattern reflects the bag-of-worms appearance of a varicocele on physical examination.	Dilatation and tortuosity of the veins of the pampiniform plexus that is most commonly observed on the left side of the scrotum. Primary varicoceles are predominantly seen in young boys. Secondary varicoceles usually result from obstruction of the renal vein, spermatic vein, or inferior vena cava.
Spermatocele	Echo-free fluid collection that can be differentiated from a hydrocele because of its anatomic location (a spermatocele is located in the epididymis and displaces the testicle anteriorly, while a hydrocele usually surrounds the testicle anteriorly).	Retention cyst of small tubules that originates at the head of the epididymis and is often bilateral. Echogenic material in a spermatocele may represent sediment composed of cellular debris, fat, or spermatozoa.
Cyst	Anechoic, well-defined structure with a sharp wall and good through-transmission of sound.	Testicular cysts are more common than previously believed and are often detected as an incidental finding. May be congenital or posttraumatic, though the precise etiology is unclear. Epididymal cysts are secondary to intrinsic cystic dilatation of the epididymal tubules and are filled with serous fluid.

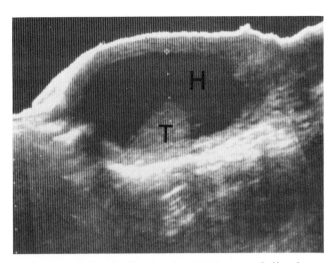

FIG GU38-1. Hydrocele. The normal testis (T) is surrounded by a large, anechoic hydrocele (H).

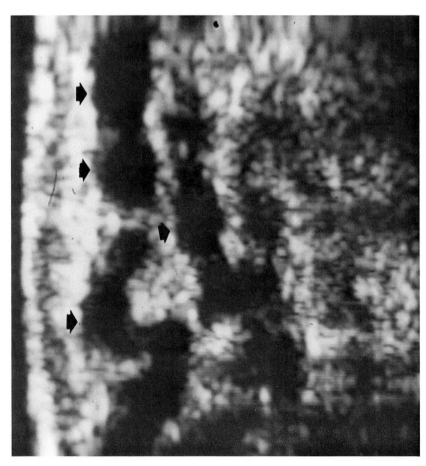

FIG GU38-2. Varicocele. Tortuous, echo-free tubular structures (arrows) are in the anatomic configuration of the spermatic vein. (The skin surface is to the left; the head is toward the top).[33]

SOURCES

1. Reprinted with permission from ''The Cortical Rim Sign in Renal Infarction'' by GJ Paul and TF Stephenson, *Radiology* (1977;122:338), Copyright © 1977, Radiological Society of North America Inc.

2. Reprinted from *Uroradiology: An Integrated Approach* by GW Friedland et al (Eds) with permission of Churchill Livingstone Inc, © 1983.

3. Reprinted with permission from ''Genitourinary Tuberculosis'' by AK Tonkin and DM Witten, *Seminars in Roentgenology* (1979;14: 305–318), Copyright © 1979, Grune & Stratton Inc.

4. Reprinted from *Radiologic Diagnosis of Renal Parenchymal Disease* by AJ Davidson with permission of WB Saunders Company, © 1977.

5. Reprinted with permission from ''Polycystic Kidney Disease'' by MA Bosniak and MA Ambos, *Seminars in Roentgenology* (1975;10: 133–143), Copyright © 1975, Grune & Stratton Inc.

6. Reprinted from *Radiographic Atlas of the Genitourinary System* by C Ney and RM Friedenberg with permission of JB Lippincott Company, © 1981.

7. Reprinted with permission from ''The Thick-Wall Sign: An Important Finding in Nephrotomography'' by MA Bosniak and D Faegenburg, *Radiology* (1965;84:692–698), Copyright © 1965, Radiological Society of North America Inc.

8. Reprinted with permission from ''The Radiology of Juxta-glomerular Tumors'' by NR Dunnick et al, *Radiology* (1983;147: 321–326), Copyright © 1983, Radiological Society of North America Inc.

9. Reprinted with permission from ''The Radiological Diagnosis of Congenital Multicystic Kidney: 'Radiological Triad'" by M Kyaw, *Clinical Radiology* (1974;25:45–62), Copyright © 1974, Royal College of Radiologists.

10. Reprinted with permission from ''Early Medullary Cystic Disease'' by FA Burgener and RF Spataro, *Radiology* (1979;130:321–322), Copyright © 1979, Radiological Society of North America Inc.

11. Reprinted with permission from ''Ultrasonic Characteristic of Chronic Atophic Pyelonephritis'' by CJ Kay et al, *American Journal of Roentgenology* (1979;132:47–53), Copyright © 1979, Williams & Wilkins Company.

12. Reprinted with permission from ''Diagnostic Value of CT Numbers in Pelvocalyceal Filling Defects'' by RA Parienty et al, *Radiology* (1982; 145:743–747), Copyright © 1982, Radiological Society of North America Inc.

13. Reprinted with permission from ''The 'Stipple Sign': Urographic Harbinger of Transitional Cell Neoplasms'' by GK McLean, HM Pollack, and MP Banner, *Urologic Radiology* (1979;1:77–83), Copyright © 1979, Springer-Verlag.

14. Reprinted with permission from ''Fungus Balls in the Renal Pelvis'' by RA Boldus, RC Brown, and DA Culp, *Radiology* (1972;102:555–557), Copyright © 1972, Radiological Society of North America Inc.

15. Reprinted with permission from ''Renal Vein Thrombosis: Occurrence in Membranous Glomerulonephropathy and Lupus Nephritis'' by WG Bradley et al, *Radiology* (1981;139:571–576), Copyright © 1981, Radiological Society of North America Inc.

16. Reprinted from *Clinical Urography* by DM Witten, GH Myers, and BC Utz with permission of WB Saunders Company, © 1977.

17. Reprinted with permission from ''Malakoplakia of the Urinary Tract'' by GB Elliott, PJ Moloney, and JG Clement, *American Journal of Roentgenology* (1972;116:830–837), Copyright © 1972, Williams & Wilkins Company.

18. Reprinted with permission from ''Lateral Ureteral Displacement: Sign of Nonvisualized Duplication'' by AD Amar, *Journal of Urology* (1971;105:638–641), Copyright © 1971, Williams & Wilkins Company.

19. Reprinted with permission from ''The Radiology of Urinary Diversions'' by MP Banner et al, *Radiographics* (1984;4:885–913), Copyright © 1984, Radiological Society of North America Inc.

20. Reprinted from *Radiology of the Urinary System* by M Elkin with permission of Little, Brown & Company, © 1980.

21. Reprinted with permission from ''Posterior Urethral Valves'' by GW Friedland et al, *Clinical Radiology* (1976;27:367–373), Copyright © 1976, Royal College of Radiologists.

22. Reprinted with permission from ''Angiomyolipoma: Ultrasonic-Pathologic Correlation'' by DS Hartman et al, *Radiology* (1981;139: 451–458), Copyright © 1981, Radiological Society of North America Inc.

23. Reprinted from *Computed Body Tomography* by JKT Lee, SS Sagel, and RJ Stanley (Eds) with permission of Raven Press, New York, © 1983.

24. Reprinted from *Computed Tomography of the Body* by AA Moss, G Gamsu, and HK Genant (Eds) with permission of WB Saunders Company, © 1983.

25. Reprinted with permission from ''Renal Ultrasound: Test Your Interpretation'' by RL Eisenberg et al, *Radiographics* (1982;2:153–178), Copyright © 1982, Radiological Society of North America Inc.

26. Reprinted with permission from ''Postoperative Urological Complications of Renal Transplantation'' by R Kumar, DD Wilson, FR Santa-Cruz, *Radiographics* (1984;3:531–547), Copyright © 1984, Radiological Society of North America Inc.

27. Reprinted from *Diagnostic Imaging in Internal Medicine* by RL Eisenberg with permission of McGraw-Hill Book Company, © 1985. Courtesy of Nolan Karstaedt, MD, and Neil Wolfman, MD.

28. Reprinted with permission from ''Computed Tomography of the Adrenal Gland'' by N Karstaedt et al, *Radiology* (1978;129:723–730), Copyright © 1978, Radiological Society of North America Inc.

29. Reprinted with permission from ''Pheochromocytoma: Value of Computed Tomography'' by TJ Welch et al, *Radiology* (1983;148: 501–503), Copyright © 1983, Radiological Society of North America Inc.

30. Reprinted from *Ultrasonography in Obstetrics and Gynecology* by PW Callen (Ed) with permission of WB Saunders Company, © 1983.

31. Reprinted with permission from ''Pediatric Gynecologic Radiology'' by CK Grimes, DM Rosenbaum, and JA Kirkpatrick, *Seminars in Roentgenology* (1982;17:284–301), Copyright © 1982, Grune & Stratton Inc.

32. Reprinted with permission from ''Ectopic Pregnancy: Sonographic-Pathologic Correlations'' by BA Spirt et al, *Radiographics* (1984;4: 821–848), Copyright © 1984, Radiological Society of North America Inc.

33. Reprinted with permission from ''High-Resolution Real-Time Sonography of Scrotal Varicocele'' by MK Wolverson et al, *American Journal of Roentgenology* (1983;141:775–779), Copyright © 1983, Williams & Wilkins Company.

Skeletal Patterns

5

B1	Localized osteoporosis	562
B2	Generalized osteoporosis	566
B3	Osteomalacia	572
B4	Solitary or multiple osteosclerotic bone lesions	576
B5	Generalized osteosclerosis	584
B6	Bubbly lesions of bone	592
B7	Moth-eaten or punched-out osteolytic destructive lesions of bone	604
B8	Localized periosteal reaction	610
B9	Widespread or generalized periosteal reaction	614
B10	Arthritides	620
B11	Sacroiliac joint abnormality	632
B12	Erosion of multiple terminal phalangeal tufts (acro-osteolysis)	638
B13	Erosion, destruction, or defect of the outer end of the clavicle	644
B14	Neuroarthropathy (Charcot's joint)	648
B15	Loose intra-articular bodies	652
B16	Chondrocalcinosis	654
B17	Periarticular calcification	658
B18	Localized calcification or ossification in muscles and subcutaneous tissues	664
B19	Generalized calcification or ossification in muscles and subcutaneous tissues	668
B20	Calcification about the fingertips	674
B21	Zones of increased density in metaphyses	676
B22	Radiolucent metaphyseal bands	680
B23	Underconstriction or undertubulation (wide diametaphysis)	682
B24	Overconstriction or overtubulation (narrow diametaphysis)	692
B25	Avascular necrosis of hip or other joints	696
B26	Rib notching	700
B27	Resorption or notching of superior rib margins	704
B28	Bone-within-a-bone appearance	708
B29	Heel pad thickening (>22 millimeters)	712
B30	Pseudoarthrosis	714
B31	Protrusio acetabuli	716
B32	Dactylitis	718
Sources		722

LOCALIZED OSTEOPOROSIS

Condition	Comments
Disuse atrophy (immobilization) (Fig B1-1)	To maintain osteoblastic activity at normal levels, bones must be subjected to a normal amount of stress and muscular activity. Within a few weeks after the fracture of a bone, localized osteoporosis becomes detectable, especially distal to the site of injury. The cortical margin of an involved bone never completely disappears (unlike bone destruction due to disease). Similar disuse atrophy due to immobilization follows neural or muscular paralysis.
Sudeck's atrophy (reflex sympathetic dystrophy) (Fig B1-2)	Rapid development of painful osteoporosis after relatively trivial injury. Probably of neurovascular origin, Sudeck's atrophy most often involves the hands and feet with a mottled, irregular osteoporosis that primarily affects the periarticular region. The juxta-articular cortex may become extremely thin but remains intact, unlike in an arthritic process.
Inflammatory disease (Fig B1-3)	Localized osteoporosis often is the first (though nonspecific) radiographic manifestation of inflammatory diseases such as osteomyelitis, tuberculosis, and rheumatoid arthritis. In pyogenic infections, bone destruction typically precedes osteoporosis, whereas in tuberculosis the reverse is true. Periarticular demineralization is a classic early sign of rheumatoid arthritis.
Burn, frostbite, electric shock (Fig B1-4)	Bone demineralization, most marked where soft-tissue damage was greatest, is an early radiographic finding that may persist for a prolonged period.
Tumor (Figs B1-5 and B1-6)	Most commonly metastases and multiple myeloma. Also primary benign and malignant bone tumors.
Shoulder-hand syndrome	Radiographic appearance simulates that of Sudeck's atrophy. Shoulder pain and stiffness combined with pain, swelling, and vasomotor phenomena in the hand after an acute illness (especially myocardial infarction, in which the left side is usually involved).
Regional migratory osteoporosis (transitory osteoporosis)	Osteoporosis after the development of severe pain about a major joint (especially the hip, knee, or ankle) in a middle-aged or elderly adult. Often termed transitory demineralization of the femoral head, since the hip is most frequently involved. Self-limited but disabling disorder that heals completely in 2 to 4 months.

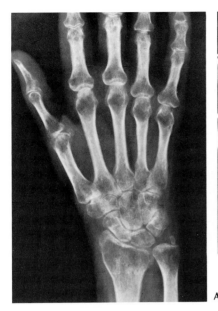

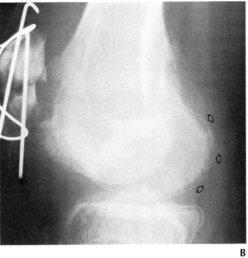

FIG B1-1. Disuse osteoporosis. (A) Severe periarticular demineralization follows prolonged immobilization of the extremity. (B) In a patient with a fractured patella, there is pronounced subcortical demineralization in the distal femur. The cortical margin (arrows) remains intact.

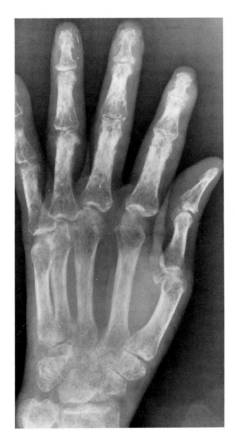

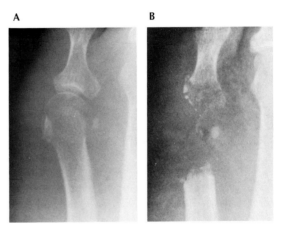

FIG B1-3. Staphylococcal osteomyelitis. (A) Initial film of the first metatarsophalangeal joint shows soft-tissue swelling and periarticular demineralization due to hyperemia. (B) Several weeks later, there is severe bony destruction about the metatarsophalangeal joint.

FIG B1-2. Sudeck's atrophy. Patchy osteoporosis predominantly affecting the periarticular regions. Endosteal scalloping and intracortical striations are evident even without magnification films.

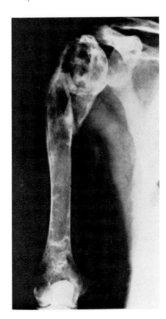

FIG B1-4. Electrical injury. Comminuted fracture of the head and shaft of the humerus associated with mottled decalcification of the humeral head. The cortex of the humerus is thin and the medullary cavity is widened. Discrete areas of rarefaction can be seen in the shaft and distal metaphyseal region.[1]

Condition	Imaging Findings	Comments
Osteoporosis circumscripta (Paget's disease) (see Fig SK1-2)		Early lytic phase of Paget's disease of the skull, in which an area of sharply demarcated radiolucency represents the destructive phase that primarily involves the outer table and spares the inner table. Deossification begins in the frontal or occipital area and slowly spreads to encompass the major portion of the calvarium. Irregular islands of sclerosis and diploic thickening during the reparative process result in the characteristic mottled, cotton-wool appearance. In long bones, the destructive phase typically begins at one edge of the bone and extends along the shaft for a variable distance to produce a sharply demarcated, V-shaped area of deossification (blade-of-grass appearance).
Diabetes mellitus (Fig B1-7)		May produce severe localized osteoporosis mimicking bone destruction. There is often a substantial amount of bone restitution after conservative therapy.
Bone infarct (Fig B1-8)		Initially, ischemic necrosis of cancellous bone causes localized demineralization. With healing, necrotic bone is replaced by new bone that is irregular in architecture and of greater density. When ischemic necrosis involves the articular surface, the initial radiographic change is a crescent of lucency.
Hemophilia		Articular hemorrhage initially results in marked periarticular osteoporosis due to local hyperemia and disuse. As cartilage is destroyed, sclerosis of adjacent bone occurs with superimposed osteophytic and other degenerative changes.

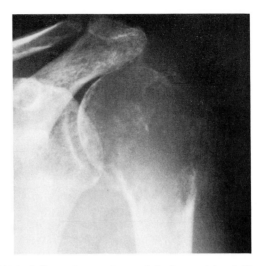

FIG B1-5. Metastases to bone. Osteolytic (blowout) metastasis to the humerus from carcinoma of the kidney.

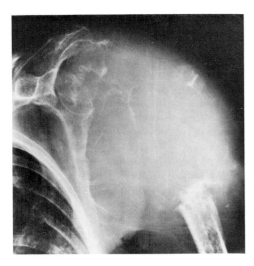

FIG B1-6. Solitary plasmacytoma of the humeral head. The highly destructive lesion has expanded the bone and broken through the cortex.

A   B

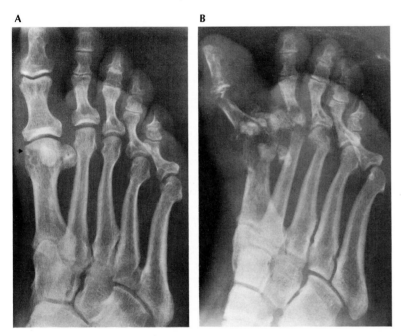

FIG B1-7. Acute osteomyelitis in diabetes. (A) Initial film of the foot in a diabetic patient with a soft-tissue infection shows minimal hyperemic osteoporosis about the head of the first metatarsal with some loss of the sharp cortical outline (arrow). (B) One month later there is severe bone destruction involving not only the head of the first metatarsal but also the rest of the big toe and the second and third metatarsophalangeal joints.

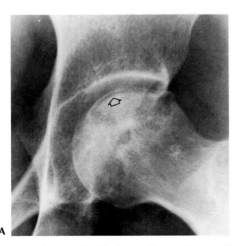

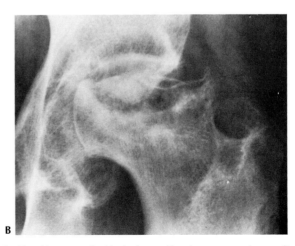

A   B

FIG B1-8. Ischemic necrosis of the femoral head. (A) An arclike radiolucent cortical band (crescent sign) in the femoral head represents a fracture line. (B) Eventually, there is a combination of lytic and sclerotic areas with severe flattening of the femoral head.

GENERALIZED OSTEOPOROSIS

Condition	Comments
Osteoporosis of aging (senile or postmenopausal osteoporosis) (Fig B2-1)	Most common form of generalized osteoporosis. As a person ages, the bones lose density and become more brittle, fracturing more easily and healing more slowly. Many elderly persons are also less active and have poor diets that are deficient in protein. Females are affected more often and more severely than males, since postmenopausal women have deficient gonadal hormone levels and decreased osteoblastic activity.
Drug-induced osteoporosis (Fig B2-2)	Patients receiving large doses of steroids over several months often develop generalized osteoporosis. Patients treated with 15,000 to 30,000 U of heparin for 6 months or longer also may develop generalized osteoporosis (possibly due to a direct local stimulating effect of heparin on bone resorption).
Deficiency states	
Protein deficiency (or abnormal protein metabolism)	Inability to produce adequate bone matrix in such conditions as malnutrition, nephrosis, diabetes mellitus, Cushing's syndrome, and hyperparathyroidism. Also patients with severe liver disease (hepatocellular degeneration, large or multiple liver cysts or tumors, biliary atresia). Pure dietary protein deficiency is rare in developed countries.
Vitamin C deficiency (scurvy) (Fig B2-3)	Deficiency of ascorbic acid causes abnormal function of osteoblasts and defective osteogenesis. Characteristic radiographic findings include widening and increased density of the zone of provisional calcification (the ''white line'' of scurvy); marginal spur formation (Pelken's spur); demineralization of epiphyseal ossification centers that are surrounded by a dense, sharply demarcated ring of calcification (Wimberger's sign); and subperiosteal hemorrhage along the shafts of long bones (calcification of elevated periosteum and hematoma is a radiographic sign of healing).
Intestinal malabsorption	Underlying mechanism in such conditions as sprue, scleroderma, pancreatic disease (insufficiency, chronic pancreatitis, mucoviscidosis), Crohn's disease, decreased absorptive surface of the small bowel (resection, bypass procedure), infiltrative disorders of the small bowel (eosinophilic enteritis, lactase deficiency, lymphoma, Whipple's disease), and idiopathic steatorrhea.
Endocrine disorders (Fig B2-4)	Hypogonadism (especially Turner's syndrome and menopause); adrenocortical abnormality (Cushing's syndrome, Addison's disease); nonendocrine steroid-producing tumor (eg, oat cell carcinoma); diabetes mellitus; pituitary abnormality (acromegaly, hypopituitarism); thyroid abnormality (hyperthyroidism and hypothyroidism).

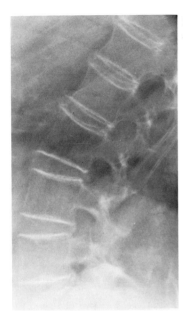

FIG B2-1. Osteoporosis of aging. Generalized demineralization of the spine in a postmenopausal woman. The cortex appears as a thin line that is relatively dense and prominent (picture-frame pattern).

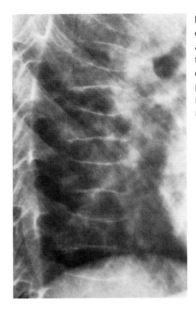

FIG B2-2. Steroid therapy. Lateral view of the thoracic spine in a patient on high-dose steroid therapy for dermatomyositis demonstrates severe osteoporosis with thinning of cortical margins and biconcave deformities of vertebral bodies.

A   B

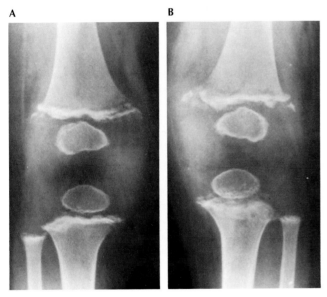

FIG B2-3. Scurvy. (A and B) Frontal views of both knees demonstrate widening and increased density of the zone of provisional calcification, producing the characteristic white line of scurvy. Note also the submetaphyseal zone of lucency and the characteristic marginal spur formation (Pelken's spur). The epiphyseal ossification centers are surrounded by a dense, sharply demarcated ring of calcification (Wimberger's sign).

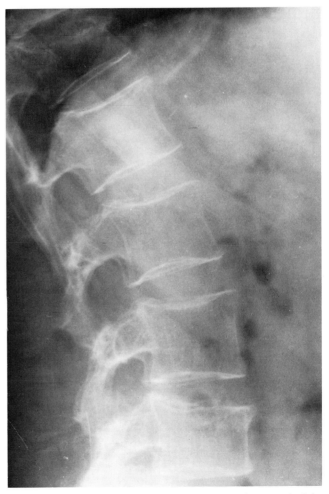

FIG B2-4. Cushing's syndrome due to adrenal hyperplasia. Marked demineralization and an almost complete loss of trabeculae in the lumbar spine. The vertebral end plates are mildly concave and the intervertebral disk spaces are slightly widened. Note the compression of the superior end plate of L4.[2]

Condition	Comments
Neoplastic disorders (Figs B2-5 and B2-6)	Diffuse cellular proliferation in the bone marrow with no tendency to form discrete tumor masses may produce generalized skeletal deossification simulating postmenopausal osteoporosis in adults with multiple myeloma or diffuse skeletal metastases and in children with acute leukemia. Pressure atrophy produces cortical thinning and trabecular resorption.
Anemia (Fig B2-7)	Extensive marrow hyperplasia widens medullary spaces and thins cortices in such conditions as thalassemia and sickle cell anemia. Severe iron deficiency can produce a similar appearance.
Collagen disease (Fig B2-8)	Rheumatoid arthritis; ankylosing spondylitis; systemic lupus erythematosus; scleroderma; dermatomyositis. Usually associated with characteristic joint changes.
Osteogenesis imperfecta (Fig B2-9)	Inherited generalized disorder of connective tissue with multiple fractures, hypermobility of joints, blue sclerae, poor teeth, deafness, and cardiovascular disorders such as mitral valve prolapse or aortic regurgitation. Osteogenesis imperfecta congenita develops in utero and appears at birth as bowing and deformity of the extremities due to multiple fractures (death in utero or soon after birth is usually caused by intracranial hemorrhage in these infants with paper-thin skulls). In the less severe tarda form, the disorder is first noted during childhood or young adulthood because of an unusual tendency for fractures, loose-jointedness, and the presence of blue sclerae. Fractures often heal with exuberant callus formation that may simulate a malignant tumor and cause bizarre deformities.
Neuromuscular diseases and dystrophies (Fig B2-10)	Decreased muscular tone leading to osteoporosis, bone atrophy with cortical thinning, scoliosis, and joint contractures occurs in congenital disorders and such acquired conditions as spinal cord disease and immobilization for chronic disease or major fracture. Lack of the stress stimulus of weight bearing is the underlying cause of the generalized disuse atrophy termed space flight osteoporosis.
Homocystinuria	Inborn error of methionine metabolism that causes a defect in the structure of collagen or elastin and a radiographic appearance similar to that of Marfan's syndrome. Striking osteoporosis of the spine and long bones (extremely rare in Marfan's syndrome).

A

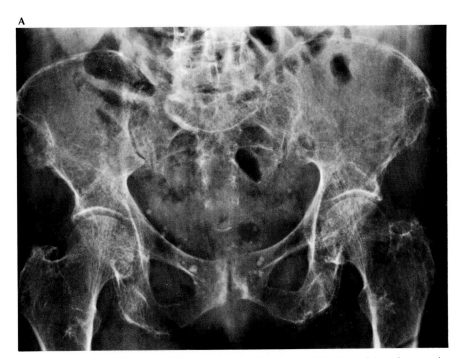

B

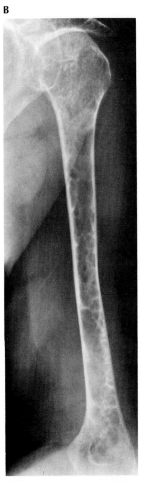

FIG B2-5. Multiple myeloma. (A) Diffuse skeletal deossification involving the pelvis and proximal femurs. (B) Generalized demineralization of the humerus with thinning of the cortices.

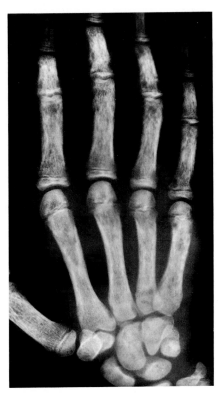

FIG B2-6. Leukemia. Patchy areas of deossification throughout the metacarpals and phalanges.

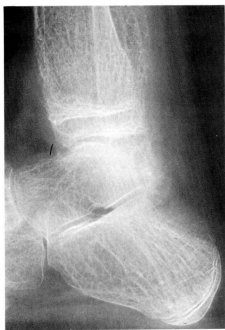

FIG B2-7. Thalassemia. Lateral view of the ankle demonstrates pronounced widening of the medullary spaces with thinning of the cortices. Note the absence of normal modeling due to the pressure of the expanding marrow space. Localized radiolucencies simulating multiple osteolytic lesions represent tumerous collections of hyperplastic marrow.

Condition	Comments
Lipid storage diseases **(Fig B2-11)**	Gaucher's disease and Niemann-Pick disease. Accumulation of abnormal quantities of complex lipids in the bone marrow produces a generalized loss of bone density and cortical thinning.
Hemochromatosis	Iron-storage disorder often associated with diffuse osteoporosis of the spine and vertebral collapse. About half the patients have a characteristic arthropathy that most frequently involves the small joints of the hand. Hepatosplenomegaly and portal hypertension are common.
Hemophilia **(see Fig B10-9)**	Multiple episodes of hemarthrosis may cause hyperemia combined with atrophy of bone and muscle, resulting in severe osteoporosis. Radiographic signs suggestive of hemophilia include abnormally large or prematurely fused epiphyses, widening and deepening of the intercondylar notch of the femur, and squaring of the inferior border of the patella.
Idiopathic juvenile **osteoporosis**	Rare condition characterized by the abrupt onset of generalized or focal bone pain in children 8 to 12 years of age. The disease is usually self-limited with spontaneous radiologic and clinical improvement.

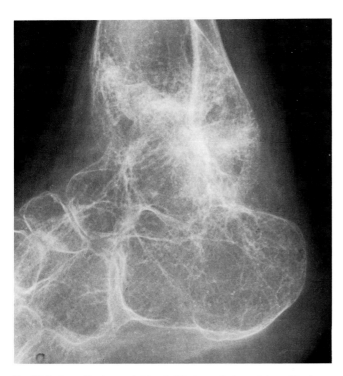

FIG B2-8. Juvenile rheumatoid arthritis. Lateral view of the ankle demonstrates severe demineralization of bone. Note the pronounced narrowing of the joints involving the talus and other tarsal bones.

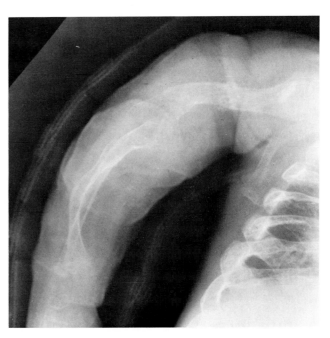

FIG B2-9. Osteogenesis imperfecta. Pronounced osteoporosis and cortical thinning of all bones with evidence of previous fractures and resultant deformities.

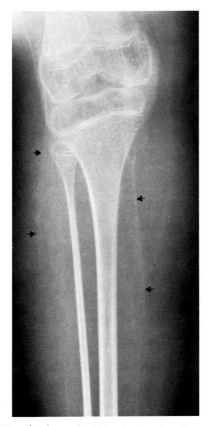

FIG B2-10. Muscular dystrophy. Thin, demineralized bones of the lower leg. The increased lucency, representing fatty infiltration in muscle bundles, makes the fascial sheaths appear as thin shadows of increased density (arrows) surrounded by fat.

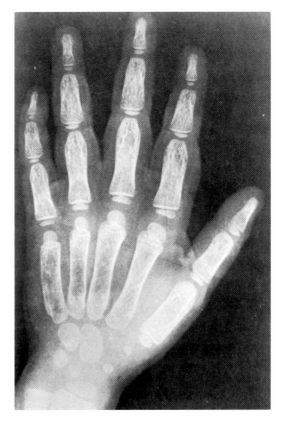

FIG B2-11. Niemann-Pick disease. Diffuse widening of the metacarpals and phalanges with thin cortices and coarsened trabeculae.[3]

OSTEOMALACIA

Condition	Comments
Deficient absorption of calcium or phosphorus	
Rickets **(Fig B3-1)**	Systemic disease of infancy and childhood in which calcification of growing skeletal elements is defective because of a deficiency of vitamin D in the diet or a lack of exposure to ultraviolet radiation (sunshine). Most common in premature infants and usually develops between 6 and 12 months of age. Classic radiographic signs include cupping and fraying of metaphyseal ends of bone with disappearance of normally sharp metaphyseal lines; delayed appearance of epiphyseal ossification centers, which have blurred margins (unlike the sharp outlines in scurvy); and excessive osteoid tissue in the sternal ends of ribs producing characteristic beading (rachitic rosary).
Malabsorption states	Primary small bowel disease (sprue, Crohn's disease, lymphoma, small bowel fistula, amyloidosis); pancreatic insufficiency (exocrine) or inflammation; hepatobiliary disease (biliary atresia or acquired chronic biliary obstruction); postoperative gastric or small bowel resection; mesenteric disease; cathartic abuse.
Dietary calcium deficiency	Extremely rare.
Excessive renal excretion of calcium or phosphorus	
Renal tubular acidosis **(Fig B3-2)**	Kidney is unable to excrete an acidic urine (below pH 5.4) because the distal nephron cannot secrete hydrogen against a concentration gradient. This can lead to cation wasting (calcium and potassium) and so-called "renal rickets." Usually there is very dense and extensive renal parenchymal calcification, often associated with staghorn calculi.
Vitamin D–resistant rickets	Hereditary disorder (X-linked dominant) with diminished proximal tubular resorption of phosphorus. May also reflect an end-organ resistance to vitamin D.
Fanconi's syndrome	Multiple defects of renal tubular resorption that may be inherited (autosomal recessive) or acquired secondary to such conditions as Wilson's disease, multiple myeloma, and lead or cadmium intoxication. Characterized by hypophosphatemia and large amounts of glucose, amino acids, and protein in the urine.

(continued page 574)

A
B

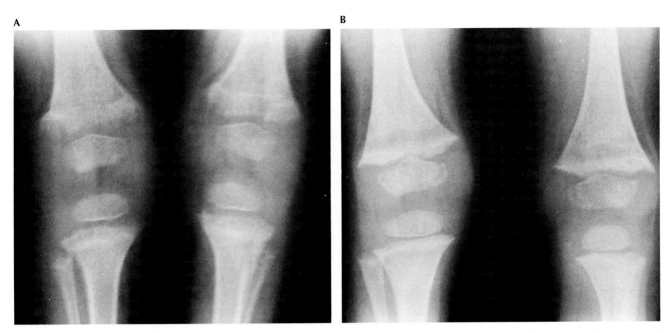

FIG B3-1. Rickets. (A) Initial film shows severe metaphyseal changes involving the distal femurs and proximal tibias and fibulas. Note the pronounced demineralization of the epiphyseal ossification centers. (B) After vitamin D therapy, there is remineralization of the metaphyses and an almost normal appearance of the epiphyseal ossification centers.

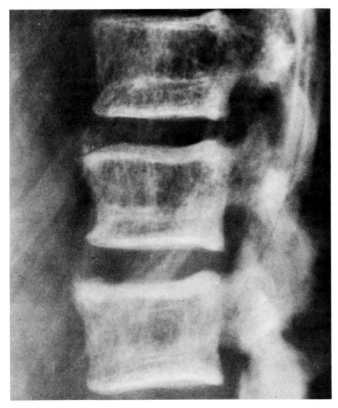

FIG B3-2. Rickets due to renal tubular disorder. Striking thickening of the cortices of the vertebral bodies with increased trabeculation of spongy bone.

Condition	Comments
Hyperparathyroidism **(Fig B3-3)**	Excessive secretion of parathyroid hormone leads to a generalized disorder of calcium, phosphorus, and bone metabolism resulting in elevated serum calcium and phosphate. May be primary (adenoma, carcinoma, or generalized hyperplasia of all glands; parathormone-like secretion by nonparathyroid tumor) or secondary (more common and most often due to chronic renal failure). Classic radiographic signs include subperiosteal bone resorption, generalized osteosclerosis (including rugger-jersey spine), brown tumors, salt-and-pepper skull, and soft-tissue calcification. Increased incidence of nephrocalcinosis, urinary tract calculi, pancreatitis, peptic ulcer, and gallstones.
Hypophosphatasia **(Fig B3-4)**	Inherited (autosomal recessive) metabolic disorder in which a low level of alkaline phosphatase leads to defective mineralization of bone. Hypophosphatasia discovered in utero or during the first few days of life is generally fatal, with the calvarium and many bones of the skeleton uncalcified. If the condition develops later, the radiographic appearance closely resembles that of rickets with large unossified areas in the skull simulating severe widening of sutures. High incidence of fractures and bone deformities.
Wilson's disease **(Fig B3-5)**	Rare familial disorder in which impaired hepatic excretion of copper results in toxic accumulation of the metal in the liver, brain, and other organs. Characteristic pigmentation of the cornea (Kayser-Fleischer ring). About half the patients demonstrate skeletal changes.
Anticonvulsant drug therapy	Prolonged use of anticonvulsants (eg, dilantin) and many tranquilizers stimulates hepatic enzymatic activity, resulting in accelerated degradation of biologically active vitamin D_3 to inactive metabolites.
Fibrogenesis imperfecta and axial osteomalacia	Extremely rare conditions of older individuals in which acquired vitamin D resistance leads to osteomalacia in both the axial and appendicular bones (fibrogenesis imperfecta) or only the axial skeleton (axial osteomalacia).

A

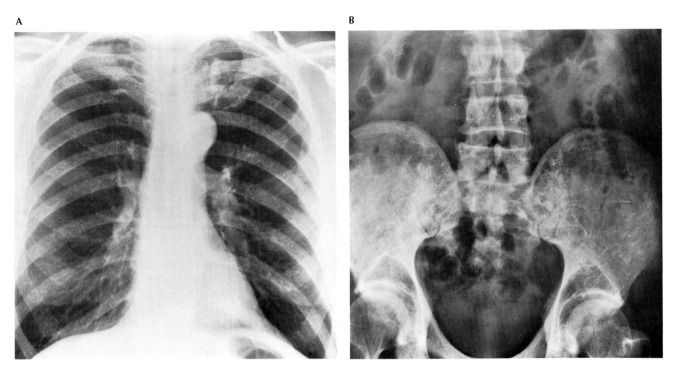

B

FIG B3-3. Hyperparathyroidism. Views of (A) the chest and (B) the abdomen show generalized bony demineralization with striking prominence of residual trabeculae (especially in the ribs).

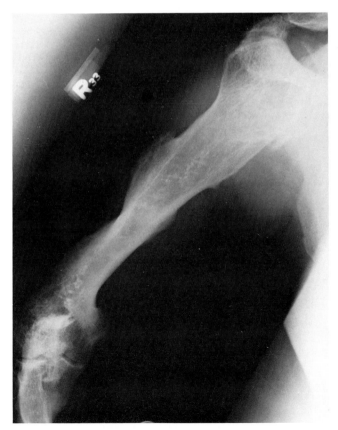

FIG B3-4. Hypophosphatasia. Osteomalacia of the arm with ossification of the deltoid and other muscle insertions. Severe manifestations of the condition in a 43-year-old man, 4 feet 9 inches tall.[4]

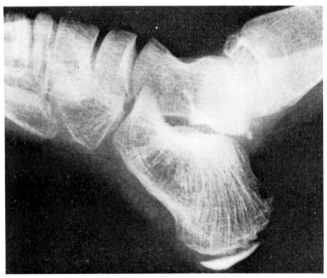

FIG B3-5. Wilson's disease. Lateral view of the ankle and foot demonstrates marked demineralization, thinning of the cortex, and coarsening of the trabecular pattern, all best seen in the os calcis.[5]

SOLITARY OR MULTIPLE OSTEOSCLEROTIC BONE LESIONS

Condition	Imaging Findings	Comments
Bone island	Single or multiple areas of dense compact bone that most commonly occur in the pelvis and upper femurs. Sharply demarcated lesion, though the margins often display thorny radiation giving a brush border appearance.	Asymptomatic and completely benign. Almost half enlarge over a period of years and many show activity on radionuclide bone scans (must be distinguished from osteoblastic metastases).
Osteoma (see Fig SK17-9)	Well-circumscribed, extremely dense round lesion (rarely larger than 2 cm). Most often arises in the outer table of the skull, paranasal sinuses (especially frontal and ethmoid), and mandible.	Benign hamartomatous lesion consisting exclusively of osseous tissue. Osteomas (often multiple) are associated with soft-tissue tumors and multiple premalignant colonic polyps in Gardner's syndrome.
Osteoid osteoma (Fig B4-1)	Small, round or oval lucent nidus (less than 1 cm in diameter) surrounded by a large, dense sclerotic zone of cortical thickening. Although usually located in the cortex, the nidus may be in an intramedullary or subperiosteal position and be difficult to detect.	Benign bone tumor that usually develops in young men. Classic clinical symptom is local pain that is worse at night and dramatically relieved by aspirin. At times, the dense sclerotic reaction may obscure the nidus on conventional radiographs and require tomography (conventional or computed) for demonstration. Surgical excision of the nidus is essential for cure (it is not necessary to remove the reactive calcification).
Osteoblastic metastases (Figs B4-2 and B4-3)	Single or multiple ill-defined areas of increased density that may progress to complete loss of normal bony architecture. Varies from a small, isolated round focus of sclerotic density to a diffuse sclerosis involving most or all of a bone (eg, ivory vertebral body).	Osteoblastic metastases are most commonly secondary to lymphoma and carcinomas of the breast and prostate. Other primary tumors include carcinomas of the gastrointestinal tract, lung, and urinary bladder. Osteoblastic metastases are generally considered to be evidence of slow growth in a neoplasm that has allowed time for reactive bone proliferation.
Osteochondroma (exostosis) (Figs B4-4 to B4-6)	Projection of bone that initially grows outward at a right angle to the host bone. As the lesion grows, the pull of neighboring muscles and tendons orients the tumor parallel to the long axis of the bone and pointed away from the nearest joint. Typically there is blending of the cortex of an osteochondroma with that of normal bone. In flat bones, an osteochondroma appears as a relatively localized area of amorphous, spotty calcification.	Benign projection of bone with a cartilaginous cap that probably represents a local dysplasia of cartilage at the epiphyseal growth plate. The lesion arises in childhood or adolescence and continues to grow until fusion of the closest epiphyseal line. Most commonly develops in the metaphyseal region of a long bone (eg, femur, tibia, or humerus). Rapid growth or the development of localized pain suggests malignant degeneration to chondrosarcoma. There are multiple and bilateral osteochondromas in hereditary multiple exostoses (diaphyseal aclasis).
Callus formation	Localized increase in bone density about a healed or healing fracture.	Callus formation about a rib fracture may simulate a pulmonary nodule and necessitate oblique views or chest fluoroscopy for differentiation.

A **B**

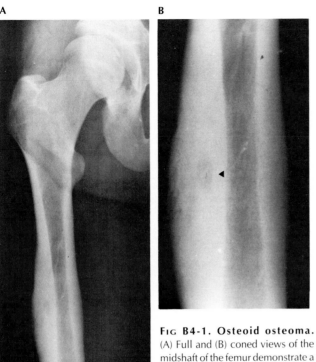

FIG B4-1. Osteoid osteoma. (A) Full and (B) coned views of the midshaft of the femur demonstrate a dense sclerotic zone of cortical thickening laterally, which contains a small oval lucent nidus.

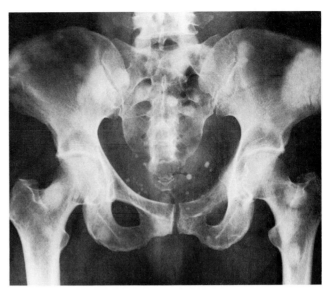

FIG B4-2. Osteoblastic metastases. Multiple areas of increased density involving the pelvis and proximal femurs representing metastases from carcinoma of the urinary bladder.

A

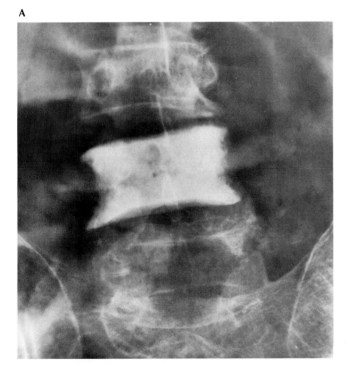

B

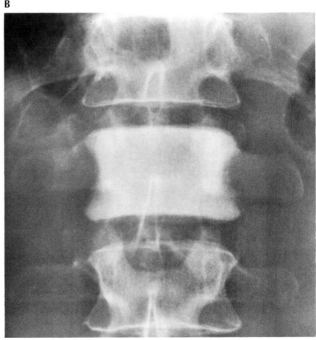

FIG B4-3. Ivory vertebrae. (A) Carcinoma of the prostate. (B) Lymphoma.

Condition	Imaging Findings	Comments
Bone infarct in shaft (Fig B4-7)	Densely calcified area in the medullary cavity. May be sharply limited by a dense sclerotic zone or be associated with serpiginous dense streaks extending from the central region of calcification.	Underlying causes include occlusive vascular disease, sickle cell anemia, collagen disease, chronic pancreatitis, Gaucher's disease, and radiation therapy.
Ischemic necrosis involving articular end of bone (Fig B4-8)	Advanced stage consisting of lytic and sclerotic areas with flattening and irregularity of joint surfaces leading to early secondary degenerative changes (especially in weight-bearing joints).	Most commonly involves the femoral head. May affect the proximal half of the navicular after a fracture. Also can occur in any disorder associated with medullary bone infarcts or be secondary to steroid therapy or Cushing's disease.
Healed or healing benign bone lesion	Initially lytic bone lesion may become sclerotic spontaneously or with appropriate therapy.	Fibrous cortical defects, nonossifying fibromas, and bone cysts may spontaneously regress. Brown tumors in primary hyperparathyroidism become sclerotic after removal of the parathyroid adenoma. Even some lytic metastases may become osteoblastic after irradiation, chemotherapy, or hormone therapy.
Osteomyelitis **Chronic or healed osteomyelitis** (Fig B4-9)	Thickening and sclerosis of bone with irregular outer margin surrounding a central ill-defined area of lucency. The cortex may become so dense that the medullary cavity is difficult to demonstrate.	Reactivation of infection may appear as recurrence of deep soft-tissue swelling, periosteal calcification, or the development of lytic abscess cavities in the bone.
Brodie's abscess (Fig B4-10)	Well-circumscribed lytic area surrounded by an irregular zone of dense sclerosis.	Chronic bone abscess of low virulence that never had an acute stage. Painful lesion often simulating an osteoid osteoma.
Garré's sclerosing osteomyelitis (Fig B4-11)	Exuberant sclerotic reaction without any bone destruction, sequestration, or periosteal response.	Rare, chronic nonsuppurative infection of bone due to an organism of low virulence.

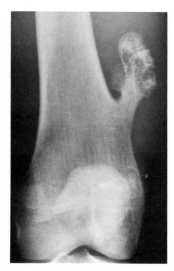

FIG B4-4. Osteochondroma of the distal femur. The long axis of the tumor is parallel to that of the femur and pointed away from the knee joint.

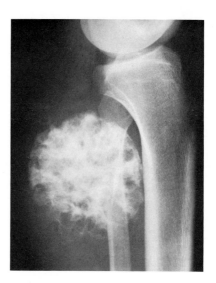

FIG B4-5. Osteochondroma. Extensive cartilaginous calcification about the proximal fibular lesion.

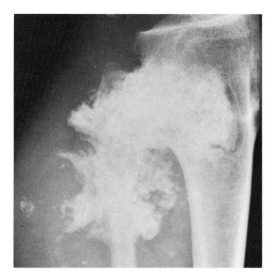

FIG B4-6. **Multiple exostoses** with sarcomatous degeneration. A chondrosarcoma arising from one of the many exostoses in this patient appears as a large soft-tissue mass with amorphous calcification.

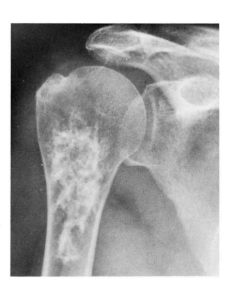

FIG B4-7. **Bone infarct.** Densely calcified area in the medullary cavity of the humerus with dense streaks extending from the central region.

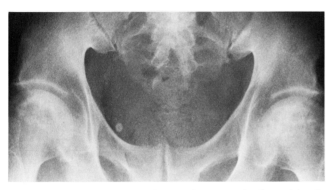

FIG B4-8. **Ischemic necrosis.** Sclerotic changes in the femoral heads bilaterally.

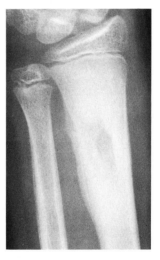

FIG B4-9. **Chronic osteomyelitis.** Ill-defined area of lucency in the distal radial shaft is almost obscured by the sclerotic periosteal new bone formation.

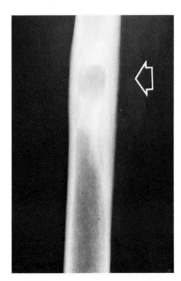

FIG B4-10. **Brodie's abscess.** Well-circumscribed lucent lesion completely fills the femoral medullary canal and is surrounded by dense endosteal sclerosis and cortical thickening (arrow).[6]

Condition	Imaging Findings	Comments
Paget's disease (see Figs SP2-2 and SK5-2)	In the reparative stage, there is a mixed lytic and sclerotic pattern with cortical thickening and enlargement of affected bone. In the sclerotic stage, there may be uniform areas of increased bone density (eg, ivory vertebra in the spine and cotton-wool appearance in the skull).	Purely sclerotic phase is less common than the combined destructive and reparative stages. Ivory vertebra may simulate osteoblastic metastases or Hodgkin's disease, though in Paget's disease the vertebra is also expanded in size.
Mastocytosis (Fig B4-12)	Scattered, well-defined sclerotic foci simulating blastic metastases. There may also be diffuse osteosclerosis mimicking myelofibrosis.	Caused by diffuse deposits of mast cells in the bone marrow. Episodic release of histamine from mast cells causes pruritus, flushing, tachycardia, asthma, and headaches and an increased incidence of peptic ulcers. There is often hepatosplenomegaly, lymphadenopathy, and pancytopenia.
Fibrous dysplasia	Dense, spotty, or linear calcification simulating medullary bone infarct.	Infrequent manifestation of long-standing disease.
Primary bone sarcoma (Figs B4-13 and B4-14)	Sclerosing forms may contain extremely dense new bone.	Osteogenic sarcoma; chondrosarcoma; Ewing's sarcoma.
Osteopoikilosis (Fig B4-15)	Multiple sclerotic foci (2 mm to 2 cm) producing a typical speckled appearance.	Rare asymptomatic hereditary condition that primarily involves the small bones of the hands and feet, the pelvis, and the epiphyses and metaphyses of long bones.
Osteopathia striata (Fig B4-16)	Dense longitudinal lines in tubular bones. Ilial involvement produces linear densities radiating from the acetabulum and fanning out to the iliac crest (sunburst pattern).	Rare, asymptomatic bone disorder reflecting an error in internal bone modeling.
Congenital stippled epiphyses (chondrodysplasia punctata) (Fig B4-17)	Multiple punctate calcifications occurring in epiphyses before the normal time for appearance of ossification centers. Most commonly involves the hips, knees, shoulders, and wrists.	Rare condition. Affected bones may be shortened or the process may regress and leave no deformity. The densities may disappear by age 3 or may gradually increase in size and coalesce to form a normal-appearing single ossification center.
Multiple myeloma (see Fig B5-13)	Generalized patchy or uniform bone sclerosis.	Very rare manifestation. Scattered, slow-growing osteoblastic lesions with dense plasmacytic infiltrates and normal laboratory findings may be termed plasma-cell granuloma.

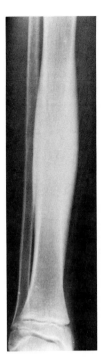

FIG B4-11. Garré's sclerosing osteomyelitis.
Exuberant sclerotic reaction in the midshaft of
the tibia without evidence of bone destruction.

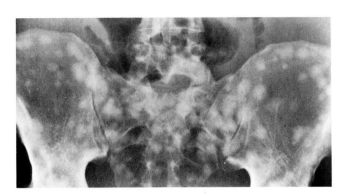

FIG B4-12. Mastocytosis. Multiple scattered, well-defined sclerotic foci
in the pelvis simulate blastic metastases.

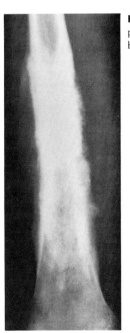

FIG B4-13. Ewing's sarcoma. Sunburst
pattern of horizontal spicules of dense
bone.

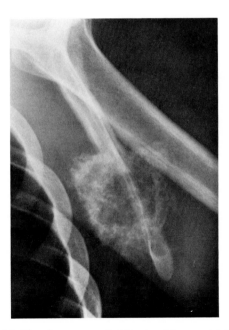

FIG B4-14. Chondrosarcoma. Ill-defined, calcium-containing mass
near the angle of the scapula.

Condition	Imaging Findings	Comments
Tuberous sclerosis	Dense sclerotic foci most often affecting the bones of the cranial vault and the pedicles and posterior portions of the vertebral bodies.	Rare inherited disorder presenting with clinical triad of convulsive seizures, mental deficiency, and adenoma sebaceum. Associated with renal and intracranial hamartomas and characteristic scattered intracerebral calcifications.
Syphilis/yaws **(Fig B4-18)**	Gumma formation causes an ill-defined lytic area surrounded by extensive dense bony proliferation and exuberant periosteal new bone formation.	Chronic osteomyelitis caused by spirochete (*Treponema*) infection.
Osteitis condensans ilii **(see Fig B11-3)**	Zone of dense sclerosis along the iliac side of the sacroiliac joint. Usually bilateral and symmetric, though there may be some variation in density between the two sides. Unlike ankylosing spondylitis, in osteitis condensans ilii the sacrum is normal and the sacroiliac joint space is preserved.	Occurs almost exclusively in women during the childbearing period, usually after pregnancy. May represent a reaction to the increased stress to which the sacroiliac region is subjected during pregnancy and delivery, since a similar type of sclerotic reaction (osteitis pubis) may be seen in the pubic bone adjacent to the symphysis in women who have borne children. The condition is usually asymptomatic and self-limited and is rarely detectable in women past 50.

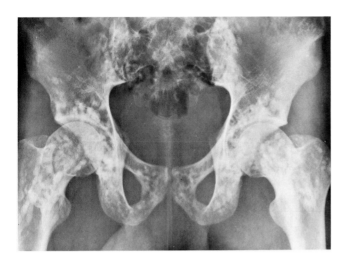

FIG B4-15. **Osteopoikilosis.** Innumerable small, well-circumscribed areas of increased density throughout the pelvis and proximal femurs.

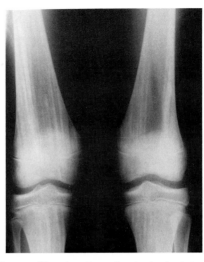

FIG B4-16. **Osteopathia striata.** Dense longitudinal striations in the distal femur and proximal tibia.

A   B

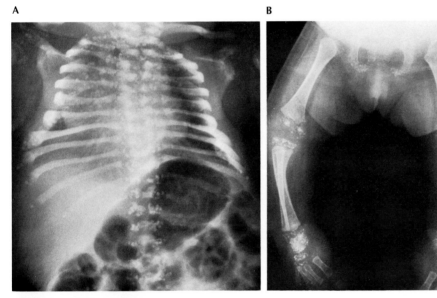

FIG B4-17. **Congenital stippled epiphyses.** Multiple small punctate calcifications of various sizes involve virtually all the epiphyses in views of (A) the chest and upper abdomen and (B) the lower extremities.

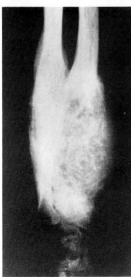

FIG B4-18. **Yaws.** Expanding inflammatory process with surrounding sclerosis involving the right forearm.[7]

GENERALIZED OSTEOSCLEROSIS

Condition	Imaging Findings	Comments
Myelosclerosis (myelofibrosis, myeloid metaplasia) (Fig B5-1)	About half the patients have a widespread, diffuse increase in bone density (ground-glass appearance) that primarily affects the spine, ribs, and pelvis but can also involve the long bones and skull. Uniform obliteration of fine trabecular margins of ribs results in sclerosis simulating jail bars crossing the thorax.	Hematologic disorder in which gradual replacement of marrow by fibrosis produces a varying degree of anemia and a leukemoid blood picture. Most commonly idiopathic, though a large percentage of patients have antecedent polycythemia vera. Extramedullary hematopoiesis causes massive splenomegaly, often hepatomegaly, and sometimes tumorlike masses in the posterior mediastinum. Patchy osteosclerosis in long bones may produce a mottled appearance suggesting a destructive malignancy.
Osteoblastic metastases (Fig B5-2)	Generalized diffuse osteosclerosis.	Primarily lymphoma and carcinomas of the prostate and breast.
Paget's disease (Fig B5-3)	Diffuse osteosclerosis may develop in advanced stage of polyostotic disease.	Although the radiographic appearance may simulate that of osteoblastic metastases, characteristic cortical thickening and coarse trabeculation should suggest Paget's disease.
Sickle cell anemia (Fig B5-4)	Diffuse sclerosis with coarsening of the trabecular pattern may be a late manifestation.	More commonly generalized osteoporosis due to marrow hyperplasia. Also characteristic "fish vertebrae" and a high incidence of acute osteomyelitis (often caused by *Salmonella* infection). Splenomegaly and extramedullary hematopoiesis are common.
Osteopetrosis (Albers-Schönberg disease, marble bones) (Fig B5-5)	Symmetric, generalized increase in bone density involving all bones. Lack of modeling causes widening of metaphyseal ends of tubular bones. In the spine, characteristic "bone-within-a-bone" appearance (a miniature bone inset in each vertebral body) and "sandwich vertebrae" (increased density at end plates).	Rare hereditary bone dysplasia in which failure of the resorptive mechanism of calcified cartilage interferes with its normal replacement by mature bone. Varies in severity and age of clinical presentation from a fulminant, often fatal condition at birth to an essentially asymptomatic form that is an incidental radiographic finding. Although radiographically dense, the involved bones are brittle and fractures are common even with trivial trauma. Extensive extramedullary hematopoiesis (hepatosplenomegaly and lymphadenopathy).
Pyknodysostosis (Fig B5-6)	Diffuse dense, sclerotic bones. Unlike osteopetrosis, the medullary cavity is preserved and there is no metaphyseal widening. Characteristically there is mandibular hypoplasia with loss of the normal mandibular angle and craniofacial disproportion.	Rare hereditary bone dysplasia. Patients have short stature but hepatosplenomegaly is infrequent. Numerous wormian bones may simulate cleidocranial dysostosis.

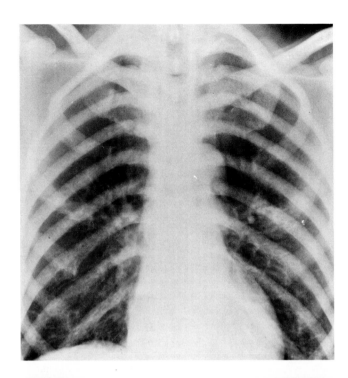

FIG B5-1. **Myelosclerosis.** Diffuse uniform sclerosis of the bones of the thorax produces an appearance of jail bars.

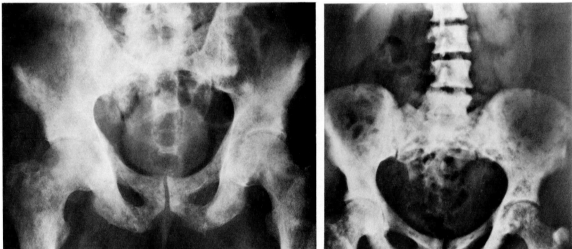

FIG B5-2. **Osteoblastic metastases.** (Left) Carcinoma of the prostate. (Right) Carcinoma of the breast.

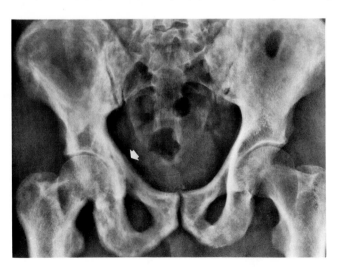

FIG B5-3. **Paget's disease.** Diffuse sclerosis with cortical thickening involving the right femur and both iliac bones. Note the characteristic thickening and coarsening of the iliopectineal line (arrow) on the involved right side.

Condition	Imaging Findings	Comments
Melorheostosis (Fig B5-7)	Irregular sclerotic thickening of the cortex, usually confined to one side of a single bone or to multiple bones of one extremity. Sclerosis begins at the proximal end of the bone and extends distally, resembling wax flowing down a burning candle.	Rare disorder, usually occurring in childhood, that typically presents with severe pain sometimes associated with limitation of motion, contractures, or fusion of an adjacent joint. Involvement of the hands and wrists may produce multiple small sclerotic islands of dense bone simulating osteopoikilosis.
Generalized cortical hyperostosis (van Buchem's syndrome) (see Fig SK5-5)	Diffuse symmetric sclerosis of the skull, mandible, clavicles, ribs, and diaphyses of long bones.	Rare dysplasia in which diaphyseal sclerosis is accompanied by thickening of the endosteal surface of the cortex, which causes widening of the cortex but does not increase the diameter of the bone.
Fluorosis (Fig B5-8)	Dense skeletal sclerosis most prominent in the vertebrae and pelvis. Obliteration of individual trabeculae may cause affected bones to appear chalky white. There is often calcification of interosseous membranes and ligaments (iliolumbar, sacrotuberous, and sacrospinous).	Fluorine poisoning may result from drinking water with a high concentration of fluorides, industrial exposure (mining, smelting), or excessive therapeutic intake of fluoride (treatment of myeloma or Paget's disease). There is usually also periosteal roughening and articular bone deposits in long bones at sites of muscular and ligamentous attachments.
Engelmann-Camurati disease (progressive diaphyseal dysplasia) (Fig B5-9)	Endosteal and periosteal cortical thickening cause fusiform enlargement and sclerosis of long bones. Primarily involves the diaphyses, sparing the epiphyses and metaphyses.	Rare bone disorder associated with a neuromuscular dystrophy that causes a peculiar wide-based, waddling gait. Encroachment on the medullary canal may cause anemia and secondary hepatosplenomegaly.
Mastocytosis (see Fig B4-12)	May present with diffuse osteosclerosis that often is not sharply demarcated from normal bone and intermingles with osteolytic areas. Another appearance is scattered, well-defined sclerotic foci simulating osteoblastic metastases.	Caused by diffuse deposits of mast cells in the bone marrow. Episodic release of histamine from mast cells causes pruritis, flushing, tachycardia, asthma, headaches, and an increased incidence of peptic ulcers. Often hepatosplenomegaly, lymphadenopathy, and pancytopenia.

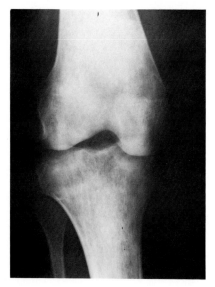

FIG B5-4. Sickle cell anemia. Diffuse sclerosis about the knee.

A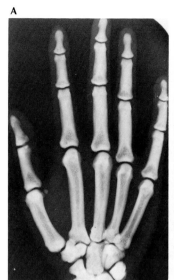

B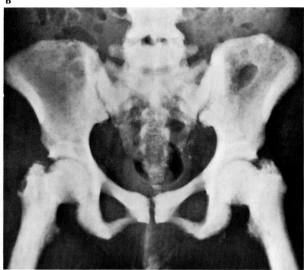

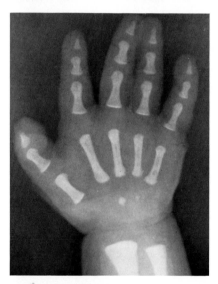

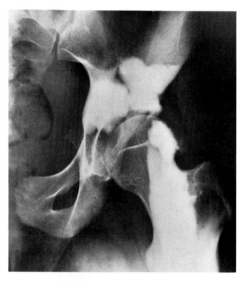

FIG B5-5. Osteopetrosis. (A) Striking sclerosis of the bones of the hand and wrist. (B) Generalized increased density of the lower spine, pelvis, and hips in a 74-year-old woman with the tarda form of the condition.

FIG B5-6. Pyknodysostosis. Generalized increase in density with cortical thickening of the bones of the hand. The distal phalanges are hypoplastic and the terminal tufts are absent.

FIG B5-7. Melorheostosis. Dense cortical sclerosis involves the proximal femur and the lower portion of the ilium.

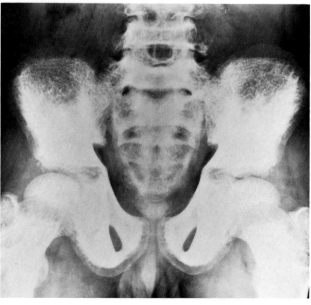

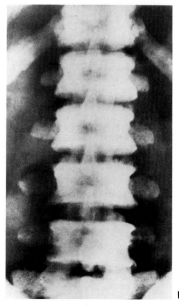

A   B

FIG B5-8. Fluorosis. (A) Dense skeletal sclerosis with obliteration of individual trabeculae causes the pelvis and proximal femurs to appear chalky white. (B) Diffuse vertebral sclerosis in another patient.[8]

Condition	Imaging Findings	Comments
Hypervitaminosis D/ idiopathic hypercalcemia	Generalized sclerosis and cortical thickening. Typically there are dense transverse metaphyseal bands (increase in depth of provisional zones of calcification).	Hypervitaminosis D results from excessive intake over a few days to several years. Idiopathic hypercalcemia is the result of excessive vitamin D intake, hypersensitivity to vitamin D, or an inborn error of cholesterol metabolism producing sterol intermediates with vitamin D–like properties. Causes renal calcification and renal failure.
Polyostotic fibrous dysplasia (Fig B5-10)	Diffuse homogeneous ground-glass density involving multiple bones. May cause marked sclerosis and thickening of facial bones, often with obliteration of sinuses and orbits, producing a leonine appearance (leontiasis ossea).	Proliferation of fibrous tissue in the medullary cavity. Often there are localized pigmentations (café au lait spots) that tend to have an irregular outline (''coast-of-Maine''), unlike the smoothly marginated lesions in neurofibromatosis. About one third of females also demonstrate precocious puberty (Albright's syndrome).
Renal osteodystrophy (Fig B5-11)	Generalized osteosclerosis, often combined with soft-tissue calcification, is one manifestation.	Represents a skeletal response to chronic renal disease of any origin. In primary hyperparathyroidism, sclerosis is generally associated with healing.
Craniometaphyseal dysplasia (see Fig SK5-5)	Generalized diaphyseal sclerosis (but metaphyseal lucency) that eventually progresses to more normal mineralization. Lack of modeling of tubular bones and often sclerosis of the base of the skull and the mandible.	Rare hereditary disorder in which failure of normal tubulation of bone is combined with hypertelorism, a broad flat nose, and defective dentition.
Congenital syphilis (Fig B5-12)	Diffuse cortical thickening and increased density of the shafts of long bones.	Most common radiographic appearance of late-stage disease that reflects periosteal reaction to underlying gummas.
Metaphyseal abnormalities (see B21)	Dense transverse metaphyseal bands.	Most commonly a manifestation of lead intoxication. Also caused by phosphorus or bismuth poisoning, cretinism, treated leukemia, and healed rickets or scurvy.
Hypoparathyroidism/ pseudohypoparathyroidism	Bandlike increase in density in long bones, usually localized to the metaphyseal area (probably reflects an abnormality in enchondral bone formation).	More frequent radiographic manifestations are cerebral calcification (especially involving the basal ganglia, the dentate nuclei of the cerebellum, and the choroid plexus) in hypoparathyroidism and shortening of the fourth and fifth metacarpals plus calcific or bony deposits in the skin or subcutaneous tissues in pseudohypoparathyroidism.

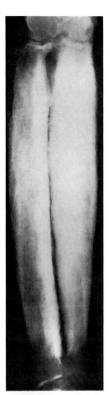

FIG B5-9. Progressive diaphyseal dysplasia. Dense endosteal and periosteal cortical thickening causes fusiform enlargement and increased density of the midshafts of the radius and ulna.

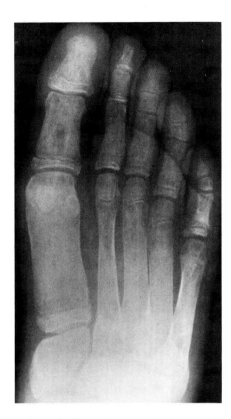

FIG B5-10. Polyostotic fibrous dysplasia. The bones of the feet show a smudgy, ground-glass appearance of the medullary cavities with failure of normal modeling.

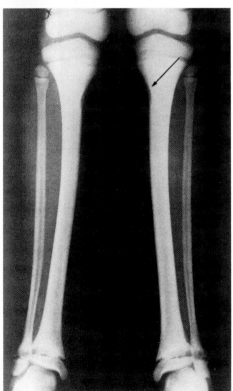

FIG B5-11. Renal osteodystrophy. Sclerosis of the long bones in a boy with chronic glomerulonephritis, renal rickets, and secondary hyperparathyroidism. In addition to the increased skeletal density, note the widened zone of provisional calcification at the ankles and the subperiosteal resorption along the medial margins of the upper tibial shafts (arrow).

Condition	Imaging Findings	Comments
Gaucher's disease	Diffuse osteosclerosis may develop in the reparative stage. More common manifestations include Erlenmeyer flask deformity with ground-glass pattern and aseptic necrosis of the femoral head.	Inborn error of metabolism characterized by accumulation of abnormal quantities of complex lipids in the reticuloendothelial cells of the spleen, liver, and bone marrow.
Multiple myeloma **(Fig B5-13)**	Uniform sclerosis of bone.	Very rare manifestation.
Hereditary hyperphosphatasia **(Fig B5-14)**	Generalized widening and increased density of bone is one manifestation (especially in adults). In children there is more commonly bowing and thickening of long bones with a varying pattern of density and thickness of the cortices.	Rare hereditary disease associated with elevated serum alkaline phosphatase. Thickening of the calvarium with patchy sclerosis may simulate the cotton-wool appearance of Paget's disease.
Infantile cortical hyperostosis (Caffey's disease) **(see Fig B8-8)**	Massive cortical thickening, widening, and sclerosis of bone with laminated periosteal reaction in the healing phase. Primarily involves the mandible, scapula, clavicle, ulna, and ribs.	Now uncommon disease characterized by hyperirritability, soft-tissue swelling, periosteal new bone formation, and cortical thickening of underlying bones. The onset is always before the age of 5 months. Scapular lesion (usually unilateral) may be mistaken for a malignant tumor.
Physiologic osteosclerosis of newborns	Extremely dense and sclerotic skeleton (may mimic osteopetrosis).	Normal variant (especially in prematures). Usually disappears within a few weeks.

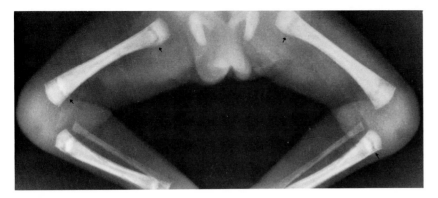

FIG B5-12. Congenital syphilis. Diffuse sclerosis with transverse bands of lucency (arrows) in the diaphyses of the femurs and tibias.

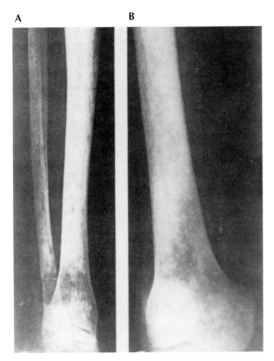

FIG B5-13. Sclerotic myeloma. Views of (A) the leg and (B) the femur demonstrate diffuse and nodular sclerosis. Cortical thickening of the tibia encroaches on the medullary canal. Similar changes were evident in the pelvis.[9]

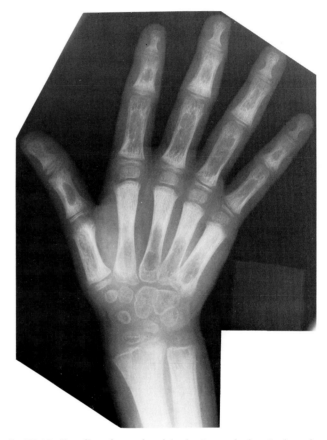

FIG B5-14. Hereditary hyperphosphatasia. Areas of sclerosis about the metacarpals and middle phalanges associated with thinning of the cortices. The proximal phalanges show diffuse deossification.

BUBBLY LESIONS OF BONE

Condition	Imaging Findings	Comments
Fibrous dysplasia (monostotic) (Fig B6-1)	Well-defined lucent area (varies from completely radiolucent to homogeneous ground-glass density depending on the amount of fibrous or osseous tissue deposited in the medullary cavity). Primarily involves long bones (especially the femur and tibia), ribs, and facial bones. Often there is local expansion of bone with endosteal erosion of the cortex (predisposes to pathologic fractures).	Proliferation of fibrous tissues in the medullary cavity, usually beginning during childhood. The most common cause of an expansile focal rib lesion. In severe and long-standing disease, affected bones may be bowed or deformed (''shepherd's crook'' deformity of the femur). Malignant degeneration is extremely rare in fibrous dysplasia.
Giant cell tumor (Figs B6-2 and B6-3)	Eccentric lucent metaphyseal lesion that may extend to the immediate subarticular cortex of a bone but does not involve the joint. Expansion toward the shaft produces a well-demarcated lucency, often with cortical expansion but without a sclerotic shell or border. Typically involves the distal femur, proximal tibia, distal radius, or ulna.	Lytic lesion in the end of a long bone of a young adult after epiphyseal closure. Usually asymptomatic, but may be associated with intermittent dull pain and a palpable tender mass and predispose to pathologic fracture. About 20% are malignant (best seen as tumor extension through the cortex and an associated soft-tissue mass on CT). There is much overlap in the radiographic appearance of benign and malignant lesions.
Fibrous cortical defect (Fig B6-4)	Small, often multilocular, eccentric lucency that causes cortical thinning and expansion and is sharply demarcated by a thin, scalloped rim of sclerosis. Initially round, the defect soon becomes oval with its long axis parallel to that of the host bone.	Not a true neoplasm, but rather a benign and asymptomatic small focus of cellular fibrous tissue causing an osteolytic lesion in the metaphyseal cortex of a long bone (most frequently the distal femur). One or more fibrous cortical defects develop in up to 40% of all healthy children. Most regress spontaneously and disappear by the time of epiphyseal closure. A persistent and growing lesion is termed nonossifying fibroma (see below).
Nonossifying fibroma (Fig B6-5)	Multilocular, eccentric lucency that causes cortical thinning and expansion and is sharply demarcated by a thin, scalloped rim of sclerosis.	Results from continued proliferative activity of a fibrous cortical defect and is seen in older children and young adults.
Simple bone cyst (Figs B6-6 and B6-7)	Expansile lucent lesion that is sharply demarcated from adjacent normal bone. May contain thin septa (scalloping of underlying cortex) that produce a multiloculated appearance. Tends to have an oval configuration with its long axis parallel to that of the host bone.	True fluid-filled cyst with a wall of fibrous tissue. Begins adjacent to the epiphyseal plate and appears to migrate down the shaft (in reality, the epiphysis has migrated away from the cyst). Bone cysts arise in children and adolescents and most commonly involve the proximal humerus and femur. Often presents as a pathologic fracture that may show the fallen fragment sign (fragments of cortical bone are free to fall to the dependent portion of the fluid-filled cyst, unlike a bone tumor that has a firm tissue consistency).

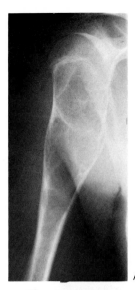

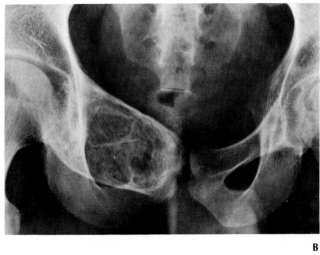

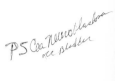

FIG B6-1. Fibrous dysplasia. Views of (A) the humerus and (B) the ischium in two different patients show expansile lesions containing irregular bands of sclerosis giving them a multilocular appearance.

B

A

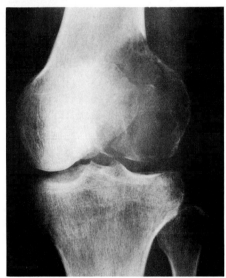

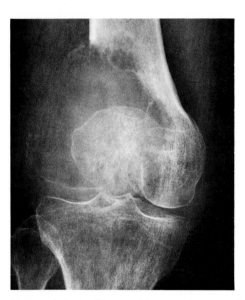

FIG B6-2. Giant cell tumor of the distal femur. Typical eccentric lucent lesion in the metaphysis extends to the immediate subarticular cortex. The surrounding cortex, though thinned, remains intact.

FIG B6-3. Malignant giant cell tumor. The tumor has caused cortical disruption, extends outside the host bone, and has an ill-defined margin.

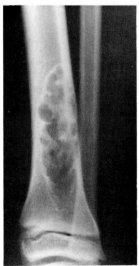

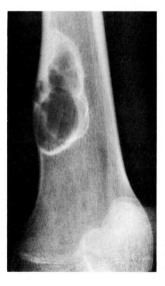

FIG B6-4. Fibrous cortical defect. Multilocular, eccentric lucency in the distal tibia. Note the thin, scalloped rim of sclerosis.

FIG B6-5. Nonossifying fibroma. Multilocular, eccentric lucency with a sclerotic rim in the distal femur.

Condition	Imaging Findings	Comments
Aneurysmal bone cyst (Fig B6-8)	Expansile, eccentric, cystlike lesion causing marked ballooning of thinned cortex. Light trabeculation and septation in the lesion may produce a multiloculated appearance. Periosteal reaction may develop. Primarily involves the metaphyses of long bones (especially the femur and tibia) and the posterior elements of vertebrae.	Not a true neoplasm or cyst, but rather numerous blood-filled arteriovenous communications. Most frequently occurs in children and young adults and presents with mild pain of several months' duration, swelling, and restriction of movement. May extend beyond the axis of the host bone and form a visible soft-tissue mass which, when combined with a cortex so thin that it is invisible on plain radiographs, may be mistaken for a malignant bone tumor.
Enchondroma (Figs B6-9 and B6-10)	Well-marginated lucency arising in the medullary canal (usually near the epiphyses) that expands bone locally and often causes thinning and endosteal scalloping of the cortex (may lead to pathologic fracture with minimal trauma). Primarily involves the small bones of the hands and feet. Characteristic calcifications (varying from minimal stippling to large, amorphous areas of increased density) develop in the lucent matrix.	Common benign cartilaginous tumor that is most frequently found in children and young adults. Usually asymptomatic and discovered either incidentally or when a pathologic fracture occurs. The development of severe pain or radiographic growth of the lesion with loss of marginal definition, cortical disruption, and local periosteal reaction suggests malignant degeneration (increased incidence the closer the tumor is to the axial skeleton). Multiple enchondromatosis is termed Ollier's disease.
Central chondrosarcoma (Fig B6-11)	Localized lucent area of osteolytic destruction in the metaphyseal end of a bone. When the rate of tumor growth exceeds that of bone repair, the margins of the lesion become irregular and ill defined and the tumor extends to cause cortical destruction and invasion of soft tissues. The cartilaginous tissue in a chondrosarcoma can be easily recognized by the amorphous punctate, flocculent, or "snowflake" calcifications that are seen in about two thirds of central tumors.	Malignant tumor of cartilaginous origin that may originate de novo or in a pre-existing cartilaginous lesion (osteochondroma, enchondroma). The tumor is about half as common as osteogenic sarcoma, develops at a later age (half the patients are more than 40 years old), grows more slowly, and metastasizes later. Central chondrosarcoma may also appear as an aggressive, poorly defined osteolytic lesion that blends imperceptibly with normal bone and can expand to replace the entire medullary cavity (may simply be a later phase of the first, benign-appearing type).

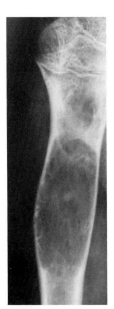

FIG B6-6. Simple bone cyst in the proximal humerus. The cyst has an oval configuration, with its long axis parallel to that of the host bone. Note the thin septa that produce a multiloculated appearance.

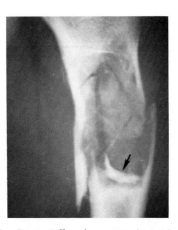

FIG B6-7. Fallen fragment sign. After pathologic fracture, a cortical bone fragment (arrow) lies free in a subtrochanteric bone cyst.[10]

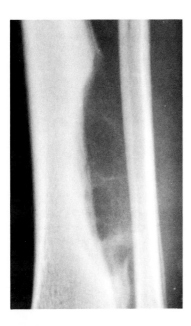

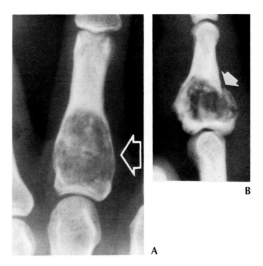

FIG B6-8. Aneurysmal bone cyst of the tibia. Expansile, eccentric, cystic lesion with multiple fine internal septa. Because the severely thinned cortex is difficult to detect, the tumor resembles a malignant process.

FIG B6-9. Enchondroma. (A) Well-demarcated tumor (arrow) expands the bone and thins the cortex. (B) Pathologic fracture (arrow).

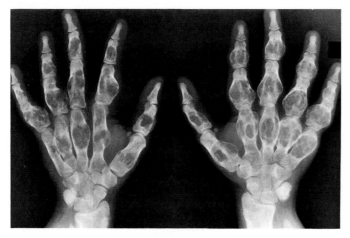

FIG B6-10. Multiple enchondromatosis. View of both hands demonstrates multiple globular and expansile lucent filling defects involving all the metacarpals and the proximal and middle phalanges.

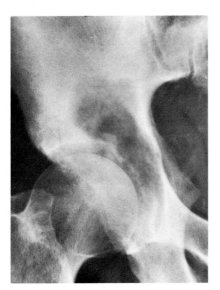

FIG B6-11. Central chondrosarcoma. Irregular and ill-defined lytic lesion of the lower ilium.

Condition	Imaging Findings	Comments
Brown tumor **(Fig B6-12)**	Single or multiple focal lytic areas that are generally well demarcated and often cause expansion of bone. Primarily involves the mandible, pelvis, ribs, and femur.	True cyst representing intraosseous hemorrhage in patients with hyperparathyroidism (especially the primary type). Usually there is other radiographic evidence of hyperparathyroidism. A large cyst may simulate malignancy or lead to pathologic fractures and bizarre deformities.
Localized myeloma **(solitary plasmacytoma)** **(Figs B6-13 and B6-14)**	Expansile, often trabeculated lucency that predominantly involves the ribs, long bones, and pelvis. A highly destructive tumor may expand or balloon bone before it breaks through the cortex. In the spine, an affected vertebral body may collapse or be destroyed.	Infrequent condition in which a single plasma cell tumor presents as an apparently solitary destructive bone lesion with no evidence of the major disease complications usually associated with multiple myeloma. Generally develops into typical multiple myeloma (diffuse lytic lesions) within 1 to 2 years.
Metastasis **(Figs B6-15 and B6-16)**	Single large metastatic focus appearing as an expansile, trabeculated lesion (blowout metastasis).	Typically secondary to carcinomas of the kidneys and thyroid. Most lytic metastases are irregular, poorly defined, and multiple.
Lymphoma **(Fig B6-17)**	Single or multiple lytic defects. There may be endosteal scalloping of the cortex.	Mottled pattern of destruction and sclerosis may simulate hematogenous metastases.
Eosinophilic granuloma **(Fig B6-18)**	Usually a well-defined medullary lucency (rapidly growing lesions may have indistinct, hazy borders) that predominantly affects the skull, pelvis, femur, and spine. There is often endosteal scalloping and local or extensive periosteal reaction. Characteristic finding is a peculiar beveled contour of the lesion that produces a ''hole-within-a-hole'' effect.	In the skull, typically produces one or more small punched-out areas that originate in the diploic space, expand and perforate both the inner and outer tables, and often contain a central bone density (button sequestrum). In the spine, generally spotty destruction in a vertebral body that proceeds to collapse the vertebra into a thin flat disk (vertebra plana).
Osteoblastoma **(Fig B6-19)**	Well-circumscribed, eccentric, and expansile lucency that may break through the cortex to produce a soft-tissue component surrounded by a thin calcific shell.	Rare bone neoplasm that most often arises in adolescence. About half involve the vertebral column (most frequently the neural arches and processes). The remainder affect the long bones or the small bones of the hands and feet. Although predominantly lytic, osteoblastomas may have some internal calcification and their aggressive appearance often simulates that of a malignant lesion. *also in distal ⅓ clavicle*
Chondroblastoma **(Fig B6-20)**	Eccentric, round or oval lucency in an epiphysis that often has a thin sclerotic rim and may contain flocculent calcification. May also involve the greater trochanter of the femur and the greater tuberosity of the humerus.	Rare, benign cartilaginous tumor of the epiphysis that occurs in children and young adults (most frequently males) before enchondral bone growth ceases.

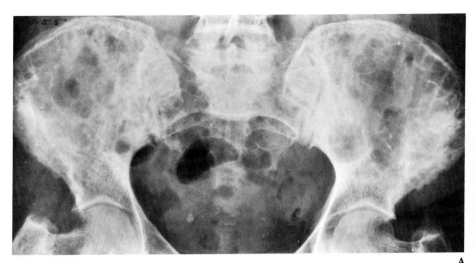
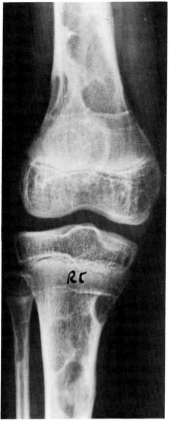

A

B

FIG B6-12. **Brown tumors.** Multiple lytic lesions (A) in the pelvis and (B) about the knee.

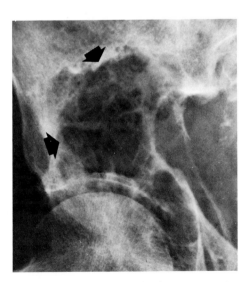

FIG B6-13. **Solitary plasmacytoma** of the ilium (arrows). Some residual streaks of bone remain in this osteolytic lesion, producing a soap-bubble appearance.

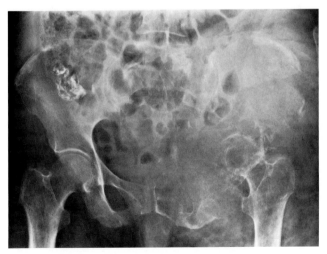

FIG B6-14. **Solitary plasmacytoma.** Highly destructive tumor that has obliterated virtually all of the left half of the pelvis.

Condition	Imaging Findings	Comments
Chondromyxoid fibroma (Fig B6-21)	Eccentric, round or oval lucency arising in the metaphysis of a long bone. The overlying cortex is usually bulging and thinned and the inner border is generally thick and sclerotic, often with scalloped margins. About 50% involve the tibia (the remainder affect the pelvis and other bones of the extremities).	Uncommon benign bone tumor originating from cartilage-forming connective tissue and predominantly occurring in young adults. Calcification is infrequent (unlike chondroblastoma and other cartilaginous bone lesions).
Epidermoid inclusion cyst	Well-circumscribed lucency in a terminal phalanx that may cause thinning, expansion, or even loss of the cortical margin.	Unlike an enchondroma, usually a history of penetrating trauma and no stippled calcification.
Intraosseous ganglion	Well-defined lucency with a sclerotic margin adjacent to the articular surface.	Most commonly involves the tibia and the head and neck of the femur.
Lipoma	Expansile lucency with a thinned cortex. May break through the cortex and have an adjacent soft-tissue component.	Rare tumor that arises in the calcaneus, skull, ribs, or extremities.

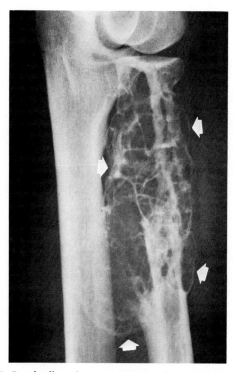

FIG B6-15. Renal cell carcinoma metastatic to bone. Typical expansile bubbly lesion (arrows) in the proximal shaft of the radius.

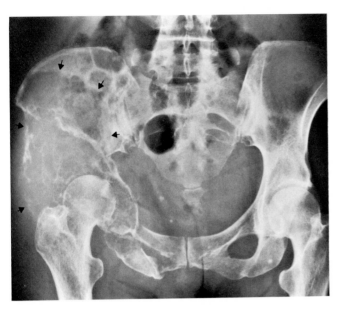

FIG B6-16. Metastatic thyroid carcinoma. Large area of entirely lytic, expansile destruction (arrows) involves the left ilium.

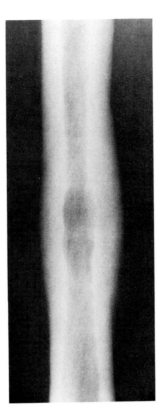

FIG B6-17. Lymphoma. Focal lytic defect with endosteal scalloping of the cortex.

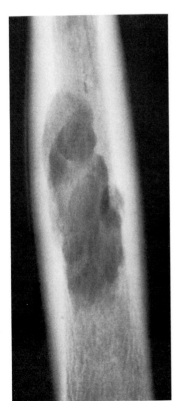

FIG B6-18. Eosinophilic granuloma. Bubbly osteolytic lesion in the femur, with scalloping of the endosteal margins and a thin layer of periosteal response.

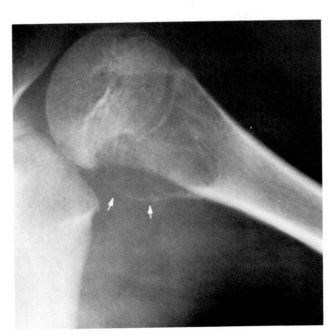

FIG B6-19. Osteoblastoma. Expansile, eccentric mass in the proximal humerus causes thinning of the cortex (arrows).

Condition	Imaging Findings	Comments
Glomus tumor	Central well-circumscribed lucency that primarily involves the distal aspect of the terminal phalanx of a finger.	May mimic an enchondroma, but a glomus tumor is painful. A subungual glomus tumor may cause pressure erosion at that site.
Ossifying fibroma (see Fig SK16-4)	Smooth, round or expansile mass involving the skull, face, or mandible.	Rare tumor that may be associated with reactive bone sclerosis or calcification of the tumor matrix.
Adamantinoma	Large loculated, expansile lucent mass that usually involves the midportion of the tibia.	Rare tumor that primarily affects adolescents and young adults. The histologic pattern resembles ameloblastoma of the mandible. Often recurs and may metastasize.
Fungal infection (Fig B6-22)	Focal area of lytic destruction (often multiple).	Coccidioidomycosis; blastomycosis. Sclerosis and periosteal reaction may develop.
Echinococcal cyst	Large central radiolucent area associated with endosteal scalloping and expansion. May show cortical breakthrough and a soft-tissue mass.	Usually monostotic and predominantly involves the pelvis, spine, and long bones.
Hemophilic pseudotumor (Fig B6-23)	Central or eccentric lucent lesion, often with a large adjacent soft-tissue hemorrhage. There may be cortical erosion suggesting a sarcoma.	Extensive local area of intraosseous hemorrhage that most commonly involves the femur, pelvis, tibia, and small bones of the hands.
Cystic osteomyelitis (tuberculosis)	Single or multiple small oval lucencies lying in the long axis of a bone and having well-defined margins with sclerosis. Primarily involves the skull, shoulder, pelvic girdles, and axial skeleton.	Rare manifestation of disseminated tuberculosis. In children (who are more commonly affected), the lesions usually affect the peripheral skeleton, are symmetric in distribution, and are unaccompanied by sclerosis.
Desmoplastic fibroma	Osteolytic lesion that destroys medullary bone with cortical erosion and expansion. Generally has an aggressive appearance simulating that of a malignant tumor.	Extremely rare benign neoplasm characterized by abundant collagen formation. Most commonly involves the pelvis, mandible, humerus, tibia, and scapula.

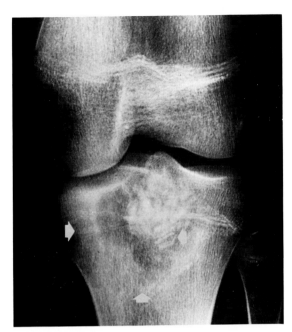

FIG B6-20. Chondroblastoma. Osteolytic lesion containing calcification (arrows) in the epiphysis. Note the open epiphyseal line.[11]

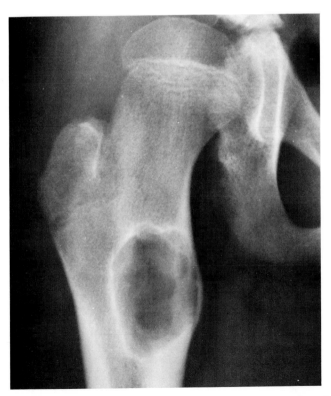

FIG B6-21. Chrondromyxoid fibroma. Ovoid, eccentric metaphyseal lucency with thinning of the overlying cortex and a sclerotic inner margin.

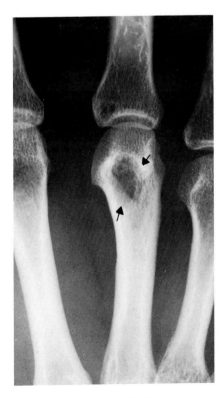

FIG B6-22. Coccidioidomycosis. Typical well-marginated, punched-out lytic defect in the head of the third metacarpal (arrows).[12]

Condition	Imaging Findings	Comments
Hemangioma (Fig B6-24; see Figs SP1-3 and SK4-7)	Lucent area with delicate bony trabeculation. Most commonly occurs near the end of a tubular or flat bone.	Rare manifestation. Much more commonly produces multiple coarse linear striations running vertically in a demineralized vertebral body or a sunburst pattern of osseous spicules radiating from a central lucency in the skull.
Angiomatous lesion	Single or (more frequently) multiple lucent metaphyseal lesions, which often have a sclerotic margin and are sometimes associated with a soft-tissue mass.	Rare congenital malformation consisting of endothelium-lined structures that may be lymphatic channels (lymphangiomatosis) or blood vascular channels (hemangiomatosis). Usually there is widespread involvement of multiple long bones, flat bones, and the skull.
Sarcoidosis (Fig B6-25)	Single or multiple sharply circumscribed, punched-out areas of lucency, primarily involving the small bones of the hands and feet. There may be cortical thinning, expansion, or destruction.	Perivascular granulomatous infiltration in the haversian canals destroys the fine trabeculae, producing a mottled or lacelike, coarsely trabeculated pattern.

A

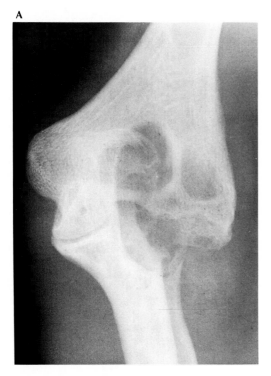

B

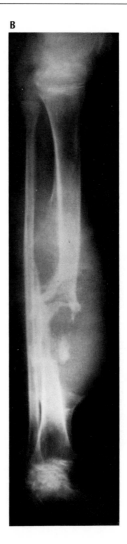

FIG B6-23. **Hemophilia.** (A) Large subchondral cysts about the elbow. (B) Destructive, expansile lesion of the lower tibial shaft.[13]

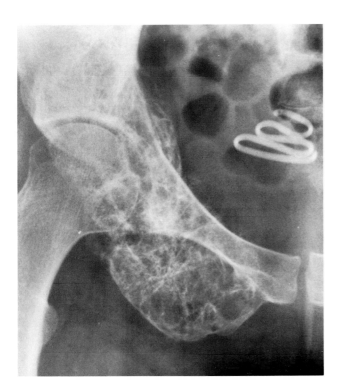

FIG B6-24. Hemangioendothelioma. Expansile lucency containing delicate bony trabeculation.

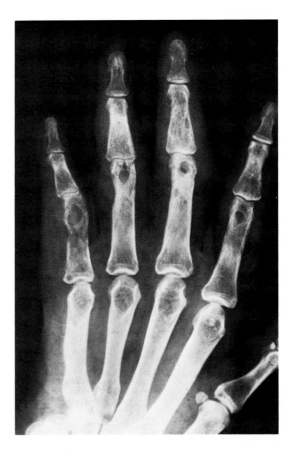

FIG B6-25. Sarcoidosis. Multiple osteolytic lesions throughout the phalanges, having a typical punched-out appearance. The apparent air density in the soft tissues is a photographic artifact.

MOTH-EATEN OR PUNCHED-OUT
OSTEOLYTIC DESTRUCTIVE LESIONS OF BONE

Condition	Imaging Findings	Comments
Osteolytic metastases (see Figs B6-15 and B6-16)	Single or multiple areas of bone destruction of variable size with irregular and poorly defined margins. Major sites of metastatic spread are bones containing red marrow, such as the spine, pelvis, ribs, skull, and the upper ends of the humerus and femur. Metastases distal to the knees and elbows are infrequent but do occur, especially with bronchogenic tumors. Periosteal reaction is rare.	Most common primary lesions causing osteolytic metastases are carcinomas of the breast, lung, kidney, and thyroid. Kidney and thyroid metastases typically produce a single large metastatic focus that may appear as an expansile trabeculated lesion (blowout metastasis). Elliptical lytic bone lesions suggest lymphoma. Metastatic neuroblastoma in children produces mottled bone destruction resembling leukemia. Spinal metastases typically destroy the pedicles, unlike multiple myeloma (in which the pedicles are infrequently involved). Because almost half the mineral content of a bone must be lost before it is detectable on plain radiographs, radionuclide bone scanning is far more sensitive for screening (false-negative bone scans occur with aggressively osteolytic lesions, especially multiple myeloma).
Multiple myeloma (Figs B7-1 and B7-2)	Multiple punched-out osteolytic lesions scattered throughout the skeletal system. Because bone destruction is due to proliferation of plasma cells distributed throughout the bone marrow, the flat bones containing red marrow (vertebrae, skull, ribs, pelvis) are primarily affected. The appearance may be indistinguishable from that of metastatic carcinoma, though the lytic defects in myeloma tend to be more discrete and uniform in size. Sharply circumscribed lytic lesions tend to eventually coalesce, destroying large segments of bone and often breaking through the cortex and periosteum to form a soft-tissue mass (especially involving a rib). Pathologic fractures are common, especially in the ribs, vertebrae, and long bones.	Disseminated malignancy of plasma cells that primarily affects persons between 40 and 70 years of age. Typical laboratory findings include an abnormal spike of monoclonal immunoglobulin and the presence of Bence Jones protein in the urine. Up to 20% of patients develop secondary amyloidosis. Extensive plasma cell proliferation in the bone marrow with no tendency to form discrete tumor masses may produce generalized skeletal deossification simulating postmenopausal osteoporosis. In the spine, there are often multiple vertebral compression fractures and usually sparing of the pedicles (lacking red marrow), which are frequently destroyed by metastatic disease. Because there is little or no stimulation of new bone formation, radionuclide bone scans may be normal even with extensive skeletal infiltration. Solitary or diffuse areas of sclerosis (simulating osteoblastic metastases) may rarely occur.
Ewing's sarcoma (Fig B7-3; see Fig B8-2)	Classic appearance (though seen in a minority of cases) is an ill-defined permeative area of bone destruction that involves a large central portion of the shaft of a long bone and is associated with a fusiform lamellated periosteal reaction parallel to the shaft. Other types of periosteal reaction include a thin periosteal elevation (Codman's triangle) or a sunburst pattern with horizontal spicules of bone extending into a soft-tissue mass.	Primary malignant tumor of children and young adults (peak incidence in the midteens) that arises in the bone marrow and most commonly involves the long bones of the extremities (especially the femur and tibia). Tends to metastasize early to the lungs and to other bones. Other appearances of Ewing's sarcoma include a purely lytic lesion or a mass of increased density (suggesting osteogenic sarcoma) in the metaphyseal region.

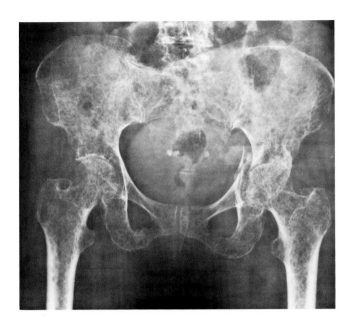

Fig B7-1. **Multiple myeloma.** Diffuse punched-out osteolytic lesions throughout the pelvis and proximal femurs.

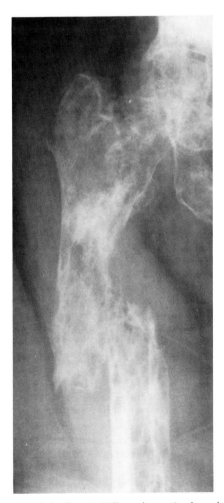

Fig B7-2. **Heavy chain disease.** Diffuse, destructive bone lesions have led to a pathologic fracture of the midshaft of the femur.

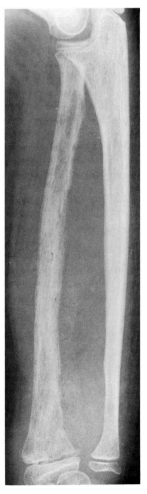

Fig B7-3. **Ewing's sarcoma.** Diffuse permeative destruction involves virtually the entire radius.

Condition	Imaging Findings	Comments
Reticulum cell sarcoma (Figs B7-4 and B7-5)	Moth-eaten pattern of permeative bone destruction that arises in the medullary cavity and then invades the cortex. There is often an amorphous or lamellated periosteal reaction. Most commonly involves a long bone (especially near the knee), but also can affect the pelvis, scapula, ribs, and vertebrae.	Primary malignant lesion of bone that is histologically similar to Ewing's sarcoma but tends to occur in older persons (average age, about 40 years). Unlike Ewing's sarcoma, reticulum cell sarcoma rarely causes systemic symptoms and the patient generally appears healthy even when local disease is extensive. The tumor tends to metastasize late to lymph nodes and the lungs and only rarely spreads to other bones.
Osteomyelitis (Figs B7-6 and B7-7)	In long bones, the earliest evidence of osteomyelitis is a localized, deep soft-tissue swelling adjacent to the metaphysis with displacement or obliteration of normal fat planes. Subtle areas of metaphyseal lucency reflecting resorption of necrotic bone are followed by more prominent bone destruction producing a ragged, moth-eaten appearance (the more virulent the organism, the larger the area of destruction). Subperiosteal spread of inflammation elevates the periosteum and stimulates the laying down of layers of new bone parallel to the shaft, producing a characteristic lamellated periosteal reaction. Eventually, a large amount of new bone surrounds the cortex in a thick, irregular bony sleeve (involucrum) and disruption of the cortical blood supply leads to bone necrosis and segments of avascular dead bone (sequestra). In vertebral osteomyelitis (see Figs SP3-3 and SP4-4), the earliest sign is subtle erosion of the subchondral bony plate with loss of the sharp cortical outline. This may progress to total destruction of the vertebral body associated with a paravertebral soft-tissue abscess. Unlike neoplastic processes, osteomyelitis usually affects the intervertebral disk space and often involves adjacent vertebrae.	Osteomyelitis is caused by a broad spectrum of infectious organisms that reach bone by hematogenous spread, by extension from a contiguous site of infection, or by direct introduction of organisms (trauma or surgery). Acute hematogenous osteomyelitis tends to involve bones with rich red marrow (metaphyses of long bones, especially the femur and tibia, in infants and children; vertebrae in adults). Because the earliest changes are usually not evident on plain radiographs until about 10 days after the onset of symptoms, radionuclide bone scanning is the most valuable imaging modality for early diagnosis (increased isotope uptake reflects the inflammatory process and increased blood flow). The radiographic findings, clinical history, and symptoms are generally sufficient to make the diagnosis of osteomyelitis, though at times aggressive bone destruction and bizarre periosteal reaction (especially in children) may suggest a malignant bone tumor and require biopsy. Chronic osteomyelitis results in a thick, irregular, sclerotic bone with central radiolucency, elevated periosteum, and often a chronic draining sinus.
Leukemia (Fig B7-8)	Patchy lytic lesions produce a permeative moth-eaten appearance or diffuse destruction with cortical erosion. Reactive response to proliferating leukemic cells can cause patchy or uniform osteosclerosis, whereas subperiosteal proliferation of tumor cells incites periosteal new bone formation. In children, the knees, ankles, and wrists are most often affected; in adults, leukemic bone lesions most commonly involve the vertebrae, ribs, skull, and pelvis.	The earliest radiographic sign of disease in children is a transverse radiolucent band at the metaphyseal ends of long bones (most commonly the knees, ankles, and wrists). Though a nonspecific indication of severe illness under age 2, its presence after this age strongly suggests acute leukemia. Diffuse skeletal demineralization (especially in the spine where it leads to vertebral compression fractures) may result from both leukemic infiltration of the bone marrow and alteration of protein and mineral metabolism. Metastatic neuroblastoma may be indistinguishable from leukemia.
Lymphoma (see Fig B4-3)	Hematogenous spread produces a mottled pattern of destruction and sclerosis that may simulate metastatic disease.	Other forms of skeletal involvement include dense vertebral sclerosis (ivory vertebra), discrete elliptical lytic lesions, and bone erosion (especially of the anterior surfaces of upper lumbar and lower thoracic vertebral bodies due to direct extension from adjacent nodes).

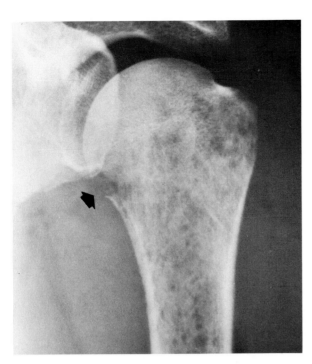

FIG B7-4. Reticulum cell sarcoma. A moth-eaten pattern of bone destruction in the proximal humerus is associated with a pathologic fracture (arrow).

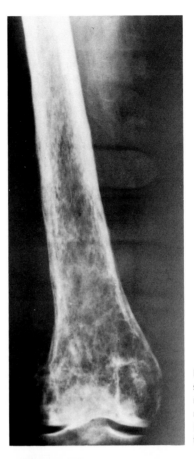

FIG B7-5. Reticulum cell sarcoma. Diffuse permeative destruction with mild periosteal response involving the distal half of the femur.

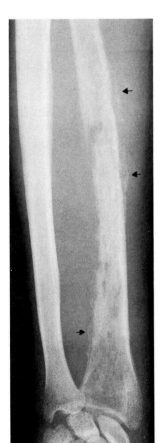

FIG B7-6. Osteomyelitis. Patchy pattern of bone destruction involves much of the shaft of the radius. Note the early periosteal new bone formation (arrows).

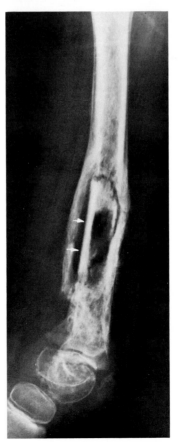

FIG B7-7. Chronic osteomyelitis. The involucrum (straight arrows), a thick, irregular, bony sleeve, surrounds the sequestrum (curved arrows), a residual segment of avascular dead bone.

Condition	Imaging Findings	Comments
Fibrosarcoma (Fig B7-9)	Initially, an irregular, destructive lesion arising in the medullary cavity that may cause thinning, expansion, and erosion of the cortex accompanied by periosteal proliferation. As the tumor develops, there may be massive invasion of the cortex and extension into the medullary canal.	Rare primary malignant tumor of fibroblastic tissue that most often involves tubular bones in young patients and flat bones in older ones. Tends to grow slowly and to have a somewhat better prognosis than osteogenic sarcoma. Unlike most primary bone tumors, fibrosarcomas tend to metastasize to lymph nodes.
Osteogenic sarcoma (Fig B7-10)	Purely lytic, destructive process is one manifestation.	More commonly a mixed form (combination of bone destruction and production) with an exuberant, irregular periosteal response.
Histiocytosis X (see Fig B6-18)	Initially, a small relatively well-defined lucent area that enlarges to produce endosteal scalloping, a multilocular appearance, and bone expansion with associated periosteal new bone formation. May produce more confluent areas of bone destruction simulating malignancy or osteomyelitis. Predominantly involves the skull, pelvis, spine, and ribs.	Bone lesions are most characteristic of eosinophilic granuloma. A calvarial defect may demonstrate a bony density in its center (button sequestrum). Spinal involvement may lead to the collapse of a vertebral body, which assumes the shape of a thin flat disk (vertebra plana).
Massive osteolysis of Gorham	Initially, radiolucent foci in intramedullary or subcortical regions with slowly progressive atrophy, dissolution, fracture, fragmentation, and disappearance of a portion of the bone. The process spreads across joints and intervertebral spaces, leading to a dramatic pattern of regional destruction that generally increases relentlessly over a period of years (may eventually stabilize).	Rare disease of unknown etiology that usually is detected before age 40. May affect the axial or appendicular skeleton. One of the "primary osteolysis syndromes," many of which affect the hands and feet.
Diffuse lymphangiomatosis (Fig B7-11)	Multiple cystic lesions throughout the skeleton causing erosions and progressive osteolytic defects in various bones.	Rare condition in children and adolescents that may be associated with widespread soft-tissue abnormalities and involvement of other organ systems.
Intraosseous hemangiomatosis	Multiple widespread bone defects.	Rare condition without the characteristic appearance seen in other forms of the disease (no vertebral or skull hemangiomas).
Weber-Christian disease	Multiple punched-out or moth-eaten lesions involving the skull, pelvis, and medullary bone.	Rare disturbance of fat metabolism resulting in diffuse panniculitis, characteristic painful nodules in subcutaneous fat, and occasional bone lesions.
Membranous lipodystrophy	Multiple radiolucent cystic lesions symmetrically distributed in the carpal and tarsal bones and the ends of long bones.	Rare hereditary disease of unknown origin that usually affects young adults and is associated with presenile mental retardation.

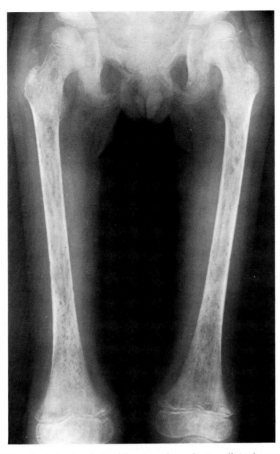

FIG B7-8. **Acute leukemia.** Proliferation of neoplastic cells in the marrow has caused extensive destruction of bone in both femurs.

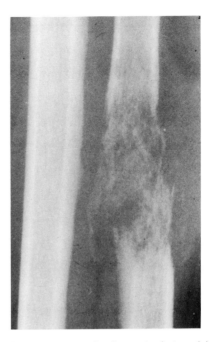

FIG B7-9. **Fibrosarcoma.** Irregular destructive lesion of the shaft of the radius.

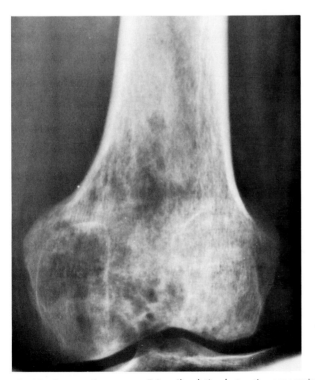

FIG B7-10. **Osteogenic sarcoma.** Primarily a lytic, destructive process in the distal femur.

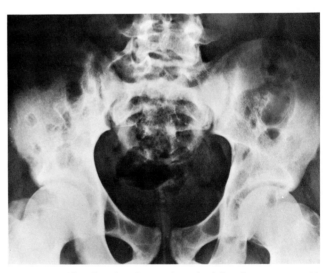

FIG B7-11. **Diffuse lymphangiomatosis.** Multiple lytic lesions, some with thin sclerotic rims, diffusely involve the pelvis.

LOCALIZED PERIOSTEAL REACTION

Condition	Imaging Findings	Comments
Fracture	Localized periosteal reaction associated with traumatic or stress fracture.	May involve multiple bones in the battered child syndrome.
Primary malignant tumor of bone (Figs B8-1 and B8-2)	Localized periosteal reaction that may be solid, laminated, spiculated (perpendicular to the shaft), or amorphous. Codman's triangle may occur.	Most commonly osteosarcoma and Ewing's sarcoma. Periosteal reaction is rare in other primary bone malignancies.
Secondary malignant tumor of bone (Fig B8-3)	Multiple areas of localized solid or laminated periosteal reaction associated with an underlying destructive process. There may be perpendicular periosteal reaction in the skull.	Common manifestation in children with leukemia and metastases from neuroblastoma.
Benign bone tumor or cyst (Fig B8-4)	Various patterns of periosteal reaction.	Solid periosteal reaction with expanding cysts or tumors, especially if there is an underlying pathologic fracture. Elliptical and dense periosteal reaction in osteoid osteoma (radiolucent intracortical nidus).
Osteomyelitis (Figs B8-5 and B8-6)	Solid or laminated periosteal reaction.	Subperiosteal spread of inflammation elevates the periosteum and stimulates the laying down of layers of new bone parallel to the shaft. Eventually, a large amount of new bone surrounds the cortex in a thick, irregular bony sleeve (involucrum). Disruption of the cortical blood supply leads to bone necrosis with dense segments of avascular dead bone (sequestra) remaining.
Subperiosteal hemorrhage	Solid or laminated periosteal reaction.	May result from trauma or hemophilia.
Eosinophilic granuloma (see Fig B6-18)	Solid or laminated periosteal reaction that may be localized or extensive.	Characteristic appearance of a sharply defined lucency with a peculiar beveled pattern and multiple undulating contours.
Arthritis (Fig B8-7)	Solid or laminated periosteal reaction.	Most common in juvenile rheumatoid arthritis and Reiter's syndrome; rare in psoriatic arthritis.
Vascular stasis	Solid, often undulating, periosteal reaction primarily along the tibial and fibular shafts.	Chronic venous or lymphatic insufficiency or obstruction. Phleboliths often occur in varicose veins.
Infantile cortical hyperostosis (Caffey's disease) (Fig B8-8)	Laminated periosteal reaction in the healing phase. Primarily involves the mandible, scapula, clavicle, ulna, and ribs.	Now uncommon disease characterized by hyper-irritability, soft-tissue swelling, periosteal new bone formation, and massive cortical thickening of underlying bones. Onset is almost always before 5 months of age.

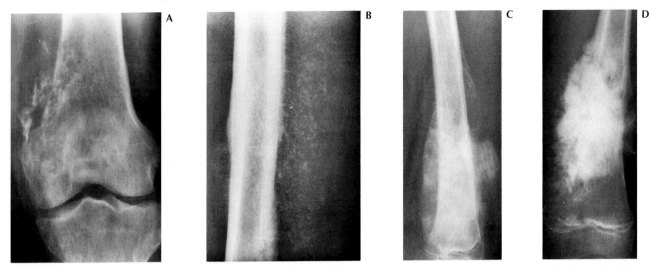

FIG B8-1. Osteogenic sarcoma. (A to D) Four examples of osteogenic sarcoma of the femur illustrate the broad spectrum of radiographic changes. There are various amounts of exuberant, irregular periosteal response and ragged bone destruction.

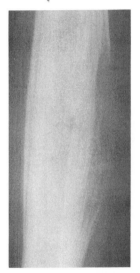

FIG B8-2. Ewing's sarcoma. Laminated periosteal reaction on one side of the bone and thin periosteal elevation (Codman's triangle) on the other.

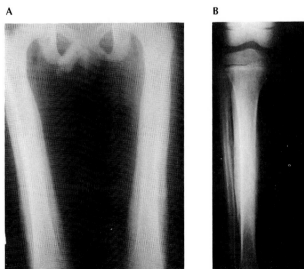

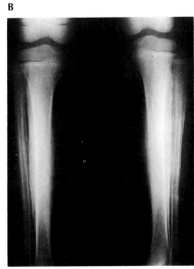

FIG B8-3. Chronic leukemia. Pronounced periosteal new bone formation cloaking (A) the femurs and (B) the tibias and fibulas.

Condition	Imaging Findings	Comments
Syphilis (acquired)/yaws (Figs B8-9 and B8-10)	Extensive solid, often undulating, periosteal reaction occurring independently or in conjunction with gummas in the bone marrow.	Diffuse, widespread, and symmetric, periosteal reaction may reflect underlying infiltration by granulation tissue in congenital syphilis.
Tropical ulcer (Fig B8-11)	Fusiform periosteal reaction localized to the bone beneath the ulcer. Periosteal new bone blends with the cortex to produce the thickened, sclerotic cortex (often exceeding 1 cm) of a classic "ivory osteoma."	Extremely common disease throughout much of Africa that is caused by the Vincent types of fusiform bacilli and spirochetes. Chronic ulcers most often affect children and young adults and are usually located in the middle or lower leg.
Bone infarct	Solid periosteal response overlying the shaft of a large tubular bone (underlying patchy lucency and sclerosis of medullary bone).	Most common in sickle cell disease. Periosteal reaction may be radiographically indistinguishable from osteomyelitis.
Secondary osteomyelitis (spread from contiguous soft-tissue infection)	Solid periosteal reaction associated with bone destruction and sclerosis.	Most frequently occurs in patients with diabetes mellitus and vascular insufficiency and predominantly involves the hands and feet or the area adjacent to a decubitus ulcer.

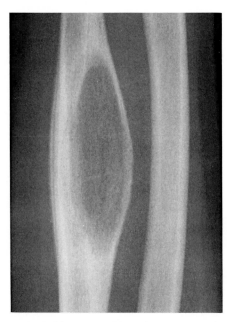

FIG B8-4. Aneurysmal bone cyst of the radius. An expansile, eccentric, cystlike lesion causes ballooning of the cortex and periosteal response.

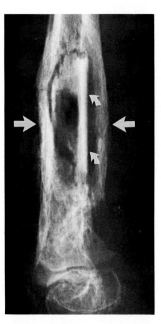

FIG B8-5. Chronic osteomyelitis. The involucrum (straight arrows) surrounds the sequestrum (curved arrows).

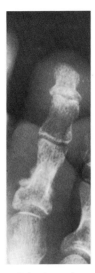

Fig B8-6. Reiter's syndrome. Typical fluffy periosteal reaction about the proximal phalanx. There is also soft-tissue swelling of the toe.[14]

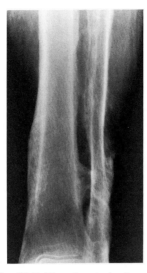

Fig B8-7. Vascular stasis. Extensive periosteal changes about the tibial and fibular shafts.

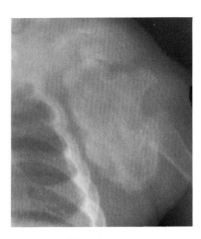

Fig B8-8. Caffey's disease. Massive periosteal new bone formation about the left scapula.

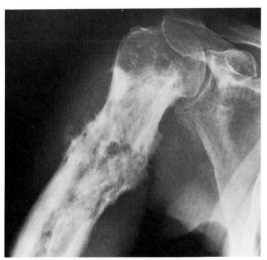

Fig B8-9. Syphilis. Diffuse lytic destruction of the proximal humerus with reactive sclerosis and periosteal new bone formation.

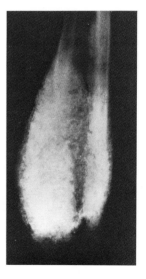

Fig B8-10. Yaws. Massive patchy new bone formation affects both bones of the forearm. Strands of new bone extend in the line of the interosseous ligament.[7]

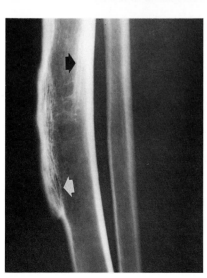

Fig B8-11. Ivory osteoma of tropical ulcer. There is cortical thickening of the tibia on the side opposite the ulcer (black arrow), which had been present for 1 year. Medullary resorption is starting at the inner margin of the osteoma and the solid cortex is beginning to show a trabecular pattern (white arrow).[15]

WIDESPREAD OR GENERALIZED PERIOSTEAL REACTION

Condition	Imaging Findings	Comments
Hypertrophic osteoarthropathy (Fig B9-1)	Thick (initially thin), irregular, undulating periosteal reaction that eventually fuses with the cortex. Symmetrically involves the diaphyses of tubular bones (especially the long bones of the forearm and leg), sparing the ends. There is often associated soft-tissue swelling of the distal phalanges (clubbing) without changes in the underlying bone.	Most frequently arises in patients with primary intrathoracic neoplasms, especially bronchogenic carcinoma. Other common causes include tumors of the pleura and mediastinum, chronic suppurative lung lesions (lung abscess, bronchiectasis, empyema), and cystic fibrosis and pulmonary metastases in infants and children. Occasionally occurs in association with extrathoracic neoplasms and gastrointestinal diseases (biliary cirrhosis, ulcerative colitis, Crohn's disease).
Arthritis (see Fig B8-6)	Generalized (or localized) solid or laminated periosteal reaction.	Juvenile rheumatoid arthritis (peripheral and axial skeleton, particularly at tendon and ligament insertions); Reiter's syndrome (calcaneus, short tubular bones of the foot, tibia, and fibula); psoriatic arthritis (infrequently).
Battered child syndrome (Fig B9-2)	Exuberant solid or laminated periosteal reaction along the shafts of long bones (associated with multiple fractures).	Repeated traumatic injuries lead to multiple fractures in various stages of healing. There are often fractures of the corners of the metaphyses (with or without associated epiphyseal displacement) and one or more fractures at otherwise unusual sites (the ribs, scapula, sternum, spine, or lateral ends of the clavicles).
Physiologic periostitis of newborns	Generalized periosteal reaction along long bones of the extremities.	Occurs during the second and third months of life in up to 50% of infants (especially prematures). Generally considered to be a normal variation due to the exuberant bone growth at this age.
Idiopathic	Multiple and often symmetric solid periosteal reaction primarily involving tubular bones.	Most frequently occurs at tendon and ligament insertions into bone.
Venous or lymphatic stasis (Fig B9-3)	Generalized (or localized) solid, thin or thick, often undulating periosteal reaction most commonly along the tibial and fibular shafts.	In venous stasis (eg, varicose veins), there may be development of phleboliths (calcified venous thrombi that appear as round densities and often contain lucent centers); there may also be plaquelike calcification in chronically congested subcutaneous tissues.
Thyroid acropachy (Fig B9-4)	Generalized and symmetric spiculated periosteal reaction that primarily involves the midportions of the diaphyses of tubular bones of the hands and feet. Multiple small radiolucencies in the irregular periosteal new bone may produce a bubbly or lacy appearance.	Rare complication of hyperthyroid disease characterized by progressive exophthalmus, relatively asymptomatic swelling of the hands and feet, clubbing of the digits, and pretibial myxedema. Develops after thyroidectomy or radioactive iodine treatment of primary hyperthyroidism (most patients are euthyroid or hypothyroid when symptoms develop).

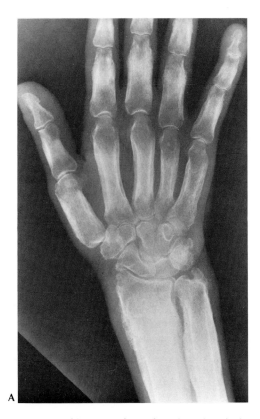

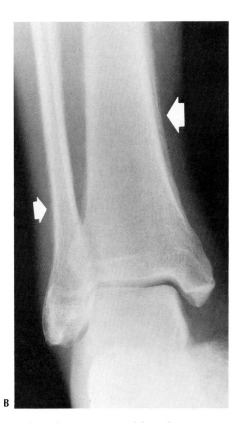

FIG B9-1. Hypertrophic osteoarthropathy. Films of (A) the lower arm and hand and (B) the lower leg in patients with bronchogenic carcinoma and mesothelioma, respectively, demonstrate characteristic plaques of periosteal new bone. Note the irregular, undulating new bone formation affecting the distal radius and ulna. In the metacarpals, the periosteal reaction involves the diaphyses and spares the ends of these tubular bones. There is some periarticular demineralization about the metacarpophalangeal and metacarpocarpal joints but no evidence of bone erosion or cartilage destruction.

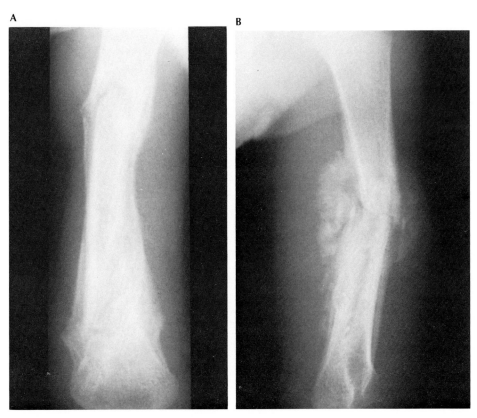

FIG B9-2. Battered child. (A and B) Periosteal reaction about healing fractures of both humeri.

Condition	Imaging Findings	Comments
Pachydermoperiostosis (primary hypertrophic osteoarthropathy) (see Fig B12-10)	Generalized and symmetric periosteal reaction that tends to blend with the cortex and primarily involves the distal ends of the radius, ulna, tibia, and fibula.	Inherited disorder characterized by marked thickening of the skin of the extremities, face, and scalp. Self-limited disease that most commonly affects adolescent males and progresses for several years before stabilizing.
Infantile cortical hyperostosis (Caffey's disease) (see Fig B8-8)	Multiple areas of laminated periosteal reaction and massive cortical thickening in the healing phase. Primarily involves the mandible, scapula, clavicle, ulna, and ribs.	Now uncommon disease characterized by hyper-irritability, soft-tissue swelling, periosteal new bone formation, and cortical thickening of underlying bones. Onset is almost always before 5 months of age. Scapular lesion (usually unilateral) may be mistaken for a malignant tumor.
Hypervitaminosis A (Fig B9-5)	Generalized solid or laminated periosteal reaction that is greatest near the center of the shaft and tapers toward the ends. Unlike Caffey's disease, periosteal thickening in hypervitaminosis A rarely involves the mandible.	Chronic excessive intake of vitamin A produces a syndrome characterized by bone and joint pain, hair loss, pruritis, anorexia, dryness and fissures of the lips, hepatosplenomegaly, and yellow tinting of the skin. The radiographic changes are most commonly seen between ages 1 and 3.
Fluorosis (see Fig B19-16)	Generalized and symmetric periosteal reaction that primarily involves tubular bones (especially at sites of muscle and ligament attachments).	Fluorine poisoning causes dense skeletal sclerosis (most prominent in vertebrae and the pelvis) with calcification of ligaments (iliolumbar, sacrotuberous, and sacrospinous).
Gaucher's disease	Generalized periosteal reaction involving long tubular bones, the spine, and the pelvis.	Inborn error of lipid metabolism characterized by a ground-glass pattern, aseptic necrosis of the femoral head, and Erlenmeyer flask deformities.
Congenital syphilis (see Fig B22-1)	Diffuse widespread, symmetric, and profound periosteal reaction primarily affecting long tubular bones.	Reflects underlying infiltration by syphilitic granulation tissue. Complete but slow resolution with treatment.
Tuberous sclerosis (see Fig B32-6)	Diffuse undulating periosteal reaction or periosteal "nodules" involving tubular bones (especially metacarpals, metatarsals, and phalanges).	Rare inherited disorder presenting with clinical triad of convulsive seizures, mental deficiency, and adenoma sebaceum. There are often renal and intracranial hematomas and characteristic scattered intracerebral calcifications.

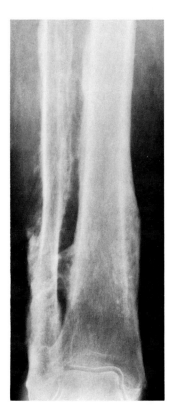

FIG B9-3. Venous stasis. Periosteal new bone formation cloaking the tibia and fibula.

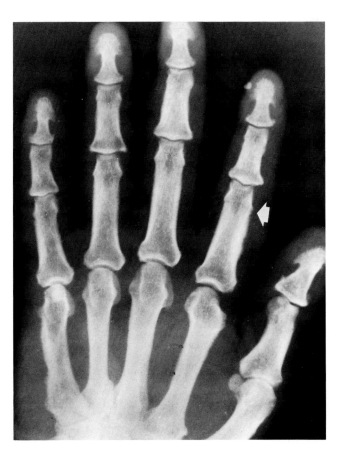

FIG B9-4. Thyroid acropachy. Spiculated periosteal new bone formation, seen best on the radial aspect of the proximal phalanx of the second digit (arrow).

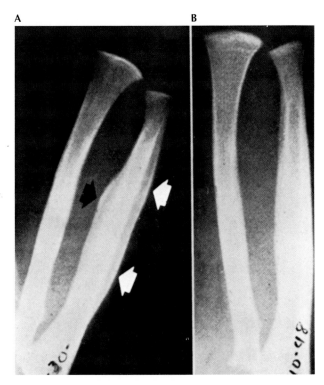

FIG B9-5. Hypervitaminosis A. (A) Thin, wavy, shelflike cortical thickening (arrows) during the active phase of poisoning. (B) Four months after stoppage of the vitamin concentrate, the hyperostosis is shrunken, smooth, and more sclerotic.[16]

Condition	Imaging Findings	Comments
Thermal burns	Periosteal reaction in bones underlying areas of severe burns (represents local response to periosteal irritation).	Generally develops within several months after injury. In tubular bones, produces a radiographic appearance similar to that of hypertrophic osteoarthropathy.
Hand-foot syndrome (sickle cell anemia) (see Fig B32-1)	Generalized periosteal reaction involving short tubular bones.	Follows infarctions in young children with sickle cell disease and produces a periosteal reaction indistinguishable from osteomyelitis.
Healing scurvy (Fig B9-6)	Generalized massive periosteal reaction during the healing phase.	Findings in acute disease include characteristic "white line," Pelken's spur, Wimberger's sign, and demineralized epiphyseal ossification centers surrounded by dense sharply demarcated rings of calcification.
Healing rickets	Generalized solid or laminated periosteal new bone formation (represents remineralization of subperiosteal osteoid).	Thin stripes of density may develop along the outer cortical margins of long bones during acute disease. Although they resemble inflammatory periosteal reaction, these shadows represent zones of poorly calcified osteoid laid down by the periosteum.
Polyarteritis nodosa	Generalized symmetric periosteal reaction, most frequently involving the shafts of bones of the lower legs.	Pattern identical to that of hypertrophic osteoarthropathy.

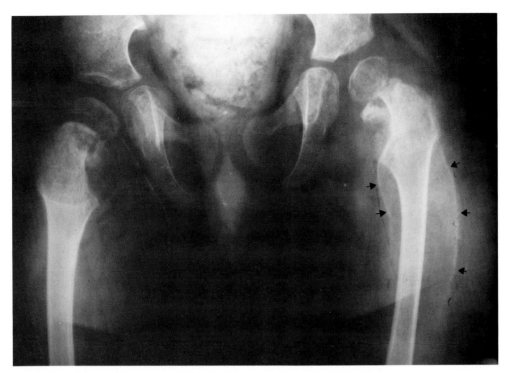

FIG B9-6. Scurvy. Large, calcifying, subperiosteal hematoma of the femoral shaft (arrows).[13]

ARTHRITIDES

Condition	Joints Commonly Involved	Radiographic and Clinical Appearance
Osteoarthritis (degenerative joint disease) (Fig B10-1)	Distal interphalangeal joints of the fingers; first carpometacarpal joint; hips; knees, first metatarsophalangeal joints; spine.	Bilateral, nonuniform joint space narrowing, subchondral sclerosis, and marginal osteophyte (spur) formation. Subchondral cysts are common while osteoporosis is typically absent. Primary osteoarthritis most frequently affects postmenopausal women and is characterized by classic Heberden's nodes (enlargement of spurs to produce well-defined bony protuberances that appear clinically as palpable and visible knobby thickening). Osteoarthritis may also be secondary to trauma, ischemic necrosis, malalignment of bony structures, and other arthritides.
Erosive (inflammatory) osteoarthritis (Fig B10-2)	Distal interphalangeal joints and first carpometacarpal joint.	Inflammatory process associated with proliferative and erosive abnormalities that predominantly involves middle-aged women. If proliferative changes (osteophytosis, sclerosis) predominate, the resulting radiographic appearance is identical to that of noninflammatory osteoarthritis. The erosions of inflammatory osteoarthritis frequently predominate in the central portion of the joint, unlike the marginal erosions of rheumatoid arthritis, psoriasis, gout, and multicentric reticulohistiocytosis.
Rheumatoid arthritis (Figs B10-3 to B10-5; see Fig SP10-1)	Bilateral, symmetric involvement of metacarpophalangeal, proximal interphalangeal, and carpal joints with similar involvement of the feet. Characteristic erosion of the ulnar styloid process. The condition often progresses toward the trunk until practically every joint in the body is involved. Atlantoaxial subluxation may develop due to weakening of the transverse ligaments from synovial inflammation.	Initially, fusiform periarticular soft-tissue swelling (due to joint effusion and hyperplastic synovitis) associated with periarticular osteoporosis (due to disuse and local hyperemia). Extension of pannus from synovial reflections onto the bones causes characteristic small foci of erosive destruction at the edges of the joint. Destruction of articular cartilage causes generalized joint space narrowing that is frequently associated with extensive bone resorption. Severe complications include opera-glass hand, solid bony ankylosis, and a variety of contractures and subluxations (boutonnière, swan neck, ulnar deviation).
Juvenile rheumatoid arthritis (Fig B10-6)	Rapidly growing joints (knees, ankles, wrists), unlike the peripheral distribution of involved joints in the adult form. Monarticular disease, especially in a knee, is more common in the juvenile type.	Initially, periarticular soft-tissue swelling and osteoporosis. Joint space narrowing and articular erosions are late findings. Periosteal calcification is much more common and severe than in the adult form, while synovial cysts infrequently occur. Ankylosis about the wrist and ankle is common. Variety of growth disturbances including initial acceleration because of local hyperemia, then delay due to epiphyseal fusion or the administration of steroids. Overgrowth of the epiphysis of an affected joint may produce a characteristic balloon appearance. Other findings include apophyseal joint ankylosis and atlantoaxial subluxation in the cervical spine, erosion of the mandibular condyles and micrognathia, and erosion of the intercondylar notch of the femur (simulates hemophilia).

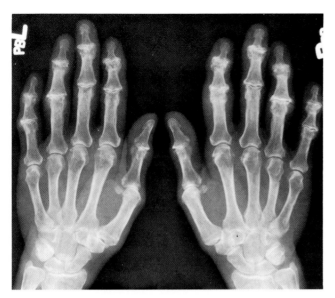

FIG B10-1. **Osteoarthritis** of the fingers.

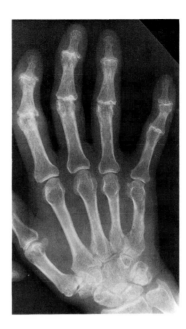

FIG B10-2. **Erosive osteoarthritis** of the hand. Narrowing of the proximal and distal interphalangeal joints with erosions and spur formation.

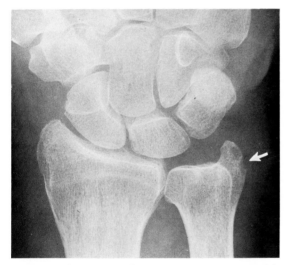

FIG B10-3. **Rheumatoid arthritis.** Characteristic erosion of the ulnar styloid process (arrow) by an adjacent tenosynovitis of the extensor carpi ulnaris tendon. Note the associated soft-tissue swelling.

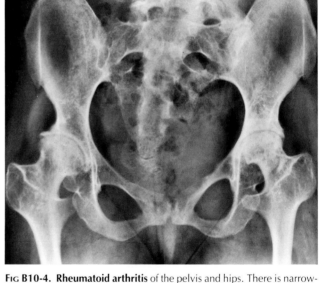

FIG B10-4. **Rheumatoid arthritis** of the pelvis and hips. There is narrowing of the hip joints bilaterally with some reactive sclerosis. Note the relative preservation of the subchondral cortical margins. In contrast to degenerative disease, the joint space narrowing in rheumatoid arthritis is symmetric and not confined to weight-bearing surfaces. Note also the obliteration of both sacroiliac joints.

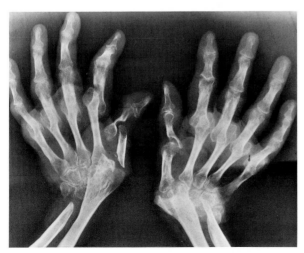

FIG B10-5. **Mutilating rheumatoid arthritis.** Opera-glass hand (main en lorgnette deformity) due to extensive destruction and telescoping of bone ends.

Condition	Joints Commonly Involved	Radiographic and Clinical Appearance
Psoriatic arthritis (Figs B10-7 and B10-8)	Bilateral, usually asymmetric, involvement of distal interphalangeal joints (may also affect proximal interphalangeal joints) of the hands and feet; sacroiliac joints; and spine.	Soft-tissue swelling, joint space narrowing, and periarticular erosions simulating rheumatoid arthritis (though psoriatic disease predominantly involves distal rather than proximal interphalangeal joints, is asymmetric, and causes little or no periarticular osteoporosis). Characteristic radiographic features include a tendency toward bony ankylosis of the interphalangeal joints, resorption of terminal tufts of the distal phalanges, fluffy periosteal reaction near joints and along shafts, and arthritis multilans with "pencil-in-cup" deformity. Unilateral or bilateral sacroiliitis and asymmetric syndesmophytes in the thoracolumbar spine.
Reiter's syndrome (arthritis, urethritis, conjunctivitis, mucocutaneous lesions) (Figs B10-9 and B10-10; see Fig B8-7)	Sacroiliac joints; heels; toes.	Primarily affects young adult males (after certain types of venereal or enteric infections). Radiographic changes often mimic rheumatoid arthritis, though in Reiter's syndrome they tend to be asymmetric and primarily involve the feet. Typical manifestations include fluffy periostitis adjacent to the small joints of the foot, ankle, and calcaneus; inferior calcaneal spurs; asymmetric sacroiliitis; and asymmetric syndesmophytes in the thoracolumbar spine.
Ankylosing spondylitis (Figs B10-11 to B10-13)	Sacroiliac joints; spine; hips; small joints of the hands and feet.	Almost always begins as bilateral, symmetric sacroiliitis that may lead to complete fibrous and bony ankylosis. In the lumbar spine, the disease tends initially to involve the lowermost levels and progress upward with characteristic squared vertebral bodies and bamboo spine (ossification in paravertebral tissues and longitudinal spinal ligaments combined with extensive lateral bony bridges [syndesmophytes] between vertebral bodies). Fractures often occur through a disk space (rather than a vertebral body) and continue through the posterior elements. Irregular proliferative new bone formation ("whiskering") often develops at sites of ligamentous or muscular attachments. Peripheral joint involvement (in up to half the patients) simulates psoriasis or Reiter's syndrome.
Jaccoud's arthritis (Fig B10-14)	Multiple joints of the hands and, less frequently, the feet.	Rare occurrence after resolution of a severe attack of rheumatic fever. Usually there is only self-limited periarticular swelling, but it may rarely cause permanent deformities (ulnar deviation, flexion contractures) without joint space narrowing or bone erosion.

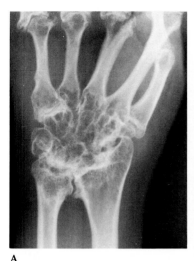

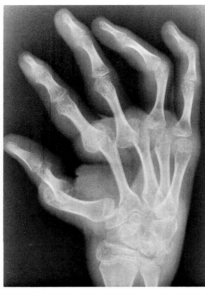

A

B

FIG B10-6. **Juvenile rheumatoid arthritis.** (A) Severe deossification of the carpal bones with joint space narrowing and even obliteration. Note the virtual ankylosis between the distal radius and the proximal carpal row. (B) Multiple subluxations, especially involving the metacarpophalangeal joints. There is diffuse periarticular soft-tissue swelling with moderate osteoporosis.

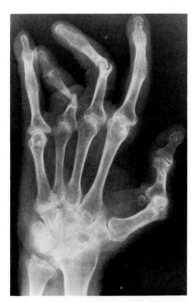

FIG B10-7. **Psoriatic arthritis.** Bizarre pattern of asymmetric bone destruction, subluxation, and ankylosis. Note particularly the pencil-in-cup deformity of the third proximal interphalangeal joint and the bony ankylosis involving the wrist and the phalanges of the second and fifth digits.

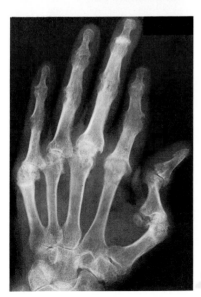

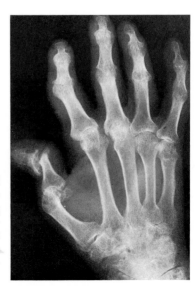

FIG B10-8. **Psoriatic arthritis.** Views of both hands and wrists demonstrate ankylosis across many of the interphalangeal joints with scattered erosive changes involving several interphalangeal joints, most of the metacarpophalangeal joints, and the interphalangeal joint of the right thumb. Note the striking asymmetry of involvement of the carpal bones, an appearance unlike that expected in rheumatoid arthritis.

Condition	Joints Commonly Involved	Radiographic and Clinical Appearance
Arthritis associated with inflammatory bowel disease (see Fig B11-2)	Sacroiliac joints; spine, knees, elbows.	Spinal involvement identical to ankylosing spondylitis. Peripheral arthritis is usually limited to soft-tissue swelling and joint effusion, which tend to be migratory, usually follow the onset of colitis, generally flare up during exacerbations of colonic disease, and usually cause no residual damage. Some form of arthritis occurs in up to 25% of patients with ulcerative or Crohn's colitis.
Gout (Figs B10-15 to B10-17)	First metatarsophalangeal joint; interphalangeal joints; elbows; knees.	Joint effusion, periarticular swelling, soft-tissue tophi, and characteristic ''rat bite'' erosions with sclerotic margins and overhanging edges adjacent to (but not involving) the articular surface. In advanced disease, severe destructive lesions are associated with joint space narrowing and even fibrous ankylosis. No osteoporosis (patients are symptom-free and without disability between acute attacks). There may be chondrocalcinosis and acro-osteolysis of terminal phalangeal tufts.
Hemophilia (Figs B10-18 and B10-19)	Knees; elbows; ankles.	Recurrent bleeding into joints initially causes joint distension with cloudy increased density (deposition of iron pigment) in the periarticular soft tissues. In chronic disease, the hyperplastic synovium causes cartilage destruction and joint space narrowing with multiple subchondral cysts. Other characteristic findings include enlargement and premature ossification of epiphyseal centers, widening and deepening of the intercondylar notch of the femur, squaring of the inferior border of the patella, and destructive expansile bone lesions (pseudotumor of hemophilia) representing extensive intraosseous hemorrhage.

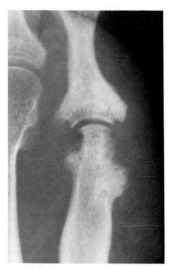

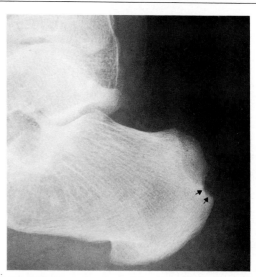

FIG B10-9. Reiter's syndrome. Erosive changes about the metatarsophalangeal joint of the fifth digit. The erosions involve the juxta-articular region, leaving the articular cortex intact.

FIG B10-10. Reiter's syndrome. Striking bony erosion (arrows) at the insertion of the Achilles tendon on the posterosuperior margin of the calcaneus.

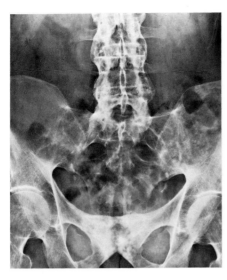

FIG B10-11. **Ankylosing spondylitis.** Bilateral symmetric obliteration of the sacroiliac joints with prominent syndesmophytes in the lower lumbar spine.

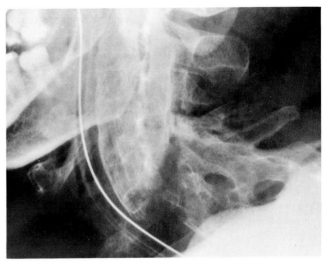

FIG B10-12. **Ankylosing spondylitis.** Oblique fracture of the midcervical spine, with anterior dislocation of the superior segment, is seen in a patient who fell while dancing and struck his head. The fracture extends through the lateral mass and lamina. Because of loss of flexibility and osteoporosis, patients with ankylosing spondylitis can suffer a fracture with relatively slight trauma.

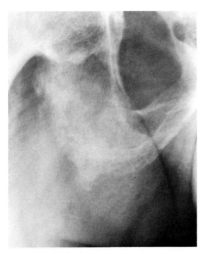

FIG B10-13. **Ankylosing spondylitis.** Irregular proliferation of new bone (whiskering) along the inferior pubic ramus.

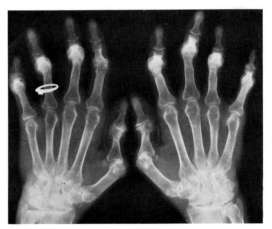

FIG B10-14. **Jaccoud's arthritis.** Frontal views of the hands and wrists demonstrate mild ulnar deviation with pronounced flexion of the proximal interphalangeal joints. There is no evidence of joint space narrowing or bone erosion.

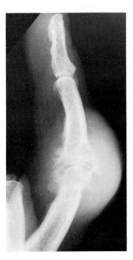

FIG B10-15. **Gout.** Severe joint effusion and periarticular swelling about the proximal interphalangeal joint of a finger. Note the associated erosion of articular cartilage.

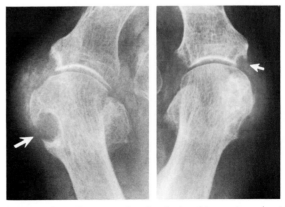

FIG B10-16. **Gout.** Two examples of typical rat-bite erosions about the first metatarsophalangeal joint (arrows). The cystlike lesions have thin sclerotic margins and characteristic overhanging edges.

Condition	Joints Commonly Involved	Radiographic and Clinical Appearance
Calcium pyrophosphate dihydrate deposition disease (pseudogout) (Fig B10-20)	Knees; wrists; elbows; hips; shoulders.	Leads to the development of secondary osteoarthritis (subchondral cyst formation, hypertrophic spurring, joint space narrowing, subchondral sclerosis). Frequent chondrocalcinosis.
Hydroxyapatite deposition disease	Shoulders; hips.	Amorphous calcifications in joints or bursae may cause inflammatory erosive changes.
Systemic lupus erythematosus (Fig B10-21)	Hands.	Subluxations and malalignment of joints in the absence of erosions. Typical deformities include ulnar deviation at the metacarpophalangeal joints and hyperextension and hyperflexion deformities (boutonnière, swan neck) at the interphalangeal joints.
Scleroderma (see Fig B20-1)	Hands and feet.	Soft-tissue swelling and periarticular osteoporosis along with characteristic terminal phalangeal resorption and soft-tissue calcifications. Erosive changes may represent coexistent rheumatoid arthritis.
Sarcoidosis (see Fig B32-5)	Hands.	In about 15% of patients, the disease presents as a transient acute polyarthritis with periarticular soft-tissue swelling. No significant osteoporosis or chronic radiographic deformities. The phalanges may show a coarsened trabecular pattern or sharply circumscribed, punched-out lucent areas.
Familial Mediterranean fever (see Fig B11-7)	Sacroiliac joints; large joints of the lower extremities.	Nonspecific transient soft-tissue swelling and osteoporosis with rare destructive changes. Bilateral, asymmetric involvement of sacroiliac joints.
Neuroarthropathies (see B14)		See page 648.
Multicentric reticulohistiocytosis (Fig B10-22)	Bilateral, symmetric involvement of interphalangeal joints of the hands and feet. Atlantoaxial subluxation.	Well-circumscribed marginal erosions (simulating gout) due to the deposition of lipid-containing macrophages. May eventually cause dramatic resorption of phalanges, foreshortening of fingers, and end-stage arthritis mutilans. Characteristic development of multiple soft-tissue masses that produce a ''lumpy-bumpy'' appearance.
Ochronosis (homogentisic acid deposition) (see Fig SP11-2)	Spine; shoulders; hips; knees.	Dense laminated calcification of multiple intervertebral disks (begins in the lumbar spine and may extend cephalad). Narrowing of intervertebral disk spaces and osteoporosis of vertebral bodies. Severe degenerative type of arthritis (joint space narrowing, marginal osteophytes, subchondral sclerosis) may develop in large peripheral joints at a young age.

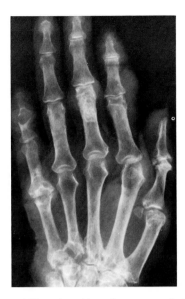

FIG B10-17. Gout. Diffuse deposition of urate crystals in periarticular tissues of the hand produce multiple large, lumpy soft-tissue swellings representing gouty tophi. Note the erosive changes that typically involve the carpal bones and the distal interphalangeal and metacarpophalangeal joints of the fifth digits.

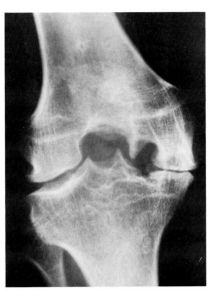

FIG B10-18. Hemophilia. The intracondylar notch is markedly widened and there are coarsened trabeculae, narrowing of the joint space, and hypertrophic spurring.

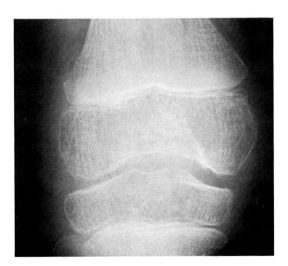

FIG B10-19. Hemophilia of the knee in a child. There is demineralization and coarse trabeculation with overgrowth of the distal femoral and proximal tibial epiphyses. The intercondylar notch is moderately widened.

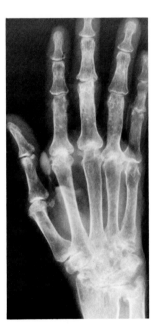

FIG B10-20. Pseudogout arthropathy. Severe joint space narrowing, erosive changes, and sclerosis about the wrist. Less marked changes involve the metacarpophalangeal joints and the proximal interphalangeal joint of the third digit.

Condition	Imaging Findings	Comments
Hemochromatosis (synovial deposition of iron) (Fig B10-23)	Metacarpophalangeal and interphalangeal joints of the hands.	Subarticular cysts and erosions, joint space narrowing, osteophytes, sclerosis, subluxation, and flattening and widening of the metacarpal heads (especially the second and third). May also produce osteoarthritic changes in large joints (knees, hips) and diffuse osteoporosis of the spine leading to vertebral collapse.
Acromegaly (excess growth hormone in adults) (Fig B10-24)	Generalized cartilage overgrowth (especially metacarpophalangeal and hip joints).	Degenerative changes with prominent hypertrophic spurring develop at an early age, but, unlike typical osteoarthritis, acromegaly results in joint spaces that remain normal or are even widened. Associated findings include overgrowth of terminal phalangeal tufts, thickened heel pads, and micrognathia.
Pigmented villonodular synovitis (Fig B10-25)	Knees; ankles; hips.	Joint effusion with multiple nodular soft-tissue masses that never calcify but may appear dense because of hemosiderin deposits. Invasion of adjacent bone may cause subchondral cystlike defects with sharp and sclerotic margins. Unlike rheumatoid or infectious arthritis, the joint space is usually preserved and there is no osteoporosis since the disorder does not cause much disability.
Infectious arthritis **Pyogenic** (Fig B10-26)	Any joint (most commonly the knees, hips, shoulders, and spine).	Soft-tissue swelling followed by rapid destruction of cartilage (joint space narrowing) and bone that first appears on plain radiographs 8 to 10 days after the onset of symptoms. Severe, untreated infection causes extensive destruction and loss of the entire cortical outline. Complete destruction of articular cartilage leads to bony ankylosis. In the spine, pyogenic arthritis rapidly involves the intervertebral disks (unlike metastatic disease).
Tuberculous (Figs B10-27 and B10-28)	Spine; hips; knees.	Insidious onset and slowly progressive course characterized by extensive juxta-articular osteoporosis that precedes bone destruction (unlike pyogenic arthritis, in which osteoporosis is a relatively late finding). Cartilage and bone destruction occur relatively late and tend initially to involve the periphery of a joint, sparing the maximum-weight–bearing surfaces that are destroyed in pyogenic arthritis. In the spine, infection begins in the vertebral body (not the disk, as in pyogenic infection) and leads to vertebral collapse and often a characteristic sharp, angular kyphosis (gibbous deformity). Extension of the infection may produce a cold abscess (fusiform soft-tissue paraspinal mass).

(continued page 630)

A B

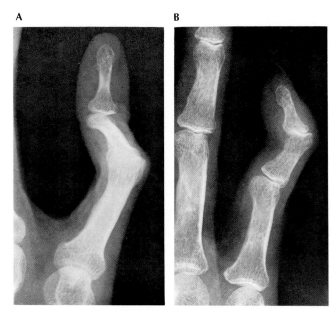

Fig B10-21. Systemic lupus erythematosus. (A) Flexion of the proximal interphalangeal joint and hyperextension of the distal interphalangeal joint result in a boutonnière deformity. (B) Hyperextension of the proximal interphalangeal joint and flexion of the distal interphalangeal joint produce a swan neck deformity.[14]

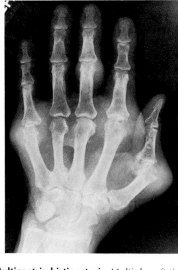

Fig B10-22. Multicentric histiocytosis. Multiple soft-tissue masses produce a "lumpy-bumpy" appearance. The soft-tissue deposits of multinucleated giant cells have produced erosions of juxta-articular bone. Although at this stage most of the joint spaces are spared, extensive involvement of the second metacarpophalangeal joint has led to total joint destruction.[14]

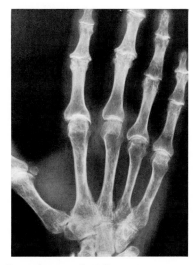

Fig B10-23. Hemochromatosis. Diffuse joint space narrowing with scattered erosions, osteophytes, and articular sclerosis.

A B

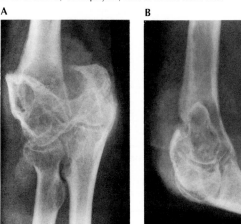

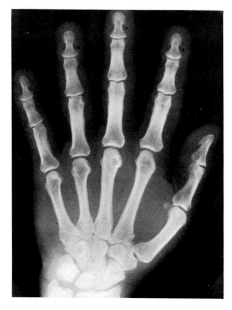

Fig B10-24. Acromegaly. Widening of the metacarpophalangeal joints, thickening of the soft tissues of the fingers, and overgrowth of the tufts of the distal phalanges (arrows).

Fig B10-25. Pigmented villonodular synovitis. (A) Frontal and (B) lateral views of the elbow demonstrate a joint effusion with nodular soft-tissue masses extending beyond the joint capsule. The soft-tissue mass appears dense because of deposits of hemosiderin in it. Large bone erosions reflect a combination of pressure effect and direct invasion by the synovial growth.

Condition	Joints Commonly Involved	Radiographic and Clinical Appearance
Fungal	Peripheral joints or the spine.	Variable radiographic manifestations requiring joint aspiration for diagnosis.
Viral	Small joints of the hands.	Transient joint effusion in rubella, mumps, or serum hepatitis that usually subsides without bone lesions.
Transient arthritides	Variable pattern.	Episodes of arthritic symptoms that usually subside without residual joint damage may occur in such conditions as Bechet's syndrome, Sjögren's syndrome, polyarteritis, dermatomyositis, and relapsing polychondritis.

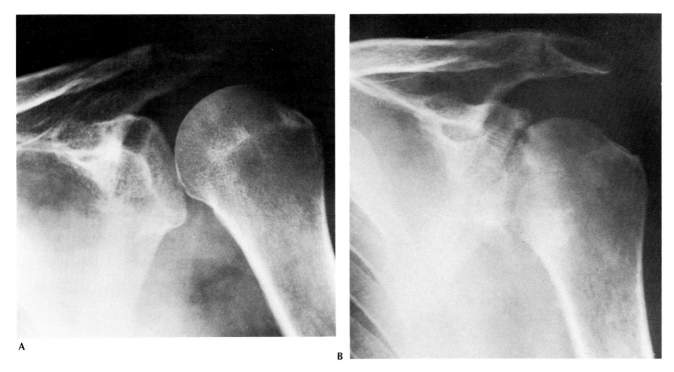

A   B

FIG B10-26. Acute staphylococcal arthritis. (A) Several days after instrumentation of the shoulder for joint pain, there is separation of the humeral head from the glenoid fossa due to fluid in the joint space. (B) Six weeks later there is marked cartilage and bone destruction, with sclerosis on both sides of the glenohumeral joint.

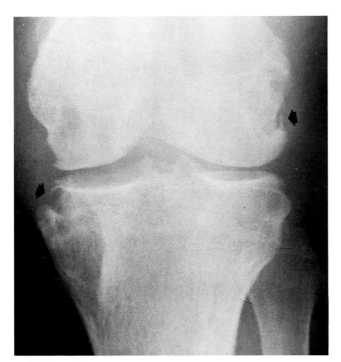

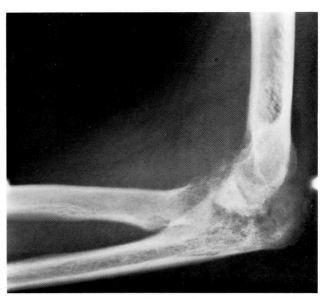

FIG B10-28. Tuberculous arthritis of the elbow. Complete destruction of the joint space. The large antecubital mass reflects marked synovial hypertrophy resulting from chronic granulomatous infection.[14]

FIG B10-27. Tuberculous arthritis of the knee. On both sides of the joint there are destructive bone lesions (arrows) involving the medial and lateral condyles and the medial aspect of the proximal tibia. Note the relative sparing of the articular cartilage and preservation of the joint space in view of the degree of bone destruction.

SACROILIAC JOINT ABNORMALITY

Condition	Comments
Bilateral, symmetric distribution	
Ankylosing spondylitis (Fig B11-1)	Sacroiliac joints are the initial site of involvement. Early findings include blurring of articular margins, irregular widening of the joints, and patchy sclerosis. This generally progresses to narrowing of the joint spaces and may lead to complete fibrosis and bony ankylosis. Dense reactive sclerosis often occurs, though it may become less prominent as the joint spaces become obliterated.
Inflammatory bowel disease (Fig B11-2)	Appearance identical in all respects to that of classic ankylosing spondylitis. Underlying conditions include ulcerative colitis, Crohn's disease, and Whipple's disease.
Hyperparathyroidism/ renal osteodystrophy	Subchondral resorption of bone (predominantly in the ilia) leads to irregularity of the osseous surface, adjacent sclerosis, and widening of the interosseous joint space. Articular space narrowing and bony fusion do not occur.
Osteitis condensans ilii (Fig B11-3)	Triangular zone of dense sclerosis along the inferior aspect of the ilia. The surfaces are well defined, the sacrum is normal, and the sacroiliac joint spaces are preserved. The condition probably represents a reaction to the increased stress to which the sacroiliac region is subjected during pregnancy and delivery (a similar type of sclerotic reaction, osteitis pubis, may occur in the pubic bones adjacent to the symphysis in women who have borne children).
Osteoarthritis	After age 40, most patients have some narrowing of the sacroiliac joint spaces, which may involve the entire articulations or appear as focal areas of abnormality at the inferior aspect of the joints. In comparison with ankylosing spondylitis, sacroiliac joint disease in osteoarthritis occurs in older patients, is often associated with prominent osteophytosis (especially at the anterosuperior and anteroinferior limits of the articular cavity) and prominent subchondral sclerosis, does not show erosions, and rarely demonstrates intra-articular bony ankylosis (though periarticular bridging osteophytes are common). Degenerative joint disease also may have a bilateral and asymmetric or a unilateral distribution.
Gout	Irregularity and sclerosis of articular margins are common (may reflect osteoarthritis in older patients). Large cystic areas of erosion in the subchondral bone of the ilia and sacrum are uncommon. Sacroiliac joint changes occur more frequently with early onset disease and tend to have a left-sided predominance. As with degenerative joint disease, sacroiliac joint involvement in gouty arthritis may be bilateral and asymmetric or unilateral.

(continued page 634)

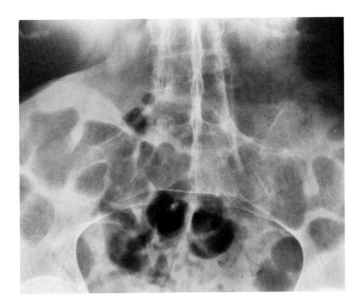

FIG B11-1. **Ankylosing spondylitis.** Bilateral, symmetric obliteration of the sacroiliac joints.

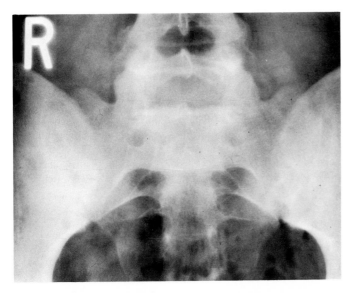

FIG B11-2. **Inflammatory bowel disease.** Bilateral, symmetric involvement of the sacroiliac joints in a patient with ulcerative colitis.

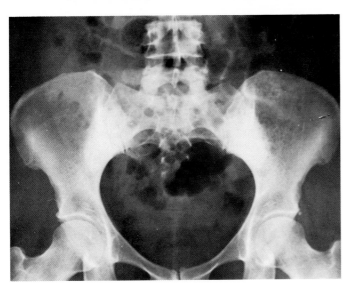

FIG B11-3. **Osteitis condensans ilii.** There is sharply demarcated sclerosis of the ilia adjacent to the sacroiliac joints. The sacrum is not affected and the margins of the sacroiliac joints are sharp and without destruction. The sclerosis that overlies the sacral wing is actually in the ilium, where it curves posteriorly behind the sacrum.[11]

Condition	Comments
Multicentric reticulohistiocytosis	Erosions and joint space narrowing leading to bony ankylosis, but no subchondral sclerosis.
Bilateral, asymmetric distribution	
Psoriatic arthritis (Fig B11-4)	Bilateral, asymmetric distribution is probably most common, though bilateral, symmetric abnormalities are frequent and even unilateral involvement may occur. The radiographic changes include erosions and sclerosis, predominantly affecting the ilium, and widening of the articular space. Although joint space narrowing and bony ankylosis can occur, this is much less frequent than in classic ankylosing spondylitis. A prominent finding may be blurring and eburnation of apposing sacral and iliac surfaces above the true joint in the region of the interosseous ligament.
Reiter's syndrome (Fig B11-5)	Bilateral, asymmetric distribution is probably most common, though bilateral, symmetric abnormalities are frequent and unilateral sacroiliac joint abnormalities may infrequently occur (especially early in the disease process). Sacroiliac joint changes are common in Reiter's syndrome, eventually developing in about 50% of patients. Osseous erosions primarily involve the iliac surface and adjacent sclerosis varies from mild to severe. Early joint space widening may later be replaced by narrowing. Although intra-articular bony ankylosis may eventually appear, it occurs much less frequently than in ankylosing spondylitis. A prominent finding may be blurring and eburnation of apposing sacral and iliac surfaces above the true joint in the region of the interosseous ligament.
Rheumatoid arthritis (Fig B11-6)	Relatively uncommon manifestation that usually produces minor subchondral erosions, mild or absent sclerosis, and either no or only focal intra-articular bony ankylosis. Infrequently has a unilateral distribution.
Familial Mediterranean fever (Fig B11-7)	Initially, widening of the articular space with loss of normal cortical definition primarily involving the ilium. Eventually, sclerosis with or without erosions and even bony ankylosis. Involvement may also be bilateral and symmetric or even unilateral.
Relapsing polychondritis	Joint space narrowing, erosion, and eburnation. Involvement may also be bilateral and symmetric or even unilateral.

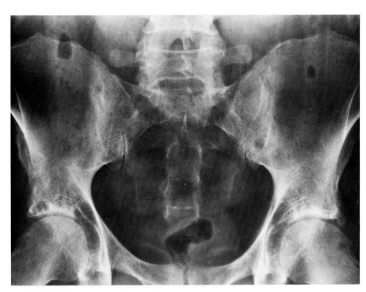

FIG B11-4. Psoriatic arthritis. Bilateral, though somewhat asymmetric, narrowing of the sacroiliac joints.

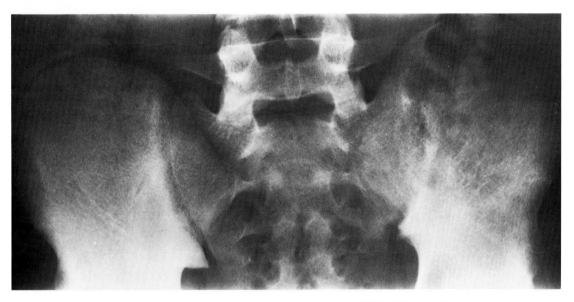

FIG B11-5. Reiter's syndrome. Bilateral, though asymmetric, sclerosis and narrowing of the sacroiliac joints with reactive sclerosis.

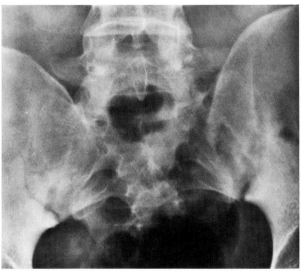

FIG B11-6. Rheumatoid arthritis. Bilateral, though asymmetric, sclerosis and narrowing of the sacroiliac joints.

Condition	Comments
Unilateral distribution	
Infection **(Fig B11-8)**	By far the most common cause of unilateral sacroiliac involvement. May be related to bacterial, mycobacterial, or fungal agents and is relatively common in drug abusers.
Paralysis	Cartilage atrophy accompanying paralysis or disuse produces diffuse joint space narrowing with surrounding osteoporosis and may even lead to intra-articular osseous fusion (perhaps related to chronic low-grade inflammation).
Osteoarthritis	May occur in conjunction with degenerative joint disease involving the contralateral hip.

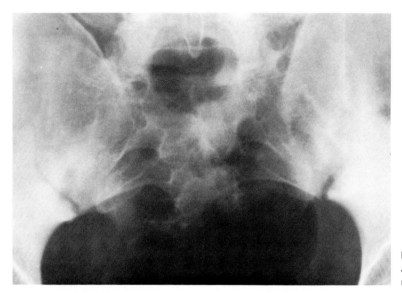

Fig B11-7. Familial Mediterranean fever. Bilateral, though asymmetric, narrowing, erosive changes, and reactive sclerosis about the sacroiliac joints.

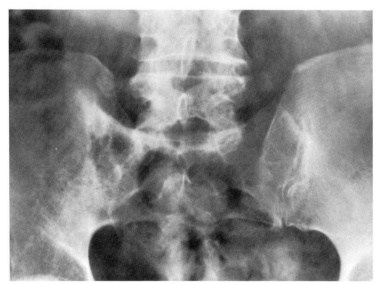

Fig B11-8. Healed tuberculosis. Obliteration of the right sacroiliac joint. The left sacroiliac joint remains intact.

EROSION OF MULTIPLE TERMINAL PHALANGEAL TUFTS (ACRO-OSTEOLYSIS)

Condition	Comments
Scleroderma (Fig B12-1)	Generalized resorption of the terminal phalanges of the hands or feet (or both), characterized by penciling of the tufts. A similar appearance may occur in other collagen vascular diseases (dermatomyositis, Raynaud's disease). Associated findings characteristic of scleroderma include skin atrophy and soft-tissue calcification.
Thermal injuries (burn, frostbite, electrical)	Resorption of the terminal tufts of the distal phalanges of the hand or foot probably reflects a combination of ischemic necrosis and secondary bacterial infection.
Diabetic gangrene (Fig B12-2)	Diffuse destruction of terminal tufts (or more extensive involvement of the phalanges and metatarsals) associated with gas in the soft tissues of the foot reflects underlying vascular disease with diminished blood supply.
Psoriatic arthritis (Fig B12-3)	Resorption of the tufts of the distal phalanges of the hands and feet is a characteristic finding. Progressive osteolysis or "whittling" of bone may eventually lead to smoothly tapered or irregular destruction of most of the phalanx. Usually associated with skin lesions and an asymmetric arthritis that primarily involves the distal interphalangeal joints of the hands and feet.
Arteriosclerosis obliterans	Vascular insufficiency leads to resorption of distal phalanges and pencil-like deformities. A similar appearance may occur in Buerger's disease (thromboangiitis obliterans).
Neurotrophic disease (Fig B12-4)	Resorption of terminal tufts occurs in such conditions as congenital indifference to pain, leprosy, diabetes mellitus, tabes dorsalis, syringomyelia, and meningomyelocele.
Hyperparathyroidism (Fig B12-5)	Tuft resorption is associated with characteristic subperiosteal resorption of the phalanges, metacarpals, and metatarsals.
Lesch-Nyhan syndrome (Fig B12-6)	Rare inherited disorder of purine metabolism in which hyperuricemia is associated with mental and growth retardation and abnormal aggressive behavior. Characteristic self-mutilation by biting of the fingers and lips.

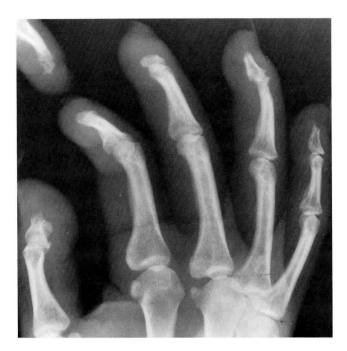

FIG B12-1. Raynaud's disease. Severe trophic changes involve the distal phalanges with resorption of the terminal tufts.

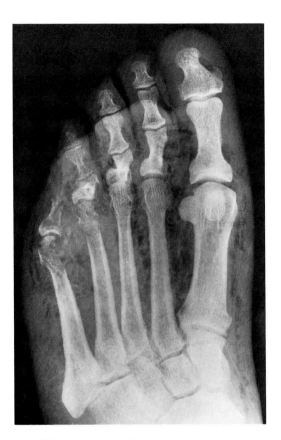

FIG B12-2. Diabetic gangrene. Diffuse destruction of the phalanges and the metatarsal head of the fifth digit. Note the large amount of gas in the soft tissues of the foot.

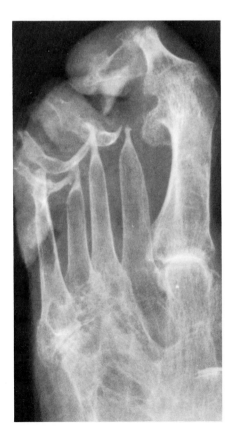

FIG B12-3. Psoriatic arthritis. Arthritis mutilans of the foot and ankle. Severe pencil-like destruction of the metatarsals and phalanges with ankylosis of almost all the tarsal joints.

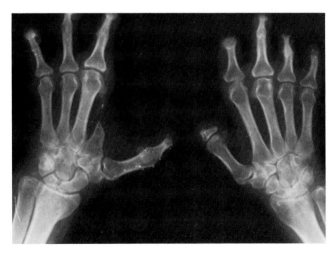

FIG B12-4. Leprosy. Severe phalangeal resorption with evidence of typical pencil-like configurations.

Condition	Comments
Epidermolysis bullosa **(Fig B12-7)**	Rare hereditary disorder in which the skin blisters spontaneously or with injury. Severe scarring causes soft-tissue atrophy and the trophic changes of shortening and tapering of the distal phalanges.
Progeria **(Fig B12-8)**	Nonhereditary congenital syndrome of dwarfism with premature aging and senility. There is typically shortening and abrupt tapering of the terminal phalanges of the hands and feet (and of the clavicles).
Familial acro-osteolysis **(Fig B12-9)**	Diverse group of idiopathic disorders, several of which cause resorption of the terminal phalangeal tufts. This is often associated with bandlike areas of lucency across the waists of the terminal phalanges.
Pachydermoperiostosis **(primary hypertrophic** **osteoarthropathy)** **(Fig B12-10)**	Soft-tissue prominence of the distal digits may rarely be associated with bone resorption of the tufts that produces tapering, pointing, or disappearance of the terminal phalanges.
Pseudoxanthoma elasticum	Vascular occlusions lead to resorption of distal phalangeal tufts. Characteristic calcification of tendons, ligaments, and large peripheral arteries and veins.
Multicentric **reticulohistiocytosis**	Rare systemic disease of unknown cause in which severe inflammation of multiple joints progresses rapidly and leads to an incapacitating and deforming arthritis. The hands (especially the distal interphalangeal joints) are most often involved, and multiple soft-tissue masses typically produce a ''lumpy-bumpy'' appearance. Resorption of the distal phalangeal tufts frequently occurs.
Sjögren's syndrome	Classic triad of dry eyes (keratoconjunctivitis sicca), dry mouth (xerostomia), and a chronic polyarthritis that occurs in half the cases and is indistinguishable from ordinary rheumatoid arthritis. Bilateral parotid gland enlargement is common. May occasionally mimic psoriatic arthritis with distal interphalangeal joint involvement and resorption of terminal tufts.

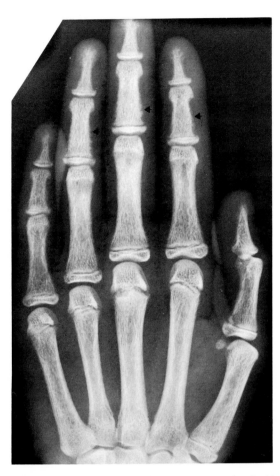

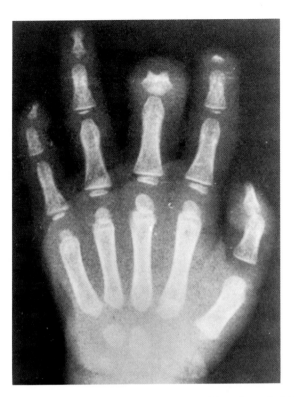

Fig B12-6. **Lesch-Nyhan syndrome.** Amputation of the index and middle fingers from a self-inflicted bite. Although the child is 5 years old, the bone age is that of a 3-year-old.[17]

Fig B12-5. **Hyperparathyroidism.** Tuft resorption associated with sub-periosteal bone resorption that predominantly involves the radial margins of the middle phalanges of the second, third, and fourth digits (arrows).

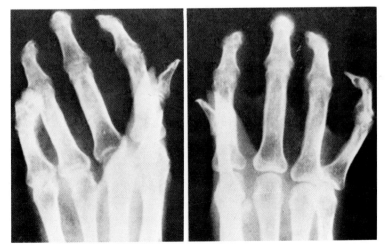

Fig B12-7. **Epidermolysis bullosa.** Diffuse trophic changes about the distal phalanges associated with bilateral contracture deformities resulting in a claw hand. Note the peculiar pointed, hooklike appearance of the terminal phalanges of the thumbs.[18]

Condition	Comments
Pyknodysostosis **(see Fig B5-6)**	Rare hereditary dysplasia characterized by short stature, diffusely dense, sclerotic bones, and mandibular hypoplasia (loss of normal mandibular angle and craniofacial disproportion). Hypoplasia of the distal phalanges and absence of the terminal tufts cause the hands to be short and stubby.
Occupational **acro-osteolysis**	Primarily due to exposure to polyvinyl chloride (acroosteolysis develops in 1% to 2% of workers involved in polymerization of vinyl chloride). Characteristic bandlike radiolucent areas across the waist of one or more terminal phalanges (most commonly the thumb) may be combined with tuft resorption and beveling and osseous fragmentation.
Rothmund's syndrome	Rare hereditary ectodermal dysplasia associated with resorption of phalangeal tufts and dystrophic soft-tissue calcification.

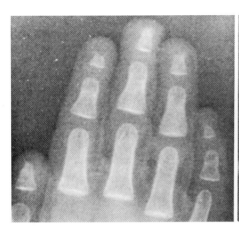

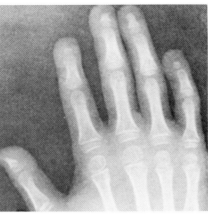

FIG B12-8. Progeria. Progressive resorption of the ungual tufts with preservation of soft tissues occurring over a 5-year period.[19]

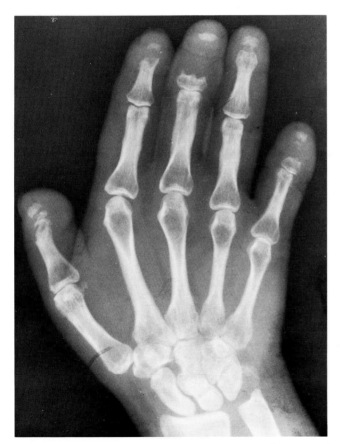

FIG B12-9. Familial acro-osteolysis. Characteristic bandlike areas of lucency crossing the waists of several phalanges.

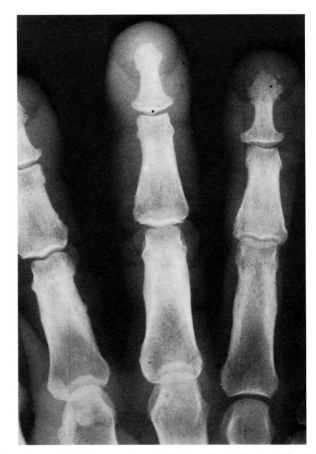

FIG B12-10. Pachydermoperiostosis. Elephantlike thickening of the skin causes clubbing of the distal fingers and exaggerated knuckle pads in addition to a generalized increase in the bulk of the soft tissues surrounding the phalanges. Loss of the tufts accompanies the increase in the overlying soft tissues.[14]

EROSION, DESTRUCTION, OR DEFECT
OF THE OUTER END OF THE CLAVICLE

Condition	Comments
Rheumatoid arthritis	Subchondral osteoporosis and erosions of the clavicle (and, to a lesser extent, the acromion) may progress to extensive osteolysis of the outer third of the clavicle, disruption of adjacent ligaments and capsular structures, and subluxation. The eroded end of the clavicle may be irregular or smoothly tapered.
Hyperparathyroidism (Fig B13-1)	Subperiosteal bone resorption primarily involves the inferior aspect of the distal clavicle (the site of tendon and ligament attachment to the bone).
Neoplasm	Myeloma; metastases; lymphoma; eosinophilic granuloma.
Cleidocranial dysostosis (Fig B13-2)	Congenital hereditary disorder of membranous bone formation characterized by partial or total absence of the clavicles. Other major anomalies include multiple accessory bones along the sutures (wormian bones) and widening of the symphysis pubis.
Scleroderma	Bone resorption of the distal clavicle (often with associated soft-tissue calcification) is an occasional finding. A far more frequent manifestation is resorption of the terminal tufts of the distal phalanges.
Gout	Erosion of the distal clavicle (occasionally with tophaceous calcification) is an uncommon appearance.
Osteomyelitis	Pyogenic or tuberculous infection can cause erosion or destruction of the distal clavicle.
Multicentric reticulohistiocytosis	Erosion of the distal clavicle is one manifestation of this rare systemic disease of unknown etiology that is characterized by severe inflammation of multiple joints and progresses rapidly to produce an incapacitating and deforming arthritis. The most common manifestations are resorption of the distal phalangeal tufts and development of multiple soft-tissue masses that typically produces a ''lumpy-bumpy'' appearance.

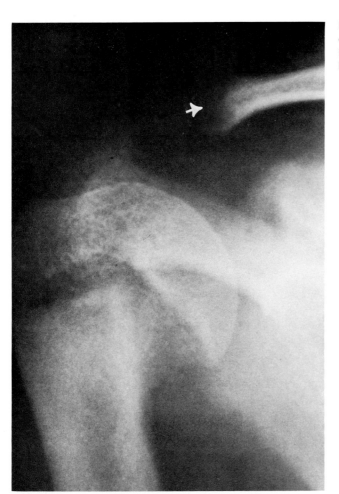

Fɪɢ B13-1. Hyperparathyroidism. Characteristic erosion of the distal clavicle (arrow). Metaphyseal subperiosteal resorption beneath the proximal humeral head has led to a pathologic fracture with slippage of the humeral head.

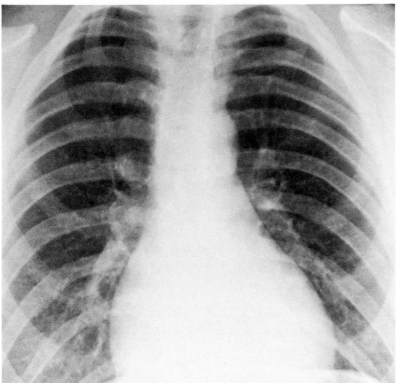

Fɪɢ B13-2. Cleidocranial dysostosis. Total absence of both clavicles.

Condition	Comments
Hurler's syndrome	Shortening and thickening of the clavicles is a manifestation of this form of mucopolysaccharidosis. The most distinctive radiographic change in this condition is hypoplasia of L2 (causing accentuated kyphosis or gibbous deformity) with inferior beaking of the anterior margin of one or more vertebral bodies.
Posttraumatic osteolysis	Progressive resorption of the outer end of the clavicle may follow single or repeated episodes of local (often minor) trauma. The osteolytic process begins several weeks to several years after injury and is associated with erosion and cupping of the acromion, soft-tissue swelling, and dystrophic calcification. After the lytic phase stabilizes, reparative changes occur over several months until the subchondral bone becomes reconstituted (though the acromioclavicular joint can remain permanently widened).
Progeria **(Fig B13-3)**	Shortening and abrupt tapering of the clavicles (and terminal phalanges of the hands and feet) is a common manifestation of this rare, nonhereditary congenital syndrome of dwarfism and premature aging and senility.
Pyknodysostosis	Hypoplasia of the lateral ends of the clavicles is a manifestation of this hereditary dysplasia that is characterized by short stature, diffusely dense sclerotic bones, and mandibular hypoplasia.
Holt-Oram syndrome	Hypoplasia of the clavicle (and radius or thumb) is among the upper extremity malformations associated with congenital heart disease (most often atrial septal defect) in this rare autosomal dominant condition.
Trisomy 13/trisomy 18	Tapering of the distal clavicles is one of multiple congenital anomalies associated with these rare syndromes.

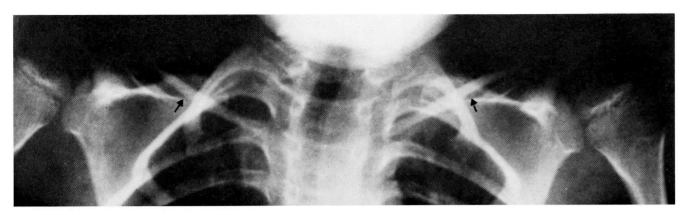

Fɪɢ **B13-3. Progeria.** Thin and dense clavicles (arrows) with absence of the lateral thirds.[19]

NEUROARTHROPATHY (CHARCOT'S JOINT)

Condition	Comments
Tabes dorsalis (syphilis) **(Fig B14-1)**	Primarily involves the weight-bearing joints of the lower extremities and lower lumbar spine. About 5% to 10% of patients with tabes dorsalis have neuroarthropathy.
Syringomyelia **(Fig B14-2)**	Primarily involves the upper extremity, especially the glenohumeral articulation, elbow, and wrist. Spinal changes are most common in the cervical region. About 20% to 25% of patients with syringomyelia develop neuroarthropathy.
Diabetes mellitus **(Fig B14-3)**	Primarily involves the metatarsophalangeal, tarsometatarsal, and intertarsal joints. Although the exact incidence of neuropathic joint disease in this condition is not clear, diabetes appears to be overtaking both syphilis and syringomyelia as the leading cause of neuroarthropathy.
Alcoholism	Primarily involves the metatarsophalangeal and interphalangeal joints. Probably an infrequent complication of the peripheral neuropathy seen in up to 30% of alcoholic patients.
Congenital indifference to pain **(Fig B14-4)**	Primarily involves the ankle and intertarsal joints. Neurologic deficit recognized in infancy or childhood in which pain sensation is decreased though there may be normal perception of touch and temperature and normal tendon reflexes. Identical skeletal abnormalities occur in familial dysautonomia (Riley-Day syndrome), which is characterized by autonomic dysfunction and sensory and motor disturbances.
Meningomyelocele/spina bifida	Most frequent cause of neuroarthropathy in childhood. Primarily affects the ankle and intertarsal joints.

A

B

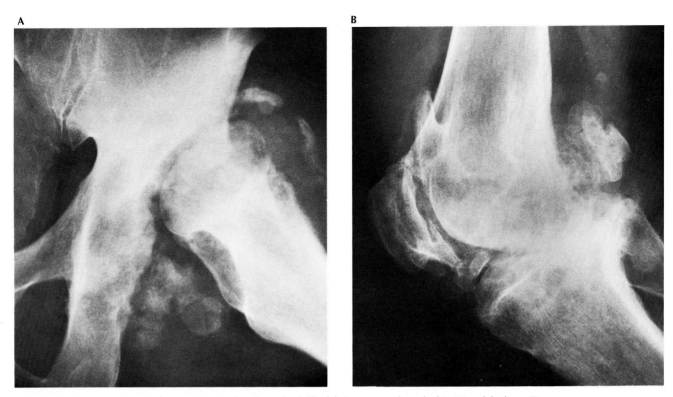

FIG B14-1. Tabes dorsalis. Joint fragmentation, sclerosis, and calcific debris are seen about the hip (A) and the knee (B).

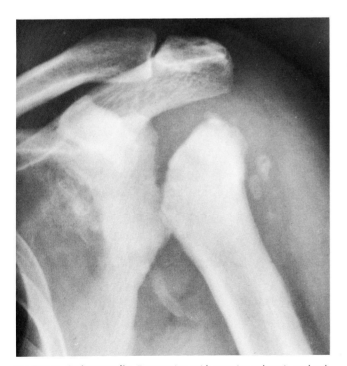

FIG B14-2. Syringomyelia. Destruction with reactive sclerosis and calcific debris about the shoulder.

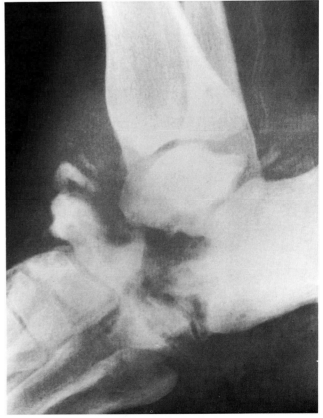

FIG B14-3. Diabetes mellitus. Severe destructive changes with calcific debris about the intertarsal joints. Note the characteristic vascular calcification posterior to the ankle joint.

Condition	Comments
Leprosy (Fig B14-5)	Chronic granulomatous mycobacterial infection that produces severe neuropathic changes in the hands and feet (due to insensitivity to pain that allows repeated trauma and infection to go untreated). Other radiographic findings include typical pencil-line tapering of the distal ends of the metatarsals and virtually pathognomic calcification of nerves in the distal extremities.
Amyloidosis	Occasional manifestation in the knees or ankles that is probably related to vascular amyloid infiltration in nerve tissue.
Steroid therapy	Systemically or locally administered steroid medication may produce a rapidly progressive, neuropathic-like joint disease characterized by severe osseous and cartilaginous destruction that most frequently involves the hips or knees.
Miscellaneous disorders	Spinal cord or peripheral nerve injury; myelopathy of pernicious anemia; inflammatory disease of the spinal cord (arachnoiditis, acute myelitis, poliomyelitis, and yaws).

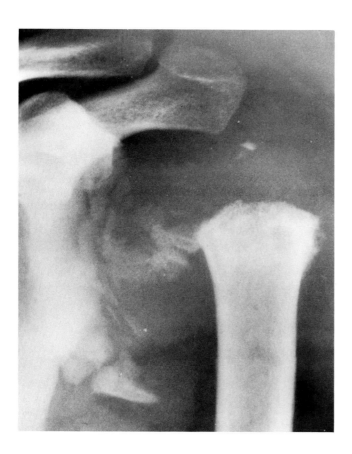

FIG B14-4. **Congenital indifference to pain.** Virtually complete disappearance of the humeral head with reactive sclerosis and calcific debris.

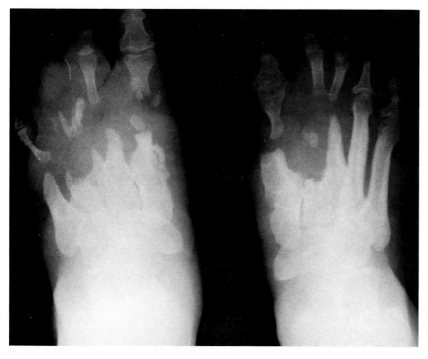

FIG B14-5. **Leprosy.** Marked bone destruction and pencil-like resorption, most severe at the metatarsophalangeal joint.[20]

LOOSE INTRA-ARTICULAR BODIES

Condition	Imaging Findings	Comments
Synovial osteochondromatosis (Fig B15-1)	Multiple calcified or ossified bodies in a single joint. The calcifications vary in size, are usually irregular, and often have a laminated appearance. Most often involves the knees, with the hips next in frequency. Rarely affects the elbows, ankles, shoulders, or wrists.	Hypertrophic synovial membrane produces multiple metaplastic growths of cartilage that are most often intra-articular but may occasionally involve bursae and tendon sheaths. The cartilaginous masses frequently calcify or even ossify in part and often become detached and lie free in the joint cavity. Usually monarticular and tends to occur in young adults or the middle-aged. If not calcified (about one third of cases), synovial chondromas cannot be detected on standard radiographs and arthrography is required to demonstrate these cartilaginous bodies.
Osteochondritis dissecans (Figs B15-2 and B15-3)	Small, round or oval necrotic segment of bone with its articular cartilage may separate to form a free joint body, leaving a residual pit in the articular surface. Primarily occurs about the knees, usually on the lateral aspect of the medial femoral condyle. Other common locations are the ankles, femoral heads, elbows, and shoulders.	Localized form of ischemic necrosis that most frequently affects young males and is probably caused by trauma. The necrotic segment of bone may remain attached and become denser and be separated from the surrounding bone by a crescentic lucent zone.
Trauma	Single or multiple joint bodies, usually associated with evidence of old trauma.	Secondary to avulsion of bone or cartilage (articular surface, meniscus). Uncalcified articular or meniscal cartilage may not be detected on plain radiographs.
Neuroarthropathy (Charcot's joint) (Fig B15-4)	Calcified intra-articular bodies in one or more joints are associated with fracture, fragmentation, and sclerosis of articular surfaces, calcific and bony debris dissecting into soft tissues and extending about the joint and along muscle planes, and severe subluxations (due to laxity of periarticular soft-tissue structures).	Severe disorganization of a joint that develops in a variety of neurologic disorders in which loss of proprioception or deep pain sensation leads to repeated trauma to an unstable joint. Causes include diabetes, syphilis, syringomyelia, and leprosy. Degeneration of cartilage, recurrent fractures of subchondral bone, and marked proliferation of adjacent bone lead to total disorganization of the joint.
Degenerative joint disease	One or more detached hypertrophic spurs, primarily involving a weight-bearing joint.	Usually occurs in elderly patients and is associated with characteristic radiographic findings of osteophytosis, sclerosis, subchondral cysts, and joint space narrowing.
Intra-articular tumor calcification	Tumor may simulate a loose body. Predominantly involves the knees.	Rare appearance in synovial sarcoma or intracapsular chondroma. There is usually an associated soft-tissue mass.
Sequestrum (osteomyelitis)	Evidence of joint destruction or deformity.	Rare manifestation of tuberculous or pyogenic arthritis.

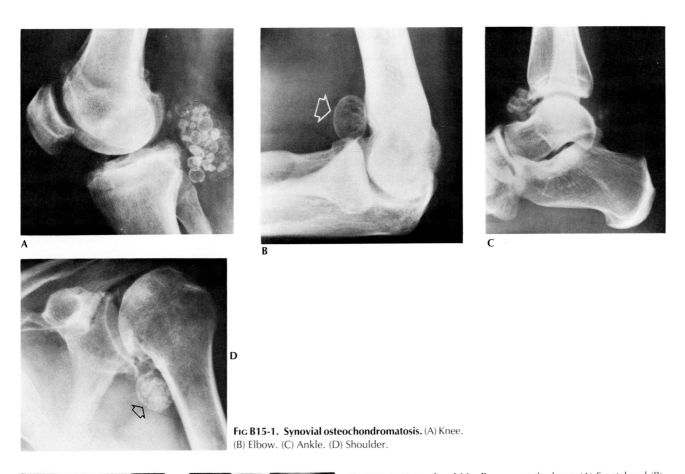

FIG B15-1. Synovial osteochondromatosis. (A) Knee.
(B) Elbow. (C) Ankle. (D) Shoulder.

◄ **FIG B15-2. Osteochondritic dissecans** at the knee. (A) Frontal and (B) lateral views of the knee demonstrate the necrotic segment (arrow) separated from the medial femoral condyle by a crescentic lucent zone.

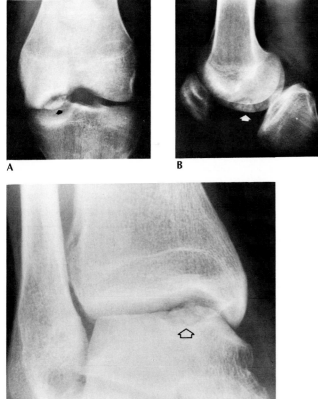

FIG B15-3. Osteochondritis dissecans at the ankle.

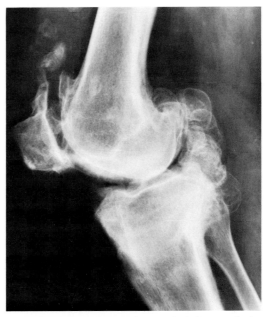

FIG B15-4. Neuroarthropathy in syphilis. Multiple free joint bodies associated with disorganization of the knee joint, bone erosion, reactive sclerosis, and soft-tissue and ligamentous calcifications.

CHONDROCALCINOSIS

Condition	Imaging Findings	Comments
Pseudogout (calcium pyrophosphate crystal deposition disease) (Figs B16-1 and B16-2)	Most commonly affects the knee joint with calcification in articular cartilage (fine linear densities parallel to subchondral bone surfaces) and menisci (dense linear deposits in the center of the knee joint). Other common sites include the triangular fibrocartilage of the wrists; vertical linear calcification of the symphysis pubis; articular cartilage in the shoulders, hips, elbows, and ankles; and the annulus fibrosis of intervertebral disks.	Inflammatory arthritis of older individuals caused by deposition of calcium pyrophosphate dihydrate crystals in the joints. May present as intermittent attacks of acute joint effusion and pain or as a progressive chronic arthritis. The acute arthritis of pseudogout may be clinically indistinguishable from gout or septic arthritis (diagnosis made by identification of calcium pyrophosphate crystals in synovial fluid). May produce a pattern of degenerative joint disease that primarily involves the radiocarpal, wrist, elbow, and shoulder joints (infrequently involved in osteoarthritis).
Degenerative joint disease/ posttraumatic/idiopathic	Calcification of cartilage in various areas.	Development of chondrocalcinosis without evidence of crystal arthropathy.
Gout (Fig B16-3)	Calcification of fibrocartilage, most commonly involving the knees. The wrists, hips, and symphysis pubis may also be affected.	Increased serum urate concentration leads to deposition of uric acid crystals in joints, cartilage, and the kidneys. Chondrocalcinosis reported in 5% to 30% of patients.
Hemochromatosis	Calcification of cartilage that most often involves the knee. The shoulders, elbows, hips, symphysis pubis, and triangular cartilage of the wrist may also be affected.	Iron storage disorder that is either inherited or, more commonly, secondary to severe anemia with abnormal erythropoiesis (eg, thalassemia), liver disease in alcoholics, or chronic excessive iron ingestion. Chondrocalcinosis develops in about 50% of patients with arthropathy.
Hyperparathyroidism	Cartilage calcification most commonly involves the wrists, knees, hips, shoulders, and elbows.	Chondrocalcinosis reported in 20% to 40% of patients. Other common manifestations include subperiosteal bone resorption, rugger-jersey spine, brown tumors, erosion of the distal clavicles, and salt-and-pepper skull.
Ochronosis	Dense laminated calcification of multiple intervertebral disks. Cartilage calcification (with a severe type of degenerative arthritis) may develop in peripheral joints, especially the shoulders, hips, and knees.	Underlying condition is alkaptonuria, a rare enzyme deficiency that results in an abnormal accumulation of homogentisic acid in blood and urine (typically turns very dark on voiding or becomes black after standing or being alkalinized). Deposition of oxidized homogentisic acid in cartilage and other connective tissue produces a distinctive form of degenerative arthritis.

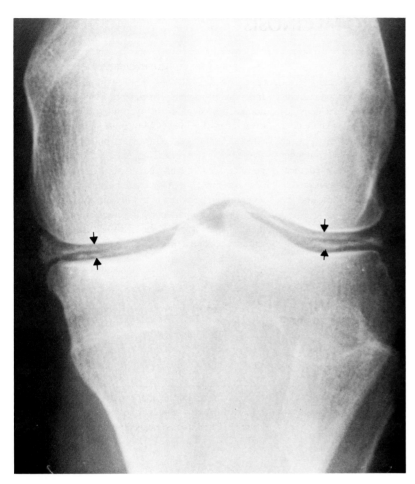

FIG B16-1. Pseudogout. Calcification of both the medial and lateral menisci of the knee (arrows).

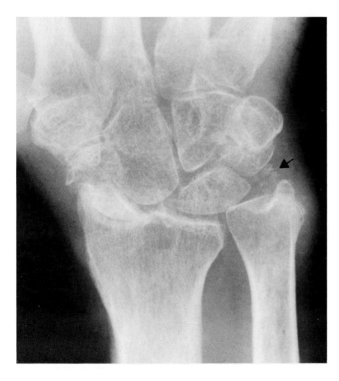

FIG B16-2. Pseudogout. Characteristic calcifications in the triangular fibrocartilage of the wrist (arrow).

Condition	Imaging Findings	Comments
Wilson's disease (Fig B16-4)	Cartilage calcification and arthropathy primarily involve the small joints of the hands and feet.	Rare familial disorder in which impaired hepatic excretion of copper results in toxic accumulation of the metal in the liver, brain, and other organs. Characteristic pigmentation of the cornea (Kayser-Fleischer ring). Skeletal changes occur in about half the patients.
Oxalosis	Deposition of calcium oxalate in cartilage.	Primary inborn error of metabolism or secondary to overabsorption of dietary oxalate (bacterial overgrowth syndromes, chronic disease of the pancreas and biliary tracts, decreased small bowel absorptive surface, Crohn's disease). Calcium oxalate is primarily deposited in the kidneys (nephrocalcinosis, nephrolithiasis), leading to recurrent urinary tract obstruction and infection, hypertension, and severe renal failure.
Acromegaly	Calcification of cartilage predominantly involving the knees.	Proliferation of articular cartilage leads to radiographically evident widening of joint spaces. Premature degenerative changes tend to develop.

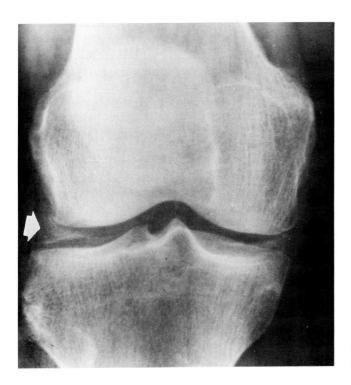

Fig B16-3. Gout. Chondrocalcinosis about the knee (arrow) simulates pseudogout.

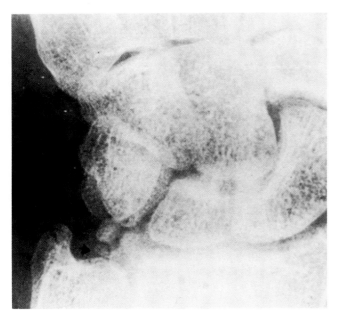

Fig B16-4. Wilson's disease. Characteristic ossicles (arrows) in the region of the triangular fibrocartilage of the wrist.[21]

PERIARTICULAR CALCIFICATION

Condition	Comments
Calcific tendinitis and bursitis (Fig B17-1)	Common cause of pain, limitation of motion, and disability about a joint. Although frequently associated with inflammation of an overlying bursa and often clinically termed ''bursitis,'' the calcium deposits (primarily calcium hydroxyapatite) usually occur in the tendon and not in the overlying bursa (a mass of calcium may rupture into a bursa). Most commonly involves the shoulders, especially the supraspinatous tendon, in which the calcification is situated directly above the greater tuberosity of the humerus. Calcification is demonstrated radiographically in about half the patients with persistent pain and disability in this region. Other affected areas include the hips (calcification in gluteal insertions into the greater trochanter and surrounding bursae), elbows, knees, and wrists. Calcification in these areas usually appears as amorphous deposits that vary from thin curvilinear densities to large calcific masses.
Pseudogout	Accumulation of calcium pyrophosphate dihydrate crystals in tendinous structures. The calcification generally appears more diffuse and elongated than that associated with hydroxyapatite crystal deposition.
Hyperparathyroidism (Fig B17-2)	Calcific deposits (hydroxyapatite crystals) in joint capsules and periarticular tissues are common (especially in renal osteodystrophy), are often dense and massive, and may be observed in multiple (and often symmetric) locations. There is usually other radiographic evidence of hyperparathyroidism (subperiosteal bone resorption, rugger-jersey spine, salt-and-pepper demineralization of the skull, brown tumors).
Other disorders of calcium and phosphate metabolism	Metastatic calcification diffusely involving periarticular and other soft tissues may occur in such conditions as hypoparathyroidism, hypervitaminosis D, milk-alkali syndrome, and idiopathic hypercalcemia.
Collagen vascular disease (Fig B17-3)	Widespread periarticular (and subcutaneous) calcification is common in scleroderma and dermatomyositis (there may be punctate, linear, or more massive ''tumoral'' calcification). Uncommon manifestation in rheumatoid arthritis, systemic lupus erythematosus, polyarteritis nodosa, and Raynaud's phenomenon.

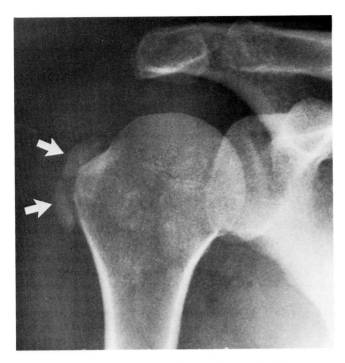

FIG B17-1. Calcific tendinitis. Frontal view of the shoulder demonstrates amorphous calcium deposits (arrows) in the supraspinatous tendon.

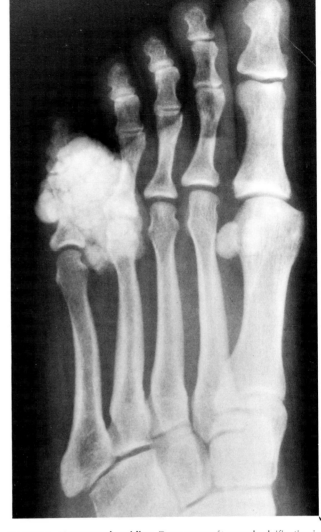

FIG B17-2. Hyperparathyroidism. Dense mass of tumoral calcification in joint capsules and periarticular soft tissues of the lateral aspect of the foot in a patient with renal osteodystrophy.

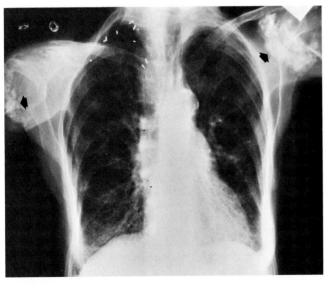

FIG B17-3. Scleroderma. Clumps of calcification about the shoulder joints. Note the reticulonodular interstitial pattern at both lung bases. The surgical clips overlying the right apex are from a cervical sympathectomy for treatment of associated Raynaud's phenomenon.

Condition	Comments
Tumoral calcinosis **(Fig B17-4)**	Localized collections of calcium in periarticular soft tissues that may involve single or multiple joints and have a predilection for the hips, elbows, shoulders, ankles, and wrists. Primarily affects young and otherwise healthy individuals. Begins as small calcified nodules that enlarge to form solid, lobulated tumors that are extremely dense and have rough, irregular borders. Pathologically, the calcific masses reflect honeycomblike clusters of cysts in a dense fibrous capsule. Because the cysts are filled with a granular, pasty, or liquid material, on upright views there may be sedimentation of calcium phosphate crystals with resulting fluid-calcium levels.
Calcinosis universalis **(Fig B17-5)**	Rare disorder of unknown etiology affecting infants and children in which calcium is initially deposited subcutaneously and later in deep connective tissues throughout the body (similar to dermatomyositis). Periarticular tissues may also be involved.
Gout **(Fig B17-6)**	Continued deposition of urate crystals in periarticular tissues causes the development of one or more characteristic large, lumpy soft-tissue swellings (gouty tophi) that may calcify. Classic sites include the first metatarsophalangeal joint, the insertion of the Achilles tendon, and the olecranon bursa (bilateral enlargement of the olecranon bursae, often with erosion or spur formation and calcified tophi, is virtually pathognomic of gout).
Myositis ossificans **(Fig B17-7)**	Osseous deposits in tendons and periarticular tissues (especially about the hips) develop in the paralyzed part in up to half of patients with paraplegia. In generalized (progressive) myositis ossificans, thick columns and plates of bone eventually replace tendons, fascia, and ligaments, causing such severe limitation of movement, contractures, and deformity that the patient becomes a virtual "stone person."
Sarcoidosis	Large periarticular soft-tissue masses, with or without calcification, is a rare manifestation.
Ochronosis	Tendinous calcification and ossification may involve the hips, knees, and shoulders. Characteristic ossification of intervertebral disks.

A

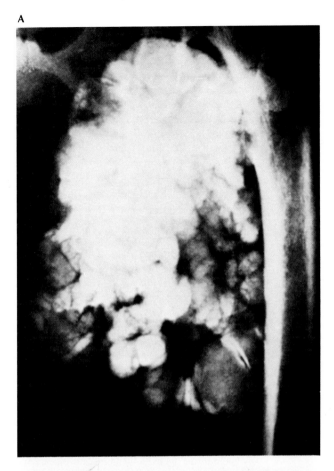

B

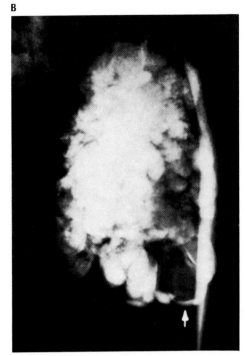

FIG B17-4. **Tumoral calcinosis.** (A) Supine view demonstrates a large, irregular calcific mass with some relatively lucent areas in the proximal thigh. (B) Upright view shows sedimentation in the liquid-filled cysts (arrow), with absence of sedimentation in the more amorphous gritty deposits.[22]

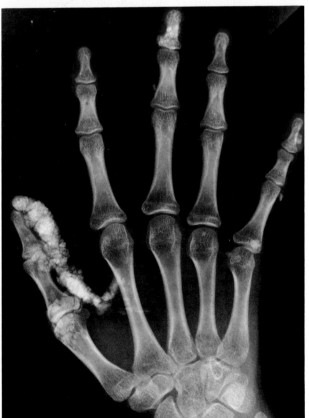

FIG B17-5. **Calcinosis universalis.** Dense calcific deposits in the soft tissues on the ulnar aspect of the thumb.

Condition	Comments
Trauma (Fig B17-8)	Posttraumatic calcification may develop after capsular or ligamentous damage (eg, Pellegrini-Stieda calcification in the proximal attachment of the medial collateral ligament of the knee). Localized periarticular calcification also commonly develops around joint replacements.
Synovial sarcoma (synovioma)	Malignant tumor that most frequently affects young adults and arises from a joint capsule, bursa, or tendon. The tumor usually develops from synovial tissue in the vicinity of a large joint (para-articular soft tissues just beyond the capsule), rather than in the synovial lining of the joint itself. Most often involves the knees, though the tumor may arise from a tendon sheath anywhere along a limb. Radiographically, a synovioma appears as a well-defined, round or lobulated soft-tissue mass adjacent to or near a joint. Amorphous punctate deposits or linear streaks of calcification frequently occur in the tumor (must be differentiated from pigmented villonodular synovitis, in which calcification does not occur though the mass may appear dense because of hemosiderin deposits).
Tuberculosis	Dystrophic calcification may follow tuberculous involvement of the synovial membranes of bursae and tendon sheaths. Primarily involves the hips and elbows.
Werner's syndrome	Rare condition characterized by symmetric growth retardation, premature aging, scleroderma-like skin changes, and cataracts. Soft-tissue calcification occurs in about one third of cases, predominantly about bony protuberances (distal ends of the tibia and fibula) and the knees, feet, and hands. Other typical findings include patchy or generalized osteoporosis, extensive arterial calcifications, and premature osteoarthritis.

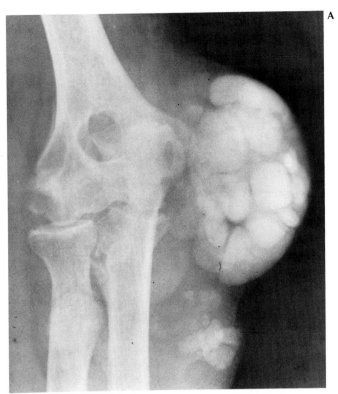

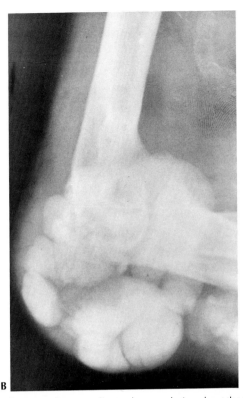

FIG B17-6. **Gout.** (A) Frontal and (B) lateral views demonstrate massive deposition of calcium in a long-standing tophaceous lesion about the elbow.

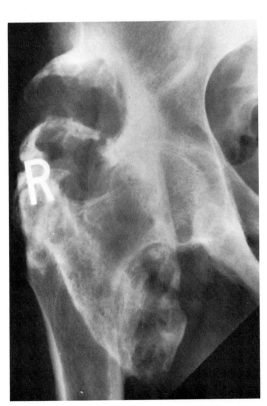

FIG B17-7. **Myositis ossificans.** Marked heterotopic bone formation about the hip joint in a patient with paralysis.

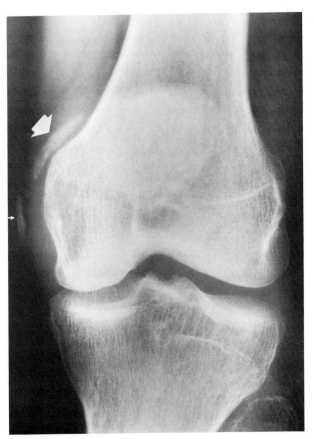

FIG B17-8. **Pellegrini-Stieda disease.** Posttraumatic ossification (arrows) along the femoral condyle.

LOCALIZED CALCIFICATION OR OSSIFICATION
IN MUSCLES AND SUBCUTANEOUS TISSUES

Condition	Comments
Idiopathic	Ligaments of the shoulder girdle and pelvis often calcify in normal individuals.
Myositis ossificans (posttraumatic) (Fig B18-1)	Development of calcification or ossification in injured muscle that is usually related to acute or chronic trauma to the deep tissues of the extremities. Heterotopic calcification or ossification typically lies parallel to the shaft of a bone or the long axis of a muscle. Although the radiographic appearance may simulate that of parosteal sarcoma (Fig B18-2), myositis ossificans is completely separated from the bone by a radiolucent zone, unlike the malignant tumor that is attached by a sessile base and has a discontinuous radiolucent zone.
Myositis ossificans associated with neurologic disorders (Fig B18-3)	Up to half the patients with paraplegia demonstrate myositis ossificans in the paralyzed part. The osseous deposits occur in muscles, tendons, and ligaments. Heterotopic bone is most pronounced around large joints, especially the hips, and may proceed to complete periarticular osseous bridging.
Postinjection (Fig B18-4)	Single or multiple irregular deposits of calcification may develop after the injection of bismuth, calcium gluconate, insulin, antibiotics, camphorated oil, or quinine. They also may occur after BCG vaccination or after the extravasation of an opaque substance.

A

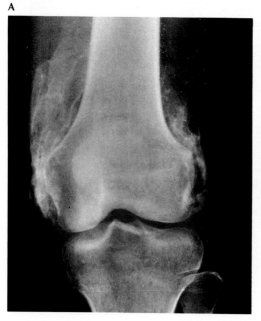

B

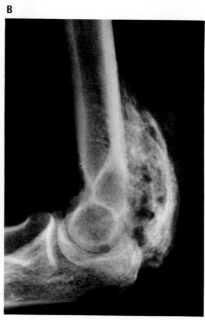

FIG B18-1. Myositis ossificans. (A) Knee. (B) Elbow.

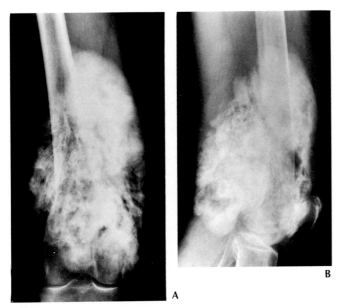

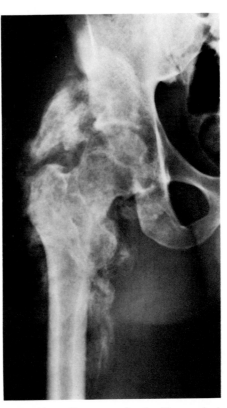

FIG B18-2. Parosteal sarcoma. (A) Frontal and (B) lateral views of the leg demonstrate a broad-based, densely ossified mass extending outward from the distal femur. The characteristic radiolucent line separating the dense mass of tumor bone from the cortex is not seen in this huge lesion.

FIG B18-3. Myositis ossificans associated with neurologic disorders. Diffuse osseous deposits in muscles, tendons, and ligaments about the hip in a patient with long-term paralysis.

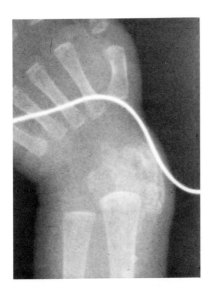

FIG B18-4. Extravasation of a calcium gluconate injection. Soft-tissue opacification in a child.

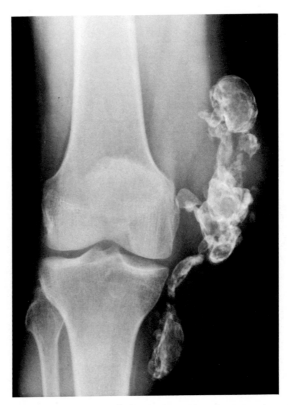

FIG B18-5. Lipoma. Bizarre calcification in an extensive tumor about the knee.

Condition	Comments
Thermal burn	Heterotopic calcification (most frequent in the periarticular region) not uncommonly becomes evident within several months.
Neoplasm (Figs B18-5 to B18-8)	Various patterns (from flecks of calcification to extensive ossification) can occur in benign neoplasms (chondroma, fibromyxoma, lipoma) and malignant neoplasms (soft-tissue osteosarcoma, chondrosarcoma, fibrosarcoma, liposarcoma, synovioma).
Postsurgical scar (Fig B18-9)	Calcification or ossification of an old surgical scar can produce linear densities on late postoperative radiographs.
Leprosy	Nerve abscesses produce soft-tissue masses that may calcify.
Healing infection or abscess	After pyogenic myositis or fibrositis.
Chronic venous stasis (Fig B18-10)	A diffuse reticular ossification pattern may develop in an affected lower extremity. More commonly, single or multiple phleboliths and periosteal reaction occur about the distal tibia and fibula.

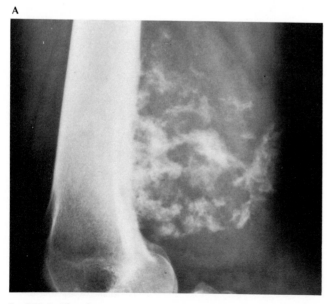

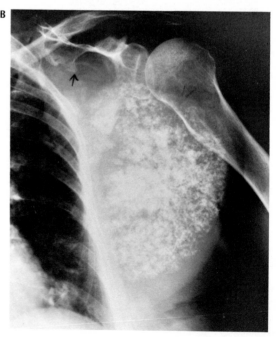

FIG B18-6. Chondrosarcoma. (A) Prominent dense calcification in a large exostotic chondrosarcoma. (B) Extensive flocculent calcification in the cartilaginous matrix. The arrow points to a small osteochondroma in this patient with multiple hereditary exostoses.

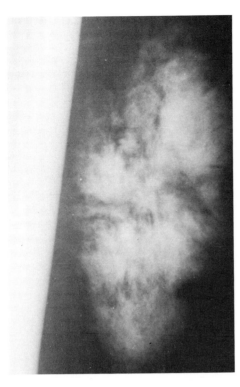

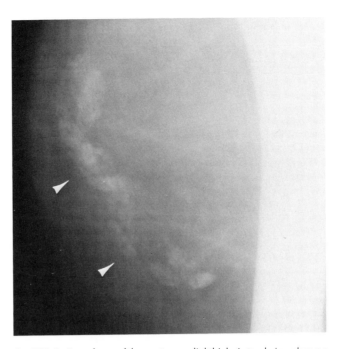

FIG B18-8. **Synovioma** of the posteromedial thigh. Lateral view shows a large soft-tissue mass with extensive calcific deposits (arrows) in it.[23]

FIG B18-7. **Extraskeletal osteosarcoma** of the posterolateral thigh.[23]

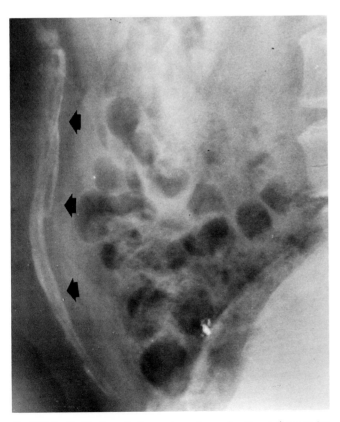

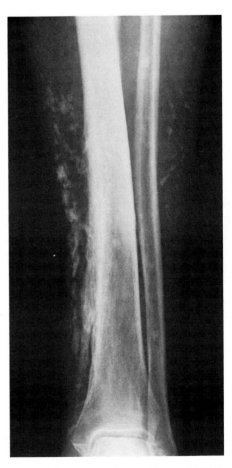

FIG B18-9. **Ossified surgical scar.** Long linear density on the anterior abdominal wall (arrows).

FIG B18-10. **Chronic venous stasis.** Soft-tissue calcification associated with periosteal reaction about the distal tibia and numerous phleboliths.

GENERALIZED CALCIFICATION OR OSSIFICATION IN MUSCLES AND SUBCUTANEOUS TISSUES

Condition	Comments
Dermatomyositis **(Fig B19-1)**	Inflammatory disease of skeletal muscles in which a lymphocytic infiltration produces muscle fiber damage and degeneration. In adults there is associated skin inflammation, a typical rash, and a relatively high incidence of underlying malignancy. Musculoskeletal changes are most severe in childhood dermatomyositis. A characteristic finding is extensive calcification in muscles and subcutaneous tissues underlying the skin lesions. The calcification may appear as superficial or deep masses, as linear deposits, or as a lacy, reticular, subcutaneous deposition of calcium encasing the torso.
Scleroderma **(Fig B19-2)**	Multisystem disorder characterized by fibrosis that involves the skin and internal organs (especially the gastrointestinal tract, lungs, heart, and kidneys). Soft-tissue calcification often occurs in the hands and over pressure areas such as the elbows and ischial tuberosities. Other typical findings include soft-tissue atrophy in the fingertips with trophic osteolysis and resorption of terminal tufts and arthritic changes in the interphalangeal joints of the hands.
Calcinosis universalis **(Fig B19-3)**	Disease of unknown etiology in which calcium is initially deposited subcutaneously and later in deep connective tissues throughout the body. Generally affects infants and children and is progressive.
Disorders of calcium and phosphorus metabolism **(Figs B19-4 to B19-6)**	Soft-tissue calcification in subcutaneous tissues, blood vessels, and periarticular regions may occur in hyperparathyroidism (especially in secondary renal osteodystrophy) as well as in other disorders of calcium and phosphorus metabolism such as hypervitaminosis D, milk-alkali syndrome, idiopathic hypercalcemia, hypercalcemia associated with bone destruction, hypoparathyroidism, and pseudohypoparathyroidism.

Vascular calcifications
  Arterial
  (Figs B19-7 and B19-8)
	Arteriosclerosis; Mönckeberg's sclerosis; aneurysm; diabetes mellitus; hyperparathyroidism (hypercalcemia); Takayasu's arteritis.

Venous **(Figs B19-9 to B19-11)**	Phleboliths may develop in association with varicose veins, hemangioma, and Maffucci's syndrome (multiple enchondromatosis) and after irradiation.

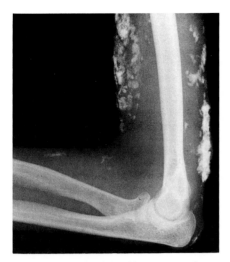

FIG B19-1. **Dermatomyositis.** Extensive deposits of calcium in the soft tissues about the humerus and elbow and loss of the sharp demarcation between the muscles and the subcutaneous tissues.

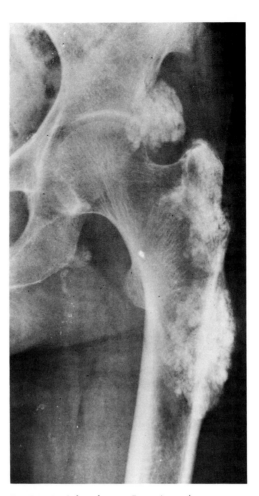

FIG B19-2. **Scleroderma.** Extensive calcifications about the hip joint and proximal femur.

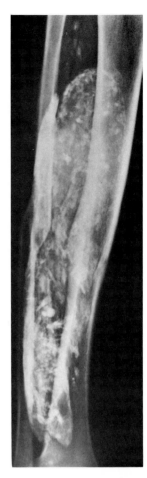

FIG B19-3. **Calcinosis universalis.** Huge calcified mass in the subcutaneous and deep connective tissues of the lower leg.

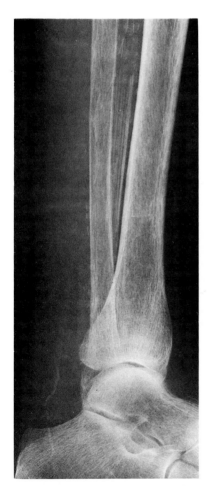

FIG B19-4. **Hypervitaminosis D.** Diffuse calcification involving the interosseous ligament between the tibia and fibula as well as vascular structures.

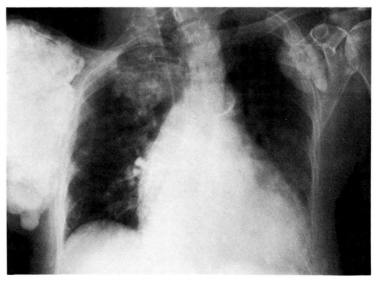

FIG B19-5. **Hypervitaminosis D.** Huge masses of calcification near the shoulder joints bilaterally.

Condition	Comments
Systemic lupus erythematosus (**Fig B19-12**)	Calcification in the soft tissues is an occasional finding that most commonly involves the lower extremities and appears as diffuse linear, streaky, or nodular calcification in subcutaneous and deeper tissues.
Ehlers-Danlos syndrome	Generalized inherited disorder of connective tissue characterized by fragile and hyperextensible skin, easy bruising, and loose-jointedness. The most typical radiographic abnormality is calcification of fatty nodules in the subcutaneous tissues of the extremities. These nodules range from 2 to 10 mm and appear as central lucent zones with ringlike calcification, simulating phleboliths (must be differentiated from calcified subcutaneous parasites, which tend to be aligned along muscular and fascial planes rather than randomly distributed in the soft tissues). Other nonspecific musculoskeletal abnormalities include scoliosis, deformities of the thoracic cage, hypermobility of joints, and subluxations.
Pseudoxanthoma elasticum (**Fig B19-13**)	Calcification typically occurs in the middle and deep layers of the dermis in this hereditary systemic disorder in which widespread degeneration of elastic fibers results in cutaneous, ocular, and vascular manifestations in children and young adults. Other sites of calcification include tendons, ligaments, and large peripheral arteries and veins.
Parasites **Cysticercosis** (*Taenia solium*) (**Fig B19-14**)	Invasion of human tissue by the larval form of the pork tapeworm typically produces multiple linear or oval calcifications in the soft tissues. The calcified cysts often have a noncalcified central area and almost always have their long axes in the plane of the surrounding muscle bundle (unlike the random distribution of soft-tissue calcifications in Ehlers-Danlos syndrome). There may also be intracranial calcification (tiny central calcification representing the scolex surrounded by an area of radiolucency and rimmed by calcium deposition in the overlying cyst capsule).
Guinea worm (*Dracunculus medinensis*)	Serpiginous or curvilinear opacification (most often in the lower extremities) that is often coiled and may be several feet long. The calcification is frequently segmented and beaded because muscle movement breaks up the underlying necrotic worm.
Loa loa (*Filaria bancrofti*)	Calcified dead worm appears curled up into a coil or as a thin, cottonlike thread of density. The calcifications are often difficult to visualize and are best seen in the web spaces of the hands or feet.

(continued page 672)

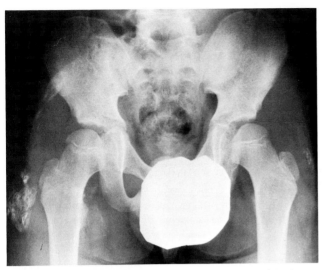

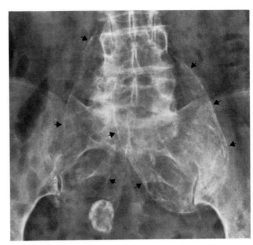

FIG B19-7. **Arteriosclerosis** of the lower extremities. There are calcified plaques in the walls of aneurysms of the lower abdominal aorta and both common iliac arteries.

FIG B19-6. **Hypoparathyroidism.** Soft-tissue calcifications lying in muscle bundles about both hip joints.

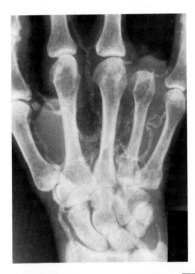

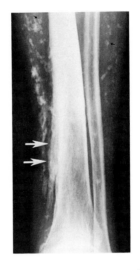

FIG B19-8. **Mönckeberg's sclerosis.** Typical calcification of the media in moderate-sized vessels of a diabetic patient. Note the prior surgical resection of the phalanges of the fourth digit.

FIG B19-9. **Varicose veins.** Multiple round and oval calcifications in the soft tissues (phleboliths) representing calcified thrombi, some of which have characteristic lucent centers (black arrows). Extensive new bone formation along the medial aspect of the tibial shaft (white arrows) caused by long-standing vascular stasis.

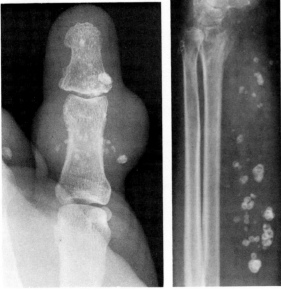

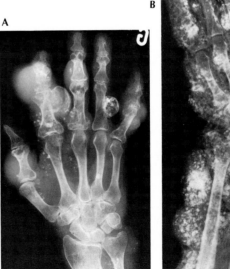

FIG B19-10. **Soft-tissue hemangiomas** with phleboliths involving (A) the thumb and (B) the forearm.

FIG B19-11. **Maffucci's syndrome.** (A) Plain radiograph demonstrates multiple soft-tissue masses and calcified thrombi in association with expansile bony lesions. (B) Late film from an arteriogram shows contrast material filling many cavernous hemangiomas of the soft tissues.

Condition	Comments
Trichinosis (*Trichinella spiralis*)	Calcification of encysted larvae is common pathologically, though their small size (1 mm or less) makes them difficult to detect radiographically.
Hydatid disease (*Echinococcus*)	Infrequent calcification in cysts within muscles or subcutaneous tissue.
Myositis ossificans progressiva (Fig B19-15)	Rare congenital dysplasia characterized by an interstitial myositis or fibrositis that undergoes cartilaginous and osseous transformation. Thick columns and plates of bone eventually replace tendons, fascia, and ligaments, causing such severe limitation of motion, contractures, and deformity that the patient becomes a virtual "stone person" and death ensues. There are usually a variety of associated congenital anomalies, most frequently hypoplasia of the great toes or thumbs.
Fluorosis (Fig B19-16)	Characteristic calcification of paraspinal, sacrotuberous, and iliolumbar ligaments as well as ligamentous calcification in the appendicular skeleton. Other skeletal findings include dense sclerosis (most prominent in the vertebrae and pelvis) and periosteal roughening and articular bone deposits arising at sites of muscular and ligamentous attachments.
Basal cell nevus syndrome	Soft-tissue calcification is occasionally seen in this inherited disorder characterized by multiple basal cell carcinomas, palmar pits, dentigerous cysts of the mandible, multiple rib and spinal anomalies, brachydactyly, and various neurologic and ophthalmologic abnormalities.
Werner's syndrome	Rare condition characterized by symmetric retardation of growth, premature aging, scleroderma-like skin changes, and cataracts. Soft-tissue calcification occurs in about one third of cases, especially about bony protuberances (especially the distal ends of the tibia and fibula) and the knees, feet, and hands.

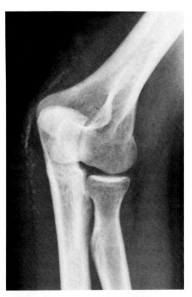

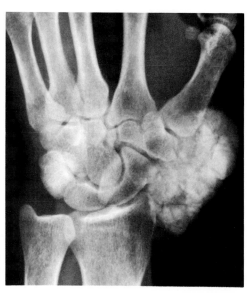

FIG B19-12. Systemic lupus erythematosus. Lacelike calcification about the elbow.

FIG B19-13. Pseudoxanthoma elasticum. Extensive calcification in soft tissues on the radial side of the wrist.

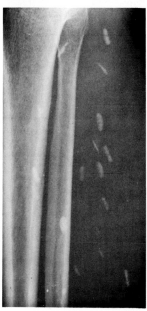

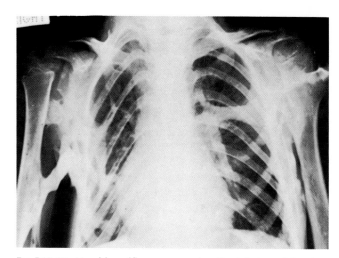

FIG B19-14. Cysticercosis. Multiple linear and oval calcifications along muscle bundles.

FIG B19-15. Myositis ossificans progressiva. Frontal view of the chest demonstrates extensive new bone formation in the soft tissues, which severely limited arm motion. Note the exostosis of the left proximal humerus due to blending of the ossific foci with the cortex of the bone.[24]

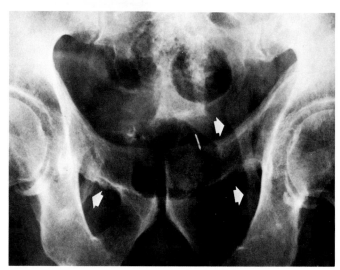

FIG B19-16. Fluorosis. Calcification of the sacrotuberous ligaments (arrows).

CALCIFICATION ABOUT THE FINGERTIPS

Condition	Comments
Scleroderma **(Fig B20-1)**	Digital calcification occurs in 10% to 20% of cases and may appear as small punctate deposits at the phalangeal tips or as more focal conglomerate calcific masses. Often associated with resorption of the terminal phalangeal tufts.
Raynaud's disease	Discrete calcium deposits may develop in the fingertips in association with soft-tissue atrophy and resorption of terminal tufts. Cold sensitivity occurs almost exclusively in women and produces symptoms of peripheral arterial spasm (especially in the upper limbs). May be either an isolated finding or a symptom of a more severe underlying condition (eg, scleroderma or other collagen vascular disease).
Dermatomyositis **(Fig B20-2)**	Calcification of the fingertips with associated terminal phalangeal erosion is one manifestation. More commonly there is extensive calcification in muscles and subcutaneous tissue underlying the associated skin lesions.
Calcinosis universalis **(Fig B20-3)**	Diffuse deposition of calcium in subcutaneous and later in deep connective tissues may involve the fingertips.
Systemic lupus erythematosus	Occasional manifestation (calcification more commonly involves the lower extremities).
Epidermolysis bullosa	Rare manifestation. Severe scarring causes soft-tissue atrophy and trophic changes involving the distal phalanges (may simulate scleroderma).
Rothmund's syndrome	Rare hereditary type of ectodermal dysplasia associated with resorption of phalangeal tufts and dystrophic soft-tissue calcification.

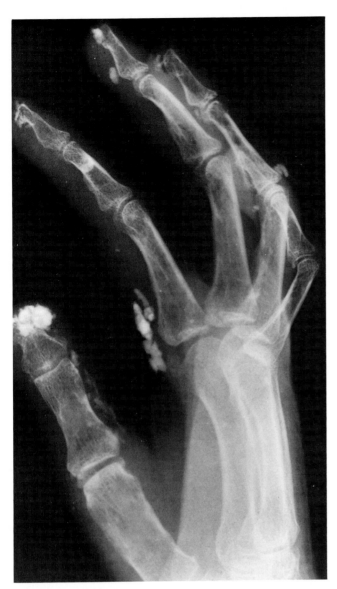

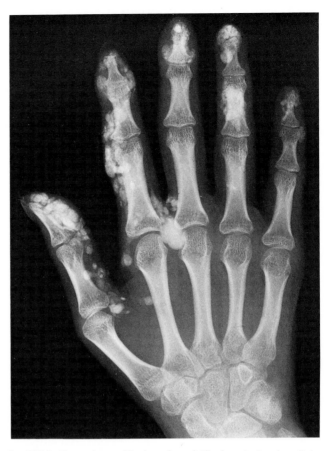

Fig B20-2. **Dermatomyositis.** Irregular calcific deposits involve all the fingers.

Fig B20-1. **Scleroderma.** Amorphous clumps of calcium in the soft tissues of the fingers. Note the trophic changes about the terminal tufts.

Fig B20-3. **Calcinosis universalis.** Coned view of the thumb demonstrates dense calcific deposits in the soft tissues on the ulnar aspect. The distal phalangeal tufts are normal, which virtually excludes scleroderma as the underlying cause of the calcification.

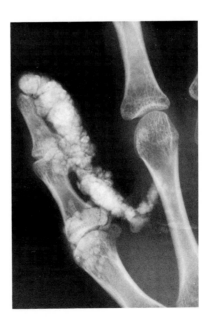

ZONES OF INCREASED DENSITY IN THE METAPHYSES

Condition	Comments
Normal variant	Normal active children less than 3 years of age often have relative whiteness of the metaphyseal ends of tubular bones.
Lead poisoning **(Fig B21-1)**	Dense transverse bands extending across the metaphyses of long bones and along the margins of flat bones such as the iliac crest. Predominantly involves the most rapidly growing portions of the skeleton (metaphyses at the distal ends of the femur and radius and both ends of the tibia). Lead lines can be observed in growing bones about 3 months after the inhalation of lead and 6 months after ingestion of the metal. Must be differentiated from the usual whiteness of the metaphyseal ends of tubular bones that is often seen in normal active children less than 3 years of age.
Other heavy metal or **chemical absorption** **(Fig B21-2)**	Bismuth; arsenic; phosphorus; fluoride; mercury; lithium; radium. May also develop in children whose mothers received high doses of estrogen or heavy metal therapy during pregnancy.
Treated leukemia **(Fig B21-3)**	Dense metaphyses (simulating lead poisoning) occur in a large percentage of patients with leukemia undergoing chemotherapy.
Transverse growth lines **(growth arrest lines)**	Fine symmetric, opaque transverse lines (single or multiple, varying in thickness and number) paralleling the contour of the provisional zone of calcification may be related to such stresses as malnutrition or chronic disease. These dense zones probably result from overproduction of, and failure to destroy, calcified cartilage matrix.
Healing rickets **(Fig B21-4)**	Represents mineralization of the zone of provisional calcification, which widens as healing progresses.
Hypervitaminosis D/ **idiopathic hypercalcemia**	Metaphyseal bands of increased density, reflecting heavy calcification of the matrix of proliferating cartilage, alternate with areas of increased lucency in the tubular bones of infants and children.

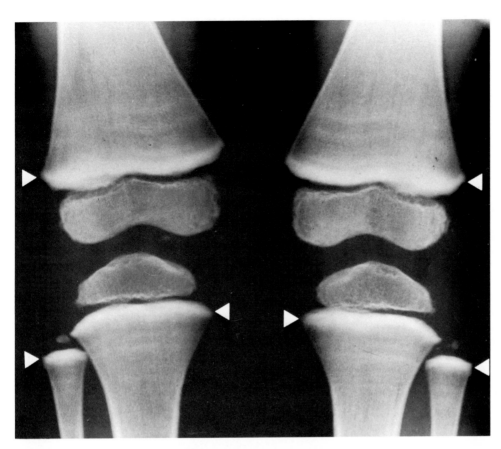

FIG B21-1. Lead poisoning.

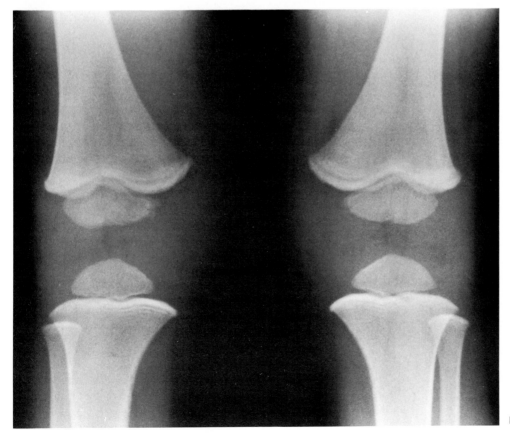

FIG B21-2. Bismuth poisoning.

Condition	Comments
Cretinism	Dense transverse metaphyseal bands may occur in association with a typical delay in the appearance and subsequent growth of ossification centers, epiphyseal dysgenesis (fragmented epiphyses with multiple ossification foci), and retarded bone age.
Healing scurvy	Increased density of the metaphyses may occur along with cortical thickening, increased density of the epiphyses, and massive subperiosteal bone formation.
Hypoparathyroidism	Zones of increased density in the metaphyseal regions of long bones may be associated with characteristic cerebral calcifications (primarily involving the basal ganglia, dentate nuclei of the cerebellum, and choroid plexus).
Osteopetrosis	Transverse radiodense metaphyseal bands often occur in the long bones and vertebrae. There may be alternating lucent transverse lines that probably reflect the intermittent nature of the pathologic process.
Congenital syphilis	Transverse metaphyseal stripes (sclerotic and lucent bands) may be an early finding. This pattern may also develop in other transplacental infections (rubella, toxoplasmosis, and cytomegalic inclusion disease).

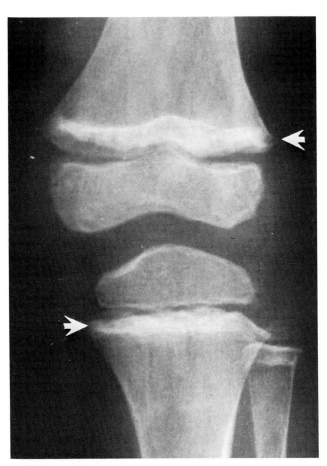

FIG B21-3. Chronic leukemia. After therapy with methotrexate, dense, irregular sclerosis has developed about the metaphyses of the distal femur and proximal tibia (arrows).

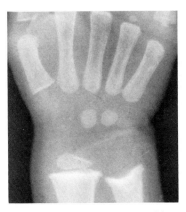

FIG B21-4. Healed rickets. Increased sharpness of the metaphyseal lines after therapy with vitamin D.

RADIOLUCENT METAPHYSEAL BANDS

Condition	Comments
Normal variant	Striated appearance of the metaphyses is common in neonates.
Transplacental infection (Figs B22-1 and B22-2)	Rubella; syphilis; herpes; toxoplasmosis; cytomegalic inclusion disease. In rubella there is a typical pattern of alternating dense and lucent longitudinal striations (celery stick sign).
Leukemia (Fig B22-3)	Symmetric bandlike lucent areas (not associated with actual leukemic cell infiltration) primarily affect sites of rapid bone growth (the distal femur, proximal tibia, proximal humerus, and distal radius). Nonspecific appearance that probably reflects a nutritional deficit that interferes with proper osteogenesis (after age 2, radiolucent metaphyseal bands strongly suggest leukemia).
Metastatic neuroblastoma	Lucent metaphyseal bands and other radiographic abnormalities (widespread osteolytic lesions, periosteal reaction) may be indistinguishable from leukemia. May be differentiated by the presence of vanillylmandelic acid (VMA) in the urine.
Scurvy	Submetaphyseal band of lucency (Trummerfeld zone) adjacent to the widened and increased density of the zone of provisional calcification (white line of scurvy). Other manifestations include Pelken's spur and Wimberger's sign.
Juvenile rheumatoid arthritis	Extensive deossification of an affected extremity may cause bands of metaphyseal lucency mimicking childhood leukemia. Primarily involves the areas of greatest bone growth (the knees, ankles, and wrists).
Craniometaphyseal dysplasia (Fig B22-4)	Rare hereditary disorder in which failure of normal tubulation of bone is combined with hypertelorism, a broad flat nose, and defective dentition. Initial metaphyseal lucency and diaphyseal sclerosis progress to more normal mineralization and lack of modeling.
Systemic illness (Fig B22-5)	Metaphyseal radiolucency is a nonspecific finding that may be encountered in various systemic illnesses of childhood (probably reflects a nutritional deficit interfering with proper osteogenesis).

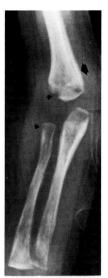

Fig B22-1. Congenital syphilis. Transverse bands of increased density across the metaphyses (small arrows) associated with patchy areas of bone destruction in the diaphyses. There is solid periosteal new bone formation (large arrow), which is best seen about the distal humerus.

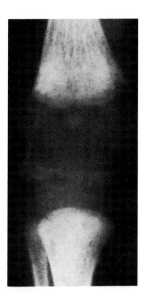

Fig B22-2. Rubella. Radiograph of the knee in a 1-day-old girl with a maternal history of rubella demonstrates alternating lucent and sclerotic longitudinal striations extending perpendicular to the epiphyseal plate and parallel to the long axis of the bone (celery stick sign).[25]

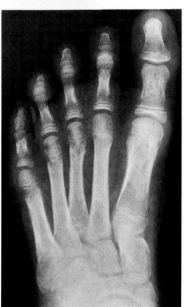

Fig B22-3. Leukemia. In addition to radiolucent metaphyseal bands, there is frank bone destruction with cortical erosion involving many of the metatarsals and proximal phalanges.

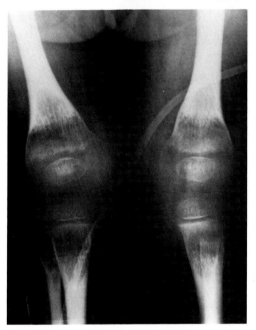

Fig B22-4. Craniometaphyseal dysplasia. Severe metaphyseal lucency with diaphyseal sclerosis about the knees.

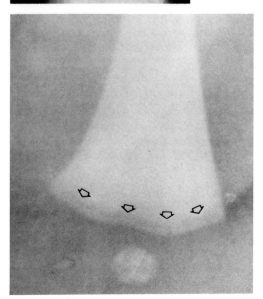

Fig B22-5. Chronic systemic illness.

UNDERCONSTRICTION OR UNDERTUBULATION
(WIDE DIAMETAPHYSIS)

Condition	Comments

Lipid storage disease
  Gaucher's disease
  (Fig B23-1)
	Inborn error of metabolism characterized by accumulation of abnormal quantities of complex lipids in the reticuloendothelial cells of the spleen, liver, and bone marrow. Skeletal infiltration causes a loss of bone density with expansion and cortical thinning of long bones, especially the femur. Marrow infiltration in the distal femur causes abnormal modeling and flaring and the characteristic Erlenmeyer flask deformity. Aseptic necrosis (especially of the femoral heads) is a common complication. The spleen is usually markedly enlarged and hepatomegaly is common.

Niemann-Pick disease **(Fig B23-2)**	Inborn error of lipid metabolism (abnormal deposition of sphingomyelin) that usually begins in infancy and is rapidly fatal. In patients with milder and more slowly progressive disease who survive until late adulthood or adolescence, the skeletal abnormalities are identical to those in Gaucher's disease. However, the early age of onset and the frequently associated nodular interstitial pulmonary infiltrates suggest Neimann-Pick disease.

Anemia
  Thalassemia
  (Fig B23-3)
	Extensive marrow hyperplasia (due to ineffective erythropoiesis and rapid destruction of newly formed red blood cells) causes pronounced widening of the medullary spaces and thinning of the cortices. Normal modeling of long bones does not occur because the expanding marrow flattens or even bulges the normally concave surfaces of the shafts. Focal collections of hyperplastic marrow cause localized radiolucencies that have the appearance of multiple osteolytic lesions. Other characteristic findings include the "hair-on-end" appearance of the skull (vertical striations in a radial pattern) and paravertebral soft-tissue masses of extramedullary hematopoiesis.

Sickle cell anemia	Marrow hyperplasia in long bones causes widening of the medullary spaces, thinning of the cortices, and coarsening of the trabecular pattern. The expanding marrow prevents normal modeling, as in thalassemia. Other characteristic changes include "fish vertebrae," bone infarcts, osteomyelitis, and papillary necrosis.

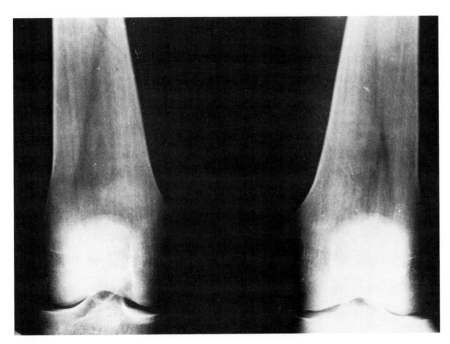

Fig B23-1. Gaucher's disease. The distal ends of the femurs show typical underconstriction and cortical thinning (Erlenmeyer flask appearance).[26]

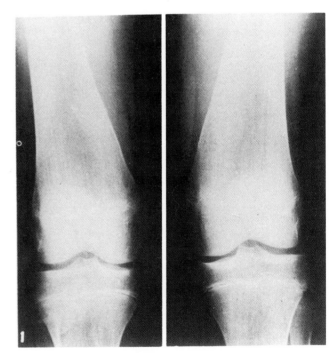

Fig B23-2. Niemann-Pick disease. Thin cortices and a lack of normal modeling of the distal femurs simulate the pattern in Gaucher's disease.[3]

Condition	Comments
Bone dysplasia **Fibrous dysplasia** **(Fig B23-4)**	Proliferation of fibrous tissue in the medullary cavity produces a well-defined area that varies from completely lucent to a homogeneous ground-glass density (depending on the amount of fibrous or osseous tissue deposited in the medullary cavity). The bone is often locally expanded, most commonly at the metaphysis but sometimes extending to involve the entire shaft. Thinning of the cortices predisposes to pathologic fracture. In severe and long-standing disease, the affected bones may be bowed or deformed (eg, shepherd's crook deformity of the femur).
Multiple exostoses **(diaphyseal acalsis)** **(Fig B23-5)**	Hereditary bone dysplasia in which multiple osteochondromas arise from the ends of the shafts of bones preformed in cartilage. Characteristic undertubulation and often bowing of long bones occurs with multiple osteochondromas in the metaphyseal regions. Frequently there is deformity of the forearm due to shortening and bowing of the ulna.
Craniometaphyseal **dysplasia**	Rare hereditary disorder in which failure of normal tubulation of bone is combined with hypertelorism, a broad flat nose, and defective dentition. Additional findings include sclerosis of the base of the skull and calvarium, lack of aeration of the paranasal sinuses and mastoids, and thickening and sclerosis of the mandible.
Metaphyseal dysplasia **(Pyle's disease)** **(Fig B23-6)**	Rare hereditary disorder in which symmetric paddle-shaped enlargement of the metaphyses and adjacent diaphyses of long bones is associated with osteoporosis and cortical thinning. No evidence of skull abnormalities (unlike craniometaphyseal dysplasia).
Multiple **enchondromatosis** **(Ollier's disease)** **(Fig B23-7)**	Bone dysplasia affecting the growth plate in which an excess of hypertrophic cartilage is not resorbed and ossified in a normal fashion. This causes proliferation of rounded masses or columns of decreased-density cartilage in the metaphyses and diaphyses of one or more tubular bones. The involvement is usually unilateral and the affected bones are invariably shortened and often deformed. In long bones, columns of radiolucent cartilage may be separated by bony septa, producing a striated appearance. In the hands and feet, the lesions are globular and expansile, often with stippled or mottled calcification.
Progressive diaphyseal **dysplasia (Camurati-** **Engelmann disease)** **(Fig B23-8)**	Rare disorder in which symmetric cortical thickening in the midshafts of long bones is associated with a neuromuscular dystrophy that causes a wide-based, waddling gait. A combination of endosteal and periosteal cortical thickening causes symmetric fusiform enlargement and undertubulation of long bones. Encroachment on the medullary canal may cause anemia and secondary hepatosplenomegaly. Amorphous increased density at the base of the skull may lead to impingement on the cranial nerves.

(continued page 686)

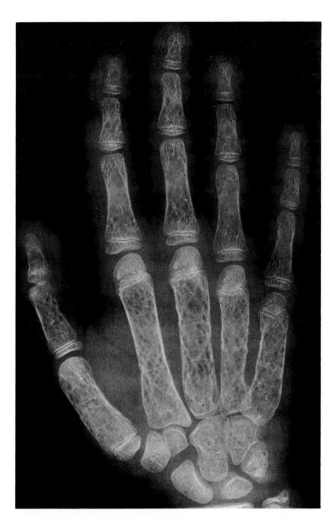

Fɪɢ **B23-3. Thalassemia.** Pronounced widening of the medullary spaces with thinning of the cortices. Note the absence of normal modeling due to the pressure of the expanding marrow space. Localized radiolucencies simulating multiple osteolytic lesions represent tumorous collections of hyperplastic marrow.

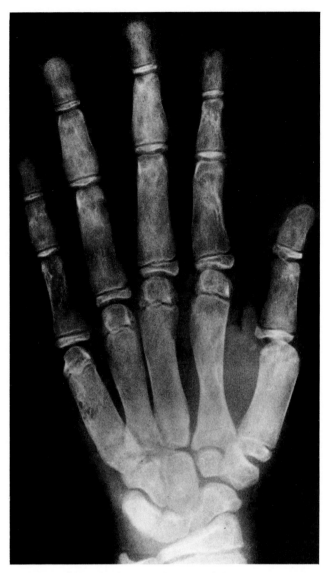

Fɪɢ **B23-4. Fibrous dysplasia.** Smudgy, ground-glass appearance of the medullary cavities with failure of normal modeling.

Condition	Comments
Osteopetrosis (Fig B23-9)	Rare hereditary bone dysplasia in which failure of the resorptive mechanism of calcified cartilage interferes with its normal replacement by mature bone. A dense, uniform, and symmetric increase in bone density is associated with undertubulation of long bones. Alternating dense and lucent transverse lines (probably reflecting the intermittent nature of the pathologic process) may develop in the metaphyses of long bones and vertebrae. Other characteristic findings include a miniature bone inset within each vertebral body (bone-within-a-bone appearance) and increased density at the end plates (sandwich vertebrae).
Hypophosphatasia	Mild form developing in adults is associated with lack of modeling of long bones, decreased stature, increased bone fragility, and various skeletal deformities.
Osteogenesis imperfecta	Inherited generalized disorder of connective tissue associated with blue sclerae, multiple fractures, and hypermobility of joints. The rarest "cystic" form is characterized by flared metaphyses that are hyperlucent and traversed by a honeycomb of coarse trabeculae. The shaft may be *over*constricted and show severe bending deformities and healed fractures in addition to generalized osteopenia.
Metatropic dwarfism	Very rare short-limbed dwarfism in which the patient is normal at birth. Progressive kyphoscoliosis with characteristic trumpetlike expansion of multiple metaphyses, especially in the femurs and tibias.
Healing fracture/ metaphyseal injury	Common cause of localized undertubulation and deformity of a long bone. During the healing phase, an elevated solid periosteal reaction may simulate a "double cortex" (especially in infants and children), but disappears with further bone remodeling.
Biliary atresia	Most common cause of persistent neonatal jaundice; usually fatal within 2 years unless corrected surgically. Undertubulation of long bones is combined with signs of osteoporosis and rickets.

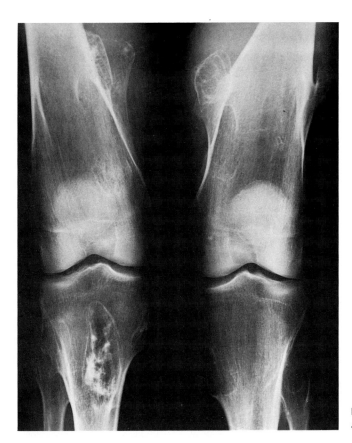

Fig B23-5. Multiple exostoses. Bilateral involvement of the distal femurs and proximal tibias.

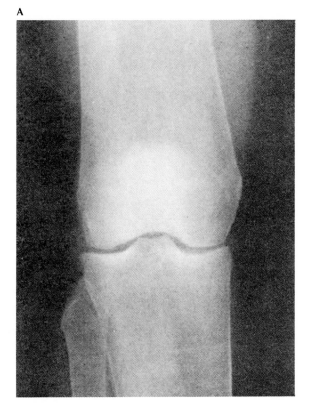

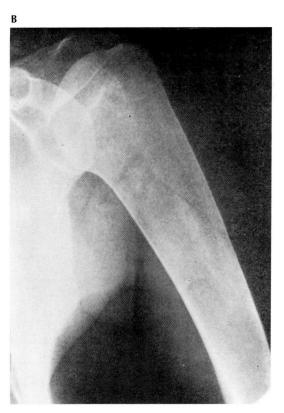

Fig B23-6. Metaphyseal dysplasia. Frontal views of (A) the knee and (B) the proximal humerus show defective modeling leading to extreme widening of the metaphyseal areas of the visualized long bones. The cortices are markedly thinned in the metaphyseal area.[27]

Condition	Comments

Metabolic and nutritional disorders
   Healing rickets and
   scurvy
   (Fig B23-10)
	Widening of the diametaphyses with cortical thickening and undertubulation occurs in the healing phase of these diseases.

Mucopolysaccharidoses	Thickening and undertubulation of the shafts of long bones, often with irregular wavy contours, is common. Metaphyseal flaring may be seen in Morquio's disease, while tapering of the ends of long bones suggests Hurler's disease.
Homocystinuria	Inborn error of methionine metabolism in which there is usually widening of the metaphyses and enlargement of the ossification centers of long bones, most commonly at the knees. There is usually striking osteoporosis of the spine that is often associated with biconcave deformities of vertebral bodies. Long bones tend to be osteoporotic with cortical thickening.
Hypervitaminosis D/ idiopathic hypercalcemia	Undertubulation, especially in the distal femurs, may occur in association with generalized sclerosis, cortical thickening, and dense transverse metaphyseal bands. Prominent renal calcification and renal failure often develop.
Congenital rubella **(see Fig B22-2)**	Undertubulation of long bones with radiolucent metaphyseal bands and characteristic alternating lucent and sclerotic longitudinal striations (celery stick pattern). Osseous changes regress in infants who grow normally, but may persist in those who fail to survive.
Bone cysts, tumors, and tumorlike conditions	Localized widening near the end of a long bone may be caused by a variety of benign expansile mass lesions (including histiocytosis X).

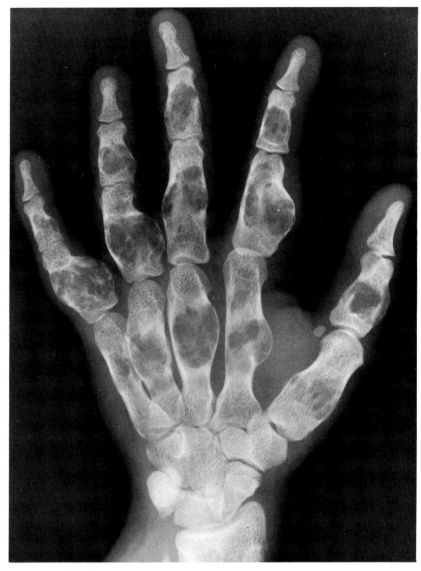

Fig B23-7. Multiple enchondromatosis. Multiple globular and expansile lucent filling defects involving virtually all the metacarpals and the proximal and distal phalanges.

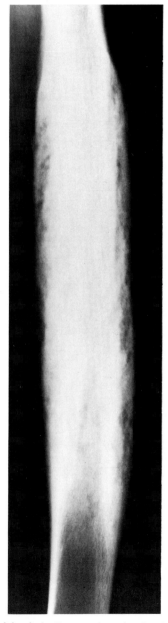

Fig B23-8. Progressive diaphyseal dysplasia. Dense endosteal and periosteal cortical thickening causes fusiform enlargement of the midshaft of the femur.

Condition	Comments
Lead poisoning	Wide sclerotic bands of lead deposited in the metaphyses can prevent normal bone remodeling and lead to residual deformity.
Infantile cortical hyperostosis (Caffey's disease)	Diffuse soft-tissue swelling, periosteal new bone formation, and massive cortical thickening cause generalized widening and undertubulation of affected bones. Primarily involves the mandible, scapula, clavicle, ulna, and ribs and almost always develops before the age of 5 months.
Chronic osteomyelitis	Sclerosis and solid periosteal new bone formation may produce marked thickening of the affected area.

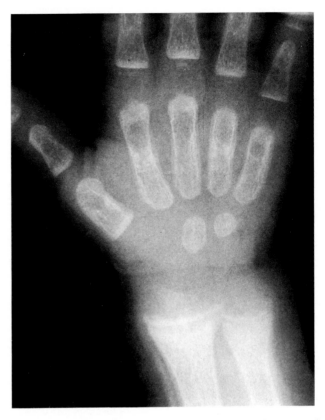

FIG B23-10. Healing rickets. Widening of the metacarpals associated with diffuse periosteal reaction. There is still some bony demineralization and residual cupping and fraying of the distal radius and ulna.

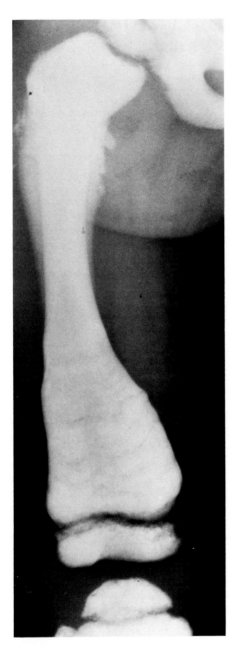

FIG B23-9. Osteopetrosis. Dense, uniform, symmetric increase in the density of the femur with failure of proper modeling.

OVERCONSTRICTION OR OVERTUBULATION
(NARROW DIAMETAPHYSIS)

Condition	Comments
Disuse atrophy	Osteoporosis with cortical thinning and a decrease in the size and number of trabeculae in the spongiosa may develop after prolonged disuse. Concentric constriction of the shaft often occurs in children (rare in adults).
Paralysis (infancy and childhood) (Fig B24-1)	Poliomyelitis, birth palsies, and congenital malformations of the spinal cord and brain result in decreased peripheral muscle tone and secondary bone atrophy. In addition to overconstriction of the shafts, there is generalized osteoporosis and cortical thinning.
Muscular disorders (Fig B24-2)	Generalized overconstriction of the shafts of long bones (similar to that in paralysis) develops in such conditions as muscular dystrophy, arthrogryposis, amyotonia congenita, and infantile muscular atrophy (Werdnig-Hoffmann disease). Replacement of muscle by fat produces a characteristic finely striated or striped appearance. The fascial sheaths may appear as thin shadows of increased density surrounded by fat.
Marfan's syndrome (Fig B24-3)	Inherited generalized disorder of connective tissue in which there is elongation and thinning (without osteoporosis) of the tubular bones that is most pronounced in the hands and feet (arachnodactyly). Most patients are tall and appear emaciated because of a decrease in subcutaneous fat. Bilateral dislocation of the lens of the eye often occurs because of weakness and redundancy of its supporting structures. Laxity of ligaments elsewhere leads to loose-jointedness, double-jointedness, and recurrent dislocations. Dissecting aneurysm is the most serious cardiovascular complication.
Homocystinuria	Inborn error of methionine metabolism that produces a Marfan-like appearance of thin and elongated tubular bones. In contrast to Marfan's syndrome, the long tubular bones in homocystinuria have widened metaphyses and enlarged ossification centers and there is often striking osteoporosis (especially in the spine).
Osteogenesis imperfecta (Fig B24-4)	Inherited generalized disorder of connective tissue in which long bones are slender and overconstricted. There is striking osteoporosis with thinning of the cortices and a marked susceptibility to fracture (from minimal trauma) that leads to bowing and other deformities.

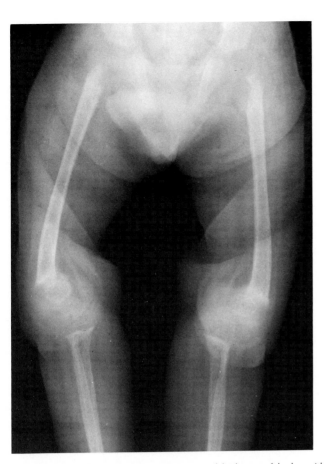

FIG B24-1. Paralysis. Generalized narrowing of the bones of the leg with cortical thinning and diffuse osteoporosis.

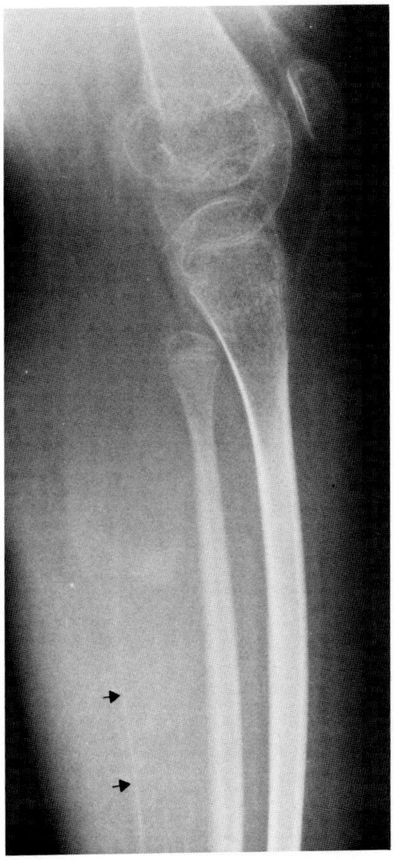

FIG B24-2. Muscular dystrophy. Generalized thinning of the bones of the lower leg. The fascial sheaths appear as thin shadows of increased density (arrows) surrounded by fatty infiltration within muscle bundles.

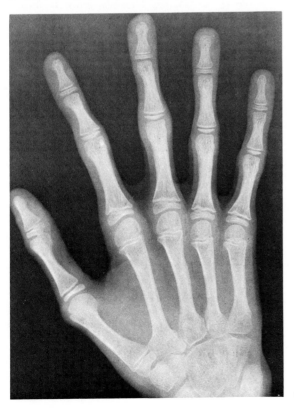

FIG B24-3. Marfan's syndrome. The metacarpals and phalanges are unusually long and slender (arachnodactyly).

Condition	Comments
Juvenile rheumatoid arthritis (Fig B24-5)	Generalized connective tissue disease of children that most frequently affects the areas of greatest bone growth (the knees, ankles, and wrists). The long tubular bones may be overconstricted with generalized osteoporosis. Periosteal new bone formation is much more common and severe than in the adult form of the disease. Growth disturbances are common and include overgrowth of the epiphyses of an affected joint (balloon epiphysis), initially accelerated bone growth because of local hyperemia, and then delayed bone growth due to early epiphyseal fusion or the administration of steroids.
Neurofibromatosis (see Figs B27-2, B30-1, SP7-2, SK2-2)	Overtubulation of bone may result in an extremely thin shaft that is usually associated with bowing deformities. Conversely, overgrowth of bone may produce elephantoid soft-tissue and bony thickening. Other major abnormalities include pseudoarthroses, "ribbon ribs," posterior vertebral scalloping, and orbital dysplasia.
Epidermolysis bullosa (see Fig B12-7)	Thin, osteoporotic tubular bones may reflect chronic muscle atrophy in this rare hereditary disorder in which the skin blisters spontaneously or with injury. Flexion contractures and webbing between the fingers may produce a clawlike hand. Severe scarring causes soft-tissue atrophy and trophic changes of shortening and tapering of the distal phalanges. Healing of esophageal mucosal lesions may progress to stenotic webs.
Dwarfism **Progeria** (Fig B24-6)	Nonhereditary congenital syndrome of dwarfism and premature aging and senility in which thin, osteoporotic long bones are associated with such findings as small facial bones and mandible; progressive resorption of terminal phalangeal tufts, clavicles, and occasionally ribs; thin calvarium with wormian bones; coxa valga; and coronary artery disease and hypertension that lead to prominent cardiomegaly.
Hypopituitarism	Proportional dwarfism that is often associated with narrowing of tubular bones and delayed epiphyseal closure. Hypogonadism and other endocrinologic disturbances commonly occur.
Tubular stenosis (Kenny-Caffey)	Proportional dwarfism characterized by overconstricted tubular bones that show symmetric internal thickening of the cortex and narrowing of the medullary cavity. Other manifestations include calvarial sclerosis and transient hypocalcemia with tetanic convulsions.

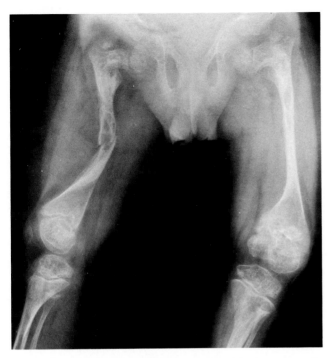

FIG B24-4. Osteogenesis imperfecta. The bones of the lower extremity are thin and deformed with evidence of previous fracture.

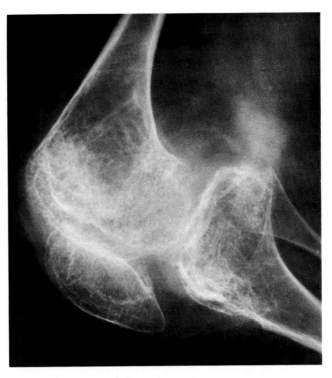

FIG B24-5. Juvenile rheumatoid arthritis. Severe demineralization of bone with expansion of the epiphyseal and metaphyseal areas and relative constriction of the underdeveloped diaphyseal portions.

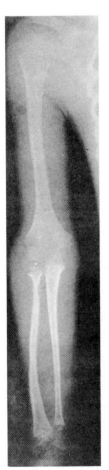

FIG B24-6. Progeria. The ulna and radius are thin and osteoporotic.[19]

AVASCULAR NECROSIS OF THE HIP OR OTHER JOINTS

Condition	Comments
Trauma	Disruption of the blood supply most commonly affects the hips and is secondary to an intracapsular femoral neck fracture, dislocation of the femoral head, or surgical correction of congenital hip dislocation or slipped femoral capital epiphysis. The carpal navicular is also frequently involved.
Sickle cell disease (Fig B25-1)	Sludging of sickled erythrocytes in the sinusoidal vascular bed results in functional obstruction.
Steroid therapy/Cushing's syndrome (Fig B25-2)	Underlying pathophysiology is unclear. May be related to microscopic fat emboli in end-arteries of bone, steroid-induced osteoporosis with microfractures, or compression of the sinusoidal vascular bed by an increase in the marrow fat cell mass.
Occlusive vascular disease	Arteriosclerosis or thromboembolic disease disrupts the blood supply.
Legg-Calvé-Perthes disease (Figs B25-3 and B25-4)	Osteochondritis of the femoral capital epiphyseal ossification center, most commonly occurring in boys between the ages of 5 and 9. There may be associated focal destructive lesions of the femoral neck (simulating an infectious or neoplastic process). Long-term complications include failure of the femoral neck to grow (with resultant shortening) and early development of degenerative arthritis.
Chronic alcoholism	Avascular necrosis, especially of the femoral head, is a fairly common complication. The underlying pathophysiologic mechanism is probably similar to that with steroid therapy. In alcoholic fatty liver disease, systemic fat emboli may lodge in bone and lead to necrosis.
Gaucher's disease (Fig B25-5)	Inborn error of metabolism in which abnormal quantities of complex lipids may accumulate in the bone marrow, causing progressive obstruction of blood flow through the sinusoids and leading to infarction.
Chronic pancreatitis	The increased incidence of avascular necrosis probably represents a complication of underlying chronic alcoholism. Circulating lipases may produce areas of fat necrosis in the bones of patients with acute pancreatitis.

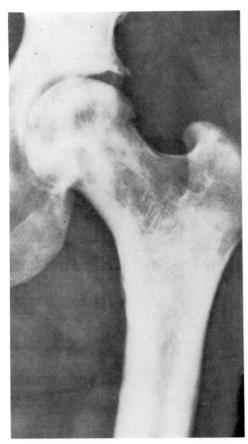

FIG B25-1. **Sickle cell disease.** Avascular necrosis of the femoral head, with mottled areas of increased and decreased density reflecting osteonecrosis without collapse. The trabeculae in the neck and intertrochanteric region are thickened by apposition of new bone. A solid layer of new bone has been laid down in continuity with the inner aspect of the cortex of the femoral shaft, with consequent narrowing of the medullary canal.[28]

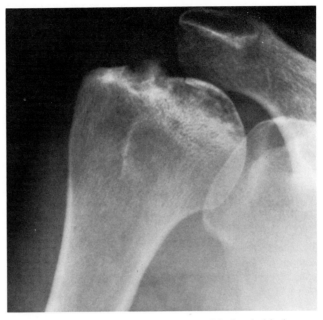

FIG B25-2. **Steroid therapy.** Aseptic necrosis of the head of the humerus in a transplant recipient.

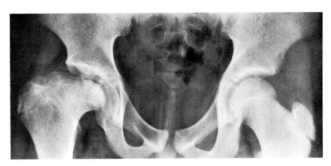

FIG B25-4. **Legg-Calvé-Perthes disease.** In a teenager with chronic disease there is severe flattening of the right femoral head with virtually complete failure of the ipsilateral femoral neck to grow. This led to shortening of the leg and a clinically obvious limp.

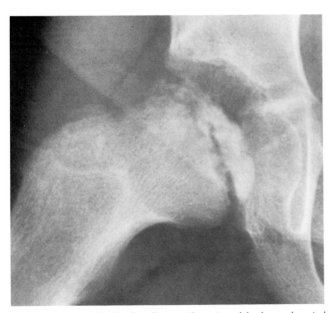

FIG B25-3. **Legg-Calvé-Perthes disease.** Flattening of the femoral capital epiphyses along with fragmentation and sclerosis.

Condition	Comments
Gout	Infrequent, but important, cause of avascular necrosis that should be considered in the older age group when no other etiology is apparent. No definite pathophysiologic explanation (other than the frequent association of chronic alcoholism and gout).
Collagen disease	Systemic lupus erythematosus; rheumatoid arthritis; polyarteritis nodosa. Ischemic bone necrosis may be related to steroid therapy or vasculitis causing interruption of the arterial blood supply.
Radiation therapy/ radium poisoning (Fig B25-6)	Direct cytotoxic effect (especially on the more sensitive hematopoietic marrow constituents) or damage to the arterial blood supply to bone.
Caisson disease (dysbaric disorders)	Result of air (nitrogen) embolization after rapid decompression. Because fat cells tend to absorb large quantities of dissolved nitrogen, rapid expansion of these cells in the marrow can cause increased intraosseous marrow pressure and vascular compromise.
Hemophilia	Hemarthrosis can occlude epiphyseal vessels and result in avascular necrosis. Most commonly involves the femoral and radial heads (both of which have a totally intracapsular epiphysis and are therefore especially vulnerable to deprivation of their vascular supply from compression by a tense joint effusion).
Osteomyelitis	Although no longer generally regarded in the context of osteonecrosis, the sequestrum of osteomyelitis is a manifestation of ischemic bone death occurring as a consequence of compressive and destructive suppuration that isolates a segment of bone from its blood supply.
Osteochondritis dissecans (Fig B25-7)	Localized form of avascular necrosis that most frequently affects young males and is probably caused by trauma. Primarily involves the knees (usually the lateral aspect of the medial femoral condyle). Other common locations are the ankles, femoral heads, elbows, and shoulders. Radiographically, a small, round or oval, necrotic segment of bone with its articular cartilage detaches and lies in a depression in the joint surface. The necrotic segment is often denser than the surrounding bone and well demarcated by a crescentic lucent zone. Separation of the necrotic segment from the joint to form a free joint body leaves a residual pit in the articular surface.

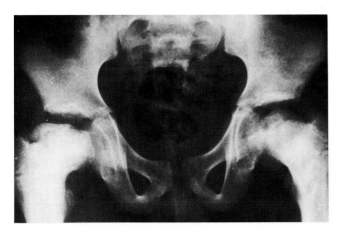

FIG B25-5. Gaucher's disease. Bilateral avascular necrosis of the femoral heads.

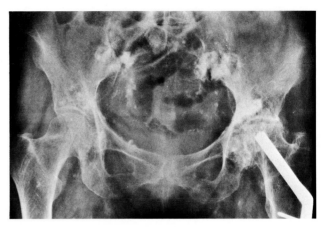

FIG B25-6. Radiation therapy. After radiation therapy for carcinoma of the cervix, there has been flattening and sclerosis of the left femoral head (reflecting avascular necrosis) and patchy areas of dense sclerosis in the pelvis.

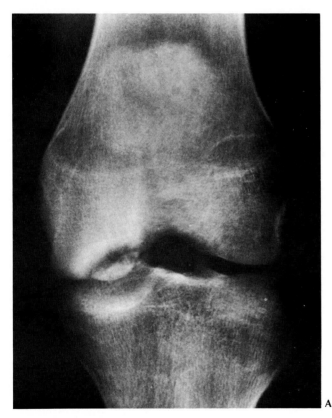

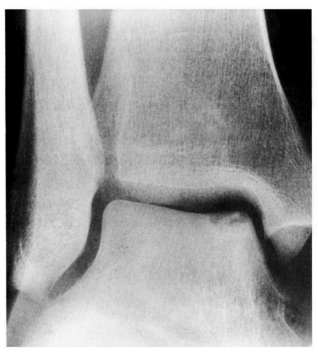

FIG B25-7. Osteochondritis dissecans. (A) Knee. (B) Ankle.

RIB NOTCHING

Condition	Comments
Arterial	
Coarctation of the aorta (Fig B26-1)	By far the most common cause of rib notching. Usually involves the posterior fourth to eighth ribs and rarely develops before age 6. Aortic narrowing typically occurs at or just distal to the level of the ductus arteriosus. Characteristic double bulge in the region of the aortic knob (figure-3 sign on plain chest radiographs and reverse figure-3, or figure-E, sign on the barium-filled esophagus) represents prestenotic and poststenotic dilatation. Collateral flow bypassing the aortic constriction to reach the abdomen and lower extremities comes almost entirely from the two subclavian arteries via the thyrocervical, costocervical, and internal mammary arteries and their subdivisions to the posterior intercostals and then into the descending aorta. The large volume of blood traversing this route causes dilatation, tortuosity, and increased pulsation of the intercostal arteries, which results in gradual erosion of the adjacent bones. Unilateral rib notching in coarctation occasionally occurs on the left side when the constriction is located proximal to an anomalous right subclavian artery and on the right side when the coarctation occurs proximal to the left subclavian artery (only the subclavian artery that arises proximal to the aortic obstruction transmits the collateral blood to the intercostals). Notching of the first two ribs does not occur because the first two intercostal arteries, arising from the supreme intercostals, do not convey blood directly to the postcoarctation segment of the aorta. The last three intercostal arteries conduct blood away from the postcoarctation aortic segment and thus do not greatly enlarge or cause rib notching.
Low aortic obstruction	Thrombosis of the lower thoracic or abdominal aorta causes collateral flow via the lower intercostal arteries to supply blood to the lower part of the body via anastomoses with arteries of the abdominal wall.
Subclavian artery obstruction	Unilateral rib notching commonly occurs secondary to interruption of a subclavian artery for the Blalock-Taussig subclavian artery–pulmonary artery anastomosis for congenital heart disease. The development of rib notching reflects increased blood flow through collateral vessels to the arm resulting from interruption of the subclavian and vertebral arteries on the involved side. Rib notching is also a rare complication of Takayasu's arteritis ("pulseless disease") causing occlusion of one or both subclavian arteries.

(continued page 702)

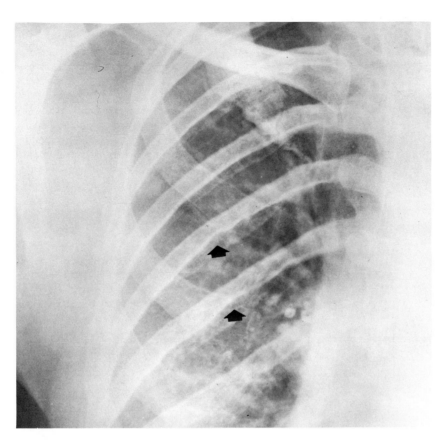

FIG B26-1. Coarctation of the aorta. Notching of the posterior fourth through eighth ribs (arrows).[29]

Condition	Comments
Decreased pulmonary blood flow	The intercostal arteries may participate in the collateral circulation to the lungs whenever there is an obstruction to pulmonary blood flow. Nevertheless, despite abundant and well-developed collateral circulation, rib notching is uncommon in this situation. Conditions with decreased pulmonary blood flow in which rib notching has been reported include tetralogy of Fallot, unilateral absence of the pulmonary artery, Ebstein's anomaly, emphysema, pseudotruncus arteriosus, and pulmonary valvular stenosis or atresia.
Venous	Chronic obstruction of the superior vena cava (as in fibrosing mediastinitis) can produce rib notching. This is a very infrequent cause, as might be expected, since dilated intercostal veins do not erode the ribs as readily as do dilated, highly pulsatile intercostal arteries.
Arteriovenous	Pulmonary arteriovenous fistula (dilated intercostal arteries carrying a systemic supply to the fistula or contributing collateral circulation to that portion of the pulmonary vascular bed bypassed by the large flow through the fistula); arteriovenous fistula of the chest wall (intercostal artery–vein communication).
Neurogenic (Fig B26-2)	Rib erosions due to multiple intercostal neurofibromas (in neurofibromatosis) or rare single intercostal nerve tumors (schwannoma or neurilemmoma). Rib deformities in neurofibromatosis frequently reflect the generalized bone dysplasia occurring in this condition.
Osseous	Periosteal irregularities mimicking rib notching rarely occur in hyperparathyroidism, tuberous sclerosis, and thalassemia. Poliomyelitis primarily causes irregularity of the superior surfaces of the ribs.
Idiopathic	Mild degrees of rib notching may develop in apparently healthy individuals with none of the above-described underlying causes.

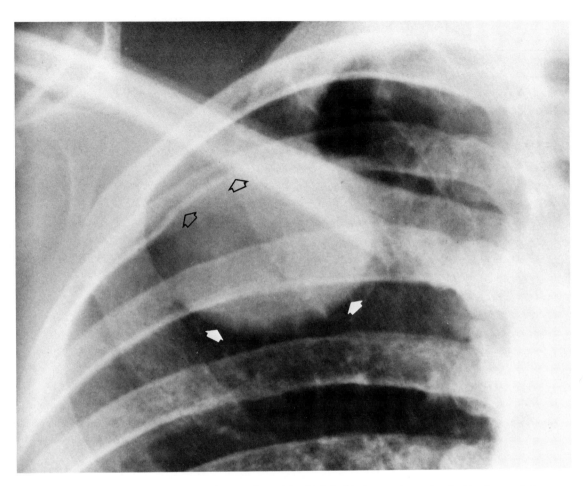

FIG B26-2. Neurofibroma. Erosion of the inferior surface of the third rib (black arrows) associated with a large soft-tissue mass (white arrows).

RESORPTION OR NOTCHING OF SUPERIOR RIB MARGINS

Condition	Comments
Disturbance of osteoblastic activity (decreased or deficient bone formation)	
Neurofibromatosis (Fig B27-1)	Irregular, notched, scalloped, and twisted ribbonlike configuration of the ribs is a manifestation of dysplastic bone formation. Rib deformities also may be secondary to mechanical pressure caused by neighboring intercostal neurofibromas.
Collagen disease	Erosions of the superior margins of the posterior aspect of the upper ribs (third, fourth, fifth, and occasionally sixth). Most commonly occurs in rheumatoid arthritis and scleroderma, but may also develop in systemic lupus erythematosus and Sjögren's syndrome.
Paralytic poliomyelitis (Fig B27-2)	Initially, a localized shallow indentation with progressive narrowing of the upper cortical margins of the ribs. As the condition progresses, the cortices of the ribs become increasingly thin and there is localized osteoporosis. A similar, though slight, indentation may occasionally occur on the inferior cortical margin, producing an hour-glass appearance. The underlying mechanism is most likely atrophy of the intercostal muscles (and their replacement by fat and fibrous tissue) at their attachment to the ribs, which decreases the normal "stress stimulus" required for osteoblastic bone production to replace the osteoid that has been lost by physiologic erosion. Another explanation is that the rib erosion is secondary to the continued pressure of the scapula against the posterior aspect of the ribs from prolonged use of a respirator. There may also be severe thinning of the humeri and usually pronounced scoliosis of the thoracic spine.
Localized pressure effect	May follow the use of rib retractors during surgery or intercostal chest drainage tubes. Also an underlying mechanism in patients with neurofibromatosis, thoracic neuroblastoma, and multiple hereditary exostoses. Severely tortuous intercostal arteries extending down from the lower border of a rib have been reported to erode the superior borders of the adjacent inferior rib.
Osteogenesis imperfecta	Systemic connective tissue disorder in which there is an inability to produce adequate amounts of osteoid to balance physiologic osteolysis. Produces a concave superior margin in multiple ribs associated with cortical thinning and abnormal rib rotation and curvature.

(continued page 706)

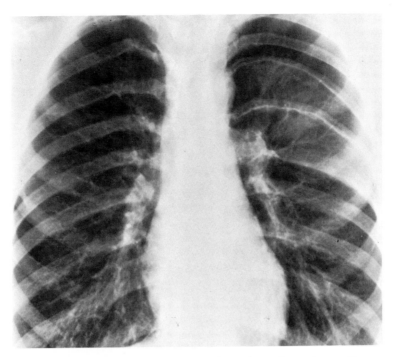

Fɪɢ B27-1. Neurofibromatosis. Narrowing and irregularity of several upper ribs.

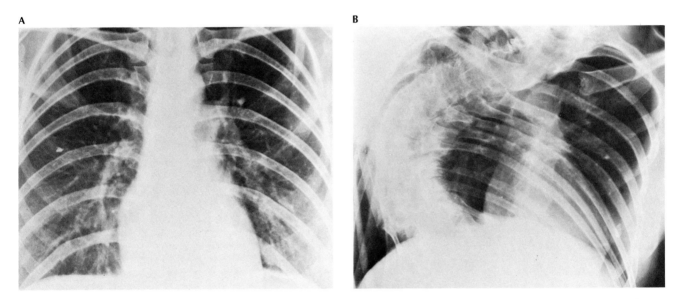

Fɪɢ B27-2. Poliomyelitis. (A) Severe thinning of the humeri and ribs bilaterally. Note the bilateral shoulder dislocations. (B) In another patient, there is severe scoliosis of the thoracic spine producing an unusual configuration of the ribs.

Condition	Comments
Marfan's syndrome **(Fig B27-3)**	Narrow ribs with thin cortices reflect poor muscle tone rather than a primary alteration in the quality of osteoid bone formation. Both superior and inferior marginal defects may occur.
Radiation therapy	Rare delayed manifestation of radiation interference with normal osteoblastic activity.
Disturbance of osteoclastic activity (increased bone resorption) Hyperparathyroidism	Subperiosteal bone resorption commonly involves the superior margins of one or more ribs (most often unilateral).
Idiopathic	Rare cases of superior marginal rib defects have been reported in patients with no demonstrable underlying cause.

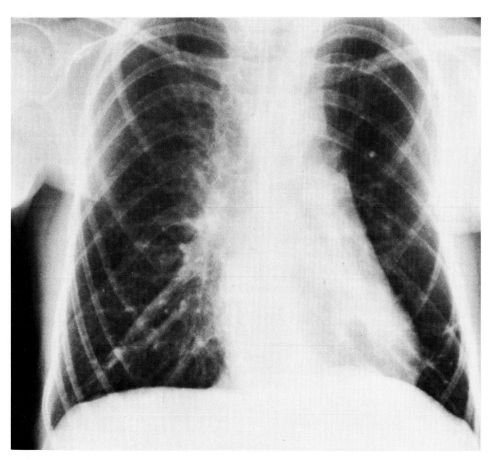

FIG B27-3. Marfan's syndrome. Pronounced generalized narrowing of the ribs with thinning of the cortices.

BONE-WITHIN-A-BONE APPEARANCE

Condition	Comments
Normal neonate **(Fig B28-1)**	Not uncommon appearance in infants 1 to 2 months of age caused by loss of bone density at the periphery of vertebral bodies (but with retention of their sharp cortical outlines). The bone subsequently assumes a normal density; thus this appearance probably reflects a normal stage in the transformation of the architecture of the neonatal vertebrae to that of later infancy.
Osteopetrosis **(Fig B28-2)**	Miniature inset in each lumbar vertebral body is a typical manifestation of this rare hereditary bone abnormality characterized by a symmetric generalized increase in bone density and lack of tubulation.
Thorotrast administration **(Fig B28-3)**	Radiographic densities of infantile vertebrae and pelvis (ghost vertebrae) in adult bones may be seen in adults who received intravenous Thorotrast during early childhood. The deposition of Thorotrast causes constant alpha radiation and temporary growth arrest so that the size of the ghost vertebrae corresponds to the vertebral size at the time of injection. Most patients also have reticular or dense opacification of the liver, spleen, and lymph nodes.
Transverse growth lines **(growth arrest lines)** **(Fig B28-4)**	Opaque transverse lines paralleling the superior and inferior margins of vertebral bodies. Underlying causes include chronic childhood diseases, malnutrition, and chemotherapy.

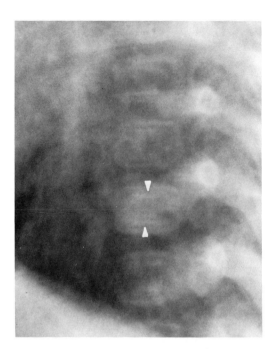

Fig B28-1. Normal neonate. The arrowheads point to one example of the bone-within-a-bone appearance.

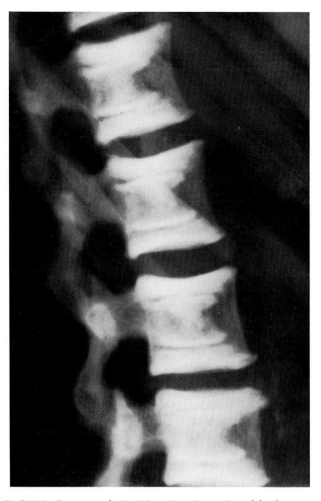

Fig B28-2. Osteopetrosis. A miniature inset is seen in each lumbar vertebral body, giving it a bone-within-a-bone appearance. There is also sclerosis at the end plates.[24]

Condition	Comments
Heavy metal poisoning	Radiodense lines paralleling the superior and inferior margins of multiple vertebral bodies are an infrequent manifestation of lead or phosphorus poisoning.
Gaucher's disease	Initial collapse of an entire vertebral body with subsequent growth recovery peripherally may be associated with horizontal and vertical sclerosis, giving the bone-within-a-bone appearance.
Paget's disease	May involve one or multiple vertebrae. More commonly produces enlarged, coarsened trabeculae with condensation of bone most prominent along the contours of a vertebral body (picture frame) or uniform increase in osseous density of an enlarged vertebral body (ivory vertebra).
Sickle cell anemia	Rare manifestation. More commonly generalized osteoporosis, localized steplike central depressions, and characteristic biconcave indentations on both the superior and inferior margins of softened vertebral bodies (fish vertebrae).
Hypervitaminosis D	The margins of the vertebral bodies are outlined by dense bands of bone that are exaggerated by adjacent radiolucent zones. The central, normal-appearing bone may simulate the bone-within-a-bone appearance.

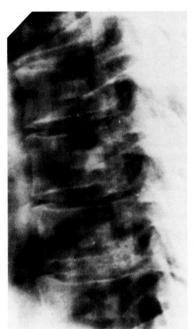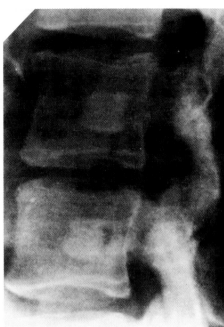

Fig B28-3. Thorotrast. Two examples of persistence of radiographic densities of infantile vertebrae in adult bones of patients who received intravenous Thorotrast during early childhood.[30]

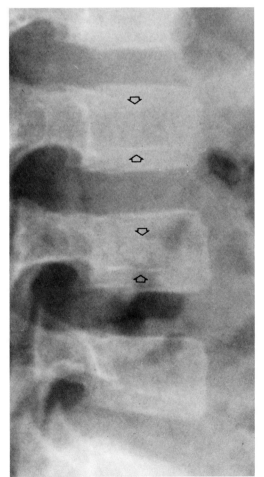

Fig B28-4. Transverse growth lines. Opaque lines paralleling the superior and inferior margins of the vertebral body in a child with severe chronic illness.

HEEL PAD THICKENING (> 22 MILLIMETERS)

Condition	Comments
Acromegaly **(Fig B29-1)**	An excess of pituitary growth hormone causes generalized overgrowth of all body tissues. Other characteristic findings include joint space widening (especially metacarpophalangeal and hip joints) due to proliferation of cartilage, overgrowth of the tips of the distal phalanges producing thick bony tufts with pointed lateral margins (square, spade-shaped hand), thickening of the calvarium with frontal bossing and enlargement of the paranasal sinuses, prognathous jaw (lengthening of the mandible and increased mandibular angle), and scalloping of the posterior aspect of vertebral bodies.
Normal variant	Apparent thickening of the heel pad without any underlying cause may be a normal variant, especially in Black males.
Obesity/high body weight	Although not directly proportional to body weight, heel pad thickening is common in people weighing more than 200 pounds.
Soft-tissue infection	Especially common in mycetoma (Madura foot), a chronic granulomatous fungal disease that affects the feet and is most prevalent in India. Pronounced soft-tissue swelling may be followed by bone destruction, deformity, and fistula formation.
Generalized edema	A manifestation of diffuse peripheral edema.
Myxedema/thyroid acropachy	Diffuse soft-tissue swelling of the hands and feet. In thyroid acropachy, a rare complication of hyperthyroid disease that develops after thyroidectomy or radioactive iodine treatment of primary hyperthyroidism, there is typically a generalized and symmetric spiculated periosteal reaction that primarily involves the midportion of the diaphyses of tubular bones of the hands and feet.
Dilantin therapy	The percentage of patients with abnormally thickened heel pads increases steadily with the length of treatment. Dilantin may also cause calvarial thickening that can be confused with acromegaly.
Trauma	Edema and bleeding in soft tissues. An associated fracture of the calcaneus may occur.

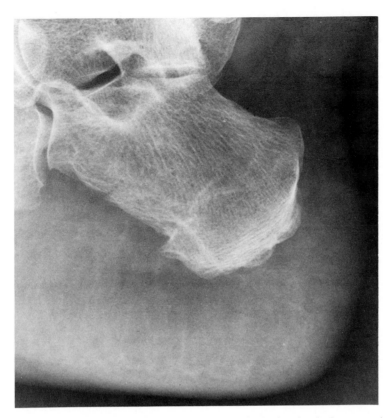

Fɪɢ **B29-1. Acromegaly.** Prominent thickening of the heel pad, which measured 32 mm on the original radiograph.

PSEUDOARTHROSIS

Condition	Comments
Neurofibromatosis **(Fig B30-1)**	Characteristic complication reflecting a fracture that failed to heal. Usually involves the junction of the middle and lower thirds of the tibia or fibula (or both) during the first year of life. Anterior bowing of the leg and severe disuse osteoporosis are typical findings. An abnormally formed, deficient, or gracile fibula is a frequent accompaniment of pseudoarthrosis of the tibia.
Nonunion of a fracture **(Fig B30-2)**	A false joint may form at the fracture site, with one fragment presenting a convex surface that fits into the concave surface of the apposing fragment.
Osteogenesis imperfecta **(see Fig B2-9)**	Inherited generalized disorder of connective tissue that causes osteoporosis with abnormal fragility of the skeleton and an unusual tendency for fractures. Although fracture healing is often normal, exuberant callus formation and bizarre deformities (including pseudoarthrosis) may occur.
Fibrous dysplasia	Proliferation of fibrous tissue in the medullary cavity causes local expansion of bone and cortical erosion from within, predisposing to pathologic fractures that may lead to pseudoarthrosis. In severe and long-standing disease, affected bones may be bowed or deformed (eg, shepherd's crook deformity of the femur).
Congenital pseudoarthrosis	Rare condition that is generally unilateral, primarily involves the tibia, and develops during the first or second year of life. Initially, there is anterior bowing of the lower half of the tibia with sclerosis, narrowing of the medullary canal, and cystic abnormalities at the apex of the curve indicating impending fracture and pseudoarthrosis. Once the fracture appears, the margins of adjacent bone become increasingly tapered. After bone grafting, healing may be expected in about 30% of patients. Congenital pseudoarthrosis of the clavicle occurs almost exclusively on the right (bilateral in 10% of patients) and presents within the first few months of life as a painless lump over the medial third of the clavicle. Radiographs show the medial end of the clavicle superior to the lateral end, osseous discontinuity, and the absence of callus formation (absence of pain and visible callus permits differentiation from posttraumatic pseudoarthrosis).

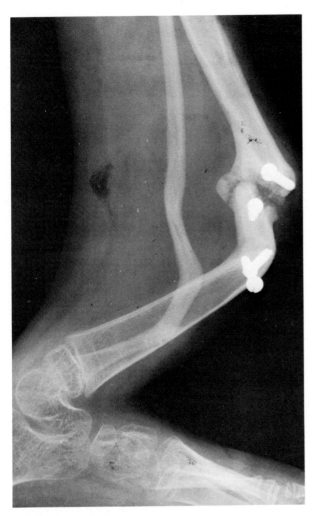

FIG B30-1. Neurofibromatosis. A false joint of the midshaft of the tibia has developed after trauma. Note the severe disuse osteoporosis of the bones of the ankle and the ribbonlike shape of the lower fibula.

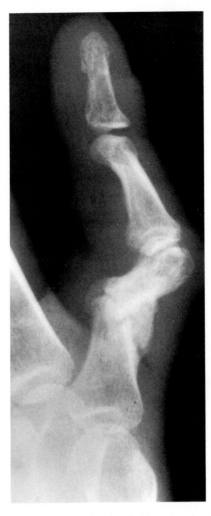

FIG B30-2. Posttraumatic pseudoarthrosis. Nonunion about a fracture of the proximal phalanx of the fifth digit. Although there is extensive callus formation, the lucent fracture line can still be clearly seen.

PROTRUSIO ACETABULI*

Condition	Comments
Normal variant	A normal phenomenon in children (4 to 12 years of age) that does not reflect any acetabular abnormality.
Rheumatoid arthritis	Common manifestation of severe rheumatoid hip disease. There is diffuse loss of the interosseous space and an eroded and often diminutive femoral head.
Rheumatoid variants	Ankylosing spondylitis; psoriatic arthritis; Reiter's syndrome; inflammatory bowel disease.
Acquired softening of bone	Paget's disease; osteomalacia or rickets; hyperparathyroidism. Rare manifestation of osteoporosis.
Osteoarthritis	Usually a mild degree of protrusion that is typically associated with medial migration of the femoral head. May be primary or secondary to hemophilia, pseudogout, hemochromatosis, or ochronosis.
Posttraumatic	May develop after an acetabular fracture with medial dislocation of the hip or after total hip replacement arthroplasty with marked thinning of the available acetabular roof.
Osteogenesis imperfecta	Caused by the osteoporotic and abnormally fragile bone in this inherited disorder of connective tissue.
Primary acetabular protrusion (Otto pelvis) (Fig B31-2)	Usually bilateral and much more frequent in women. Associated loss of the joint space usually results in axial or medial migration of the femoral head with respect to the acetabulum. Although the etiology is unknown, postulated causes include failure of ossification or premature fusion of the Y cartilage or a direct consequence of normal stress on the Y cartilage (normally, the protrusion is reversible due to diminished stress after age 8; failure of correction of the protrusio resulting in its persistence into adult life may be due to premature fusion and coxa vera).
Miscellaneous causes	Destruction of the acetabulum resulting from septic arthritis, neoplasm, or radiation therapy.

*Pattern: Projection of the acetabular line (the medial wall of the acetabulum) medial to the ilioischial line (a portion of the quadrilateral surface) by 3 mm or more in adult men and by 6 mm or more in adult women (Fig B31-1).

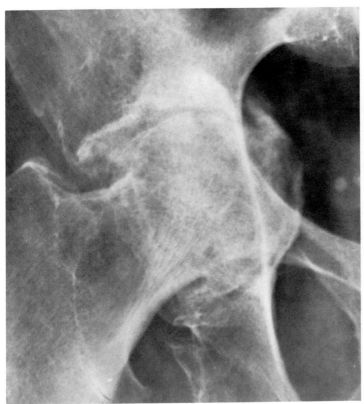
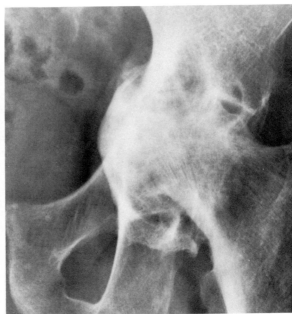

Fɪɢ B31-1. **Protrusio acetabuli.** Two typical examples.

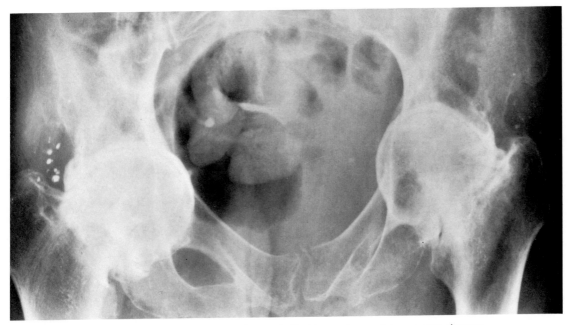

Fɪɢ B31-2. **Otto pelvis.** Bilaterally symmetric protrusio acetabuli with superimposed degenerative changes.

DACTYLITIS*

Condition	Comments
Sickle cell anemia **(hand-foot syndrome)** **(Fig B32-1)**	The small bones of the hands and feet are the most common site of infarction in children. The peak incidence is between 6 and 24 months of age (children less than 6 months may still have the protection of their fetal hemoglobin). Differentiation from osteomyelitis is difficult both clinically and radiographically, though the lack of systemic symptoms and fever suggests infarction without osteomyelitis).
Pyogenic osteomyelitis	Most commonly represents *Salmonella* infection in a child with sickle cell anemia. Usually involves several bones in each hand. May be extremely difficult to differentiate from the hand-foot syndrome in this condition.
Tuberculosis **("spina ventosa")** **(Fig B32-2)**	Most often occurs in children, in whom it may be multiple. Sequestrum formation is uncommon, though it may be associated with small sinus tracts through which bony fragments may be extruded.
Leprosy	Most frequently produces acro-osteolysis. More destructive lesions may lead to neuroarthropathy and a classic "licked candy stick" appearance and progress to a virtually fingerless hand.
Other infections **(Figs B32-3 and B32-4)**	Yaws; syphilis; smallpox; atypical mycobacteria; fungal disease.
Sarcoidosis **(Fig B32-5)**	About 15% of patients have bone involvement, predominantly in the middle and distal phalanges of the hand. Usually associated with characteristic hilar and paratracheal adenopathy, interstitial pulmonary disease, or both.
Leukemia	Leukemic changes are generally more diffuse than in osteomyelitis or sickle cell anemia, though the radiographic differentiation may be difficult.

*Pattern: Soft-tissue swelling, periosteal reaction, and variable degrees of bone destruction and expansion involving one or multiple bones of the hands or feet or both.

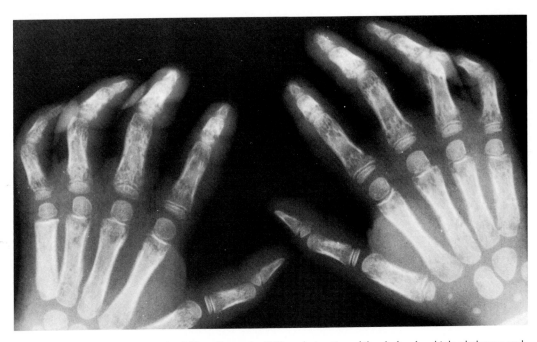

FIG B32-1. Hand-foot syndrome in sickle cell anemia. Diffuse destruction of the shafts of multiple phalanges and metacarpals is due to infarction. There are reactive bone changes with sclerosis and periosteal thickening.

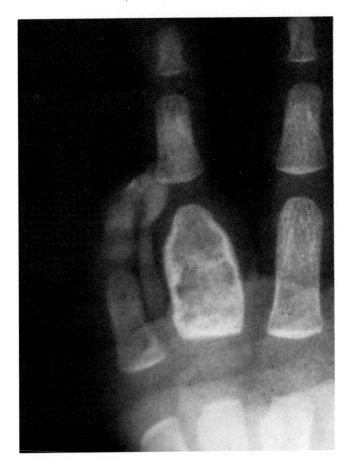

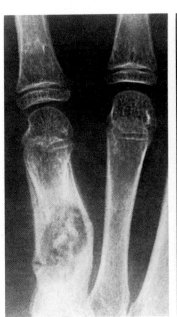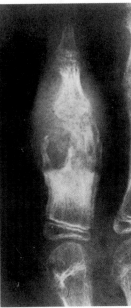

FIG B32-3. Yaws. Examples of cortical and medullary granulomas along with intense periosteal new bone formation.[8]

FIG B32-2. Tuberculosis. Typical expansion of a phalanx along with irregular destruction of bone architecture. Note the absence of periosteal reaction, which differentiates the appearance from that of syphilitic dactylitis.[31]

Condition	Comments
Tuberous sclerosis (Fig B32-6)	Characteristic abnormalities in the hands and feet are wavy periosteal new bone formation along the shafts of the metatarsals and metacarpals and cystlike changes in the phalanges.
Pancreatic fat necrosis	Infrequent manifestation that probably results from elevated levels of lipase during the acute phase of the disease. In children, the lesions must be distinguished from those caused by infection or sickle cell dactylitis.

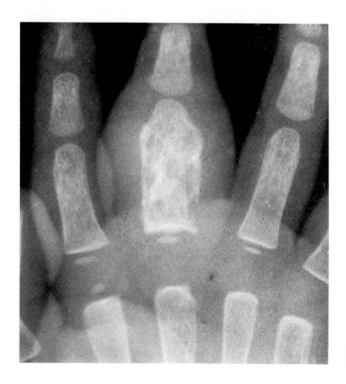

FIG B32-4. **Congenital syphilis.** Typical destructive expansion of a phalanx with periosteal calcification forming a dense shell around the lesion.

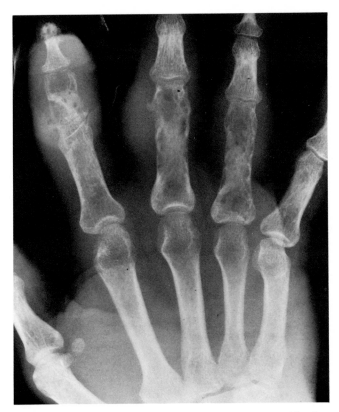

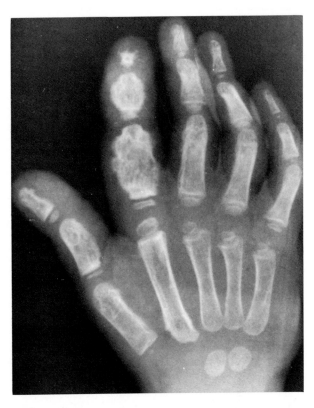

FIG B32-5. Sarcoidosis. Destructive changes involving the middle phalanx of the second finger, with soft-tissue swelling about the third proximal interphalangeal joint and cortical thinning and a lacelike trabecular pattern affecting the proximal phalanges of the third and fourth digits.

FIG B32-6. Tuberous sclerosis. Cystlike expansion and characteristic wavy periosteal new bone formation about the proximal and middle phalanges of the second digit. Periosteal new bone formation is also seen along the shaft of the second metacarpal.

SOURCES

1. Reprinted with permission from "Bone Changes Following Electrical Injury" by LB Brinn and JE Moseley, *American Journal of Roentgenology* (1966;97:682–686), Copyright © 1966, Williams & Wilkins Company.

2. Reprinted with permission from "Radiologic Diagnosis of Metabolic Bone Disease" by WA Reynolds and JJ Karo, *Orthopedic Clinics of North America* (1972;3:521–532), Copyright © 1972, WB Saunders Company.

3. Reprinted with permission from "Radiologic Findings in Niemann-Pick Disease" by R Lachman et al, *Radiology* (1973;108:659–664), Copyright © 1973, Radiological Society of North America Inc.

4. Reprinted with permission from "The Radiologic Assessment of Short Stature" by JP Dorst, CI Scott, and JG Hall, *Radiologic Clinics of North America* (1972;10:393–414), Copyright © 1972, WB Saunders Company.

5. Reprinted with permission from "Skeletal Changes in Wilson's Disease" by R Mindelzun et al, *Radiology* (1970;94:127–132), Copyright © 1970, Radiological Society of North America Inc.

6. Reprinted with permission from "Brodie's Abscess: Reappraisal" by WB Miller, WA Murphy, and LA Gilula, *Radiology* (1979;132:15–23), Copyright © 1979, Radiological Society of North America Inc.

7. Reprinted with permission from "Tumoural Gummatous Yaws" by WB Cockshott and AGM Davies, *Journal of Bone and Joint Surgery* (1960; 42B:785–791), Copyright © 1960, Journal of Bone and Joint Surgery Inc.

8. Reprinted from *Clinical Radiology in the Tropics* by WP Cockshott and H Middlemiss (Eds) with permission of Churchill Livingstone Inc, © 1979.

9. Reprinted with permission from "The Many Facets of Multiple Myeloma" by WT Meszaros, *Seminars in Roentgenology* (1974;9:219–228), Copyright © 1974, Grune & Stratton Inc.

10. Reprinted with permission from "The 'Fallen Fragment Sign' in the Diagnosis of Unicameral Bone Cysts" by J Reynolds, *Radiology* (1969;92: 949–953), Copyright © 1969, Radiological Society of North America Inc.

11. Reprinted from *Roentgen Diagnosis of Diseases of Bone* by J Edeiken with permission of Williams & Wilkins Company, © 1981.

12. Reprinted with permission from "Classic and Contemporary Imaging of Coccidioidomycosis" by JP McGahan et al, *American Journal of Roentgenology* (1981;136:393–404), Copyright © 1981, Williams & Wilkins Company.

13. Reprinted with permission from "Skeletal Changes in Hemophilia and Other Bleeding Disorders" by DJ Stoker and RO Murray, *Seminars in Roentgenology* (1974;9:185–193), Copyright © 1974, Grune & Stratton Inc.

14. Reprinted from *The Radiology of Joint Disease* by DM Forrester, JC Brown, and JW Nesson with permission of WB Saunders Company, © 1978.

15. Reprinted with permission from "Ulcer Osteoma: Bone Response to Tropical Ulcer" by TM Kolawole and SP Bohrer, *American Journal of Roentgenology* (1970;109: 611–618), Copyright © 1970, Williams & Wilkins Company.

16. Reprinted with permission from "Chronic Poisoning Due to Excess of Vitamin A" by J Caffey, *Pediatrics* (1950;5:672–688), Copyright © 1950, American Academy of Pediatrics.

17. Reprinted with permission from "Congenital Hyperurecosuria" by MH Becker and JK Wallin, *Radiologic Clinics of North America* (1968; 6:239–243), Copyright © 1968, WB Saunders Company.

18. Reprinted with permission from "Epidermolysis Bullosa with Characteristic Hand Deformities" by LB Brinn and MT Khilnani, *Radiology* (1967;89:272–277), Copyright © 1967, Radiological Society of North America Inc.

19. Reprinted with permission from "Progeria" by FR Margolin and HL Steinbach, *American Journal of Roentgenology* (1968;103:173–178), Copyright © 1968, Williams & Wilkins Company.

20. Reprinted from *Diagnostic Imaging in Internal Medicine* by RL Eisenberg with permission of McGraw-Hill Book Company, © 1985. Courtesy of Robert R Jacobson, Pearl Mills, and Tanya Thomassie.

21. Reprinted with permission from "Calcium Deposition Diseases" by MK Dalinka, AJ Reginato, and DA Golden, *Seminars in Roentgenology* (1982;17:39–48), Copyright © 1982, Grune & Stratton Inc.

22. Reprinted with permission from "Tumoral Calcinosis with Sedimentation Sign" by I Hug and J Guncaga, *British Journal of Radiology* (1974; 47:734–736), Copyright © 1974, British Institute of Radiology.

23. Reprinted with permission from "Tumors of the Soft Tissues of the Extremities" by RC Cavanagh, *Seminars in Roentgenology* (1973; 8:83–89), Copyright © 1973, Grune & Stratton Inc.

24. Reprinted from *Radiology of Bone Diseases* by GB Greenfield, JB Lippincott Company, with permission of the author, © 1986.

25. Reprinted with permission from "The Roentgenographic Manifestations of the Rubella Syndrome in Newborn Infants" by EB Singleton et al, *American Journal of Roentgenology* (1966;97:82–91), Copyright © 1966, Williams & Wilkins Company.

26. Reprinted with permission from "Gaucher's Disease" by B Levin, *American Journal of Roentgenology* (1961;85:685–696), Copyright © 1961, Williams & Wilkins Company.

27. Reprinted with permission from "Familial Metaphyseal Dysplasia" by MB Hermel, J Gershon-Cohen, and DT Jones, *American Journal of Roentgenology* (1953;70:413–421), Copyright © 1953, Williams & Wilkins Company.

28. Reprinted with permission from "Skeletal Changes in the Anemias" by JE Moseley, *Seminars in Roentgenology* (1974;9:169–184), Copyright © 1974, Grune & Stratton Inc.

29. Reprinted from *Plain Film Interpretation in Congenital Heart Disease* by LE Swischuk with permission of Williams & Wilkins Company, © 1979.

30. Reprinted with permission from "Ghost Infantile Vertebrae and Hemipelves within Adult Skeletons from Thorotrast Administration in Childhood" by JG Teplick et al, *Radiology* (1978;129:657–660), Copyright © 1978, Radiological Society of North America Inc.

31. Reprinted with permission from "Tuberculosis of the Bones and Joints" by M Chapman, RO Murray, and BJ Stoker, *Seminars in Roentgenology* (1979;14:266–282), Copyright © 1979, Grune & Stratton Inc.

Spine Patterns

6

SP1   Cystlike lesion of a vertebral body or
       posterior elements   **726**

SP2   Increase in size of one or more vertebrae   **730**

SP3   Loss of height of one or more vertebral
       bodies   **732**

SP4   Narrowing of intervertebral disk space
       and adjacent sclerosis   **740**

SP5   Localized widening of interpedicular
       distance   **742**

SP6   Anterior scalloping of a vertebral body   **744**

SP7   Posterior scalloping of a vertebral body   **744**

SP8   Squaring of one or more vertebral bodies   **748**

SP9   Enlarged cervical intervertebral foramen   **750**

SP10 Atlantoaxial subluxation   **752**

SP11 Calcification of intervertebral disks   **754**

SP12 Beaked, notched, or hooked vertebrae in
       a child   **758**

SP13 Intramedullary lesion on myelography
       (widening of the spinal cord)   **762**

SP14 Intradural, extramedullary lesion on
       myelography   **766**

SP15 Extradural lesion on myelography   **770**

Sources   **774**

CYSTLIKE LESION OF A VERTEBRAL BODY
OR POSTERIOR ELEMENTS

Condition	Imaging Findings	Comments
Osteoblastoma (Figs SP1-1 and SP1-2)	Expansile lucent (or opaque) lesion that grows rapidly, readily breaking through the cortex and producing a sharply defined soft-tissue component that is often circumscribed by a thin calcific shell.	Rare bone neoplasm that involves the vertebral column (most frequently the neural arches and spinous processes) in about half of patients. Most frequently occurs in the second decade and produces a dull aching pain, tenderness, and soft-tissue swelling. May contain some internal calcification.
Hemangioma (Fig SP1-3)	Demineralized and occasionally expanded vertebral body with characteristic multiple coarse linear striations running vertically.	Benign, slow-growing tumor composed of vascular channels. Usually asymptomatic and identified in middle-aged patients. The coarse vertical trabecular pattern may extend into the pedicles and laminae. Soft-tissue and intraspinal extension of the tumor or secondary hemorrhage can produce a paraspinal mass.
Aneurysmal bone cyst (Fig SP1-4)	Expansile, trabeculated, lucent lesion that primarily involves the posterior elements. There may be extension into or primary involvement of a vertebral body.	Consists of numerous blood-filled arteriovenous communications, rather than being a true neoplasm. Most frequently occurs in children and young adults and presents as mild pain of several months' duration, swelling, and restriction of movement. May cross a vertebral interspace and involve adjacent vertebrae.
Giant cell tumor (Fig SP1-5)	Slowly growing lucent lesion that often has ill-defined margins and may progress to vertebral collapse.	Most giant cell tumors of the spine occur in the sacrum, where the tumor has an expansile appearance.
Chordoma (see Figs SK9-4 and SK10-4)	Bulky mass causing ill-defined bone destruction or cortical expansion. Flocculent calcifications may develop in a large soft-tissue mass.	Arises from remnants of the notocord and primarily involves the sacrococcygeal region (50%) and clivus (30%). The remainder of the tumors occur elsewhere in the spine. Locally invasive, but does not metastasize.
Fibrous dysplasia	Expansile lesion with a ground-glass or purely lytic appearance.	Infrequent manifestation. Vertebral collapse or a posteriorly expanding fibrous-tissue mass can result in cord compression.
Hydatid (echinococcal) cyst	Single or multiple expansile lytic lesions containing trabeculae. May be associated with cortical erosion and a soft-tissue mass.	Bone involvement occurs in about 1% of patients and most commonly affects the vertebral bodies, pelvis, and sacrum. Infiltration of daughter cysts into the bone produces a multiloculated appearance that resembles a bunch of grapes. Rupture into the spinal canal may produce neurologic abnormalities, including paraplegia.

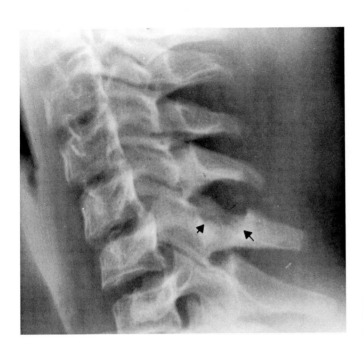

Fig SP1-1. Osteoblastoma of the cervical spine. Sharply defined, erosive lesion (arrows) involves the superior margin of a lower cervical spinous process.

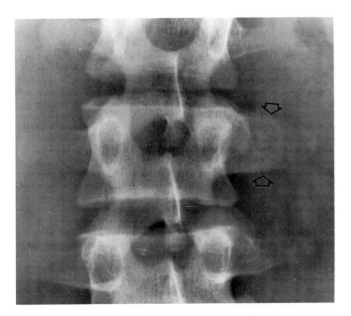

Fig SP1-2. Osteoblastoma of the lumbar spine. Well-circumscribed, expansile lesion (arrows) involves the left transverse process of a midlumbar vertebra.

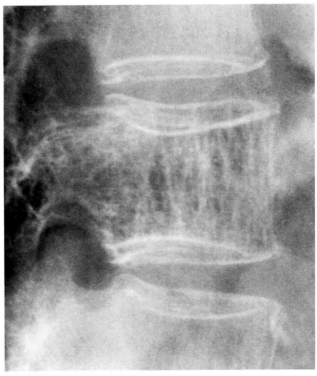

Fig SP1-3. Hemangioma of a vertebral body. Multiple coarse, linear striations run vertically in the demineralized vertebral body.

Condition	Imaging Findings	Comments
Metastases	Lytic destructive process.	Expansile lesions may occur with melanoma and carcinomas of the kidney or thyroid.
Plasmacytoma	Multicystic expansile lesion with thickened trabeculae. Primarily involves the vertebral body.	Involved vertebral body may collapse and disappear completely or the lesion may extend across the intervertebral disk to invade the adjacent vertebral body (simulating infection). Multiple myeloma causes generalized decreased bone density and destructive changes involving multiple vertebral bodies and often results in multiple vertebral compression fractures (see Fig SP3-2).

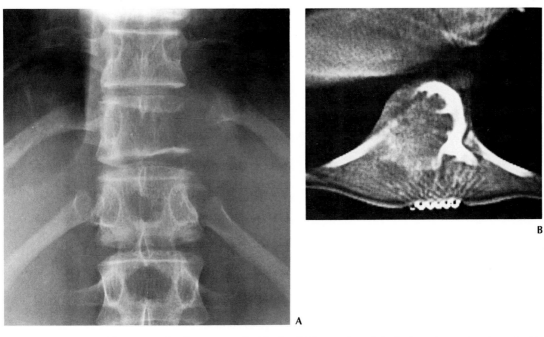

FIG SP1-4. **Aneurysmal bone cyst** of a thoracic vertebral body. (A) Destruction of the body and posterior elements. No peripheral shell of bone can be recognized. (B) CT scan shows irregular destruction suggesting a malignant process.[1]

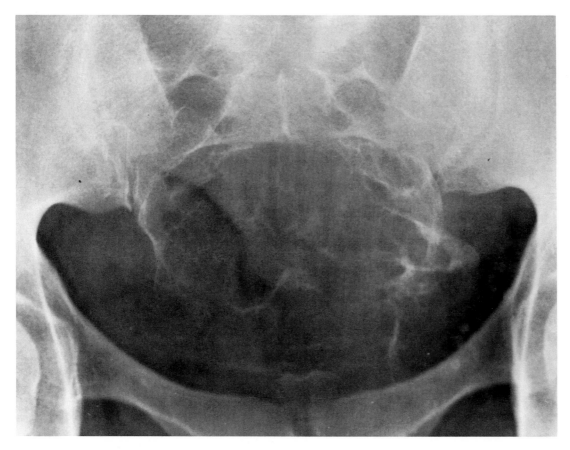

FIG SP1-5. **Giant cell tumor** of the sacrum. Huge expansile lesion.

INCREASE IN SIZE OF ONE OR MORE VERTEBRAE

Condition	Comments
Acromegaly **(Fig SP2-1)**	Appositional bone growth results in a generalized increase in the size of the vertebral bodies. Hypertrophy of cartilage widens the intervertebral disk spaces, while hypertrophy of soft tissue may lead to an increased concavity (scalloping) of the posterior aspects of the vertebral bodies.
Paget's disease **(Fig SP2-2)**	Generalized enlargement of affected vertebral bodies. Increased trabeculation, which is most prominent at the periphery of the bone, produces a rim of thickened cortex and a picture-frame appearance. Dense sclerosis of one or more vertebral bodies (ivory vertebrae) may present a pattern simulating osteoblastic metastases or Hodgkin's disease, though in Paget's disease the vertebrae are also enlarged.
Congenital **(Fig SP2-3)**	Fusion or partial fusion of two or more vertebral bodies (block vertebra) is a frequent occurrence. The underlying bone is otherwise normal. Congenital fusion can usually be differentiated from that resulting from disease because the total height of the combined fused bodies is equal to the normal height of two vertebrae less the intervertebral disk space.
Neuromuscular deficit	Increased height of the vertebral bodies related to the absence of normal vertical stress may develop in patients who cannot bear weight (eg, paralysis, Down's syndrome, rubella syndrome).
Benign bone tumor	Expansion of a vertebral body may result from hemangioma, aneurysmal bone cyst, osteoblastoma, or giant cell tumor.
Fibrous dysplasia	Proliferation of fibrous tissue in the medullary cavity may infrequently involve the spine and cause one or more vertebral bodies to expand. Complications include vertebral collapse and spinal cord compression.

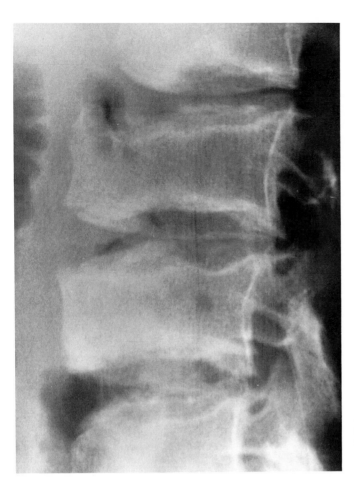

Fig SP2-1. Acromegaly. Enlargement of all vertebral bodies, especially in the anteroposterior direction. Note the mild posterior scalloping.

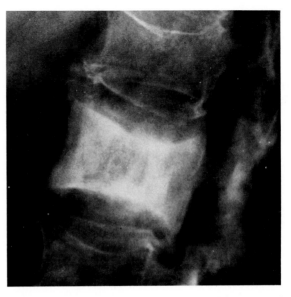

Fig SP2-2. Paget's disease. Enlargement and cortical thickening of a vertebral body, producing an ivory vertebra.[2]

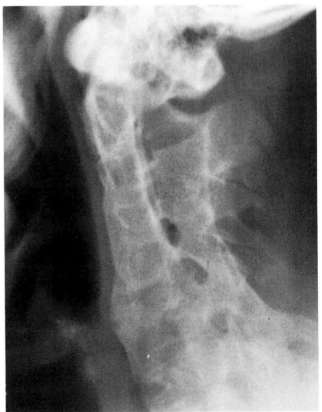

Fig SP2-3. Block vertebrae. Essentially complete fusion of the cervical spine into a solid mass in a patient with Klippel-Feil deformity.

LOSS OF HEIGHT OF ONE OR MORE VERTEBRAL BODIES

Condition	Imaging Findings	Comments
Osteoporosis **(Fig SP3-1)**	Smooth, archlike indentations of the vertebral end plates that are most marked centrally in the region of the nucleus pulposus. Primarily involves the lumbar and lower thoracic spine (where weight-bearing stress is directed toward the axes of the vertebral bodies).	Regardless of the cause (most commonly senile or postmenopausal osteoporosis, steroid therapy), as the bone density of the vertebral body decreases the cortex appears as a thin line that is relatively dense and prominent, producing a picture-frame pattern. In addition to the typical ''fish vertebrae'' appearance, osteoporotic vertebral bodies may demonstrate anterior wedging and compression fractures. The characteristic concave contours of the superior and inferior disk surfaces result from expansion of the nucleus pulposus into the weakened vertebral bodies.
Hyperparathyroidism	Generalized demineralization of the vertebral bodies produces archlike contour defects of the superior and inferior vertebral surfaces, simulating osteoporosis.	Subchondral resorption at the discovertebral junctions produces areas of structural weakening that allow herniation of disk material into the vertebral body (cartilaginous or Schmorl's nodes). In patients with hyperparathyroidism secondary to renal failure, thick bands of increased density adjacent to the superior and inferior margins of vertebral bodies produce the characteristic ''rugger jersey'' spine.
Osteomalacia	Archlike contour defects of the superior and inferior surfaces of multiple vertebral bodies, simulating osteoporosis.	Insufficient mineralization of the vertebral bodies. In osteomalacia secondary to renal tubular disorders, hyperostosis may be more prominent than deossification. This results in a striking thickening of the cortices and increased trabeculation of spongy bone. Nevertheless, the bony architecture is abnormal and is prone to fracture with relatively minimal trauma.
Multiple myeloma **(Fig SP3-2)**	Generalized skeletal deossification simulating osteoporosis or destructive changes mimicking metastases. Severe loss of bone substance in the spine often results in multiple vertebral compression fractures.	Decreased bone density and destructive changes are usually limited to the vertebral bodies, sparing the pedicles (lacking red marrow) that are frequently destroyed by metastatic disease. Because multiple myeloma causes little or no stimulation of new bone formation, radionuclide bone scans may be normal even with extensive skeletal infiltration.
Metastases	Destructive process involving not only the vertebral bodies but also the pedicles and neural arches. Pathologic collapse of vertebral bodies frequently occurs in advanced disease.	Destruction of one or more pedicles may be the earliest sign of metastatic disease and aids in differentiating this process from multiple myeloma (pedicles are much less often involved). Because cartilage is resistant to invasion by metastases, preservation of the intervertebral disk space may help to distinguish metastases from an inflammatory process.

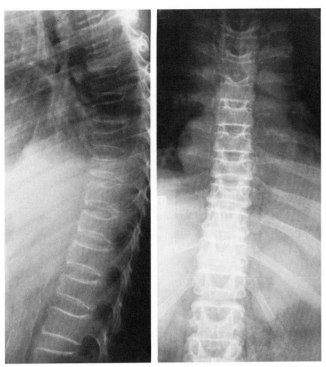

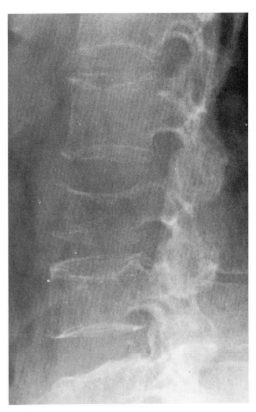

FIG SP3-1. Severe osteoporosis. (A) Lateral and (B) frontal views of the thoracolumbar spine show striking demineralization and compression of multiple vertebral bodies in a 14½-year-old girl treated with steroids for 5 years for chronic glomerulonephritis. The height age of the girl was only 9 years at this time.[3]

FIG SP3-2. Multiple myeloma. Diffuse myelomatous infiltration causes generalized demineralization of the vertebral bodies and a compression fracture of L2.

A

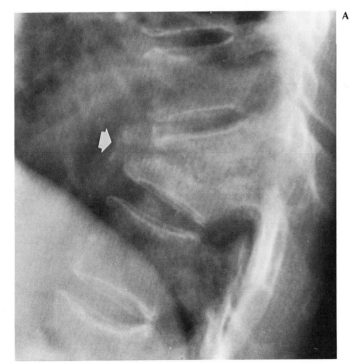

B

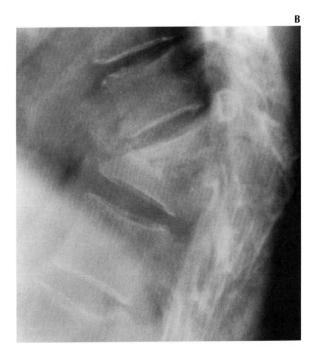

FIG SP3-3. Tuberculous osteomyelitis of the thoracic spine. (A) Initial film demonstrates vertebral collapse and anterior wedging of adjacent midthoracic vertebrae (arrow). The residual intervertebral disk space can barely be seen. (B) Several months later there is virtual fusion of the collapsed vertebral bodies, producing a characteristic sharp kyphotic angulation (gibbous deformity).

Condition	Imaging Findings	Comments
Osteomyelitis **Pyogenic**	Various radiographic patterns including disk space narrowing, loss of the normally sharp adjacent subchondral plates, areas of cortical demineralization, vertebral body destruction and even collapse, and sclerotic new bone formation.	Rapid involvement of the intervertebral disks (loss of disk spaces and destruction of adjacent end plates), in contrast to the vertebral body involvement and preservation of disk spaces in metastatic disease.
Tuberculous **(Fig SP3-3)**	Irregular, poorly marginated bone destruction in a vertebral body, with narrowing of the adjacent intervertebral disk and extension of infection and bone destruction across the disk to involve the contiguous vertebral body.	Most commonly involves the anterior part of vertebral bodies in the thoracic and lumbar region. Often associated with a paravertebral abscess, an accumulation of purulent material that produces a soft-tissue mass about the vertebra. Unlike pyogenic infection, tuberculous osteomyelitis is rarely associated with periosteal reaction or bone sclerosis. In the untreated patient, progressive vertebral collapse and anterior wedging lead to the development of a characteristic sharp kyphotic angulation and gibbous deformity. Healed lesions may demonstrate mottled calcific deposits in a paravertebral abscess and moderate recalcification and sclerosis of the affected bones.
Brucellosis **(Fig SP3-4)**	In the less common central type of vertebral lesion, lytic destruction of the vertebral body leads to vertebral collapse with various degrees of wedging and often the development of a paraspinal abscess (overall pattern closely simulates that of tuberculous infection).	Primarily a disease of animals (cattle, swine, goats, sheep) that is transmitted to humans by the ingestion of infected dairy products or meat or through direct contact with animals, their carcasses, or their excreta. In the more common peripheral form, loss of cortical definition or frank erosions of the anterior and superior margins of the vertebral bodies and disk space narrowing is followed by reactive sclerosis and hypertrophic spur formation.
Fungal infections	Generally produce spinal involvement mimicking tuberculosis.	Infrequent manifestation of actinomycosis, blastomycosis, coccidioidomycosis, cryptococcosis, or aspergillosis. The diagnosis depends on biopsy and culture of the organism.
Fractures **(Fig SP3-5)**	Primarily anterior wedging of the superior end plate of a vertebral body. Severe compressive forces may drive the nucleus pulposus into the vertebral body, resulting in a burst fracture with the posterosuperior fragment often driven into the spinal canal. In patients who have jumped from great heights, compression fractures of the thoracolumbar junction are frequently associated with a fracture of the calcaneus.	Primarily involve the T11 to L4 region. In older patients it may be difficult to distinguish an acute spinal fracture from the vertebral compression that is frequently associated with osteoporosis. In acute trauma there is often evidence of cortical disruption, a paraspinal soft-tissue mass, or an ill-defined increase in density beneath the end plate of an involved vertebra, indicating bone impaction. In osteoporosis, vertebral compression is often associated with osteophytic spurs arising from the apposing margins of the involved and adjacent vertebral bodies. An acute spinal fracture may be difficult to distinguish from a pathologic fracture caused by metastases or multiple myeloma (the presence of bone destruction, especially involving the cortex, indicates a pathologic fracture).

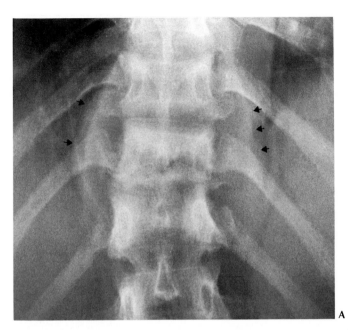

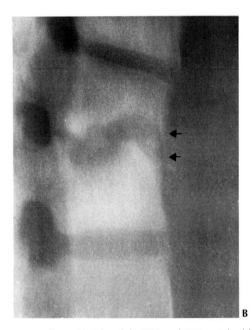

FIG SP3-4. Brucellosis. (A) Frontal plain film of the lower thoracic spine demonstrates loss of height of the T11 and T12 vertebral bodies with destruction of end plates and swelling of the paravertebral soft tissues (arrows). (B) A lateral tomogram of the lower thoracic spine demonstrates cortical destruction with sclerosis of the inferior end plate of T11 and the superior end plate of T12. There is a mild degree of anterior wedging. The overall radiographic appearance is indistinguishable from that of tuberculous spondylitis.

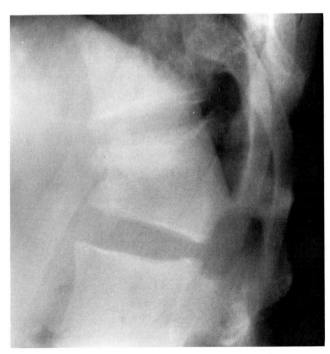

FIG SP3-5. Fracture. Characteristic anterior wedging of the superior end plate of the L1 vertebral body.

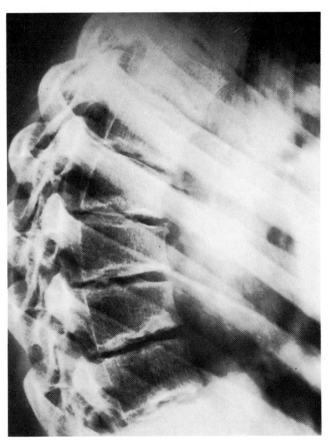

FIG SP3-6. Scheuermann's disease. Irregularity of the vertebral end plates and wedging of the vertebral bodies, which causes an arcuate kyphosis.[4]

Condition	Imaging Findings	Comments
Scheuermann's disease (vertebral epiphysitis) (Fig SP3-6)	Irregularity and loss of the sharp outline of the ringlike epiphyses along the upper and lower margins of vertebral bodies that is followed by fragmentation and sclerosis, causing the adjacent border of the vertebral body to become irregular. The affected vertebrae tend to become wedge-shaped (they decrease in height anteriorly).	Occurs in both sexes between the ages of 12 and 17. Although the cause of this familial condition is unclear, possible contributing factors include circulatory disturbances, early disk degeneration, and faulty ossification. Wedging of vertebral bodies produces a dorsal kyphosis, which persists even after the disease has healed.
Eosinophilic granuloma (Fig SP3-7)	Spotty destruction in a vertebral body that proceeds to collapse. The vertebra assumes the shape of a thin flat disk (vertebrae plana).	Most commonly occurs in children under age 10. The intervertebral disk spaces are preserved.
Morquio's syndrome (Fig SP3-8)	Universal flattening of vertebral bodies (vertebrae plana).	Characteristic central anterior beaking in this form of mucopolysaccharidosis.
Spondyloepiphyseal dysplasia (Fig SP3-9)	Generalized flattening of lumbar vertebral bodies, often with a distinctive hump-shaped mound of bone on their superior and inferior surfaces.	Rare hereditary dwarfism that affects both the extremities and the vertebrae. Characteristic findings include flattening of the femoral capital epiphyses with early degenerative changes, a small pelvis, and a general delay in ossification of the skeleton.
Paget's disease	Archlike contour defects of the superior and inferior vertebral surfaces or a pathologic fracture.	Although there is typically enlargement of the vertebral body with increased trabeculation that is most prominent at the periphery, the weakened bone permits expansion of the nucleus pulposus and results in an increased incidence of pathologic fracture.
Sickle cell anemia (Fig SP3-10)	Localized steplike central depression of multiple vertebral end plates. There may also be biconcave indentations on the superior and inferior margins of the softened vertebral bodies due to expansile pressure of the adjacent intervertebral disks.	Probably caused by circulatory stasis and ischemia, which retard growth in the central portion of the vertebral cartilaginous growth plate while the periphery of the growth plate (with a different blood supply) continues to grow at a more normal rate.
Gaucher's disease	Localized steplike central depression of multiple vertebral end plates.	Probably caused by circulatory stasis and ischemia, which retard growth in the central portion of the vertebral cartilaginous growth plate while the periphery of the growth plate (with a different blood supply) continues to grow at a more normal rate. This inborn error of metabolism is characterized by the accumulation of abnormal quantities of complex lipids in the reticuloendothelial cells of the spleen, liver, and bone marrow.
Primary bone neoplasm	Various patterns of bone destruction and pathologic fracture.	Benign tumor (hemangioma, giant cell tumor, aneurysmal bone cyst); lymphoma; sarcoma; chordoma (sacrum).

A

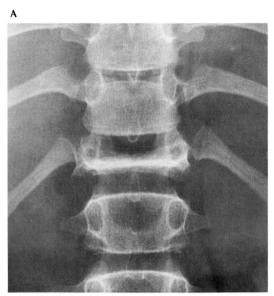

B

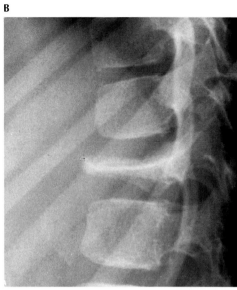

FIG SP3-7. Eosinophilic granuloma. (A) Frontal and (B) lateral views of the spine show complete collapse with flattening of the T12 vertebral body (vertebra plana).

FIG SP3-8. Morquio's syndrome. Generalized flattening of vertebral bodies in the (A) cervical and (B) lumbar regions.

A

B

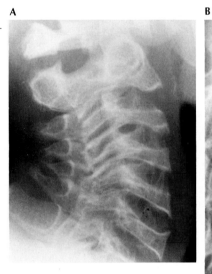

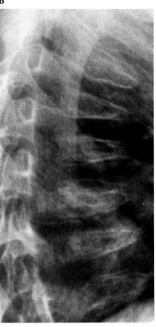

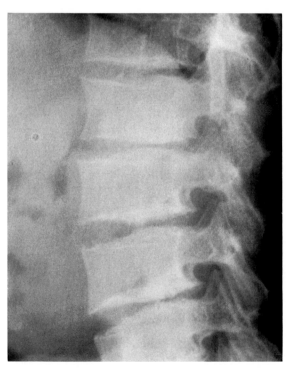

FIG SP3-9. Spondyloepiphyseal dysplasia. Generalized flattening of vertebral bodies (platyspondyly).

Condition	Imaging Findings	Comments
Osteogenesis imperfecta (Fig SP3-11)	Flattening of vertebral bodies, which are either biconcave or wedge-shaped anteriorly.	Inherited generalized disorder of connective tissue causing thin, brittle bones. Severe kyphoscoliosis results from a combination of ligamentous laxity, osteoporosis, and posttraumatic deformities.
Convulsions (Fig SP3-12)	Multiple compression fractures, primarily involving the midthoracic vertebrae.	Tetanus (*Clostridium tetani*); tetany; hypoglycemia; shock therapy. Although the degree of compression may be substantial, the fractures infrequently cause pain and usually do not lead to neurologic sequelae.
Vanishing bone disease	Diffuse destruction of multiple vertebral bodies.	Rare condition that most often involves the pelvis, ribs, spine, and long bones. No sclerotic or periosteal reaction.
Amyloidosis	Loss of bone density and collapse of one or more vertebral bodies.	Rare manifestation caused by diffuse infiltration of the bone marrow by the amorphous protein. Generalized demineralization with collapse of vertebral bodies is usually a manifestation of underlying multiple myeloma.
Hydatid (echinococcal) cyst	Expanding lytic lesion causing a pathologic fracture.	Bone involvement occurs in about 1% of patients and most commonly affects the vertebral bodies, pelvis, and sacrum.
Traumatic ischemic necrosis (Kümmell's spondylitis)	Delayed posttraumatic reaction characterized by rarefaction of the vertebral body, intravertebral vacuum cleft, and vertebral collapse.	The existence of this condition is controversial. Most authorities believe that significant trauma to the spine occurred at the time of the initial injury in instances of alleged Kümmell's spondylitis.

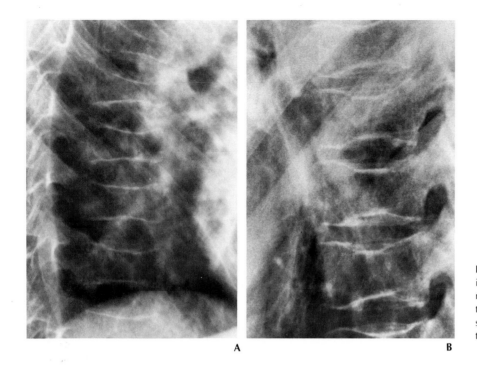

Fig SP3-10. Sickle cell anemia. (A) Biconcave indentations on both the superior and inferior margins of the soft vertebral bodies produce the characteristic fish vertebrae. (B) Localized steplike central depressions of multiple vertebral end plates.

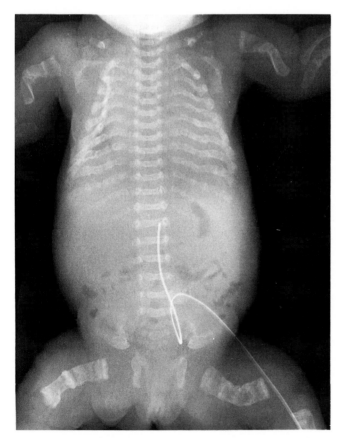

Fig SP3-11. Osteogenesis imperfecta. Generalized flattening of vertebral bodies associated with fractures of multiple ribs and long bones in an infant.

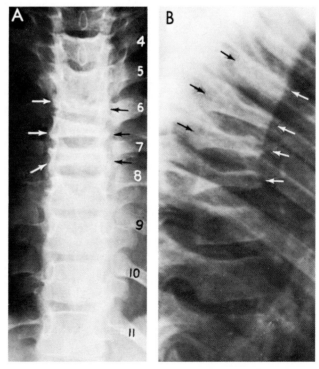

Fig SP3-12. Tetanus. (A) Frontal and (B) lateral projections show residual fractures and compression deformities of vertebral bodies.[5]

NARROWING OF THE INTERVERTEBRAL DISK SPACE AND ADJACENT SCLEROSIS

Condition	Imaging Findings	Comments
Intervertebral osteochondrosis (degenerative disk disease) (Fig SP4-1)	Well-defined sclerosis of vertebral margins and characteristic "vacuum" phenomenon.	Degeneration of the nucleus pulposus and the cartilaginous endplate.
Infection (Figs SP4-2 to SP4-4)	Ill-defined vertebral margins and often a soft-tissue mass. Reactive sclerosis is common with pyogenic inflammation but infrequent with tuberculosis.	Depending on the site of disease, anterior extension of vertebral osteomyelitis may cause retropharyngeal abscess, mediastinitis, pericarditis, subdiaphragmatic abscess, psoas muscle abscess, or peritonitis. Posterior extension of inflammatory tissue can compress the spinal cord or produce meningitis if the infection penetrates the dura to enter the subarachnoid space.
Trauma	Well-defined sclerotic vertebral margins, soft-tissue mass, and evidence of fracture.	Disk injury and degeneration is the underlying mechanism.
Neuroarthropathy (Fig SP4-5)	Extensive sclerosis of the vertebrae associated with osteophytosis, fragmentation, and malalignment.	Caused by repetitive trauma in patients with loss of sensation and proprioception due to such conditions as diabetes, syphilis, syringomyelia, leprosy, and congenital insensitivity to pain.
Pseudogout	Ill- or well-defined sclerotic vertebral margins associated with fragmentation, subluxation, and calcification.	Degenerative process secondary to the deposition of calcium pyrophosphate dihydrate crystals in cartilaginous endplates and intervertebral disks.
Ochronosis (see Fig SP11-2)	Well-defined sclerotic vertebral margins with "vacuum" phenomena and pathognomonic diskal calcification.	Degenerative change resulting from the deposition of the black pigment of oxidized homogentisic acid in cartilaginous endplates and intervertebral disks.
Rheumatoid arthritis	Ill- or well-defined sclerotic vertebral margins associated with subluxations and apophyseal joint abnormalities.	Loss of the intervertebral disk space (usually in the cervical region) may reflect apophyseal joint instability with recurrent diskovertebral trauma or extension of inflammatory tissue from neighboring articulations.

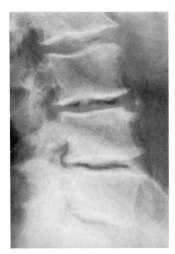

Fig SP4-1. Degenerative disk disease. Hypertrophic spurring, intervertebral disk space narrowing, and reactive sclerosis. Note the linear lucent collections (vacuum phenomenon) overlying several of the intervertebral disks.

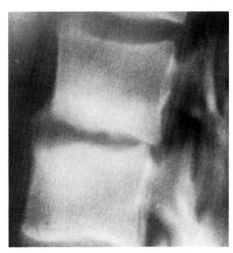

Fig SP4-2. Pyogenic vertebral osteomyelitis. Narrowing of the intervertebral disk space with irregularity of the end plates and reactive sclerosis.

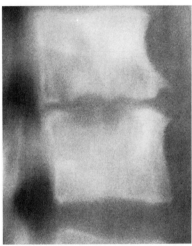

Fig SP4-3. *Pseudomonas* osteomyelitis. Tomogram shows the destructive process in L2 and L3, irregular narrowing of the intervertebral disk space, and reactive sclerosis.

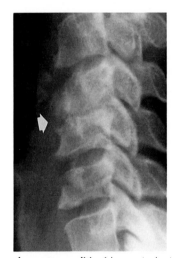

Fig SP4-4. Tuberculous osteomyelitis of the cervical spine. Narrowing of the intervertebral disk space (arrow) is accompanied by diffuse bone destruction involving the adjacent vertebrae. Note the lack of sclerotic reaction.

A   B

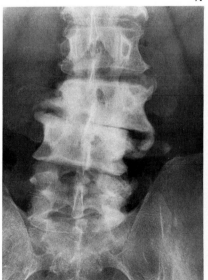 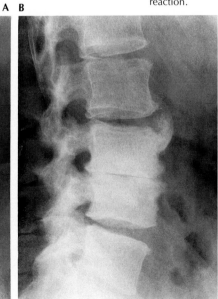

Fig SP4-5. Neuroarthropathy. (A) Frontal and (B) lateral views of the lumbosacral spine in a patient with tabes dorsalis show marked hypertrophic spurring with virtual obliteration of the intervertebral disk space between L3 and L4. Note the reactive sclerosis of the apposing end plates and the subluxation of the vertebral bodies seen on the frontal view.

LOCALIZED WIDENING OF THE INTERPEDICULAR DISTANCE

Condition	Comments
Intramedullary neoplasm of spinal cord	Large tumors can cause localized thinning and remolding of the pedicles, most commonly at the L1 to L3 level. The most common cause is an ependymoma of the cord, especially of the conus or filum terminale. Also may occur with astrocytoma, oligodendroglioma, glioblastoma multiforme, and medulloblastoma.
Meningocele/ myelomeningocele (Fig SP5-1)	Large posterior spinal defect through which there is herniation of the meninges (meningocele) or of the meninges and a portion of the spinal cord or nerve roots (myelomeningocele). The posterior defect is marked by absence of the spinous processes and laminae and widening of the interpedicular distance, as well as a soft-tissue mass representing the herniation itself.
Diastematomyelia (Fig SP5-2)	Fusiform widening of the spinal canal with an increase in the interpedicular distance that extends over several segments is a characteristic finding in this rare malformation in which the spinal cord is split by a midline bony, cartilaginous, or fibrous spur extending posteriorly from a vertebral body. If the septum dividing the cord is ossified, it may appear on frontal views as a pathognomonic thin vertical bony plate lying in the middle of the neural canal. The condition most commonly occurs in the lower thoracic and upper lumbar regions and is often associated with a variety of skeletal and central nervous system anomalies.

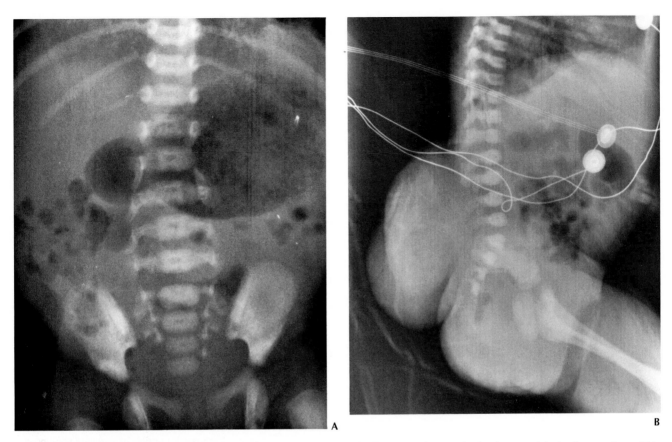

FIG SP5-1. Meningomyelocele. (A) Frontal view of the abdomen shows the markedly increased interpedicular distance of the lumbar vertebrae. (B) In another patient, a lateral view demonstrates the large soft-tissue mass (arrows) situated posterior to the spine. Note the absence of the posterior elements in the lower lumbar and sacral regions.

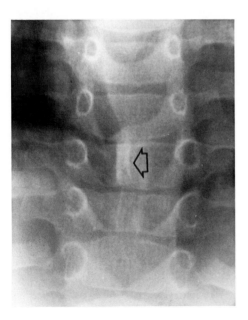

FIG SP5-2. Diastematomyelia. Note the pathognomonic ossified septum (arrow) lying in the midline of the neural canal.

ANTERIOR SCALLOPING OF A VERTEBRAL BODY

Condition	Comments
Lymphoma/chronic leukemia	Erosion of the anterior surfaces of upper lumbar and lower thoracic vertebral bodies is caused by direct neoplastic extension from adjacent lymph nodes. Other skeletal abnormalities include paravertebral soft-tissue masses, dense vertebral sclerosis (ivory vertebrae), and a mottled pattern of destruction and sclerosis with hematogenous spread that may simulate metastatic disease.
Other causes of lymphadenopathy	Metastases or inflammatory processes (especially tuberculosis).
Aortic aneurysm	Continuous pulsatile pressure can rarely cause erosions of the anterior aspect of one or more vertebral bodies. The concomitant demonstration of the calcified wall of the bulging aneurysm is virtually pathognomonic.

POSTERIOR SCALLOPING OF A VERTEBRAL BODY

Condition	Comments
Normal variant (physiologic scalloping)	Minimal to moderate posterior scalloping limited to the lumbar spine can be demonstrated in about half of normal adults. The appearance is identical to that of a mild degree of pathologic scalloping, but there is no associated pedicle abnormality or widening of the interpedicular distance.
Increased intraspinal pressure	Posterior scalloping most commonly occurs with local expanding lesions that are situated in the more caudal portion of the spinal canal, are relatively large and slow growing, and originate during the period of active growth and bone modeling. Generally reflects an intraspinal neoplasm (ependymoma, dermoid, lipoma, or neurofibroma). Intraspinal meningiomas rarely produce even minor bone changes since they are situated above the level of the conus and tend to produce cord symptoms while still relatively small. Other rare underlying causes include spinal cysts, syringomyelia and hydromyelia, and severe generalized communicating hydrocephalus.

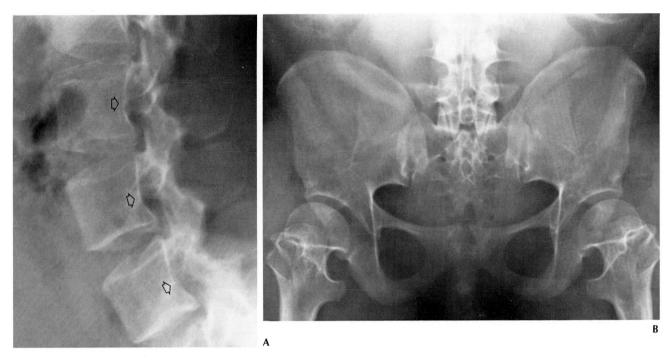

FIG SP7-1. Achondroplasia. (A) Posterior scalloping of multiple vertebral bodies (arrows). (B) Characteristic short, broad pelvis with small sacrosciatic notch.

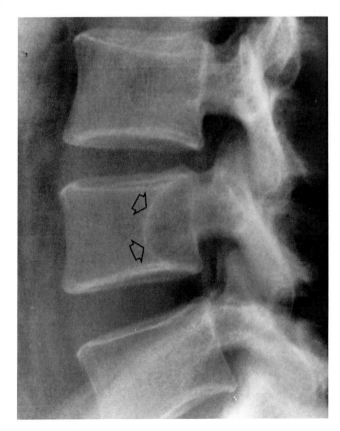

FIG SP7-2. Neurofibromatosis.

Condition	Comments
Achondroplasia **(Fig SP7-1)**	Decreased endochondral bond formation causes the pedicles to be short and the interpedicular spaces to narrow progressively from above downward (opposite of normal), thus reducing the volume of the spinal canal. This is postulated to limit the normal posterior enlargement of the vertebral canal during the early growth period, with the result that the growing sub-arachnoid space must gain room for expansion through scalloping of the posterior aspects of the vertebral bodies.
Neurofibromatosis **(Fig SP7-2)**	Posterior scalloping may reflect an osseous dysplasia, weakness of the dura (permitting transmission of cerebrospinal fluid pulsations to the bone), or an associated thoracic meningocele.
Hereditary connective tissue disorders **(dural ectasia)**	Posterior scalloping is secondary to loss of the normal protection afforded the posterior surfaces of the vertebral bodies by an intact, strong dura. The underlying mesodermal dysplasia causes dural ectasia or weakness that permits transmission of cerebrospinal fluid pulsations to the bone. Occurs in such congenital syndromes as Ehlers-Danlos, Marfan's, and osteogenesis imperfecta tarda.
Mucopolysaccharidoses **(Fig SP7-3)**	Inborn disorders of mucopolysaccharide metabolism in Hurler's and Morquio's syndromes may produce abnormal vertebral bodies that are unable to resist the normal cerebrospinal fluid pulsations over their posterior surfaces (even though the dura is normal).
Acromegaly **(Fig SP7-4)**	Hypertrophy of soft tissue may produce posterior scalloping.

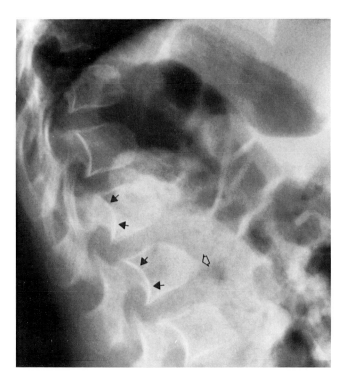

FIG SP7-3. Hurler's syndrome. In addition to the posterior scalloping (closed arrows), there is typical inferior beaking (open arrow) of the anterior margin of the vertebral body.

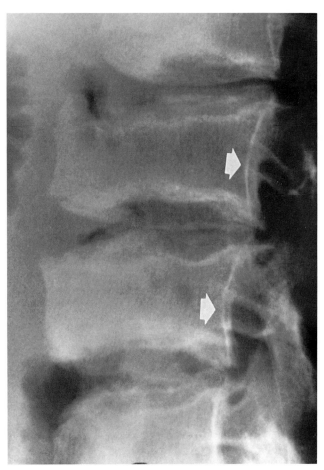

FIG SP7-4. Acromegaly. Posterior scalloping (arrows) associated with enlargement of vertebral bodies (especially in the anteroposterior dimension).

SQUARING OF ONE OR MORE VERTEBRAL BODIES

Condition	Comments
Ankylosing spondylitis (Fig SP8-1)	Erosive osteitis of the corners of the vertebral bodies produces a loss of the normal anterior concavity and a characteristic squared vertebral body. Spinal involvement initially involves the lower lumbar area and progresses upward to the dorsal and cervical regions. Characteristic bilateral and symmetric sacroiliitis and a "bamboo" spine (ossification in paravertebral tissues and longitudinal spinal ligaments combined with extensive lateral bony bridges, or syndesmophytes).
Paget's disease	Enlargement of affected vertebral bodies with increased trabeculation that is most prominent at the periphery of the bone and produces a rim of thickened cortex and a squared, picture-frame appearance. Dense sclerosis may produce an ivory vertebra.
Rheumatoid variants	Uncommon manifestation of rheumatoid arthritis, psoriatic arthritis, or Reiter's syndrome.
Down's syndrome (mongolism)	Manifestations include a decrease in the acetabular and iliac angles with hypoplasia and marked lateral flaring of the iliac wings, multiple manubrial ossification centers, the presence of 11 ribs, and shortening of the middle phalanx of the fifth finger.

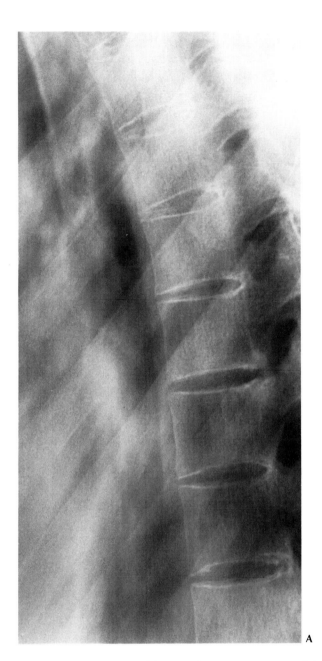

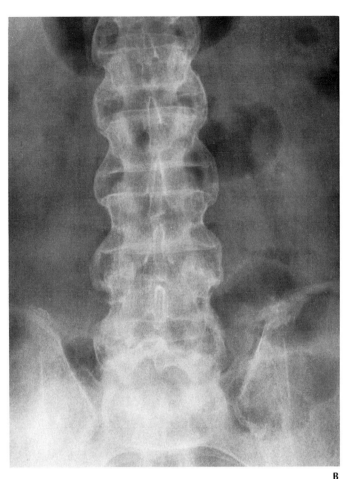

FIG SP8-1. Ankylosing spondylitis. (A) Characteristic squaring of thoracic vertebral bodies. (B) Extensive lateral bony bridges (syndesmophytes) connect all the lumbar vertebral bodies to produce a bamboo spine.

ENLARGED CERVICAL INTERVERTEBRAL FORAMEN

Condition	Comments
Neurofibroma **(Fig SP9-1)**	The most common cause of an enlarged cervical intervertebral foramen is the "dumbbell" type of neurofibroma (intradural and extradural components) that erodes the superior or inferior margins of the pedicles. Enlargement of an intervertebral foramen may also develop because of protrusion of a lateral intrathoracic meningocele in a patient with generalized neurofibromatosis.
Other spinal tumors	Rare manifestation of dermoid, lipoma, lymphoma, meningioma, and neuroblastoma.
Congenital absence of pedicle	Produces the radiographic appearance of an enlarged cervical intervertebral foramen.
Vertebral artery aneurysm or tortuosity **(Fig SP9-2)**	Erosion is caused by pulsatile flow as the vertebral artery passes through the foramina transversarium of the upper six cervical vertebrae between its origin from the subclavian artery and its entrance into the cranial vault through the foramen magnum.
Traumatic avulsion of nerve root **(Fig SP9-3)**	On myelography, a brachial root avulsion produces a pouchlike appearance of the root sleeve, which is blunted and distorted and extends for a variable distance into the intervertebral foramen. Nerve root avulsions can be readily differentiated from diverticula of the subarachnoid space, which have smooth, delicately rounded contours and exhibit the normal radiolucent outlines of intact nerve roots within the opaque, contrast-filled pocket.

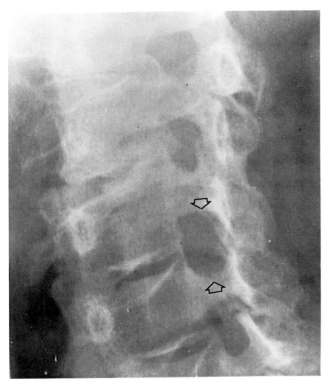

FIG SP9-1. Neurofibroma. Smooth widening (arrows) due to the contiguous mass, without evidence of bone destruction.

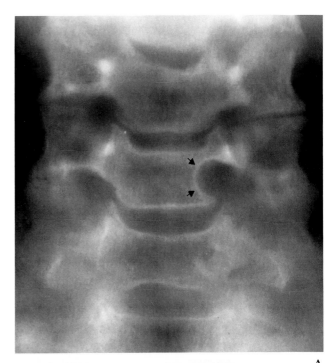

A

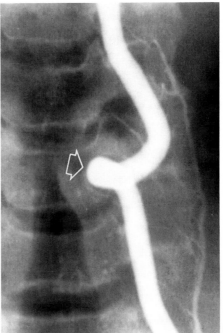

B

FIG SP9-2. Tortuous vertebral artery. (A) Frontal tomogram shows the enlarged foramen (arrows). (B) Arteriogram shows the tortuous vertebral artery (arrow) entering the enlarged foramen.

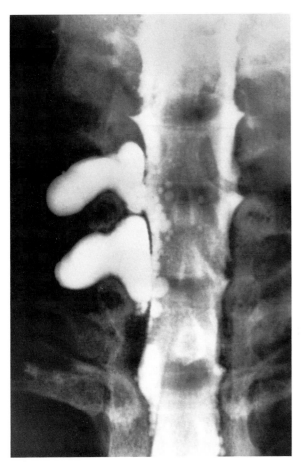

FIG SP9-3. Traumatic avulsion of nerve roots. Note the pouchlike appearance of the blunted nerve roots that extend into the cervical foramina.

ATLANTOAXIAL SUBLUXATION

Condition	Comments
Rheumatoid arthritis (Fig SP10-1)	Synovial inflammation causes weakening of the transverse ligaments. The odontoid process is often eroded and the dens may be completely destroyed. Upward displacement of C2 may permit the dens to impinge on the upper cervical cord or medulla, producing acute neurologic symptoms requiring immediate traction or decompression. Atlantoaxial subluxation also occurs in juvenile rheumatoid arthritis.
Rheumatoid variants	Ankylosing spondylitis; psoriatic arthritis. Inflammatory changes of the synovial and adjacent ligamentous structures can lead to erosion of the dens.
Trauma	Almost always accompanied by a fracture of the odontoid process resulting from hyperflexion (dens and atlas displaced anteriorly) or hyperextension (posterior displacement). Isolated atlantoaxial subluxation (without fracture) indicates tearing of the transverse ligaments.
Congenital cervicobasilar anomaly	Absent anterior arch of the atlas; absent or separate odontoid process; atlanto-occipital fusion.
Retropharyngeal abscess (child)	Presumably causes laxity of the transverse ligaments due to the hyperemia associated with the inflammatory process.
Down's syndrome	Results from laxity of the spinal ligaments and has been reported in up to 20% of cases. Although usually mild and asymptomatic, a few patients develop symptoms ranging from discomfort in the neck to quadriparesis.
Morquio's syndrome	Hypoplasia of the dens in this condition predisposes to atlantoaxial subluxation with consequent damage to the spinal cord. This risk is so high that some authors recommend early prophylactic posterior cervical fusion for patients with this disease.

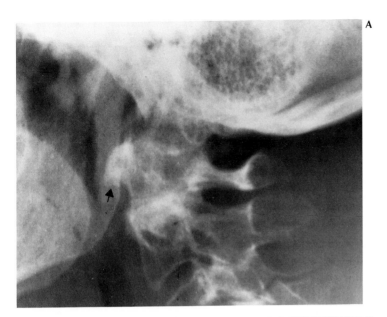

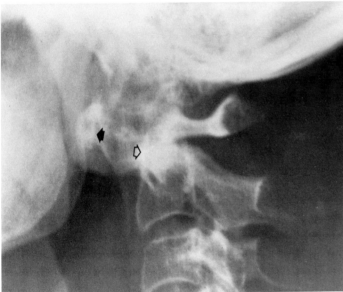

Fɪɢ SP10-1. Rheumatoid arthritis. (A) Routine lateral film of the cervical spine shows a normal relation between the anterior border of the odontoid process and the superior portion of the anterior arch of the atlas (arrow). (B) With flexion, there is wide separation between the anterior arch of the atlas (closed arrow) and the odontoid (open arrow).

CALCIFICATION OF INTERVERTEBRAL DISKS

Condition	Comments
Degenerative disk disease (Fig SP11-1)	Radiographic manifestations include osteophytosis, narrowing of intervertebral disk spaces with marginal sclerosis, and the vacuum phenomenon (linear lucent collection overlying one or more intervertebral disks).
Transient calcification in children	Unlike most other causes of intervertebral disk calcification, in children the cervical region is most commonly involved and there is a high frequency of associated clinical signs and symptoms. A self-limited condition requiring only conservative symptomatic treatment.
Posttraumatic	Associated findings of previous spinal injury.
Ochronosis (Fig SP11-2)	Dense laminated calcification of multiple intervertebral disks (beginning in the lumbar spine and extending to the dorsal and cervical regions) is virtually pathognomonic of this rare inborn error of metabolism in which deposition of the black pigment of oxidized homogentisic acid in cartilage and other connective tissue produces a distinctive form of degenerative arthritis. The intervertebral disk spaces are narrowed, the vertebral bodies are osteoporotic, and limitation of motion is common. Severe degenerative arthritis may develop in peripheral joints, especially the shoulders, hips, and knees (an infrequent manifestation of osteoarthritis, especially in young patients).
Ankylosing spondylitis (Fig SP11-3)	Central or eccentric, circular or linear calcific collections may appear in the intervertebral disks at single or multiple sites along the spinal column. Usually associated with apophyseal joint ankylosis at the same vertebral levels and adjacent syndesmophytes. The development of similar calcific deposits in other conditions affecting the vertebral column that are characterized by ankylosis (diffuse idiopathic skeletal hyperostosis, juvenile rheumatoid arthritis) suggests that immobilization of a segment of the spine may interfere with diskal nutrition and lead to degeneration and calcification.
Pseudogout	Calcification frequently affects the intervertebral disks and may be associated with back pain. The deposits involve the annulus fibrosis (not the nucleus pulposus, as in ochronosis). Disk space narrowing often occurs.

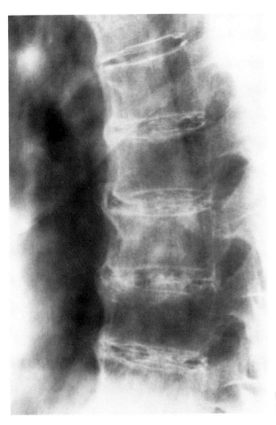

FIG SP11-1. Degenerative disk disease. Note the anterior osteophytes, narrowing of intervertebral disk spaces, and calcification in the anterior longitudinal ligament.

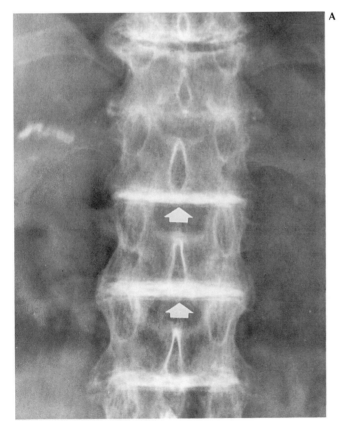

A

FIG SP11-2. Ochronosis. (A) Frontal and (B) lateral views of the lumbar spine in two different patients show dense laminated calcification of multiple intervertebral disks (arrows).

B

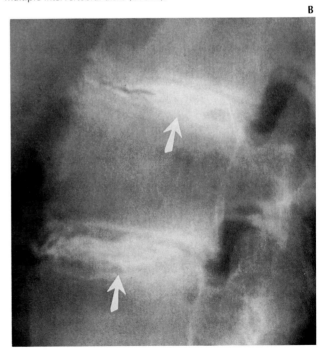

Condition	Comments
Hemochromatosis	Deposition of calcium pyrophosphate dihydrate crystals occurs in the outer fibers of the annulus fibrosis, as in pseudogout. Other radiographic manifestations include diffuse osteoporosis of the spine associated with vertebral collapse and a peripheral arthropathy that most commonly involves the small joints of the hands (especially the second and third metacarpophalangeal joints).
Hypervitaminosis D	Calcification of the annulus fibrosis is an uncommon finding. More often causes generalized osteoporosis with extensive masses of soft-tissue calcification.

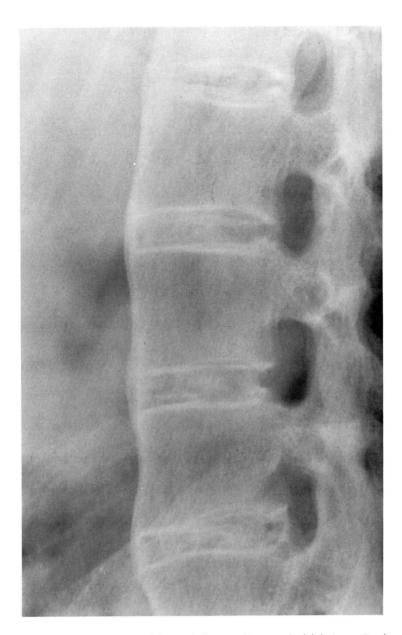

FIG SP11-3. Ankylosing spondylitis. Calcification of intervertebral disks is associated with squaring of vertebral bodies and dense calcification of the anterior longitudinal ligament.

BEAKED, NOTCHED, OR HOOKED VERTEBRAE IN A CHILD

Condition	Imaging Findings	Comments
Normal variant	Variable pattern of vertebral notching.	Vertebral notching can be seen in infants who are presumably normal. This incidental finding is probably secondary to subclinical hyperflexion trauma or to the exaggerated thoracolumbar kyphosis that is seen in all young infants who are unable to remain erect in the sitting position because of normal muscular immaturity.
Mucopolysaccharidoses		Genetically determined disorders of mucopolysaccharide metabolism that result in a broad spectrum of skeletal, visceral, and mental abnormalities.
Hurler's syndrome (gargoylism) (Fig SP12-1)	Inferior beaking. The centrum of the second lumbar vertebra is usually hypoplastic and displaced posteriorly, giving rise to an accentuated kyphosis, or gibbous, deformity.	Other radiographic manifestations include swelling of the central portions of long bones (due to cortical thickening or widening of the medullary canal), "canoe-paddle" ribs, and J-shaped sella (shallow, elongated sella with a long anterior recess extending under the anterior clinoid processes).
Morquio's syndrome (Fig SP12-2)	Generalized flattening of the vertebral bodies with central anterior beaking. There is often hypoplasia and posterior displacement of L1 or L2, resulting in a sharp, angular kyphosis.	Other radiographic manifestations include tapering of long bones (less marked than in Hurler's syndrome) and flaring, fragmentation, and flattening of the femoral heads combined with irregular deformity of the acetabula (often results in subluxations at the hip).
Cretinism (hypothyroidism)	Inferior beaking.	Radiographic manifestations include delay in appearance and subsequent growth of ossification centers, epiphyseal dysgenesis (fragmented epiphyses with multiple foci of ossification), retarded bone age, increased thickness of the cranial vault, and widened sutures with delayed closure.
Achondroplasia (Fig SP12-3)	Central anterior wedging of vertebral bodies. Progressive narrowing of the interpedicular distances from above downward (opposite of normal) and scalloping of the posterior aspects of the vertebral bodies.	Radiographic manifestations include symmetric shortening of all long bones, ball-and-socket epiphyses, trident hand, and a characteristic short, broad pelvis with short and square ilia and decreased acetabular angles.
Down's syndrome (mongolism)	Variable pattern of vertebral notching.	Radiographic manifestations include a decrease in the acetabular and iliac angles with hypoplasia and marked lateral flaring of the iliac wings, squaring of vertebral bodies, multiple manubrial ossification centers, the presence of only 11 ribs, and shortening of the middle phalanx of the fifth finger.

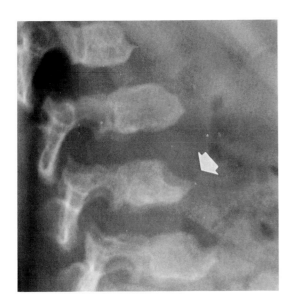

Fɪɢ **SP12-1. Hurler's syndrome.** Typical inferior beaking (arrow) of the anterior margin of a vertebral body.

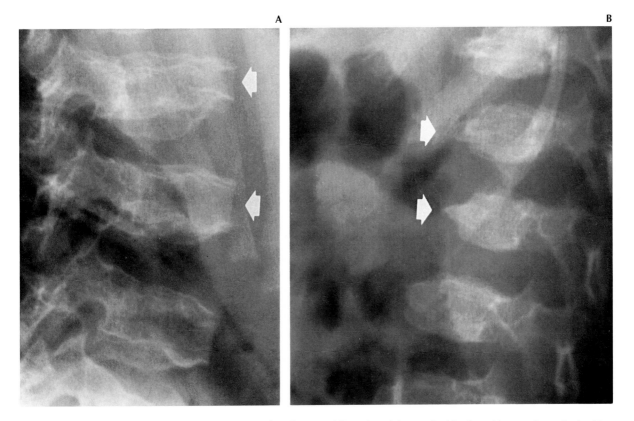

A   B

Fɪɢ **SP12-2. Morquio's syndrome.** (A and B) Two examples of universal flattening of the vertebral bodies with central anterior beaking (arrows).

Condition	Imaging Findings	Comments
Neuromuscular disease with generalized hypotonia	Variable pattern of vertebral notching.	Niemann-Pick disease, phenylketonuria. Werdnig-Hoffmann disease, mental retardation. Probably related to an exaggerated kyphotic curvature of the thoracic spine.
Trauma	Variable pattern of vertebral notching.	Hyperflexion-compression spinal injuries. Repeated hyperflexion of the spine is postulated to be the underlying cause of vertebral notching in battered children.

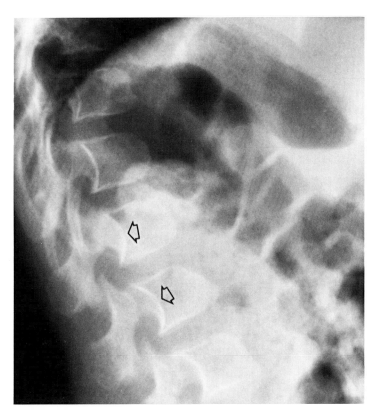

Fɪɢ **SP12-3. Achondroplasia.** Central anterior wedging of several vertebral bodies. Note the characteristic posterior scalloping (arrows).

INTRAMEDULLARY LESION ON MYELOGRAPHY
(WIDENING OF THE SPINAL CORD)*

Condition	Imaging Findings	Comments
Primary intramedullary neoplasm (Fig SP13-1)	Fusiform widening of the spinal cord, often with localized thinning and remolding of the pedicles.	About two thirds are ependymomas, particularly of the conus and filum terminale. Other intramedullary tumors include astrocytoma, glioblastoma, hemangioblastoma, lipoma, dermoid, epidermoid, teratoma, and metastases.
Syringomyelia/hydromyelia (Fig SP13-2)	Fusiform widening of the spinal cord that is indistinguishable from an intramedullary tumor. In patients with hydromyelia who undergo air myelography in the semierect or erect position, fluid in the dilated central canal migrates caudally and permits the apparently enlarged cord to collapse (collapsing-cord sign), indicating the presence of a cystic lesion rather than a solid intramedullary neoplasm.	Syringomyelia is an intraspinal cystic cavity that may extend over many segments and is independent of, but may be connected with, the central canal. When the cavity is a distended central canal, the condition is termed hydromyelia. Usually associated with the Arnold-Chiari I malformation. CT shows low-density fluid in a syrinx (some intramedullary gliomas may also have low density, though they have a serrated border unlike the smooth margin of a syrinx). A delayed CT scan obtained hours after a myelogram permits filling of the syrinx cavity by direct connection from the subarachnoid space or by diffusion of contrast material across the spinal cord. MRI may be able to detect cavities in normal-sized or diminished spinal cords.
Diastematomyelia (Fig SP13-3)	Fusiform widening of the spinal canal with increased interpedicular distance extending over several segments. The contrast material is split around a round or oval midline defect representing the septum (septum and two hemicords about it can be well demonstrated by CT).	Rare malformation in which the spinal cord is split by a midline bony, cartilaginous, or fibrous spur extending posteriorly from a vertebral body. Most commonly occurs in the lower thoracic and upper lumbar regions and is often associated with a variety of skeletal and central nervous system anomalies. If the septum dividing the cord is ossified, it may appear on frontal views as a pathognomonic vertical, thin bony plate lying in the midline of the neural canal.
Arteriovenous malformation/angioma (Fig SP13-4)	Focal mass or, more commonly, multiple parallel or serpiginous filling defects representing dilated, tortuous vessels.	May vary in size from a few insignificant vessels to huge intertwined masses of abnormal vasculature reaching from one end of the spinal cord to the other.
Hematoma/contusion	Intramedullary lesion.	Intramedullary bleeding may be related to trauma, neoplasm, or vascular malformation.
Granulomatous lesion	Intramedullary lesion.	Very rare manifestation of tuberculosis or sarcoidosis.

*Pattern: Fusiform widening of the spinal cord with symmetric narrowing of the surrounding contrast-filled subarachnoid space. Complete obstruction causes an abrupt concave termination of the contrast column, which appears similar in all radiographic projections.

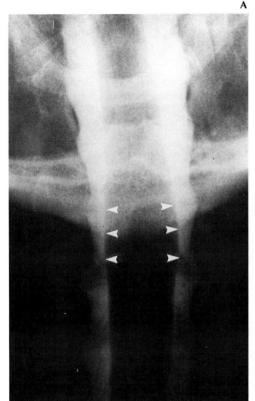

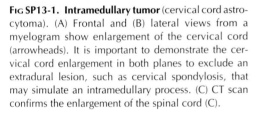

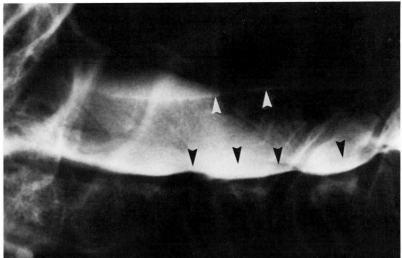

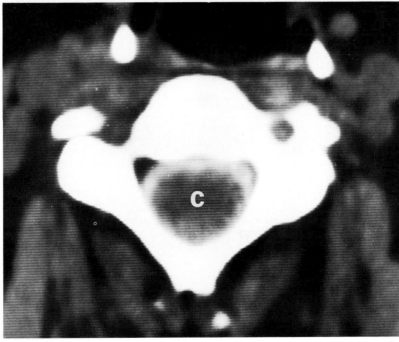

FIG SP13-1. Intramedullary tumor (cervical cord astrocytoma). (A) Frontal and (B) lateral views from a myelogram show enlargement of the cervical cord (arrowheads). It is important to demonstrate the cervical cord enlargement in both planes to exclude an extradural lesion, such as cervical spondylosis, that may simulate an intramedullary process. (C) CT scan confirms the enlargement of the spinal cord (C).

Condition	Imaging Findings	Comments
Infection	Intramedullary lesion.	Isolated infection is rare (usually spread from vertebral infection, trauma, lumbar puncture, or via a congenital skin sinus).
Neurenteric cyst	Intramedullary lesion.	May be associated with developmental vertebral anomalies and tethering of the cord.

A

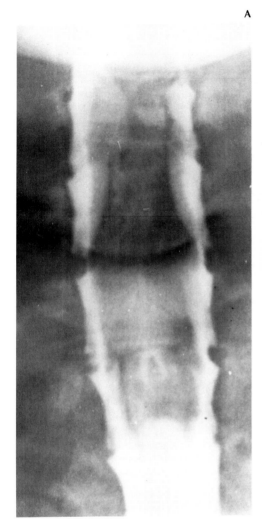

B

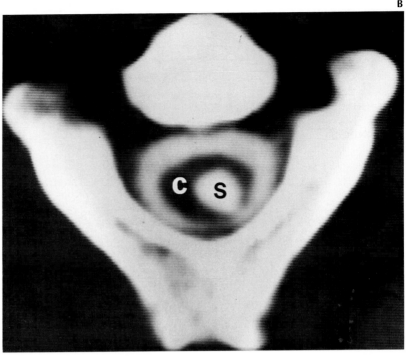

FIG SP13-2. **Syringomyelia/hydromyelia.** (A) Fusiform widening of the spinal cord in syringomyelia. (B) Hydromyelia. CT scan after the subarachnoid injection of metrizamide shows enlargement of the cervical spinal cord (C) with the high-density contrast material filling the central cavity (S).

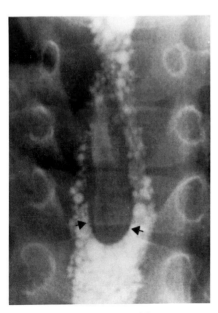

FIG SP13-3. **Diastematomyelia.** Splitting of the contrast material around an oval midline defect (arrows), which represents the septum.

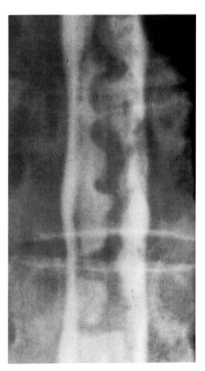

FIG SP13-4. **Arteriovenous malformation.** Serpiginous filling defect representing dilated, tortuous vessels.

INTRADURAL, EXTRAMEDULLARY LESION
ON MYELOGRAPHY*

Condition	Imaging Findings	Comments
Meningioma (Fig SP14-1)	Intradural, extramedullary mass.	Typically occurs in middle-aged or elderly females. About 80% are located in the thoracic portion of the spinal canal, while most of the remainder are situated in the region of the foramen magnum.
Neurofibroma (Figs SP14-2 and SP14-3)	Intradural, extramedullary mass.	More evenly distributed along the course of the spinal canal than are meningiomas; there is no age or sex predominance. Because of their very slow growth and (in about 30%) their location partially or completely in the extradural space, neurofibromas tend to erode the bony margins of the spinal canal (especially the inner borders of the pedicles and the posterior margins of the vertebral bodies).
Metastases ("seeding") (Fig SP14-4)	Multiple spherical lesions (1 mm to 2 cm) that generally arise on individual nerve roots and thus do not usually displace the cord.	Multiple metastases, which tend to attach to the lower lumbar and sacral roots by spreading from primary intracerebral tumors, are becoming more common since primary tumors are now better controlled with radiation and chemotherapy. The most common brain tumors giving rise to spinal metastases are medulloblastoma and pinealoma. Occasional metastases from glioblastoma multiforme and ependymoma.
Other tumors (Fig SP14-5)	Intradural, extramedullary lesion.	Dermoid; epidermoid; lipoma.
Arachnoiditis (Fig SP14-6)	Thickened and tortuous nerve roots that appear fixed in position. Associated epidural and peridural inflammatory changes may lead to irregular constriction of the thecal sac with obliteration of nerve-root sheaths.	Chronic inflammation in the dural sac that causes the normal gentle netlike pattern of the arachnoid to become dense and thickened with crisscrossing arachnoid septa producing pockets and cysts. The most frequent cause is the introduction of foreign substances (antibiotics, radiopaque contrast media, spinal anesthetics). Trauma and chronic infection may cause similar changes. Lumbar puncture may be painful, and in severe cases a "dry tap" may be obtained because of obliteration of the thecal sac.
Arachnoid cyst	Intradural, extramedullary lesion.	Usually posterior, may extend over several vertebral segments, primarily involves the thoracic region, and may be multiple. CT shows the cerebrospinal fluid density of the cyst.

*Pattern: Spinal cord appears to be displaced and compressed against the opposite wall, causing narrowing of the contralateral subarachnoid space with widening of the space on the ipsilateral side.

A

B

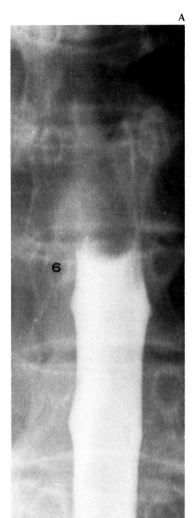

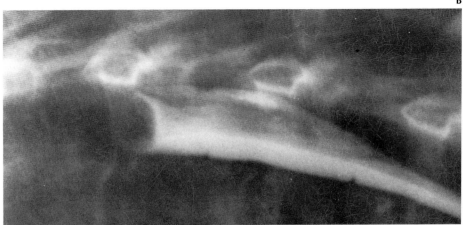

FIG SP14-1. Meningioma. (A) Frontal view shows the spinal cord displaced to the right (reader's right) at the level of T6. At the upper margin of T6, the lower edge of the tumor produces a cuplike defect in the contrast column. A thin layer of contrast material ascends along the right lateral aspect of the tumor (arrow). (B) Cross-table lateral view shows that the tumor arises anteriorly and displaces the spinal cord posteriorly. Note the characteristic cupping of the upper margin of the subarachnoid contrast column.[6]

B

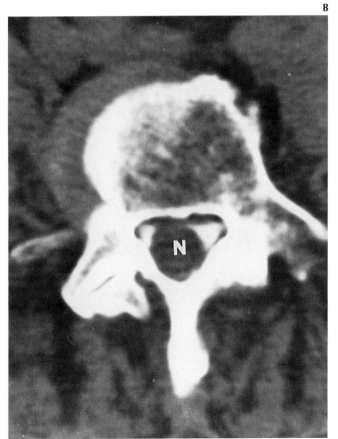

A

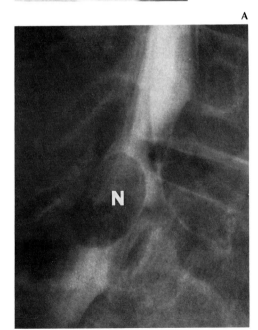

FIG SP14-2. Neurofibroma. (A) Oblique film from a myelogram shows a well-demarcated lesion (N) in the lower lumbar thecal sac. (B) A CT scan confirms that the neurofibroma (N) is intradural. Because the spinal cord ended at T12, the mass must represent an extramedullary, intradural process.

Condition	Imaging Findings	Comments
Vascular malformation/ angioma	Focal mass or, more commonly, multiple parallel or serpiginous filling defects representing dilated, tortuous vessels.	May vary in size from a few insignificant vessels to huge intertwined masses of abnormal vasculature reaching from one end of the spinal cord to the other.
Subdural abscess	Intradural, extramedullary lesion.	Rare occurrence that represents infection of the subdural space by direct extension, spinal puncture, or, more commonly, hematogenous spread from a distant focus.

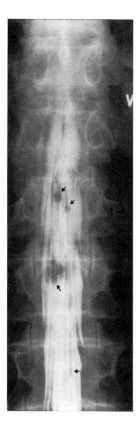

FIG SP14-3. Metastases. Multiple small lesions (arrows) arising from nerve roots.

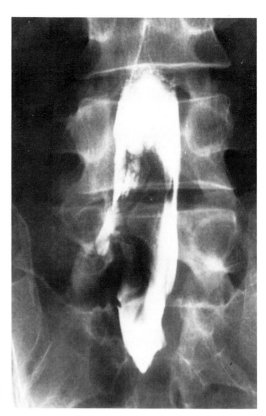

FIG SP14-4. Lipoma. Intradural, extramedullary mass with extradural extension.

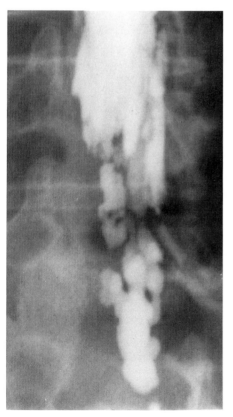

FIG SP14-5. Arachnoiditis. Collections of subarachnoid myelographic contrast material in irregular pockets that are separated by the radiolucent shadows of thickened nerve roots and arachnoid septa.

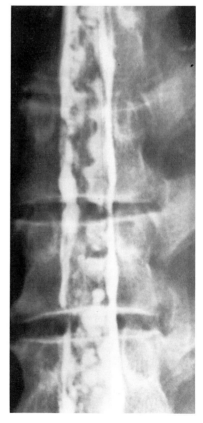

FIG SP14-6. Arteriovenous malformation. Multiple serpiginous filling defects representing dilated, tortuous vessels.

EXTRADURAL LESION ON MYELOGRAPHY*

Condition	Imaging Findings	Comments
Herniated disk (Fig SP15-1)	Smooth extradural defect at the anterior or lateral portion of the contrast column at the level of an intervertebral disk space. There is often amputation of the nerve root at the disk space and incomplete filling of the nerve-root sheath.	Protrusion of a lumbar intervertebral disk is the major cause of severe acute, chronic, or recurrent low back and leg pain. Most frequently occurs at the L4-L5 and L5-S1 levels.
Osteophyte (Fig SP15-2)	Bony spurs arising from the posterior margins of the vertebral bodies can cause anterior compression of the contrast column at the level of an intervertebral disk space.	Multiple irregularities on the ventral aspect of the radiopaque column frequently occur in patients with osteoarthritis of the spine. To produce symptoms, the spurs must be sufficiently large to obliterate the ventral subarachnoid space and reach the anterior surface of the spinal cord.
Thickening of ligamentum flavum	Extradural impression on the dorsal aspect of the subarachnoid space.	Thickening of the dorsolateral structures that connect the laminae of successive vertebrae represents a degenerative process with resulting fibrosis. Although rarely of any significance in itself, ligamentous thickening can impede the posterior displacement of the dural sac by a large ventral mass (eg, a herniated intervertebral disk) and thus contribute to further nerve root compression.
Metastases (Fig SP15-3)	Asymmetric extradural defect with a smooth or lobular margin. May extend along the spinal canal for a variable distance. There is usually evidence of bone destruction.	Hematogenous metastases to the bodies or pedicles of one or several vertebrae may be caused by almost any malignant neoplasm of epithelial origin (about two thirds are secondary to carcinomas of the lung or breast). As the metastasis enlarges, it breaks through the bony cortex and spreads into the spinal canal, compressing and displacing the thecal sac.
Lymphoma	Extradural defect that is typically longer, smoother, and more often circumferential than carcinomatous metastases.	Lymphoma usually involves the extradural soft tissues without producing recognizable changes in the adjacent vertebral bodies.
Vertebral neoplasm with intraspinal extension	Smooth or irregular extradural defect associated with vertebral destruction.	Myeloma; chordoma; sarcoma; hemangioma.

*Pattern: Extrinsic displacement of the entire thecal sac and its contents that causes the distance between the lateral margin of the sac and the medial margin of the pedicle to be widened on the side of the mass and narrowed on the opposite side. The margins of the sac remain smooth unless the lesion has invaded through the dura to produce a concomitant intradural component. Large masses compress the subarachnoid space on the side of the lesion and displace the spinal cord away from the mass.

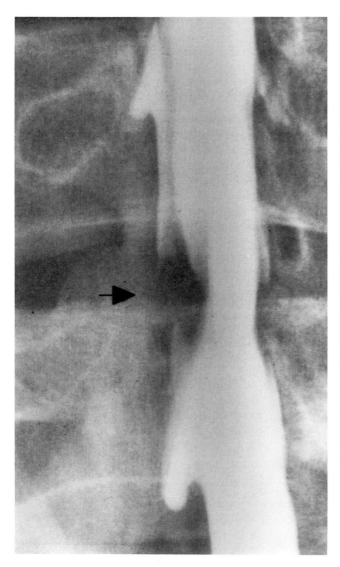

FIG SP15-1. **Lumbar disk herniation.** Extradural lesion at the level of the intervertebral disk space. Note the amputation of the nerve root by the disk compression.

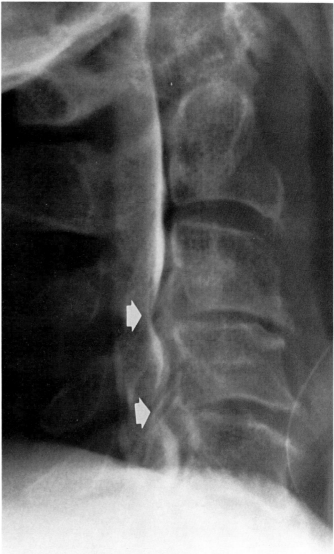

FIG SP15-2. **Osteophyte.** Posterior spurs cause impingement on the contrast column (arrows).

Condition	Imaging Findings	Comments
Benign extradural tumor	Extradural lesion that may be associated with vertebral erosion resulting from local pressure by the tumor.	Neuroma; meningioma; lipoma; fibroma; dermoid; epidermoid. Extradural neuromas frequently extend through and enlarge one or more intervertebral foramina and may be contiguous with a large mass in the paraspinal region. Extradural meningiomas are much less common but may produce local erosion of vertebral pedicles, laminae, or bodies. Lipomas are often associated with spina bifida or other anomalies of the vertebral column.
Fracture or dislocation	Extradural lesion.	Displaced and comminuted fragments of vertebral bodies or neural arches, lacerated ligaments, and hematoma may all contribute to the extradural mass.
Hematoma (Fig SP15-4)	Extradural lesion.	Posttraumatic or spontaneous (defect in blood coagulation due to anticoagulant therapy or a bleeding diathesis).
Scar tissue	Extradural lesion.	Usually a sequela of disk surgery.
Epidural abscess	Extradural lesion that is often associated with vertebral destruction.	Most commonly the result of extension of vertebral osteomyelitis. An epidural infection may occasionally follow spinal or pelvic surgery, trauma, or even lumbar puncture. The initial site of infection is usually the posterior epidural space, where the loose fatty tissue permits the development of rapid inflammatory change.
Arachnoid cyst	Extradural lesion that is usually posterior and occasionally multiple.	An extradural arachnoid cyst is frequently accompanied by dysraphism. It fills slowly or not at all and usually causes a partial or complete block of contrast flow. The cerebrospinal fluid density of the cyst can be shown by CT.
Paget's disease	Extradural defect mimicking the extension of tumor from a vertebral body.	The combination of flattening of a vertebral body, proliferation of uncalcified osteoid tissue on all sides, and enlargement of the pedicles may constrict the vertebral canal and intervertebral foramina, resulting in compression of the spinal cord and nerve roots.

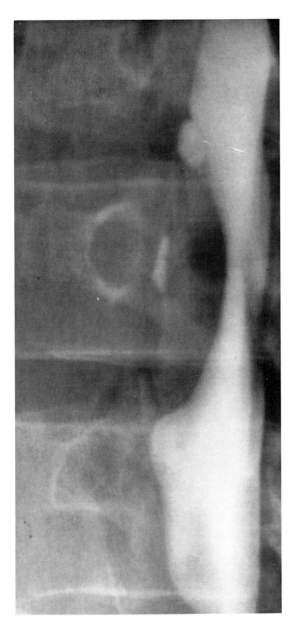

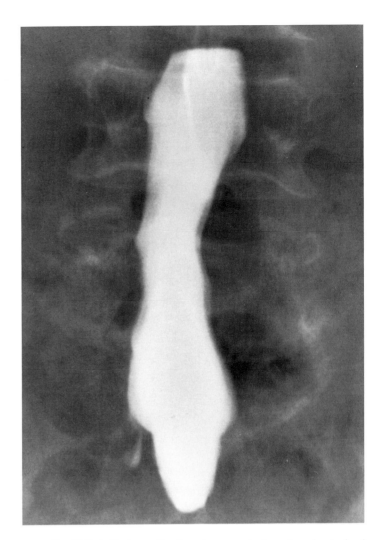

FIG SP15-4. **Postoperative hematoma** producing a broad extradural defect.

FIG SP15-3. **Metastasis** from carcinoma of the lung. Broad extradural defect.

SOURCES

1. Reprinted with permission from ''Benign Tumors'' by JW Beabout, RA McLeod, and DC Dahlin, *Seminars in Roentgenology* (1979;14:33–43), Copyright © 1979, Grune & Stratton Inc.

2. Reprinted from *Roentgen Diagnosis of Diseases of Bone*, ed 3, by J Edeiken with permission of Williams & Wilkins Company, © 1981.

3. Reprinted with permission from ''The Radiologic Assessment of Short Stature'' by JP Dorst, CI Scott, and JG Hall, *Radiologic Clinics of North America* (1972;10:393–414), Copyright © 1972, WB Saunders Company.

4. Reprinted from *Radiology of Bone Diseases* by GB Greenfield, JB Lippincott Company, with permission of the author, © 1986.

5. Reprinted from *Caffey's Pediatric X-Ray Diagnosis*, ed 8, by FN Silverman with permission of Year Book Medical Publishers Inc, © 1985.

6. Reprinted from *Introduction to Neuroradiology* by HO Peterson and SA Kieffer with permission of JB Lippincott Company, © 1972.

Skull Patterns
7

SK1 Diffuse demineralization or destruction of the skull 778

SK2 Single or multiple lytic defects in the skull 780

SK3 Button sequestrum 788

SK4 Localized increased density or hyperostosis of the calvarium 790

SK5 Generalized increased density or thickness of the calvarium 794

SK6 Normal (physiologic) intracranial calcifications 798

SK7 Solitary intracranial calcifications 802

SK8 Multiple intracranial calcifications 808

SK9 Sellar or parasellar calcifications 812

SK10 Enlargement, erosion, and destruction of the sella turcica 816

SK11 Erosion and widening of the internal auditory canal 818

SK12 Dilated cerebral ventricles 820

SK13 Multiple wormian bones 824

SK14 Basilar impression 826

SK15 Cystlike lesions of the jaw 828

SK16 Radiopaque lesions of the jaw 832

SK17 Mass in a paranasal sinus 836

SK18 Hypodense supratentorial mass on computed tomography 840

SK19 High-attenuation mass in a cerebral hemisphere on computed tomography 846

SK20 Ring-enhancing lesion on computed tomography 848

SK21 Cerebellar lesions on computed tomography 852

SK22 Multiple enhancing cerebral and cerebellar nodules on computed tomography 856

SK23 Sellar and juxtasellar masses on computed tomography 860

SK24 Masses in the pineal region on computed tomography 864

SK25 Cerebellopontine angle masses on computed tomography 866

SK26 Low-density mass in the brainstem on computed tomography 870

SK27 Enhancing ventricular margins on computed tomography 872

SK28 Computed tomography of periventricular calcification in a child 874

SK29 Thickening of the optic nerve on computed tomography 876

SK30 Thickening of the rectus muscles on computed tomography 878

Sources 880

DIFFUSE DEMINERALIZATION OR DESTRUCTION OF THE SKULL

Condition	Imaging Findings	Comments
Osteoporosis	Generalized demineralization of the skull.	Most commonly a condition of aging (senile or postmenopausal osteoporosis). Also a manifestation of deficiency states, endocrine disorders, and steroid therapy.
Hyperparathyroidism (Fig SK1-1)	Diffuse granular pattern of skull demineralization.	Irregular demineralization produces the characteristic salt-and-pepper skull. Individual brown tumors and hemorrhagic cysts may occur (best seen after the removal of a parathyroid adenoma because of remineralization of the surrounding bone).
Paget's disease (osteoporosis circumscripta) (Fig SK1-2)	Sharply defined lucent zone that is usually large and may involve more than half the calvarium. Primarily involves the outer table, sparing the inner table.	Represents the destructive phase of the disease that usually begins in the frontal or occipital area. The development of irregular islands of sclerosis during the reparative process results in a mottled, cotton-wool appearance.
Osteogenesis imperfecta (see Fig SK13-2)	Diffusely thin and lucent bones with abnormally wide sutures simulating increased intracranial pressure.	As calvarial ossification proceeds, a number of wormian bones may develop in the sutural gaps. Multiple fractures may occur in the paper-thin skull.
Hypophosphatasia (Fig SK1-3)	Large unossified areas in the skull simulate severe widening of the sutures.	If the infant survives and calvarial recalcification occurs, there may be premature closure of the sutures.
Rickets	Thin, lucent skull in infants with severe disease.	Fine lucent lines traversing the calvarium may mimic multiple fractures.

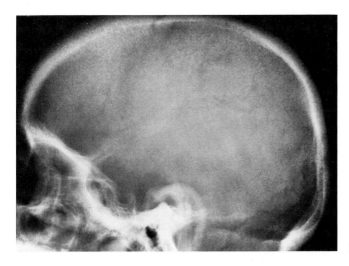

Fɪɢ **SK1-1.** **Hyperparathyroidism.** Characteristic salt-and-pepper skull.

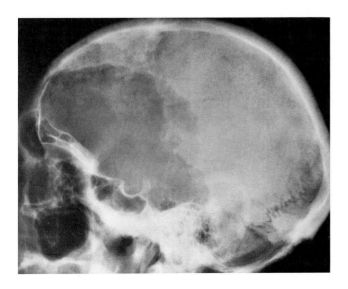

Fɪɢ **SK1-2.** **Paget's disease** (osteoporosis circumscripta).

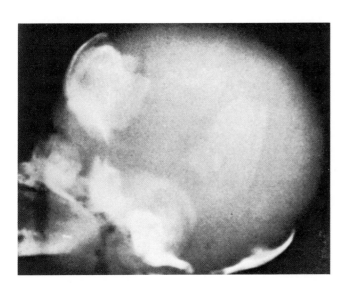

Fɪɢ **SK1-3.** **Hypophosphatasia.** Large areas of uncalcified osteoid in the membranous bones in the region adjoining the sutures and, to a lesser extent, at the base.[1]

SINGLE OR MULTIPLE LYTIC DEFECTS IN THE SKULL

Condition	Imaging Findings	Comments
Neoplasm		
Metastases	Multiple irregular, ill-defined lucent areas of various sizes. A solitary metastasis may occasionally present as a larger area of bone destruction.	Lytic metastases may arise from a wide spectrum of malignant neoplasms, most commonly carcinomas of the breast and lung. Solitary metastases are most likely to arise from carcinomas of the thyroid and kidney.
Multiple myeloma (Fig SK2-1)	Multiple sharply circumscribed (''punched-out'') osteolytic lesions that are scattered throughout the skull and are relatively uniform in size.	Although often indistinguishable from metastatic carcinoma, the lytic defects in multiple myeloma tend to be more discrete and uniform in size. A solitary lytic defect (plasmacytoma) may occasionally exist for years and be the only osseous manifestation of a plasma-cell dyscrasia.
Lymphoma/leukemia	Multiple poorly defined lytic areas that may become confluent.	Most common in childhood leukemia. Spreading of cranial sutures indicates increased intracranial pressure secondary to central nervous system involvement.
Neuroblastoma	Widespread punctate areas of destruction.	Elevation of the periosteum causes radial bone spiculation extending into the soft tissues. A similar process occurring between the inner table and the dura with invasion of the sutures results in marked sutural spreading.
Primary sarcoma of bone	Large lytic area with poorly defined margins.	Rare site of osteosarcoma, chondrosarcoma, or fibrosarcoma. There may occasionally be radiating bony spicules in osteosarcoma or stippled calcifications in chondrosarcoma.
Meningioma	Purely lytic lesion with irregular margins and a faint reticular or spiculated internal architecture (on tangential view).	Unusual manifestation that occurs when a tumor infiltrating the bone causes erosion rather than the much more common hyperostosis. The association of enlarged dural arterial grooves or tumor calcification aids in making the diagnosis.
Hemangioma (see Fig SK4-7)	Expansile lytic lesion that arises in the diploic space.	Usually contains characteristic osseous spicules that radiate from the center to produce a sunburst pattern.
Direct extension of tumor	Destructive process involving the base of the skull.	Contiguous spread into adjacent areas of the skull from carcinoma of the paranasal sinuses or nasopharynx.
Erosion by other intracranial tumors	Indistinct, patchy area of lucency.	Rare manifestation of carcinoma metastatic to the brain and meninges. The underlying intracranial tumor dominates the clinical picture.
Neurofibromatosis (Fig SK2-2)	Irregular lytic defects in the occipital and temporal bones.	Rare manifestation. Neurofibromatosis more commonly produces orbital dysplasia, in which unilateral absence of a large part of the greater wing of the sphenoid and hypoplasia and elevation of the lesser wing result in a markedly widened superior orbital fissure.
Skin malignancy (Fig SK2-3)	Ill-defined lucent defect that initially affects the outer table.	Rare manifestation of extension of a malignant skin tumor to destroy the underlying skull.

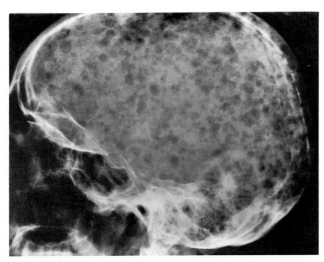

A

B

Fɪɢ **SK2-1. Multiple myeloma.** Diffuse punched-out osteolytic lesions scattered throughout the skull.

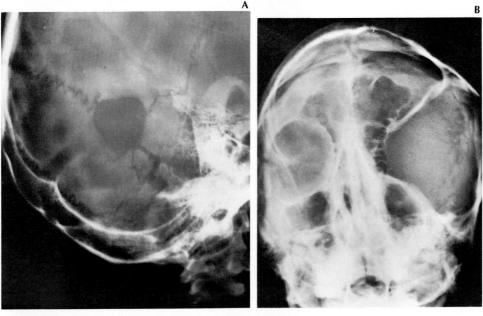

Fɪɢ **SK2-2. Neurofibromatosis.** (A) Mesenchymal defect in the lambdoid suture. (B) Severe orbital dysplasia with virtual absence of the posterolateral walls of the orbit.

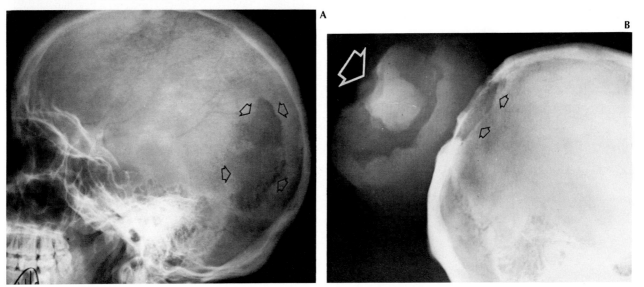

A

B

Fɪɢ **SK2-3. Scalp malignancy.** (A) Ill-defined lucency (arrows) representing erosion of the underlying skull. (B) Huge soft-tissue mass (white arrow) eroding the skull (black arrows).

Condition	Imaging Findings	Comments
Congenital or developmental defect		
Lacunar skull (Fig SK2-4)	Large radiolucent areas of calvarial thinning in newborns and infants, producing a pattern simulating exaggerated convolutional impressions.	Usually an underlying meningocele of the skull or spine or hydrocephalus due to aqueductal stenosis or an Arnold-Chiari malformation. There may even be a complete calvarial defect (fenestra).
Parietal foramina (Fig SK2-5)	Small, symmetric, smoothly marginated openings situated posteriorly on both sides of the sagittal suture and through which emissary veins pass.	Normal finding with no pathologic significance. Although these foramina are usually small, they may be as large as 2 to 3 cm in diameter.
Parietal thinning	Crescentic lucencies over the middle and upper parts of the parietal bones.	Normal variant consisting of marked thinning of the superior portion of the parietal bones.
Pacchionian depressions (Fig SK2-6)	Multiple smooth erosions of the inner table representing underlying dural venous pools. Usually located parasagittally within 3 cm of the midline.	Arachnoid granulations (pacchionian bodies) for the absorption of cerebrospinal fluid fill the parasagittal venous lakes, which receive blood laterally from hemispheric veins and communicate medially with the superior sagittal sinus.
Epidermoid (primary cholesteatoma) (Fig SK2-7)	Generally round, frequently lobulated, lytic lesion with a thin, well-defined sclerotic border.	Benign lesion caused by the congenital inclusion of ectoderm in the diploic space. The keratinizing epithelium proliferates and desquamates, resulting in slow expansion of the tumor with erosion of diploic bone and displacement of the inner and outer tables. Erosion of the tumor through the inner table occasionally results in a large intracranial component.
Arachnoid cyst (Fig SK2-8)	Smooth lucency, often with a thin sclerotic rim.	Localized pressure causes outward bowing of the inner table and thinning of the diploic space. Although usually congenital, may be due to trauma or inflammation.
Dermoid	Small round lucency without surrounding sclerosis. Usually occurs near the midline.	Benign lesion arising in the diploic space as a result of the congenital inclusion of ectoderm and mesoderm.
Meningocele/ encephalocele	Midline bone defect that is generally round with smooth, well-defined, slightly sclerotic margins.	Herniation of brain, meninges, or both through a variably sized skull defect. Most commonly involves the occipital bone, followed by the frontal bone and the base of the skull.
Arteriovenous malformation	Localized area of skull thinning.	Infrequent manifestation overlying a superficial intracranial angioma.
Fibrous dysplasia (Fig SK2-9)	Blister-like expansion of bone with relative lucency in the center. There usually are areas of formless sclerosis lying in the lucent region and abnormally dense bone about the periphery of the lesion.	Radiolucency of the fibrous ''cysts'' is only relative because they are always surrounded by disorganized, densely woven bone. A mixed lytic and sclerotic pattern is the major calvarial manifestation.

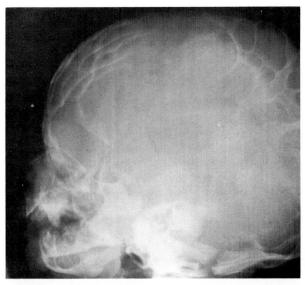

Fig SK2-4. Lacunar skull. Pattern resembling pronounced convolutional impressions.

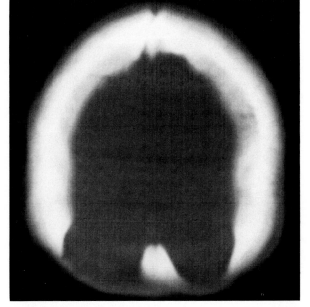

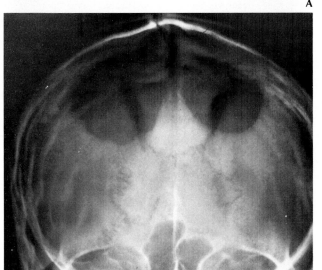

Fig SK2-5. Parietal foramina. (A) Plain skull radiograph. (B) CT scan.

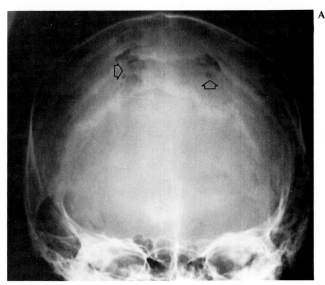

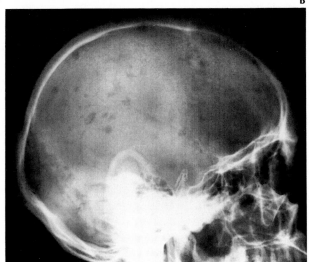

Fig SK2-6. Paccionian depressions. (A) Frontal and (B) lateral views of the skull show multiple lucent venous lakes (arrows).

Condition	Imaging Findings	Comments
Trauma		
Burr hole/ craniotomy	Lytic defect of variable size.	Margins are initially beveled and smooth, but may become irregular with new bone formation.
Skull fracture (Figs SK2-10 and SK2-11)	Sharp lucent line that is often irregular or jagged and occasionally branches.	Must be distinguished from suture lines (which generally have serrated edges and tend to be bilateral and symmetric) and vascular grooves (which usually have a smooth curving course and are not as sharp or distinct as a fracture line). Fractures involving the sinuses or mastoid air cells may result in posttraumatic pneumocephalus. Fractures intersecting a suture and coursing along it (diastatic fractures) cause sutural separation.
Leptomeningeal cyst (growing fracture) (Fig SK2-12)	Enlarging bone defect that typically has smooth, scalloped, well-defined margins.	Complication of skull fracture in infants and children. Soft tissue or a pouch of arachnoid membrane interposed between the fracture edges prevents healing and leads to widening of the fracture line.
Inflammation		
Osteomyelitis (Fig SK2-13)	Multiple irregular, poorly defined lytic areas that may enlarge and coalesce centrally with an expanding perimeter of small satellite foci. As elsewhere in the skeleton, the radiographic changes often lag 1 to 2 weeks behind the clinical symptoms and signs.	Most commonly due to direct extension of a suppurative process from the paranasal sinuses, mastoids, or scalp. May also develop after direct contaminating trauma. Pyogenic calvarial osteomyelitis may remain a predominantly lytic process until treated and may closely resemble a malignant lesion. The appearance of a host response (poorly defined reactive sclerosis superimposed on the initial lytic changes) is characteristic of chronic osteomyelitis caused by syphilis, tuberculosis, or fungal infection.
Hydatid (echinococcal) cyst	Large expanding lesion causing thinning and destruction of bone.	Multilocular cysts usually break through the bone, resulting in erosion and destruction of bone and invasion of the cranial cavity. A unilocular cyst may become an enormous expanding lesion with walls covered by impressions as in convolutional atrophy.
Cholesteatoma	Well-circumscribed lytic defect centered on the attic and often extending into the mastoid antrum.	Complication of chronic otomastoiditis that usually arises in the presence of sclerotic, poorly pneumatized mastoid air cells. Typically causes displacement or erosion of the ossicles, blunting of the scutum, and erosion of Korner's septum.
Sarcoidosis	Smooth lytic defect without marginal sclerosis.	Infrequent and nonspecific manifestation of this granulomatous disease of unknown etiology.
Miscellaneous		
Parietal thinning of aging	Symmetric thinning of the middle and upper parts of the parietal bones.	Although occurring as a normal variant in younger individuals, there is evidence that parietal thinning may increase, become more obvious, or turn into true defects with advancing age.
Histiocytosis X (Fig SK2-14)	Solitary or multiple small punched-out areas that originate in the diploic space and expand to perforate the inner and outer tables.	Margins of an eosinophilic granuloma are usually well defined and often beveled. The calvarial defect may have a bony density in its center (button sequestrum). The more malignant forms of the disease can produce multiple larger and more irregular skull defects in young children.

(continued page 786)

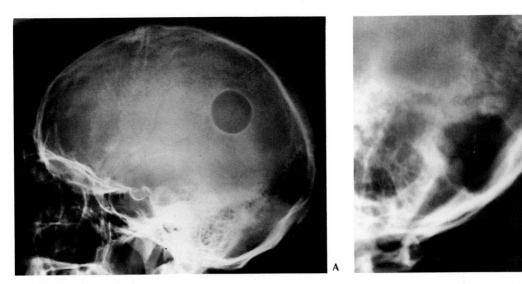

Fig SK2-7. Epidermoid. (A) Round lucent lesions with a smooth dense peripheral ring of sclerosis at the margin. (B) In another patient, there is erosion of the inner table of the posterior fossa.

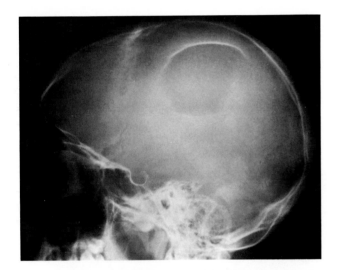

Fig SK2-8. Arachnoid cyst. Large parietal lucency with a thin sclerotic rim along its superior border.

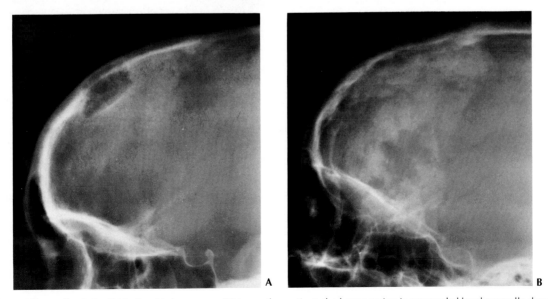

Fig SK2-9. Fibrous dysplasia. (A) Isolated lytic process. (B) In another patient, the lucent region is surrounded by abnormally dense bone.

Condition	Imaging Findings	Comments
Hyperparathyroidism (see Fig SK1-1)	Solitary or multiple poorly defined lesions surrounded by granular demineralization (salt-and-pepper skull).	Individual brown tumors and hemorrhagic cysts may be better seen after the removal of a parathyroid adenoma because of remineralization of the surrounding bone. After treatment, brown tumors heal by filling in with bone and may persist as sclerotic foci.
Radiation necrosis	Multiple lytic foci that coalesce. No evidence of sclerosis or periosteal new bone formation.	Aseptic necrosis of the skull, particularly a bone flap, may occur after the irradiation of an intracranial tumor. The appearance often mimics that of osteomyelitis, though it develops very slowly. The skull may return to an almost normal appearance after healing.
Paget's disease (osteoporosis circumscripta) (see Fig SK1-2)	Sharply circumscribed area of lucency representing the destructive phase of the disease. Primarily involves the outer table, sparing the inner table.	Deossification begins in the frontal or occipital area and spreads slowly to encompass the major portion of the calvarium. During the reparative process, the development of irregular islands of sclerosis in the inner table combined with thickening of the diploë and later the outer table results in the characteristic mottled, cotton-wool appearance.

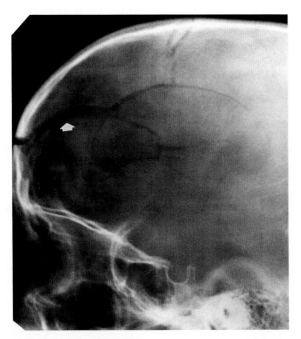

FIG SK2-10. **Skull fracture.** Widely diastatic fracture (arrow) extending to a stellate array of linear fractures.

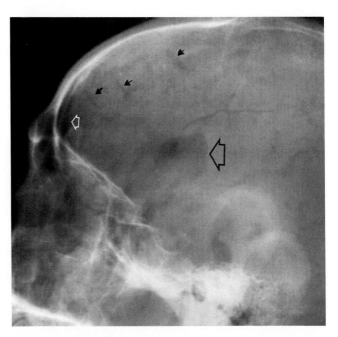

FIG SK2-11. **Posttraumatic pneumocephalus.** Lateral view of the skull made with a horizontal beam and the patient supine demonstrates air in the anterior recesses of the lateral ventricle (open black arrow), anterior to the frontal lobe (open white arrow), and in the subarachnoid space outlining the sulci (closed black arrows). The patient had sustained multiple facial fractures, some of which involved the walls of the sinuses.

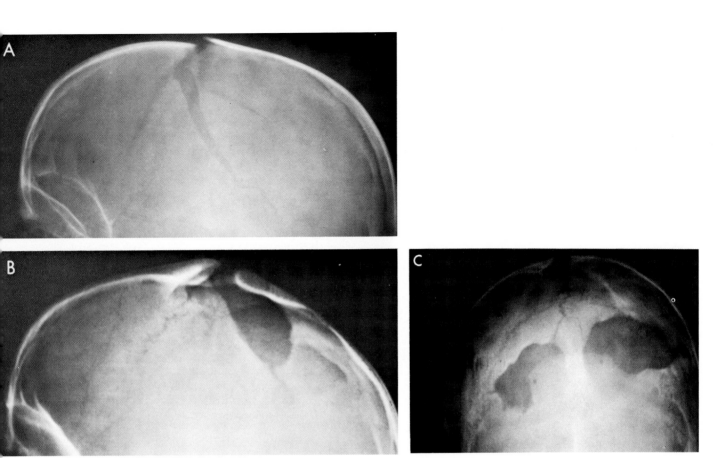

Fɪɢ SK2-12. Pulsating leptomeningeal cyst with residual bilateral large defects in the calvarium. (A) An initial lateral view shows diastatic bilateral comminuted parietal fractures after head injury during infancy. (B) Lateral and (C) frontal views 5 years later show large bilateral defects at the sites of the earlier parietal fractures. At surgery, the dura beneath the fractures was found to be torn. The bone on the margins of the defect is sclerotic and thickened.[2]

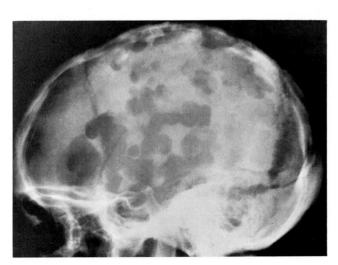

Fɪɢ SK2-13. Blastomycosis osteomyelitis. Diffuse areas of osteolytic destruction affect most of the calvarium.

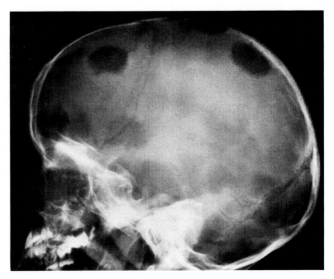

Fɪɢ SK2-14. Histiocytosis X. Multiple punched-out lytic lesions in the skull. Note the beveled appearance of the inner margins.

BUTTON SEQUESTRUM*

Condition	Comments
Eosinophilic granuloma **(Fig SK3-1)**	Most common cause and usually associated with pain or tenderness over the area. The lesion originates in the diploic space and expands to perforate both the inner and outer tables. The margins are usually well defined and often beveled.
Neoplasm **(Fig SK3-2)**	Meningioma; metastases; dermoid cyst; epidermoid; hemangioma.
Infection **(Fig SK3-3)**	Tuberculous osteitis; staphylococcal abscess of the scalp.
Radiation necrosis	More commonly produces purely lytic areas of destruction in the skull that do not develop until at least 5 years after therapy.
Iatrogenic	Appearance mimicking that of a button sequestrum due to a superficially placed polyethylene shunt reservoir within a burr hole.
Calvarial "doughnut" **(Fig SK3-4)**	Lucent region containing densities of various sizes that is an incidental finding on routine skull radiographs. This entity invariably has a sclerotic outer border and is benign and asymptomatic, unlike button sequestra, which are frequently associated with localized pain or soft-tissue abnormalities in the region of the bony lesion.

*Pattern: Round, lucent calvarial defect with a bony density or sequestrum in its center.

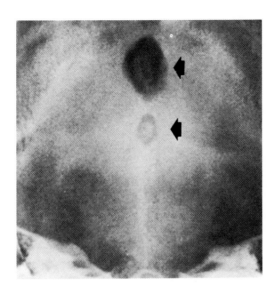

FIG SK3-1. Eosinophilic granuloma. Central retained bone is seen in each of two midline parietal lesions.[3]

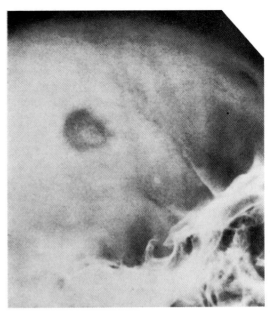

FIG SK3-2. Meningioma. The lucent lesion is irregularly marginated and residual bone remains in the center.[3]

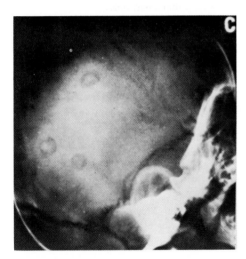

FIG SK3-3. Staphylococcal osteomyelitis. A central nidus is seen in each of the multiple round lytic lesions.[3]

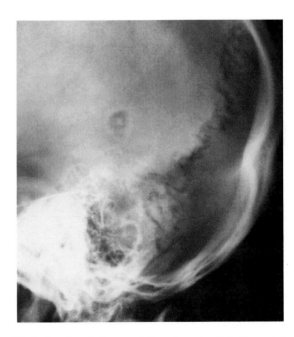

FIG SK3-4. Doughnut lesion containing a large density in the central area of a lucency.[4]

LOCALIZED INCREASED DENSITY OR HYPEROSTOSIS
OF THE CALVARIUM

Condition	Imaging Findings	Comments
Hyperostosis frontalis interna (Fig SK4-1)	Bilateral, symmetric bony overgrowth that thickens the inner table of the frontal bone.	Almost always found in women, especially those over age 35, and generally considered to be of no clinical significance. Because the irregular thickening surrounds the venous sinuses but does not obliterate them, on frontal views the superior sagittal sinus and the veins draining into it stand out as prominent radiolucent zones surrounded by dense hyperostosis.
Meningioma (Fig SK4-2)	Localized thickening of the inner table produces an area of increased calvarial density. Dense calcification or granular psammomatous deposits may be seen in the tumor.	Benign tumor that arises from arachnoid lining cells and is attached to the dura, most commonly over the convexities of the calvarium, olfactory groove, tuberculum sellae, parasagittal region, sylvian fissure, and cerebellopontine angle. Hyperostosis is caused by an invasion of the skull vault by tumor cells that simulates osteoblastic activity. Associated radiographic findings include prominence of meningeal vascular margins and enlargement of the foramen spinosum.
Fibrous dysplasia (Fig SK4-3)	Sclerotic ground-glass appearance (more common at the base of the skull and in the facial bones than as isolated involvement of the vault).	Involvement of the facial bones causes a marked sclerosis and thickening, often with obliteration of the sinuses and orbits, that creates a leonine appearance (leontiasis ossea). May also cause multiple irregular areas of lucency with expansion of the outer table of the skull.
Metastases (Figs SK4-4 and SK4-5)	Ill-defined, often multiple areas of increased density in the calvarium.	Most originate from carcinoma of the prostate or breast carcinoma (after therapy). Tangential radiographs may show localized thickening of bone due to subperiosteal reaction. Metastases to the skull more commonly produce multiple lytic areas.
Cephalhematoma (Fig SK4-6)	Shell-like deposition of calcium beginning around the periphery of and finally bridging a well-localized soft-tissue mass under the scalp.	Result of subperiosteal hemorrhage that usually occurs over the parietal area, is limited by sutural margins, and at times is associated with a fissure fracture of the skull. Primarily found in newborns, especially those with high birth weight and following forceps delivery. The entire mass eventually may become ossified, remodeled, and assimilated into the rest of the skull, usually leaving no residual signs.
Chronic osteomyelitis	Single or multiple areas of poorly defined bone sclerosis surrounding areas of rarefaction.	Low-grade bone infections (fungus, syphilis, tuberculosis) of long duration may occasionally provoke an osteoblastic reaction in which the vault is increased by periosteal new bone. Osteomyelitis much more commonly causes lytic bone destruction. Sequestra are rare because the skull has such a rich blood supply.

A
B

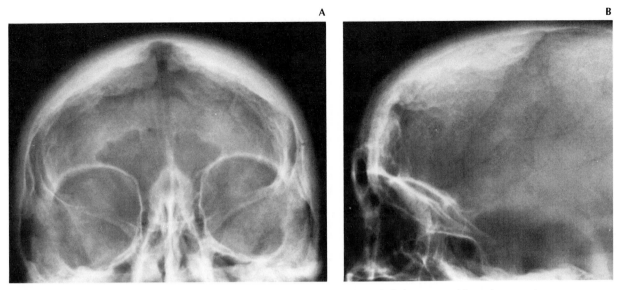

FIG SK4-1. Hyperostosis frontalis interna. (A) Frontal and (B) lateral views of the skull demonstrate bilateral symmetric osseous overgrowth that thickens the inner table of the frontal bone (open arrows). Note the prominent midline lucency representing the superior sagittal sinus.

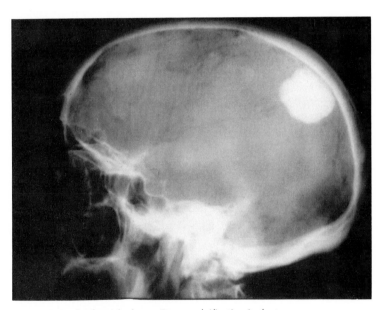

FIG SK4-2. Parietal meningioma. Dense calcification in the tumor.

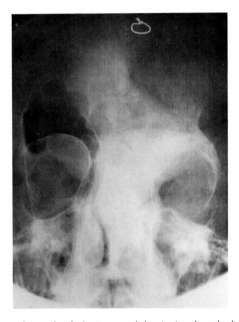

FIG SK4-3. Fibrous dysplasia. Increased density involves the left orbital region and extends to adjacent bones.[5]

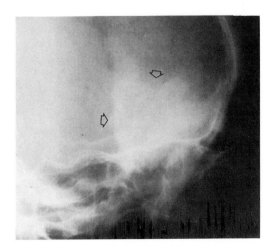

FIG SK4-4. Metastatic prostate carcinoma. Ill-defined area of increased density in the supraorbital region.

Condition	Imaging Findings	Comments
Cerebral hemiatrophy	Affected half of the skull vault is thicker and smaller than the contralateral side.	Probably due to a lack of the stimulus to bone remolding that is usually provided by the growth of the underlying cerebrum. The ipsilateral convolutional impressions of the inner table are few and shallow or are absent.
Hemangioma (Fig SK4-7)	Osseous spicules radiating from the center of a round, lucent lesion produce a typical sunburst pattern.	Pathognomonic appearance of this benign, slow-growing tumor involving the skull.
Other bone tumors (Fig SK4-8)	Various patterns of sclerosis.	Osteoma; osteochrondroma; osteosarcoma.
Radiation necrosis	Extensive area of thickened, featureless, and dense bone (often with associated lytic destruction).	Rare manifestation. Almost all the bone changes after therapeutic irradiation of an intracranial tumor are radiolucent.
Neurofibromatosis	Single or multiple areas of increased density.	Rare manifestation. Meningiomas associated with neurofibromatosis may be the cause of the hyperostosis.
Paget's disease	Localized area of dense expanded bone containing abnormally thick trabeculae.	Unusual manifestation in patients in whom the disease has remained localized but has progressed beyond the stage of lucent destruction. Most commonly a diffuse cotton-wool appearance.
Ischemic bone flap	Sclerosis may be superimposed on coalescing lytic areas at the center or margins of the flap.	May develop after surgical disruption of the blood supply to a craniotomy flap. The radiographic pattern resembles that of osteomyelitis, but the slow course and the absence of clinical signs and symptoms of infection help in making the distinction.

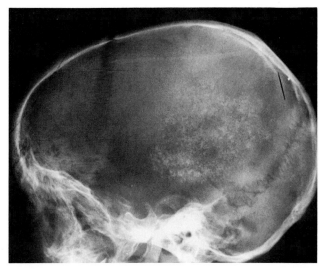

Fig SK4-5. Metastatic neuroblastoma. Diffuse granular calcific deposits in a metastatic lesion in the calvarium. Note the sutural widening, consistent with increased intracranial pressure.

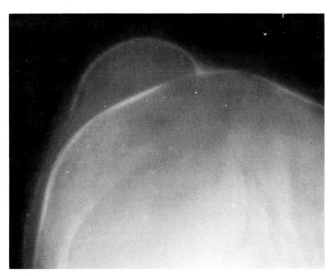

Fig SK4-6. Calcified cephalhematoma.

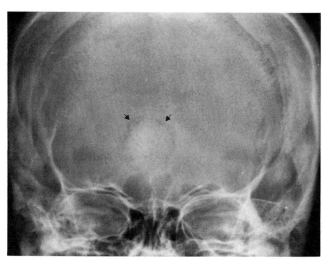

Fig SK4-7. Hemangioma (arrows).

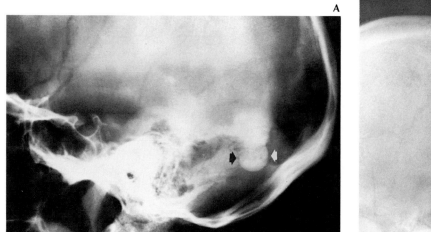

Fig SK4-8. Osteoma. (A) Lateral and (B) tangential views of the skull show sclerotic lesions (arrows) in two patients.

GENERALIZED INCREASED DENSITY OR THICKNESS
OF THE CALVARIUM

Condition	Imaging Findings	Comments
Severe anemia (Fig SK5-1)	Hyperplastic marrow proliferating under the periosteum causes spicules of new bone to be laid down perpendicular to the inner table (characteristic hair-on-end appearance of vertical striations in a radial pattern). There is widening of the diploic space and thinning or obliteration of the outer table.	Congenital hemolytic anemias (thalassemia, sickle cell anemia, hereditary spherocytosis); less commonly, iron-deficiency anemia or long-standing cyanotic congenital heart disease. The occipital bone inferior to the internal occipital protuberance is not involved because of the lack of bone marrow in this area. In thalassemia, marrow hyperplasia in the facial bones causes lack of pneumatization of the paranasal sinuses and mastoid air cells as well as lateral displacement of the orbits and forward displacement of the upper central incisors that produce malocclusion and overbite (rodent facies).
Hyperostosis interna generalisata	Generalized calvarial thickening with irregularity of the inner table.	Condition of unknown significance that affects the entire supratentorial portion of the skull.
Paget's disease (Fig SK5-2)	Development of irregular islands of reparative sclerosis in the inner table followed by thickening of the diploë and later the outer table, resulting in a mottled, cotton-wool appearance.	Downward thrust of the heavy head on the softened bone of the spine may cause basilar invagination of the skull, compression of the brainstem, and numerous cranial nerve deficits.
Fibrous dysplasia (Fig SK5-3)	Sclerosis and thickening of the facial bones, often with obliteration of the sinuses and orbits, produce a leonine appearance (leontiasis ossea).	In the calvarium, there are usually multiple irregular areas of lucency with expansion of the outer table of the skull and only minimal involvement of the inner table.
Osteoblastic metastases (Fig SK5-4)	Multiple, fairly discrete, dense bony nodules of various sizes throughout the skull.	Usually secondary to carcinoma of the prostate, though almost any metastatic neoplasm may rarely produce this appearance.
Acromegaly	Generalized thickening and increased density of the bones of the skull. Most prominent in the frontal and occipital regions, leading to characteristic frontal bossing and enlargement of the occipital protuberance.	Other characteristic findings include enlargement of the sella turcica, excessive pneumatization of the paranasal sinuses (especially the frontal) and mastoids, lengthening of the mandible, and an increase in the mandibular angle (prognathous jaw).
Cerebral atrophy in childhood	Generalized calvarial thickening with few and shallow convolutional impressions in the inner table.	The greater than normal thickness is more easily recognized when it affects only half of the calvarium (cerebral hemiatrophy).
Chronic increased intracranial pressure	Generalized calvarial thickening may develop in adults.	Usually related to an intermittent congenital obstruction. Abnormal calvarial thickness may occur in children after successful relief of increased intracranial pressure (surgery for hydrocephalus).

A

B

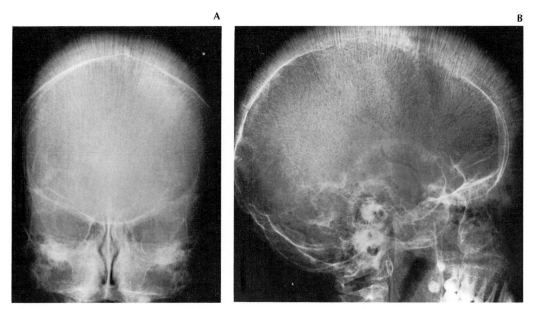

FIG SK5-1. **Thalassemia.** (A) Frontal and (B) lateral views of the skull demonstrate the hair-on-end appearance. Note the normal appearance of the calvarium inferior to the internal occipital protuberance and the poor pneumatization of the visualized paranasal sinuses.

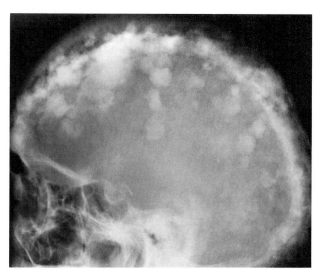

FIG SK5-2. **Paget's disease.** Typical cotton-wool appearance of the skull.

A

B

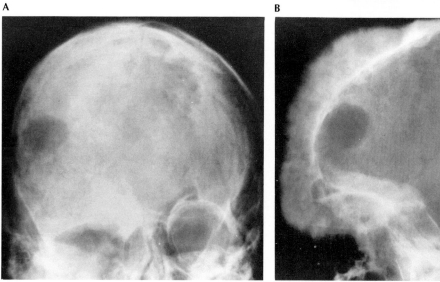

FIG SK5-3. **Fibrous dysplasia.** (A) Frontal and (B) lateral films show generalized sclerosis of the skull with a lucent area in the right frontal region. Note that the thickening primarily involves the outer table, unlike Paget's disease or osteoblastic metastases.

Condition	Imaging Findings	Comments
Dilantin therapy	Generalized calvarial thickening.	Develops after prolonged treatment with this anti-epileptic agent.
Myelosclerosis (myelofibrosis, myeloid metaplasia)	Replacement of the diploic space by dense amorphous bone.	Gradual replacement of the marrow by fibrosis produces a diffuse increase in bone density that primarily affects the spine, ribs, and pelvis.
Congenital syndromes (Fig SK5-5)	Generalized increase in calvarial density with variable amounts of bone thickening.	Osteopetrosis; pyknodysostosis; generalized cortical hyperostosis (van Buchem's disease); Engelmann-Camurati disease (progressive diaphyseal dysplasia); craniometaphyseal dysplasia; melorheostosis; dystrophia myotonica; hyperphosphatasia.
Abnormalities of calcium and phosphorus metabolism	Generalized or patchy increase in calvarial density.	Hypervitaminosis D; idiopathic hypercalcemia; hypoparathyroidism and pseudohypoparathyroidism; patients under treatment for hyperparathyroidism and rickets.
Fluorosis	Generalized increase in calvarial density.	Dense skeletal sclerosis is most prominent in the vertebrae and pelvis.
Congenital syphilis	Generalized increase in calvarial density.	Infrequent manifestation of chronic syphilitic osteitis due to congenital infection.

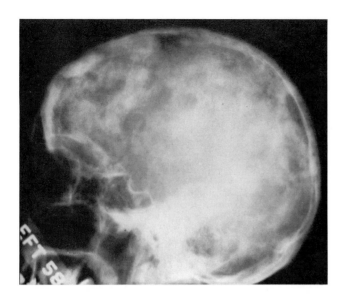

FIG SK5-4. Osteoblastic metastases. Multiple sclerotic lesions secondary to metastases from carcinoma of the breast.

A

B

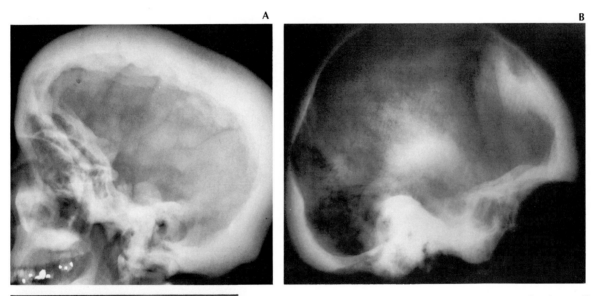

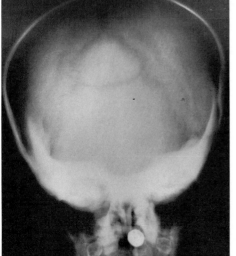

C

FIG SK5-5. Congenital syndromes. (A) Osteopetrosis. (B) Generalized cortical hyperostosis (van Buchem's disease). (C) Craniometaphyseal dysplasia. Note the unusual dense sutural bone.

NORMAL (PHYSIOLOGIC) INTRACRANIAL CALCIFICATIONS

Condition	Comments
Pineal gland **(Fig SK6-1)**	Pineal calcification is visible on lateral skull radiographs in 50% to 70% of adults (and even in 5% of children under age 10). CT scanning shows calcification in almost all pineal glands of adults and in a high percentage of children. The calcification is more difficult to detect on frontal views and varies from a single faint speck to a ring up to 1 cm in diameter (larger calcification in this region is probably pathologic and suggests a pinealoma or aneurysm of the vein of Galen). Pineal calcification appears about 3 cm above the highest posterior elevation of the petrous pyramids on lateral views and in the midline on frontal projections (displacement of the calcification more than 3 mm to one side of the midline suggests an intracranial mass).
Habenula **(Fig SK6-1)**	Calcification of the choroid plexus in the posterior portion of the third ventricle along the anterior surface of the habenular commissure. The typical C-shaped configuration is open posteriorly and located a few millimeters anterior and superior to the pineal gland. Although less common than pineal calcification, habenular calcification may occur in the absence of the former and provide an alternative midline indicator.
Choroid plexus **(Fig SK6-2)**	The glomus of the choroid plexus, which is located at the junction of the body of the lateral ventricle with the posterior and temporal horns, calcifies in about 20% of patients. There is a variable pattern of calcification ranging from curvilinear peripheral rings to amorphous "popcorn" nodules to a fine granularity. In lateral views the calcification is situated just posterior and superior to the pineal gland. On frontal views it is usually bilateral and reasonably symmetric, at the same level, and 2.5 to 3 cm from the midline.
Dura **(Figs SK6-3 to SK6-6)**	Dural calcification may occur along the superior sagittal sinus, falx, tentorium, petroclinoid ligaments, and interclinoid ligaments. Calcification of the falx most commonly occurs anteriorly and appears as a thin, linear opacification seen "end on" on frontal views. Calcification in the free edge of the tentorium has an inverted-V shape on frontal views, while a V-shaped appearance at the vertex reflects dural calcification around the sagittal sinus. Elderly patients often have calcification of the petroclinoid ligaments (connecting the tip of the dorsum sellae to the apex of the petrous bone) and the interclinoid ligaments (causing apparent bridging across the sella).

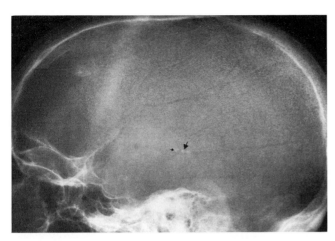

FIG SK6-1. **Pineal and habenula.** Lateral view of the skull shows calcification in the pineal gland (large arrow). Calcification in the habenular commissure (small arrow) lies a few millimeters anterior to the pineal gland and has a typical C-shaped configuration that opens posteriorly.

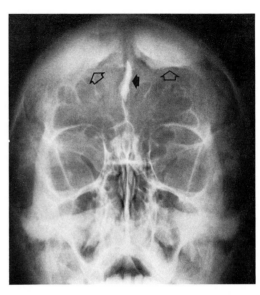

FIG SK6-3. **Falx.** Dense linear calcification in the midline (black arrow). Of incidental note is bilateral hyperostosis frontalis interna (open arrows).

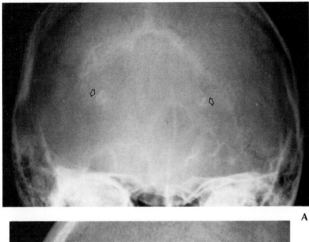

A

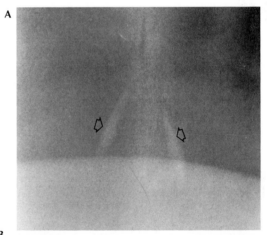

A

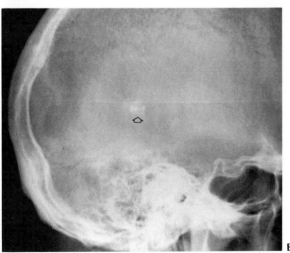

B

FIG SK6-2. **Choroid plexus.** (A) Frontal and (B) lateral views of the skull show the typical calcification (arrows).

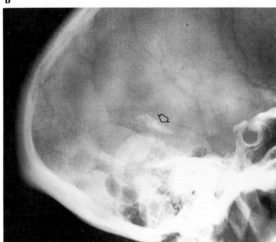

B

FIG SK6-4. **Tentorium.** (A) Frontal view shows the characteristic inverted-V shape of calcification in the free edge of the tentorium. (B) Lateral view of the calcification (arrow).

Condition	Comments
"Physiologic" calcifications **Internal carotid artery** **(Fig SK6-7)**	Curvilinear streaks or dense tubular S-shaped calcification in the region of the sella turcica. Arteriosclerotic calcification is common in the internal carotid artery as it passes through the cavernous sinus. On frontal views the calcification appears as a circular ring on either side of the sella.
Basal ganglia and **dentate nucleus** **(Figs SK6-8 and** **SK6-9)**	Basal ganglia calcification appears as punctate to conglomerate densities that are symmetric and parasagittal on frontal views and may assume a gentle curve that roughly parallels the squamosal suture on lateral views. Dentate nucleus calcification is often obscured by the mastoid air cells on lateral views and is best seen on the occipital (Towne) view as symmetric crescentic densities. Calcification in the basal ganglia and, less commonly, the dentate nucleus of the cerebellum may be a normal variant or a manifestation of such conditions as hypoparathyroidism, pseudohypoparathyroidism, infections, birth anoxia, carbon monoxide poisoning, and Cockayne's syndrome (a rare form of truncal dwarfism with retinal atrophy).

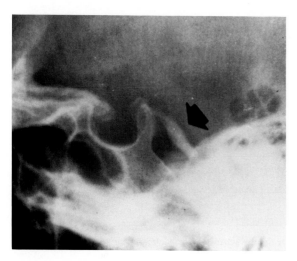

FIG SK6-5. **Petroclinoid ligament** (arrow).

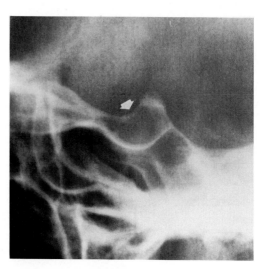

FIG SK6-6. **Interclinoid ligament** (arrow).

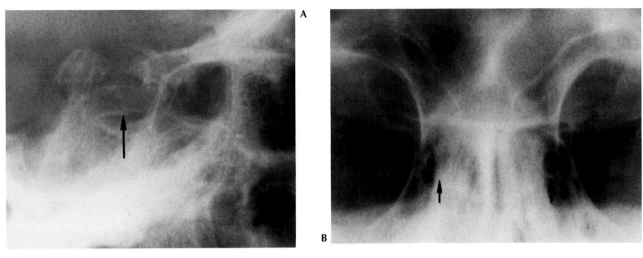

FIG SK6-7. **Calcification in the carotid siphon.** (A) On the lateral view the calcification appears tubular and S-shaped (arrow). (B) On an inclined posteroanterior projection, there is calcification bilaterally (arrows) that appears as circular ringlike densities lateral to and slightly above the floor of the sella.[6]

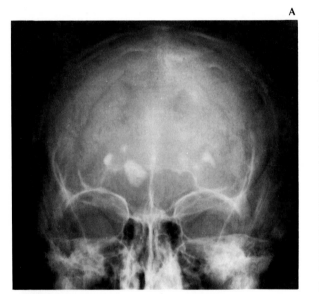

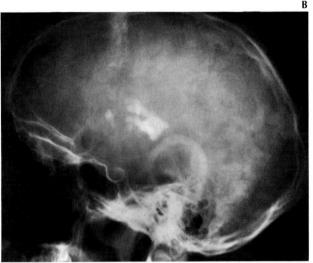

FIG SK6-8. **Basal ganglia.** (A) Frontal and (B) lateral views of the skull demonstrate calcification in the basal ganglia in a patient with hypoparathyroidism.

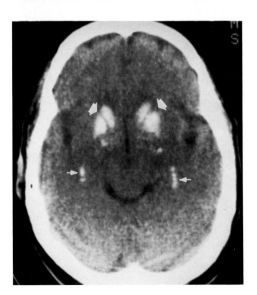

FIG SK6-9. **Basal ganglia.** CT scan shows characteristic bilateral calcification (broad arrows). Note also the small calcific deposits in the tail of the caudate nuclei (thin arrows).

SOLITARY INTRACRANIAL CALCIFICATIONS

Condition	Imaging Findings	Comments
Normal (physiologic) calcification (see SK6)	Various patterns and positions.	Pineal gland; habenula; choroid plexus; dura (falx, tentorium, sagittal sinus); petroclinoid and interclinoid ligaments (see page 798).
Vascular		
Arteriosclerosis	Curvilinear streaks or dense tubular S-shaped calcification, primarily in the parasellar area.	Common appearance in the intracavernous portion (siphon) of the internal carotid artery. Appears as a circular ring of calcification on either side of the sella on frontal views.
Aneurysm (see Fig SK9-1)	Curvilinear ringlike calcification in the region of the circle of Willis.	Calcification is most common in atherosclerotic aneurysms of the intracavernous segment of the internal carotid artery (may be associated with erosion of the sidewall of the sella and the margins of the superior orbital fissure). There is usually partial or complete thrombosis of the aneurysm.
Vein of Galen aneurysm	Thin crescents of calcification producing a characteristic eggshell pattern.	Actually represents a variceal expansion of this vessel caused by increased blood flow from an adjacent arteriovenous malformation. The calcification is more delicate than that seen in a pineal region tumor.
Arteriovenous malformation (angioma)	Amorphous small calcific patches or flakes or a more strikingly curvilinear pattern of calcification.	About 25% of arteriovenous malformations show calcification on skull radiographs. The calcium deposits may be in the walls of component vessels (arteries and veins) or in the intervening dystrophic brain tissue.
Neoplasm		
Craniopharyngioma (Fig SK7-1)	Nodular, amorphous, or cloudlike calcification in mixed or solid lesions. Shell-like calcification along the periphery of cystic lesions. Calcification occurs in 80% to 90% of childhood tumors and 30% of tumors in adults.	Benign congenital, or ''rest-cell,'' tumor with cystic and solid components. Usually originates above the sella turcica, depressing the optic chiasm and extending up into the third ventricle. Less commonly, a craniopharyngioma lies in the sella, where it compresses the pituitary gland and may erode adjacent bony walls.
Glioma (Fig SK7-2)	Various patterns of calcification ranging from a few punctate deposits or irregular linear streaks to a densely calcified nodule.	Calcification is most commonly seen in slow-growing gliomas. Oligodendrogliomas (typically involving the frontoparietal white matter in young adults) calcify in about 50% of cases. Although low-grade astrocytomas calcify less frequently (about 20%) than oligodendrogliomas, they are much more common and therefore account for most instances of calcified gliomas.
Ependymoma	Granular or flocculent calcification, often near a ventricular surface, occurs in about 15% of cases.	Most commonly arises from the wall of the fourth ventricle in children and from a lateral ventricle in adults.

(continued page 804)

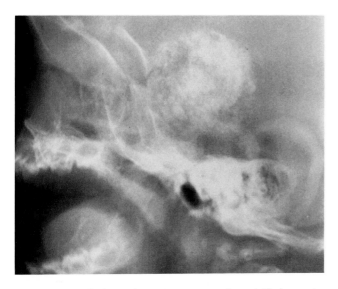

FIG SK7-1. Craniopharyngioma. Large suprasellar calcified mass in a child.

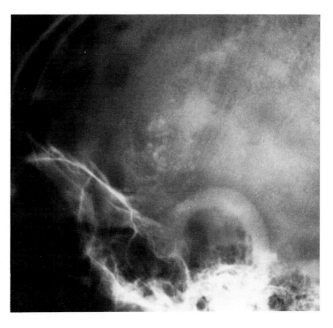

FIG SK7-2. Oligodendroglioma. Clusters of small stippled calcifications in a tumor in the inferior frontal region.[6]

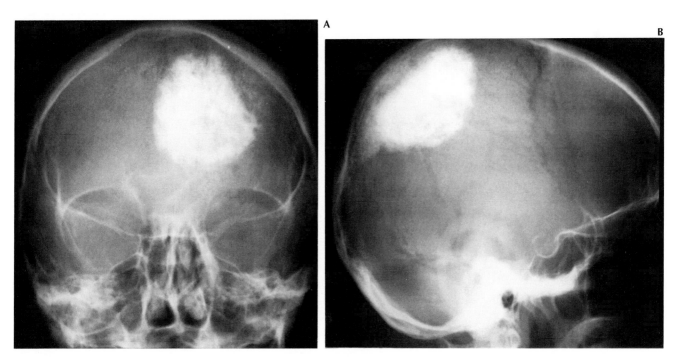

FIG SK7-3. Meningioma. (A) Frontal and (B) lateral views of the skull show dense calcification in a large left parieto-occipital tumor.

Condition	Imaging Findings	Comments
Meningioma (Fig SK7-3)	Dense calcification or granular psammomatous deposits may be visible in the tumor in about 10% of cases. Invasion of bone by tumor cells that stimulate osteoblastic activity causes hyperostosis of the calvarium.	Benign tumor that arises from arachnoid lining cells and is attached to the dura. The most common sites are the convexities of the calvarium, olfactory groove, tuberculum sellae, parasagittal region, sylvian fissure, and cerebellopontine angle. Associated radiographic findings include prominence of meningeal vascular markings and enlargement of the foramen spinosum.
Pinealoma (Fig SK7-4)	Central punctate calcification or peripheral calcific shell (> 1 cm) in about 50% of cases.	Most common tumors of the pineal region are germinomas and teratomas, both of which occur predominantly in males under 25 years of age and may be associated with precocious puberty. "Ectopic pinealomas" develop elsewhere in the brain, especially in the anterior aspect of the third ventricle or in the suprasellar cistern.
Pituitary adenoma	Flakes, curvilinear lines, or even complete shells of calcification develop in about 5% of cases.	Calcification occurs in large chromophobe adenomas (rarely eosinophilic adenomas) and is usually associated with ballooning or erosion of the sella. Symptoms of pituitary tumors may result from a mass effect causing compression of parasellar structures or from an alteration in pituitary trophic hormone production (increased levels with secreting adenomas; decreased levels caused by compression of the pituitary gland by a nonsecreting tumor).
Chordoma (see Fig SK9-4)	Flocculent or dense calcification in the parasellar region associated with destruction of the clivus and often extension to the sella.	Tumor arising from remnants of the notochord that most commonly involves the clivus and lower lumbosacral region. Although locally invasive, the tumors do not metastasize. Chordomas arising at the base of the skull produce the striking clinical picture of multiple cranial nerve palsies on one or both sides combined with a retropharyngeal mass and erosion of the clivus.
Lipoma of corpus callosum (Fig SK7-5)	Two symmetric curvilinear calcifications with their concavities facing the midline.	Pathognomonic appearance with the calcification actually located in adjacent cerebral tissue.
Choroid plexus papilloma (Fig SK7-6)	Intraventricular calcification in about 25% of cases.	Uncommon tumor that primarily occurs in children under 5 years of age. Unlike most tumors, choroid plexus papillomas most commonly occur in the lateral ventricles in children and in the fourth ventricle in adults. Hydrocephalus may be caused by overproduction of cerebrospinal fluid or obstruction of cerebrospinal fluid pathways.
Other brain tumors	Extremely rare calcification.	Metastases (especially osteogenic sarcoma and mucinous adenocarcinoma of the colon), angioma, neurofibroma, hamartoma.

(continued page 806)

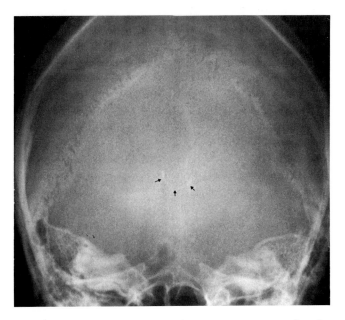

Fig SK7-4. Pinealoma. Shell of calcification (arrows) surrounding the inferior half of this 1.5-cm tumor.

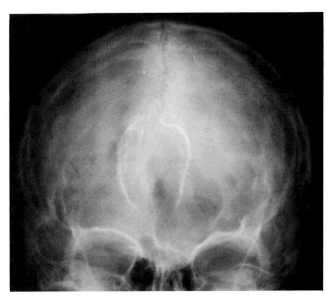

Fig SK7-5. Lipoma of the corpus callosum. Dense curvilinear calcification at the margins of a rounded midline mass anteriorly. Between the calcifications, the skull appears slightly rarefied due to the fat content of the lipoma.

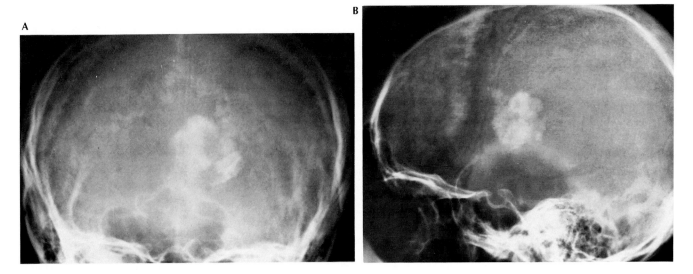

Fig SK7-6. Choroid plexus papilloma. (A) Frontal and (B) lateral views show dense calcification in the intraventricular mass.

Condition	Imaging Findings	Comments
Calvarial tumor (see Fig SK4-7)	Calcification may mimic meningioma or chordoma.	Enchondroma, osteochondroma, osteoma, hemangioma.
Infection		
Tuberculoma	Dense, coarsely granular calcification similar to that found in tuberculous lymph nodes. There may be multiple calcific foci.	Tuberculous infection of the brain parenchyma most commonly involves the cerebellum (especially in children) or cerebral cortex. Calcification may also develop after streptomycin treatment of tuberculous meningitis.
Healed brain abscess	Dense, irregular calcification.	Uncommon manifestation that is the end result of organization of the septic process.
Meningitis (Fig SK7-7)	Collections of small, not very dense, amorphous calcific nodules.	Infrequent occurrence following bacterial or tuberculous meningitis (especially after streptomycin therapy).
Hydatid (echinococcal) cyst	Peripheral rim or central clump of calcification.	Involvement of the brain is relatively common in endemic areas. Cerebral hydatid cysts may attain considerable size.
Torulosis	Irregular calcification in a cerebral granuloma or brain abscess.	Infection by the yeastlike fungus *Cryptococcus neoformans*, which lives in the soil, particularly that contaminated by pigeon droppings. Most frequently an opportunistic invader that infects debilitated patients or those undergoing steroid or antibiotic therapy.
Miscellaneous		
Hematoma (Fig SK7-8)	Large curvilinear sheets or plaques of calcification that follow the curvature of the skull.	Chronic subdural hematomas may have calcification in their membranes and margins. A nonspecific amorphous pattern of calcification rarely occurs in old intracerebral hematomas. This complication of neglected head injury is now rare because of improved diagnosis and treatment.
Radiation necrosis	Fine amorphous calcification.	Infrequent manifestation that may develop long after irradiation of the brain.
Scarring (gliosis)	Dense area of calcification (occasionally multiple) of variable size.	Incidental finding that may represent the end result of birth trauma or an injury later in life that has produced an intracerebral hematoma.
Cerebral infarct	Calcification that is usually in the distribution of the anterior or medial cerebral artery.	Rare manifestation that is probably related to necrosis or hemorrhage.

A

B

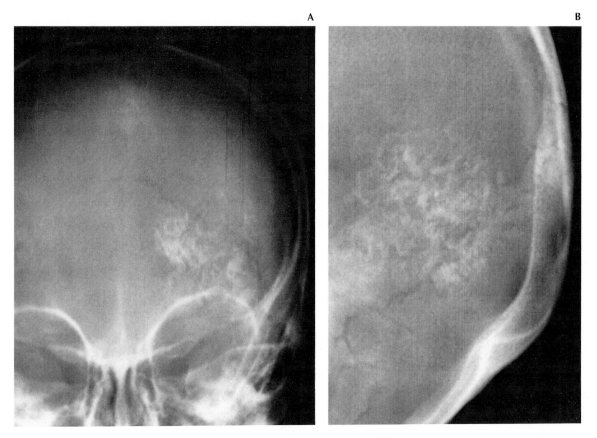

FIG SK7-7. Meningitis. (A) Frontal and (B) coned lateral views show amorphous calcification after meningococcal meningitis.

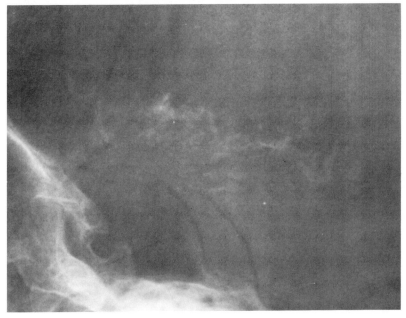

FIG SK7-8. Hematoma. Amorphous plaques of calcification after intracerebral hemorrhage.

MULTIPLE INTRACRANIAL CALCIFICATIONS

Condition	Imaging Findings	Comments
Normal (physiologic) calcification	Various patterns and positions (see page 798).	Pineal gland; habenula; choroid plexus; dura (falx, tentorium, sagittal sinus); petroclinoid and interclinoid ligaments.
Basal ganglia calcification (Fig SK8-1)	Punctate to conglomerate densities that are symmetric and parasagittal on frontal views and may assume a gentle curve that roughly parallels the squamosal suture on lateral views.	May be a normal variant or a manifestation of such conditions as hypoparathyroidism, pseudohypoparathyroidism, infections, birth anoxia, carbon monoxide poisoning, and Cockayne's syndrome (a rare form of truncal dwarfism with retinal atrophy).
Vascular calcification	Various patterns of ringlike, curvilinear, and amorphous calcification (see page 780).	Arteriosclerosis in the intracavernous portion (siphon) of the internal carotid artery; aneurysms; and arteriovenous malformations.
Infection		
Cytomegalic inclusion disease (Fig SK8-2)	Stippled or curvilinear calcifications outlining an enlarged ventricular system.	Viral disorder that predominantly affects neonates and small infants and produces a clinical syndrome that includes jaundice, hepatosplenomegaly, purpura, and respiratory distress. In addition to the typical calcifications, there is usually marked atrophy of the brain with dilatation of the ventricular system.
Toxoplasmosis (Fig SK8-3)	Small granulomatous calcifications diffusely scattered throughout the brain parenchyma. Meningeal calcifications are plaquelike, while calcifications in the basal ganglia or thalamus tend to be striated or curvilinear.	Protozoan infection that is the most common cause of scattered intracranial calcifications in the neonate (may be indistinguishable from cytomegalic inclusion disease). In up to 80% of patients, obstruction of the aqueduct or one of the foramina by toxoplasmic granulomas causes hydrocephalus. Postinflammatory scarring with cerebral atrophy may result in microcephaly.
Viral encephalitis (Fig SK8-4)	Various patterns of calcification that may mimic toxoplasmosis or cytomegalic inclusion disease.	Rubella; neonatal herpes simplex; poliomyelitis; chickenpox; measles.
Cysticercosis (Fig SK8-5)	Multiple small oval calcifications. Dense central calcification of the larval scolex may be surrounded by an area of lucency and rimmed by calcium deposition in the overlying cyst capsule.	Infestation by the larval form of the pork tapeworm (*Taenia solium*). Central nervous system involvement commonly occurs and can produce epilepsy, mental disturbances, loss of vision, and even a fulminating disease that resembles acute encephalitis. Large cysts may mimic cerebral tumors, while cysts in the ventricles may cause hydrocephalus.
Trichinosis	Multiple small calcifications (virtually identical to cysticercosis).	Infestation by encysted larvae of *Trichinella spiralis*. Calcification in skeletal muscles is unusual in trichinosis, unlike cysticercosis, in which muscles frequently show prominent linear or oval calcifications.
Paragonomiasis (Fig SK8-6)	Intracranial calcifications appear as amorphous punctate densities, ill-defined small nodules, or aggregates of round or oval cysts that have characteristic peripheral areas of increased density ("soap bubbles"). Although individual cysts are often small, when grouped together a cluster may measure up to 10 cm in diameter.	Infestation by the liver fluke *Paragonimus westermani,* which is common in the Orient in persons who eat raw, or poorly cooked, infected crabs or crayfish. Intracranial calcifications are almost always unilateral and usually occur in the parietal and occipital lobes. Other manifestations include increased intracranial pressure, space-occupying lesions (large cysts or abscesses), subcortical atrophy, and arachnoiditis.

(continued page 810)

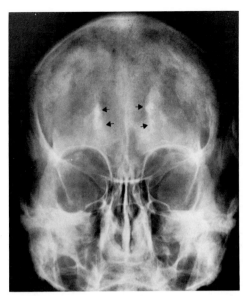

FIG SK8-1. **Basal ganglia calcification** (arrows) in lead poisoning.

FIG SK8-2. **Cytomegalovirus.** (A) Frontal and (B) lateral views of the skull of a young infant demonstrate multiple intracranial calcifications with a typical periventricular distribution.

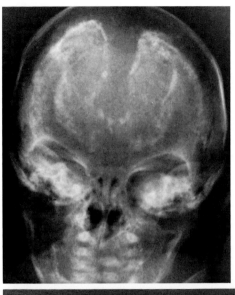

A

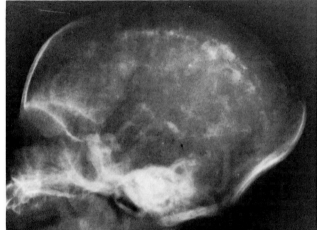

B

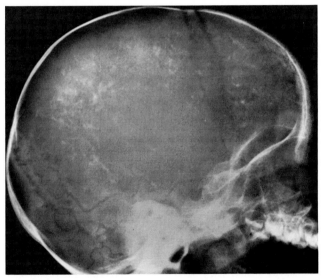

FIG SK8-3. **Toxoplasmosis.** Diffuse flecks, plaques, and nodules of calcification scattered throughout the brain parenchyma and meninges.

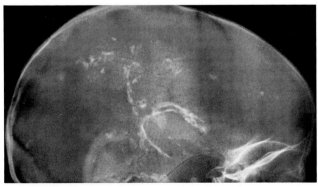

FIG SK8-4. **Viral encephalitis** mimicking cytomegalic inclusion disease.

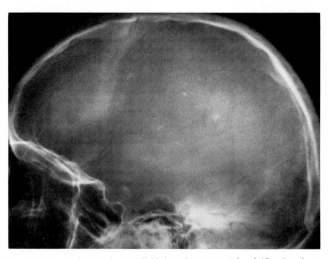

FIG SK8-5. **Cysticercosis.** Small blebs of intracranial calcification in a young Guatamalan immigrant with headaches and seizures.

Condition	Imaging Findings	Comments
Hydatid (echinococcal) cysts	Central clumps of calcification or calcification of the peripheral rims of cysts.	Involvement of the brain is relatively common in endemic areas. Cerebral hydatid cysts may attain considerable size.
Torulosis	Irregular calcification in cerebral granulomas or brain abscesses.	Infection by the yeastlike fungus *Cryptococcus neoformans,* which lives in the soil, particularly that contaminated by pigeon droppings. Most frequently an opportunistic invader that infects debilitated patients or those undergoing steriod or antibiotic therapy.
Tuberculomas	Dense, coarsely granular calcification similar to that found in tuberculous lymph nodes.	Tuberculous infection of the brain parenchyma most commonly involves the cerebellum (especially in children) or cerebral cortex. A more plaquelike pattern of calcification may develop after streptomycin treatment of tuberculous meningitis.
Healed brain abscesses	Dense, irregular calcifications.	Uncommon manifestation that is the end result of organization of the septic process.
Tuberous sclerosis	Clusters of calcified hamartomatous nodules develop in about 75% of patients, primarily in the walls of the lateral ventricles.	Inherited disorder manifested by the clinical triad of convulsive seizures, mental deficiency, and adenoma sebaceum. The brain is typically involved with hyperplastic nodules of malformed glial-neuroglial tissue. Large lesions may obstruct the aqueduct or ventricular foramina and produce hydrocephalus. Renal angiomyolipomas occur in about half the patients.
Sturge-Weber syndrome (encephalotrigeminal angiomatosis) (Fig SK8-7)	Undulating parallel plaques of calcification in the brain cortex that appear to follow the cerebral convolutions and most often develop in the parieto-occipital area.	Congenital vascular anomaly in which a localized meningeal venous angioma occurs in conjunction with an ipsilateral facial angioma (port wine nevus). The clinical findings include mental retardation, seizure disorders, and hemiatrophy and hemiparesis. Hemiatrophy leads to elevation of the base of the skull and enlargement and increased aeration of the ipsilateral mastoid air cells.
Von Hippel–Lindau disease (cerebelloretinal hemangioblastomatosis)	Calcifications in retinal and, less frequently, intracranial angiomas.	Vascular malformations of the retina (usually multiple capillary angiomas) combined with one or more slow-growing hemangioblastomas of the cerebellum and spinal cord (in which calcification is rare). There may be angiomas of the liver, pancreas, and kidneys; renal tumors; and pheochromocytomas.
Multiple tumors	Various patterns of calcification (see page 802).	Meningiomas, gliomas, rare metastases.
Scarring (gliosis)	Dense calcified areas of various sizes.	Incidental finding that may represent the end result of birth trauma or injuries later in life that have produced intracerebral hematomas.
Hematoma	Large curvilinear sheets or plaques of calcification that follow the curvature of the skull.	Chronic subdural hematomas may show calcification in their membranes and margins. A nonspecific amorphous pattern of calcification rarely occurs in old intracerebral hematomas.

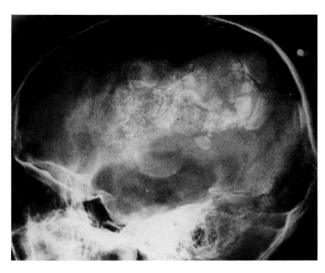

Fig SK8-6. Paragonomiasis. Characteristic soap-bubble appearance of calcification in the parietal area and posterior part of the frontal lobe. The dorsum sellae is not visible, a result of increased intracranial pressure.[7]

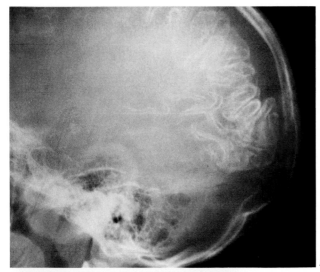

A   **Fig SK8-7. Sturge-Weber syndrome.** (A) Plain film. (B) CT scan.

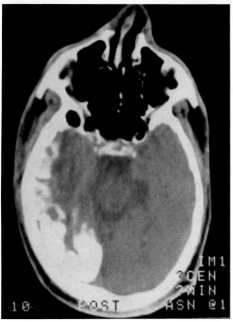

B

SELLAR OR PARASELLAR CALCIFICATIONS

Condition	Imaging Findings	Comments
Normal structures (see Fig SK6-5)	Ligamentous calcification between the tip of the dorsum sellae and the apex of the petrous bone. Also interclinoid bridging (see Fig SK6-6).	Calcification of the petroclinoid or interclinoid ligaments commonly occurs in elderly patients.
Internal carotid artery	Calcification of the carotid siphon produces small curvilinear streaks or dense S-shaped tubular densities.	Common manifestation of arteriosclerosis involving the internal carotid artery as it passes through the cavernous sinus.
Aneurysm (Fig SK9-1)	Curvilinear or complete ring of calcification.	Most commonly in arteriosclerotic aneurysms of the cavernous portion of the internal carotid artery. May erode the sidewall of the sella and the margins of the superior orbital fissure.
Craniopharyngioma (Fig SK9-2)	Suprasellar calcification that may be nodular, amorphous, or cloudlike in mixed or solid lesions or shell-like along the periphery of cystic lesions. About 80% to 90% of childhood craniopharyngiomas show calcification (30% of adult tumors).	Benign congenital, or rest-cell, tumor with cystic and solid components. Usually originates above the sella turcica, depressing the optic chiasm and extending up into the third ventricle. Less commonly, the tumor may lie in the sella, where it compresses the pituitary gland and may erode adjacent bony walls.
Optic chiasm glioma	Speckled calcification may develop in large tumors.	Although the sella is usually normal, there may be undercutting of the anterior clinoid processes with deepening of the chiasmatic groove.
Meningioma (Fig SK9-3)	Calcification in the mass or reactive hyperostosis of adjacent bone.	Parasellar meningiomas may arise from the tuberculum sellae, diaphragma sellae, cerebellopontine angle cistern, cavernous sinus, or medial sphenoidal ridge.
Chordoma (Fig SK9-4)	Retrosellar flocculent calcification may infrequently develop in a large soft-tissue mass in association with ill-defined bone destruction or cortical expansion of the clivus.	Rare tumor, arising from remnants of the notocord, that primarily involves the clivus and lower lumbosacral region. May produce multiple cranial nerve palsies on one or both sides combined with a retropharyngeal mass and erosion of the clivus. The tumor may be locally invasive but does not metastasize.
Ectopic pinealoma	Punctate calcification in the mass.	Tumor with the histologic appearance of a pinealoma but developing elsewhere in the brain at some distance from the normal pineal gland. Generally occurs in the anterior aspect of the third ventricle or in the suprasellar cistern. The clinical triad of bitemporal hemianopsia, hypopituitarism, and diabetes insipidus may simulate a craniopharyngioma.

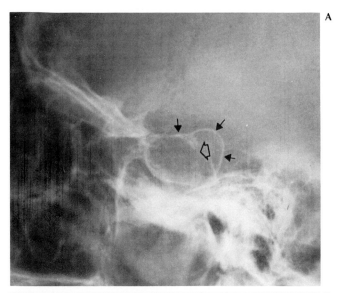

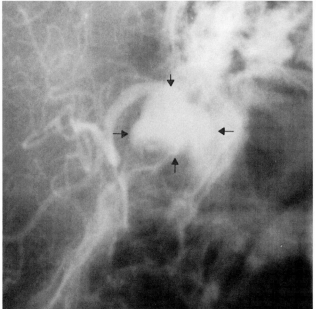

FIG SK9-1. **Aneurysm** simulating pituitary tumor. (A) Plain lateral view of the skull shows marked expansion of the sella turcica, with calcification (closed arrows) rimming the lesion. The open arrow points to the dorsum sellae. (B) Film from a carotid arteriogram shows the large juxtasellar aneurysm (arrows).

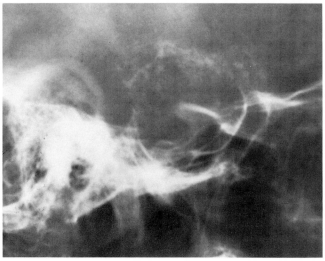

FIG SK9-2. **Craniopharyngioma.** Amorphous suprasellar calcification associated with enlargement and erosion of the sella turcica.

Condition	Imaging Findings	Comments
Pituitary adenoma	Calcification may develop in large chromophobe or, less frequently, eosinophilic adenomas. There is almost always associated expansion or destruction of the sella.	Pituitary adenomas, almost all of which arise in the anterior lobe, constitute more than 10% of all intracranial tumors. Symptoms may result from a mass effect causing compression of parasellar structures or from an alteration in pituitary trophic hormone production (increased levels with secreting adenomas; decreased levels caused by compression of the pituitary gland by a nonsecreting tumor).
Healed tuberculous meningitis	Collections of small, not very dense, amorphous calcific nodules.	Calcification commonly occurs in the exudate after tuberculous meningitis has been treated with streptomycin. Generally occurs in the suprasellar region, sylvian fissures, and interpeduncular cistern.
Arteriovenous malformation	Curvilinear streaks or lacelike punctate collections of calcification situated in the vessel walls.	About 25% of arteriovenous malformations exhibit calcification on skull films, though this is a rare finding in the parasellar region.
Pituitary "stones"	Small, densely calcified masses in the sella.	Calcified nodules in the sella may rarely be seen in asymptomatic persons and are thought to be the residua of small adenomas that have undergone autonecrosis.

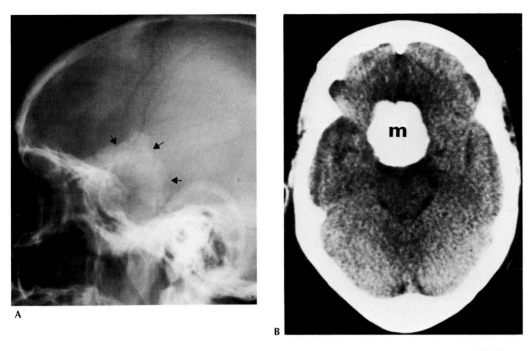

FIG SK9-3. Parasellar meningioma mimicking pituitary tumor. (A) Plain skull radiograph demonstrates a calcified mass (arrows) and destruction of the sella turcica. (B) CT scan shows the large calcified mass (m).

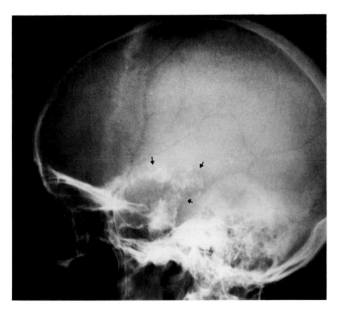

FIG SK9-4. Chordoma. Dense calcification (arrows) in a large soft-tissue mass that has eroded the dorsum sellae and the upper portion of the clivus.

ENLARGEMENT, EROSION, AND DESTRUCTION
OF THE SELLA TURCICA

Condition	Imaging Findings	Comments
Chronic increased intracranial pressure	Initially, diffuse demineralization of cortical bone on the anterior aspect of the dorsum sellae and floor of the sella. Eventually, the dorsum is eroded from the top down and there may even be complete dissolution of the dorsum. The anterior and posterior clinoid processes may also be thinned or eroded.	Causes include intracranial masses, cerebral edema, hydrocephalus, and meningitis. Long-standing increased intracranial pressure (especially in children) may cause enlargement of the sella, simulating a neoplasm. If the pressure subsides to normal levels, a demineralized sella will recalcify and may appear normal on subsequent studies. Downward bulging of an expanded third ventricle acts as a pulsatile mass that causes direct sellar erosion superimposed on the bony demineralization.
Pituitary tumor (Fig SK10-1)	Ballooned sella with erosion, backward bowing, or complete destruction of the dorsum. Also unequal downward displacement of the sellar floor ("double floor") and undercutting of the anterior clinoid processes.	Pituitary adenomas primarily arise in the anterior lobe and constitute more than 10% of all intracranial tumors. Chromophobe adenomas and eosinophilic adenomas (causing acromegaly) usually produce substantial sellar enlargement, while basophilic adenomas (causing Cushing's syndrome) and prolactin-secreting microadenomas (causing amenorrhea and galactorrhea) usually do not cause any sellar abnormality. The rare carcinomas of the pituitary produce extremely rapid sellar enlargement and destruction.
Craniopharyngioma (Fig SK10-2)	Truncation or amputation of the dorsum sellae (typical of any suprasellar mass). Less commonly the tumor is intrasellar, where it compresses the pituitary gland and may erode adjacent bony walls and be indistinguishable from a pituitary tumor.	Benign congenital, or rest cell, tumor with cystic and solid components that usually originates above the sella turcica, depressing the optic chiasm and extending up into the third ventricle. Characteristic nodular, amorphous, or cloudlike suprasellar calcification (mixed or solid lesions) or shell-like calcification along the periphery of cystic lesions is seen in 80% to 90% of childhood craniopharyngiomas (30% of adult tumors).
Other juxtasellar or suprasellar tumors	Truncation or amputation of the dorsum sellae. Occasional enlargement of the sella.	Parasellar or tuberculum sellae meningioma (calcifies in 5% to 15% of cases); optic chiasm glioma; tumor of the optic nerve sheath or hypothalamus.
Metastases	Destruction of the sella.	Rare metastases to the pituitary gland or adjacent dura and bone are usually secondary to carcinomas of the breast or lung.
Sphenoid sinus carcinoma/ mucocele (Fig SK10-3)	Soft-tissue mass in the sphenoid sinus with destruction of the sellar floor.	Rare lesions. Sphenoid sinus carcinoma develops only in elderly patients, while mucoceles may occur at any age.
Chordoma (Fig SK10-4)	Secondary invasion of the posterior aspect of the sella from a destructive lesion of the clivus.	Rare tumor arising from remnants of the notocord. There may infrequently be flocculent calcification in the retrosellar soft-tissue mass.

Condition	Imaging Findings	Comments
Aneurysm of internal carotid artery (cavernous or suprasellar segment)	Enlargement and erosion of the dorsum sellae with undercutting of the anterior clinoid processes (may mimic a pituitary tumor).	Usually asymmetric or unilateral involvement. The wall of the aneurysm frequently calcifies.
Empty sella syndrome	Slight to moderate globular enlargement of the sella without erosion, destruction, or posterior displacement of the dorsum (usually an incidental finding on plain skull radiographs).	Developmental defect in (or absence of) the diaphragma sellae that permits downward extension of the subarachnoid space into the pituitary fossa. Pulsations of cerebrospinal fluid cause remodeling and symmetric expansion of the sella that may simulate a pituitary tumor.
Generalized osteoporosis	Demineralization of the sellar floor and dorsum sellae.	Osteoporosis of aging (senile or postmenopausal osteoporosis); Cushing's disease; hyperparathyroidism.

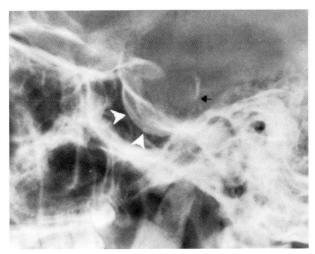

FIG SK10-1. Pituitary adenoma. Ballooning of the sella turcica with downward displacement of the floor (arrowheads) into the posterior portion of the sphenoid sinus. Note the thinning and erosion of the dorsum sellae (arrow) by the intrasellar tumor.

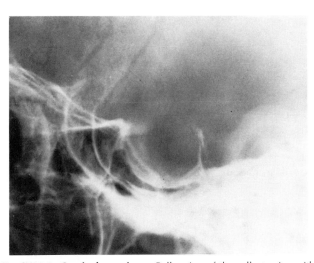

FIG SK10-2. Craniopharyngioma. Ballooning of the sella turcica with downward displacement of the floor, undermining of the anterior clinoids, and backward angulation of the dorsum.

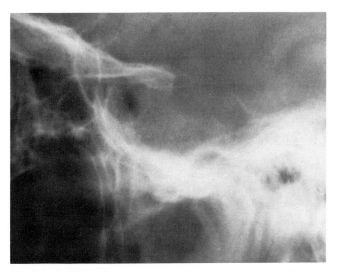

FIG SK10-3. Sphenoid sinus carcinoma. Large soft-tissue mass with complete destruction of the floor and posterior part of the sella turcica.

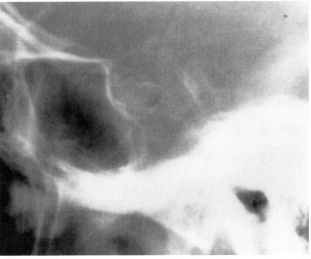

FIG SK10-4. Chordoma. Destruction of the clivus with extension into the posterior aspect of the sella.

EROSION AND WIDENING OF THE INTERNAL AUDITORY CANAL

Condition	Comments
Normal variant (patulous canal)	Bilateral symmetry, maximum enlargement in the midportion of the canal, preservation of the porus, and a well-defined cortical margin are indicative of the true nature of the enlargement.
Acoustic neuroma (Figs SK11-1 and SK11-2)	Almost invariably the cause of pathologic widening of the internal auditory meatus and erosions near the medial aspect of the canal. Slow-growing benign tumor arising from Schwann cells in the vestibular portion of the eighth cranial nerve that represents about 85% of cerebellopontine angle tumors (usually originates in the internal auditory meatus and extends into the cerebellopontine angle cistern). CT shows a uniformly enhancing mass causing enlargement and erosion of the internal auditory canal. Small intracanalicular tumors may require CT examination after the intrathecal administration of contrast material (metrizamide or air).
Neurofibromatosis	A single enlarged auditory canal may occasionally be seen in neurofibromatosis, reflecting the widespread dural ectasia and bony malformations that can occur in this condition. More commonly, unilateral or bilateral enlargement of the internal auditory meatus in neurofibromatosis is due to an often-associated acoustic neuroma.
Other cerebellopontine angle tumors	Erosion or widening of the internal auditory canal is a rare manifestation of meningioma, epidermoid, brainstem glioma, choroid plexus papilloma, hemangioma, or other neuroma (cranial nerves V and VII).
Long-standing hydrocephalus	Rare cause of bilateral, often asymmetric, enlargement of the internal auditory canal.
Vascular	Extremely rare manifestation of an arteriovenous malformation or an aneurysm of the internal auditory canal artery.

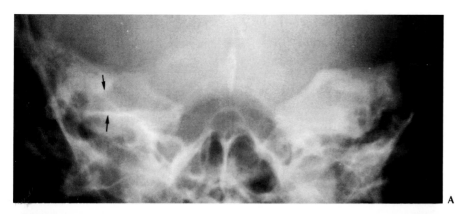

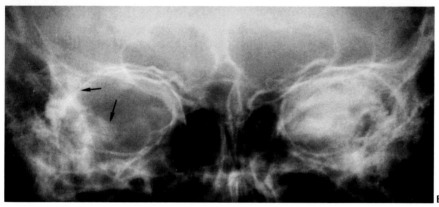

Fig SK11-1. Acoustic neuroma. (A) Anteroposterior (Towne) projection. There is erosion of the superior and inferior margins of the right internal auditory canal laterally (arrows). The canal, which normally has a barrel shape in this projection (note the left side), assumes the configuration of a funnel or trumpet. The angular midline density projected above the upper margin of the foramen magnum represents a calcified plaque in the falx anteriorly. (B) Posteranterior view of an acoustic neuroma in another patient. Destruction of the medial aspect of the petrous pyramid is more advanced than in (A). The superior aspect of the medial third of the petrous pyramid has been eroded (arrows), and only the extreme lateral portion of the internal auditory canal is recognized.[6]

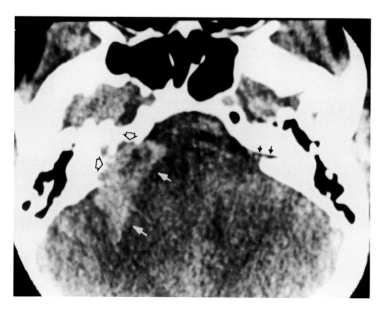

Fig SK11-2. Acoustic neuroma. CT scan shows widening and erosion of the right internal auditory canal (open arrows) associated with a large extra-axial mass (white arrows) in the right cerebellopontine angle. The solid black arrows point to the normal internal auditory canal on the left.

DILATED CEREBRAL VENTRICLES

Condition	Imaging Findings	Comments
Noncommunicating (obstructive) hydrocephalus	Symmetric distension of the ventricular system proximal to the obstruction and a ventricular system of normal or less than normal size distal to the obstruction.	Possible site of obstruction should be examined in detail with thin CT slices and, if necessary, overlapping cuts to establish the pathogenesis of the obstruction.
Level of foramen of Monro (Fig SK12-1)	Enlargement of the lateral ventricles with normal-sized third and fourth ventricles.	Colloid cyst; suprasellar tumors (especially craniopharyngioma); intraventricular tumors; arachnoid cysts of the suprasellar cistern; intraventricular hemorrhage (trauma, arteriovenous malformation, hemophilia). Unilateral tumors, such as those arising in the hypothalamus, basal ganglia, or cerebral parenchyma, may obstruct only one side and cause dilatation of the opposite ventricle and mass compression of the ipsilateral ventricle.
Level of aqueduct (Fig SK12-2)	Enlargement of the lateral and third ventricles with a normal-sized fourth ventricle.	Most common causes are congenital aqueduct stenosis or occlusion (most commonly associated with the Arnold-Chiari malformation) and neoplasm (pinealoma, teratoma). Other underlying conditions include cyst of the quadrigeminal cistern, brainstem edema, aneurysmal dilatation of the vein of Galen, hemorrhage, and acute infection.
Level of outlet of fourth ventricle (Fig SK12-3)	Enlargement of the entire ventricular system (with the fourth ventricle often dilated out of proportion).	Atresia of fourth ventricle foramina (Dandy-Walker cyst); Arnold-Chiari malformation; basilar arachnoiditis (eg, tuberculous meningitis); tonsilar herniation; neoplasm (medulloblastoma, ependymoma); basilar impression (eg, Paget's disease); arachnoid cyst.
Communicating hydrocephalus (Fig SK12-4)	Generalized ventricular enlargement with normal or absent sulci.	Obstruction of the normal cerebrospinal fluid pathway distal to the fourth ventricle (usually involves the subarachnoid space at the basal cisterns, cerebral convexity, or foramen magnum). Causes include infection (meningitis, empyema), subarachnoid or subdural hemorrhage, congenital anomalies, neoplasm, and dural venous thrombosis. A similar pattern is seen in "normal-pressure" hydrocephalus, a syndrome of gait ataxia, urinary incontinence, and dementia associated with ventricular dilatation and relatively normal cerebrospinal fluid pressure.

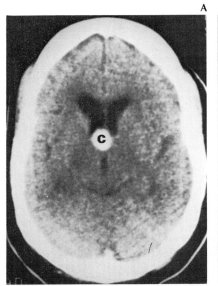

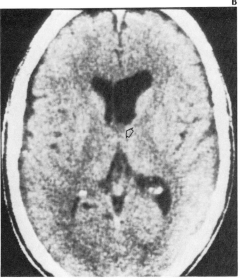

FIG SK12-1. Level of the foramen of Monro.
(A) Bilateral enlargement of the frontal horns with a normal-sized third ventricle in a patient with a hyperdense colloid cyst (c). (B) Unilateral enlargement of the left frontal horn caused by a tiny hypodense unilateral tumor (arrow).

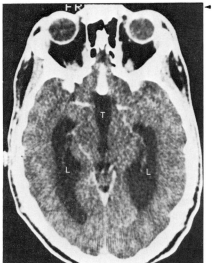

◄ **FIG SK12-2. Level of the aqueduct.** Dilatation of the lateral (L) and third (T) ventricles in a patient with congenital hydrocephalus. The symptoms of headache and papilledema resolved after ventricular shunting.

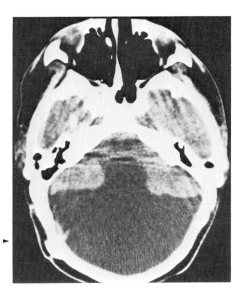

FIG SK12-3. Dandy-Walker cyst. Huge low-density cyst that occupies most of the enlarged posterior fossa and represents an extension of the dilated fourth ventricle. ►

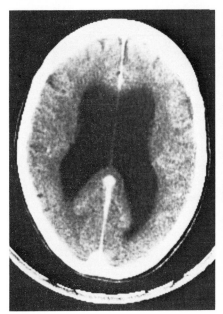

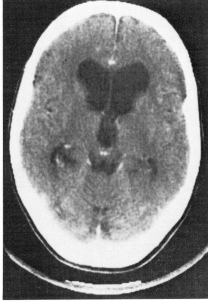

FIG SK12-4. Communicating hydrocephalus. Generalized ventricular enlargement in a 69-year-old patient with ataxia, dementia, and incontinence. Note the absence of the dilated sulci seen in obstructive hydrocephalus.[8]

Condition	Imaging Findings	Comments
Overproduction of cerebrospinal fluid (Fig SK12-5)	Generalized enlargement of the ventricular system.	Choroid plexus papilloma or carcinoma that causes overproduction of cerebrospinal fluid. This rare tumor usually occurs in the fourth ventricle in adults and the lateral ventricle in children. Differentiation from other intraventricular masses is made by the CT demonstration of its choroid location and the typical choroidal pattern of contrast enhancement.
Atrophy (atrophic hydrocephalus) (Figs SK12-6 to SK12-8)	Diffuse dilatation of the lateral and third ventricles as well as the cisterns. The sulci over the surfaces of the cerebral hemispheres are prominent and appear as wide linear lucent stripes.	Multiple causes including normal aging, degenerative diseases (Alzheimer's, Pick's, Jakob-Creutzfeldt, Binswanger's), Huntington's disease, congenital inflammatory disease (eg, toxoplasmosis, torulosis, cytomegalic inclusion disease), vascular disease (multifocal infarct, arteriovenous malformation).
Atrophy of one cerebral hemisphere (Fig SK12-9)	Enlargement of the ipsilateral lateral ventricle and sulci and a shift of midline structures to the affected side.	Usually the result of complete occlusion of the ipsilateral middle cerebral artery. If the occlusion occurs in early childhood, the affected half of the skull is underdeveloped.
Localized atrophy (Fig SK12-10)	Focal enlargement of a part of one ventricle or a group of sulci.	Usually a late residual of previous insult to the brain (eg, infarct, hematoma, severe contusion, abscess).

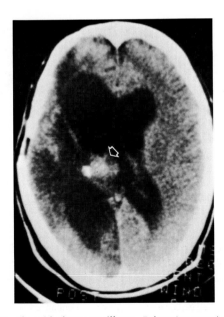

FIG SK12-5. **Choroid plexus papilloma.** Enhancing ventricular mass (arrow) causing pronounced generalized enlargement of the ventricular system.

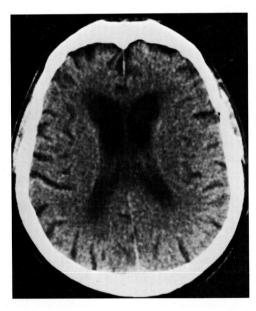

FIG SK12-6. **Normal aging.** CT scan of a 70-year-old man shows generalized ventricular dilatation with prominence of the sulci over the surfaces of the cerebral hemispheres.

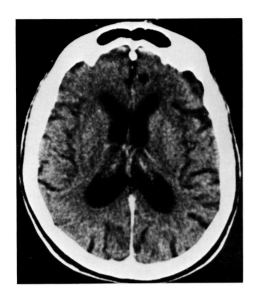

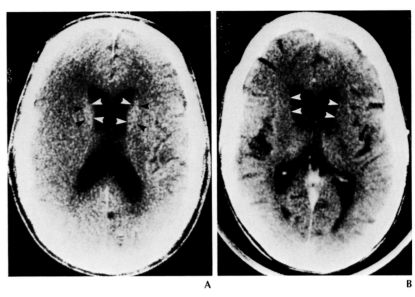

Fig SK12-7. Alzheimer's disease. Noncontrast scan of a 56-year-old woman with progressive dementia shows generalized enlargement of the ventricular system and sulci.

Fig SK12-8. Huntington's disease. (A) CT scan in a normal patient shows the heads of the caudate nucleus (black arrows) producing a normal concavity of the frontal horns (white arrows). (B) In a patient with Huntington's disease, atrophy of the caudate nucleus causes a characteristic loss of the normal concavity (white arrowheads) of the frontal horns.

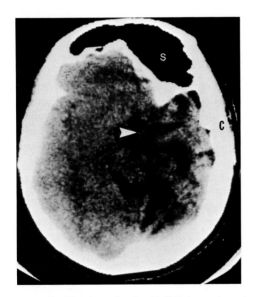

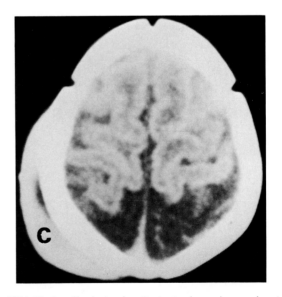

Fig SK12-9. Cerebral hemiatrophy (Davidoff-Dyke syndrome). CT scan of a 5-year-old boy who had intrauterine difficulties demonstrates extensive loss of brain volume in the left hemisphere. There is also enlargement of the left hemicalvarium (C), enlargement of the left frontal sinus (S), and a shift of midline structures such as the third ventricle (arrowhead) from right to left. The low density in the remainder of the hemisphere represents encephalomalacia.

Fig SK12-10. Localized atrophy. Contrast-enhanced scan of an infant with intrauterine infection shows bilateral occipital atrophy. Note the cephalhematoma (C) on the right.

MULTIPLE WORMIAN BONES

Condition	Comments
Normal variant	A few sutural bones may be seen in normal skulls, usually in the lambdoid suture.
Cleidocranial dysostosis (Fig SK13-1)	Congenital hereditary disorder of membranous bone formation that principally involves the calvarium, clavicles, and pelvis. In the skull, there is also defective ossification of the calvarium, widening of sutures (maldevelopment of bone rather than a manifestation of increased intracranial pressure), and persistence of the metopic suture.
Osteogenesis imperfecta (Fig SK13-2)	Inherited generalized disorder of connective tissue characterized by blue sclerae, thin bones, and multiple fractures. An infant with severe disease has a paper-thin skull, and death in utero or soon after birth is usually caused by intracranial hemorrhage. If the infant survives, ossification of the skull progresses slowly, leaving wide sutures (delayed closure) with multiple wormian bones producing a mosaic appearance.
Cretinism	Hypothyroidism dating from birth that results in multiple developmental anomalies. Other skull changes are common and include increased thickness of the cranial vault, underpneumatization of the sinuses and mastoids, widened sutures with delayed closure, and a delay in the development and eruption of the teeth.
Hypophosphatasia	Inherited metabolic disorder in which a low level of alkaline phosphatase leads to defective mineralization of bone. The skull contains large unossified areas simulating severe widening of the sutures. If the infant survives and calvarial recalcification occurs, there may be premature closure of the sutures.
Pyknodysostosis	Rare hereditary dysplasia in which patients have short stature and diffusely dense, sclerotic bones. In the skull, there is failure of the cranial sutures and fontanelles to close, lack of pneumatization of the sinuses and mastoids, sclerosis and thickening of the cranial and facial bones, and characteristic mandibular hypoplasia with loss of the normal mandibular angle.

Condition	Comments
Rickets	Defective calcification of growing skeletal elements due to a deficiency of vitamin D in the diet or a lack of exposure to ultraviolet radiation. Softening of the skull bones (craniotabes) is an early finding that may be followed by frontal and parietal bossing, giving the head a boxlike appearance. The cranial sutures are widened and fontanelle closure is often delayed.
Infantile hydrocephalus	Result of ossification in the separated suture margins.

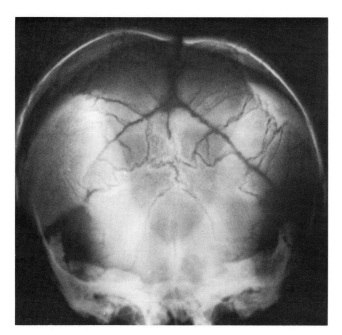

FIG SK13-1. Cleidocranial dysostosis.

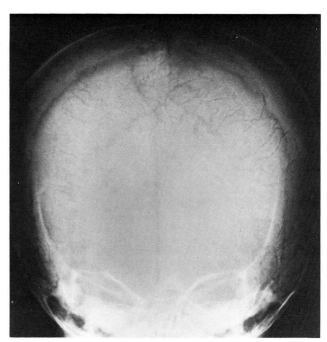

FIG SK13-2. Osteogenesis imperfecta.

BASILAR IMPRESSION

Condition	Comments
Congenital basilar impression (Fig SK14-1)	Infrequently occurs as an isolated abnormality. Usually found in association with one or more of the following defects: failure of the posterior arch of the atlas to fuse, assimilation of part or all of the atlas to the occiput, Klippel-Feil deformity, atlantoaxial dislocation, and stenosis of the foramen magnum.
Arnold-Chiari malformation	Caudal projection of the medulla and inferior-posterior portions of the cerebellar hemispheres through the foramen magnum, often to the level of the second cervical vertebra. Associated neurologic anomalies include spinal meningocele or myelomeningocele and deformities of the cervical spine and cervico-occipital junction. Occlusion of the foramina of Luschka and Magendie leads to obstructive hydrocephalus, which dominates the clinical picture in infants.
Softening of bone at the skull base (Fig SK14-2)	Paget's disease; rickets; osteomalacia; hyperparathyroidism; osteogenesis imperfecta. In these conditions the weight of the skull on the soft base permits invagination of the cervical spine.
Cleidocranial dysostosis	Congenital hereditary disorder in which faulty membranous bone formation primarily involves the calvarium, clavicles, and pelvis. Other skull anomalies include widening of the sutures, persistence of the metopic suture, and the presence of multiple accessory bones along the sutures (wormian bones).
Trauma	Trauma causing basilar impression is usually fatal.

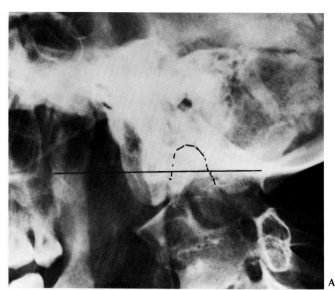

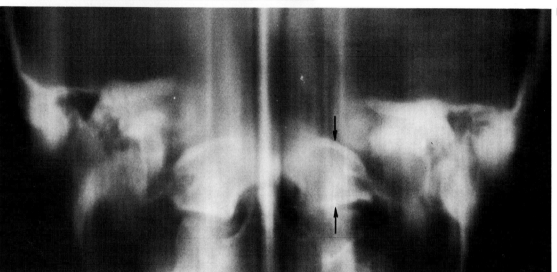

Fig SK14-1. **Congenital basilar impression** associated with assimilation of the atlas. (A) Lateral view of the skull shows fusion of C1 with the base of the occiput posteriorly (arrow) and anteriorly. The odontoid process of C2 (interrupted line) projects upward into the foramen magnum and compresses its contents. Almost the entire odontoid lies above Chamberlain's line (solid horizontal line), which is drawn from the posterior margin of the hard palate to the posterior margin of the foramen magnum. (B) Frontal tomogram of the region of the craniovertebral junction shows complete fusion of the lateral mass of C1 (lower arrow) with the occipital condyle (upper arrow) bilaterally. Note the upward angulation of the petrous pyramids.[6]

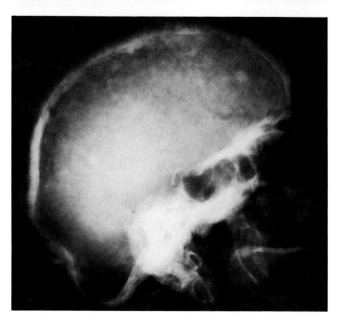

Fig SK14-2. **Basilar impression** secondary to Paget's disease. The calvarium shows a mottled thickening with nodular densities scattered throughout. Portions of the base of the skull are also sclerotic and thickened. The floor of the posterior cranial fossa is markedly depressed and slants sharply upward toward the foramen magnum. The odontoid process of C2 protrudes into the foramen magnum (arrow).[6]

CYSTLIKE LESIONS OF THE JAW

Condition	Imaging Findings	Comments
Radicular cyst (dental cyst, periodontal cyst) (Fig SK15-1)	Round or oval lucency with well-defined, discrete margins. Large lesions may exert uniform outward pressure on the buccal and lingual cortical plates.	Most common cyst of the mandible. Develops as a result of infection of the dental pulp and occurs at the root apex of a necrotic, nonvital tooth that has typically been gutted by caries. The radiopaque lamina dura that normally surrounds the root apex is absent. The cyst forms from epithelial remnants or cell rests in the periodontal ligament space that proliferate when stimulated by a dental inflammation.
Dentigerous cyst (follicular cyst) (Fig SK15-2)	Smooth, round, well-circumscribed unilocular radiolucent lesion containing the crown of an unerupted tooth. Varies in size from less than 1 cm to a huge expansile mass that fills much of the body or ramus of the mandible and expands the cortical plates.	Most commonly involves the canine and molar regions of the mandible. The cyst is derived from the dental lamina and outer enamel epithelium of developing teeth. Most are discovered in young persons during routine dental radiographic surveys or in a deliberate search for an unerupted permanent tooth.
Primordial cyst	Purely radiolucent lesion containing no tooth crown (unlike dentigerous cysts). Most commonly develops in the third molar region of the mandible and expands posteriorly into the ramus or superiorly toward the coronoid process.	Arises from special odontogenic epithelial cells that ordinarily do not participate directly in tooth development. Cysts containing keratin have a high rate of recurrence. Multiple keratin-containing primordial cysts in the mandible are a principal feature of Gorlin's syndrome (basal cell nevus syndrome).
Traumatic cyst (hemorrhagic bone cyst, solitary bone cyst) (Fig SK15-3)	Unilocular lucent cavity with no internal trabeculation that is fairly well defined at its periphery but is usually without a complete cortical border. A characteristic feature is its tendency to extend upward between the teeth toward the alveolar crest without causing splaying, movement, or erosion of the teeth (the scalloped superior border seems to undulate around the roots and up into the intradental bone).	Fluid-containing structure without an epithelial lining. Generally found in older children and adolescents (rare over age 35). Usually asymptomatic and an incidental radiographic finding.
Periapical rarefying osteitis (periapical granuloma, periapical abscess) (Fig SK15-4)	Localized round lucency at the apex of a nonvital tooth with associated discontinuity of the opaque lamina dura. Usually fairly well circumscribed, though it may be ill defined in an acute infection.	General term that includes periapical abscess and periapical granuloma, both of which may produce the same radiographic appearance and are treated identically (root canal filling or tooth extraction).
Ameloblastoma (adamantinoma) (Fig SK15-5)	Initially, a round unilocular cavity in the interdental or periapical bone. With increasing size, a characteristic multiloculated mass containing multiple round cystic cavities with curved septa. Large lesions cause irregular and undulating expansion of the adjacent cortex. Resorption of tooth roots is common.	Most common benign tumor of the mandible. Usually develops in the body of the mandible at its junction with the ramus. Lesions larger than 5 cm often contain one or two larger central cavities surrounded by numerous small daughter cysts. Adenoameloblastoma and ameloblastic fibroma are rare tumors occurring in the first two decades of life that are clinically less aggressive than ameloblastomas and may contain clusters of calcification and retained teeth.

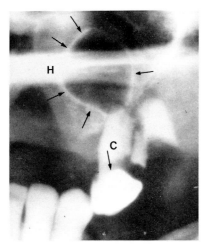

FIG SK15-1. Radicular cyst. Regular, well-circumscribed lucent lesion (arrows). The involved tooth has gross caries (C). The shadow of the hard palate (H) is superimposed across the cyst.[9]

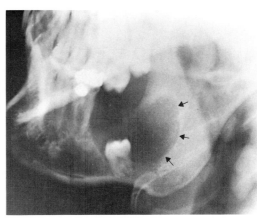

FIG SK15-2. Dentigerous cyst. Smooth, well-circumscribed lucent cavity (arrows) containing the crown of an unerupted tooth.

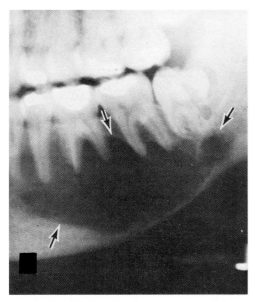

FIG SK15-3. Traumatic cyst. Note the thinning of the inferior border of the mandible and the characteristic scalloping of the superior border of the lesion around the roots of the teeth.[9]

FIG SK15-4. Periapical rarefying osteitis. The lamina dura can be seen around the canine root apex but not around the apex of the lateral incisor (arrows). Radiographically, it is impossible to distinguish among granuloma, cyst, or abscess in this lesion.[9]

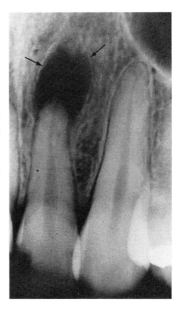

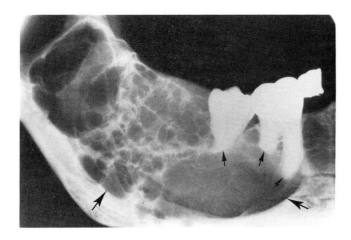

FIG SK15-5. Ameloblastoma. Plain radiograph of an excised specimen shows a lesion extending from the molar region to the superior portion of the ramus (upper left). Note particularly the multilocularity of the lesion, the heterogeneity in the size of various loculations, the well-defined margins (large arrows), and the resorption of tooth roots (small arrows).[9]

Condition	Imaging Findings	Comments
Fibrous dysplasia (Figs SK15-6 and SK15-7)	Expansile, lytic to sclerotic, fairly well-circumscribed lesion. Usually unilateral and most commonly involves the posterior portion of the maxilla.	Jaw involvement occurs in about 10% of cases (more common in the polyostotic form). In children, bilateral lesions (frequently with a familial pattern) can produce a multiloculated and bubbly cystic expansion of the mandible, termed cherubism.
Fissural developmental cyst	Lucent lesion that most commonly arises in the midline of the mandible or maxilla (incisive canal or nasopalatine cyst). Infrequently located laterally (globulomaxillary cyst) between the lateral incisor and canine tooth.	Arises from epithelial remnants at lines of embryonic fusion of the frontonasal process and the two maxillary processes.
Cementoma (cementifying fibroma) (see Fig SK16-3)	Initially, a radiolucent periapical lesion resembling a radicular cyst (though the involved tooth is usually healthy). Primarily involves the mandible and is often multiple.	Mesodermal tumor that arises from proliferation of connective tissue of the periodontal membrane and may reflect a localized form of fibrous dysplasia. In the late stage of development, complete calcification of the lesion results in an ovoid or round radiopaque mass surrounded by a lucent space that separates it from surrounding normal bone.
Giant cell (reparative) granuloma (Fig SK15-8)	Unilocular or multilocular expansile lesion that occurs twice as frequently in the mandible as the maxilla and usually arises anterior to the first molars.	Nonneoplastic reactive type of bone disease that is initiated by some unknown stimulus and is virtually identical histopathologically to giant cell tumor of the skeleton. Primarily affects adolescents and young adults.
Paget's disease	Diffuse lytic, mixed, or sclerotic process with gross enlargement of the entire mandible (unlike fibrous dysplasia, which is almost always unilateral).	Jaw involvement (most commonly in the maxilla) occurs in about 15% of patients. There is almost always concomitant involvement of the skull.
Histiocytosis X	Osteolytic area in or near the alveolar process. Characteristic "floating teeth" appearance.	Eosinophilic granuloma (often multiple) destroys the bony support of one or more teeth (especially in the posterior alveolar ridge) while leaving the tooth structures intact.
Hyperparathyroidism (Fig SK15-9)	Generalized loss of the lamina dura without widening of the periodontal membrane. Brown tumors (often multiple) appear as well-defined, round cystic lucencies that may expand the affected bone.	Resorption of the lamina dura is a much less sensitive radiographic indicator of hyperparathyroidism than the basically analogous subperiosteal cortical resorption of the phalanges. This appearance is also nonspecific, since it can occur in Paget's disease, fibrous dysplasia, and osteomalacia.
Metastases and nonodontogenic benign and primary malignant tumors	Variable appearance similar to the counterparts of these processes occurring elsewhere.	Metastases may be hematogenous or may spread directly from tumors of the oral or nasal cavity, salivary glands, or skin. Rare instances of aneurysmal bone cyst, hemangioma, neurofibroma, fibrosarcoma, osteosarcoma (see Fig SK16-6), chondrosarcoma, and multiple myeloma.

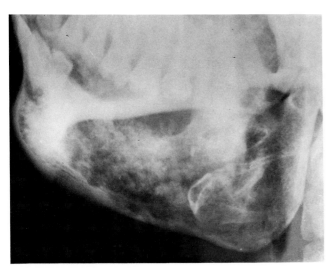

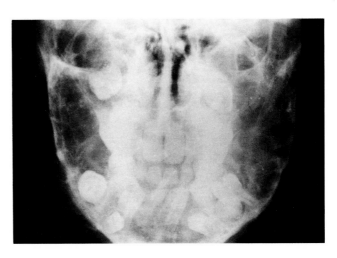

FIG SK15-6. **Fibrous dysplasia.** Large mixed lytic and sclerotic lesion involving most of one mandibular ramus.

FIG SK15-7. **Cherubism.** Typical multiloculated appearance and associated malpositioning of teeth in a patient with bilateral fibrous dysplasia.[9]

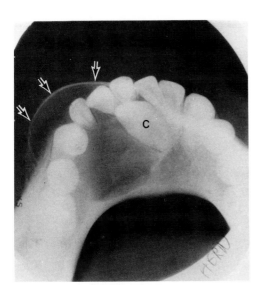

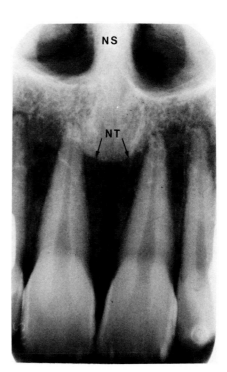

FIG SK15-8. **Giant cell granuloma.** Occlusal view demonstrates an expansile radiolucency in the anterior portion of the mandible producing even, regular swelling of the buccal cortical plate (arrows) and intrusion of a canine tooth (C).[9]

FIG SK15-9. **Primary hyperparathyroidism.** The overall bone density between the teeth is overly radiolucent, indicating severe demineralization. There was loss of lamina dura from around the roots, which causes the roots to have the appearance of accentuated tapering. (NT, tip of nose and NS, nasal septum)[9]

RADIOPAQUE LESIONS OF THE JAW

Condition	Imaging Findings	Comments
Odontoma (Fig SK16-1)	*Compound* odontoma appears as a small bundle of numerous dwarfed, misshapened rudimentary teeth surrounded by a thin radiolucent line representing the fibrous capsule. *Complex* odontoma appears as a uniformly opaque, irregular mass surrounded by a thin but intact radiolucent line.	More common *compound* type originates from proliferation of fetal dental lamina and usually contains 3 to 36 (up to 2,000) tiny teeth. *Complex* odontoma is generally a single tumor mass composed of two or more hard dental tissues (enamel, dentin, or cementum) in various proportions. The jumbled mass does not even remotely resemble normal teeth.
Torus mandibularis and palatinus (Fig SK16-2)	Opaque exostosis or bony protuberance that occurs along the midline of the palate or along the lingual surface of the mandible. Almost always bilateral and usually symmetric.	Benign, static growths that do not become malignant and have no clinical significance (unless denture construction is contemplated). *Torus mandibularis* occurs on the lingual surface of both sides of the mandible above the myelohyoid ridge, primarily in the canine-premolar region. *Torus palatinus* occurs on both midline margins of the hard palate of the maxilla.
Paget's disease	Various patterns of sclerosis in the later stages.	Round, radiopaque foci of abnormal bone may produce a "cotton wool" appearance. As the fluffy, opacified areas enlarge and become more numerous, they tend to coalesce.
Fibrous dysplasia (see Fig SK15-6)	May produce a unilateral, primarily sclerotic, fairly well-circumscribed lesion.	Jaw involvement occurs in about 10% of cases and may produce an expansile, lytic appearance.
Cementoma (cementifying fibroma) (Fig SK16-3)	In the late stage of development, there is almost complete opacification of the previously lucent lesion. This results in an ovoid or round dense mass surrounded by a lucent space separating it from normal bone.	Mesodermal tumor that is initially completely lucent and may reflect a localized form of fibrous dysplasia. Often multiple and most frequently involves the mandible.
Ossifying fibroma (Fig SK16-4)	Various amounts of calcified material in a unilocular, well-marginated mass.	Probably arises from primitive mesenchymal tissue surrounding the tooth. The dense material formed by the tumor may be typical bone or resemble cementum.
Osteoma (Fig SK16-5)	Island of dense bone that grows very slowly. Primarily involves the mandible below the lower molars and protrudes inferiorly.	Generally does not produce symptoms or signs until its size causes notable deformity. May be multiple in the skull, face, or jaw and associated with multiple colonic polyps in Gardner's syndrome.
Osteosarcoma (Fig SK16-6)	Central, ill-defined area of bone destruction with variable amounts of opacification that may resemble a mass of cotton wool.	Represents about 7% of all osteosarcomas. The most common symptoms are bone swelling and bleeding around the necks of the teeth. A bizarre pattern of periosteal response occasionally occurs.

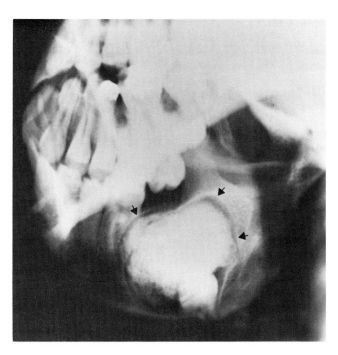

Fig SK16-1. Odontoma. Densely calcified mandibular mass surrounded by a thin radiolucent line (arrows) representing the fibrous capsule.

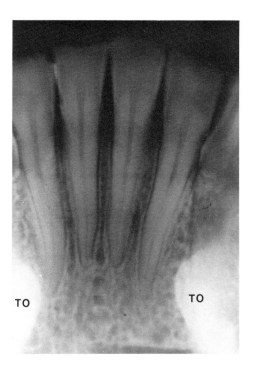

Fig SK16-2. Torus mandibularis. On this periapical view of the anterior teeth, tori (TO) appear bilaterally as convex radiopaque protuberances pointing medially from the sides of the film. These bony exostoses could be easily seen and palpated intraorally.[9]

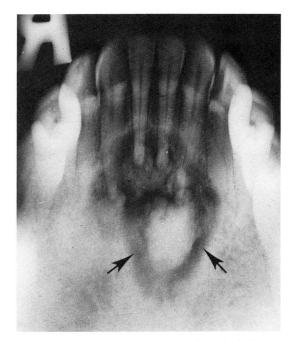

Fig SK16-3. Cementoma. Occlusal view reveals a calcified mass with a lucent zone separating it from the surrounding palate (arrows). Note the small radiopaque densities surrounding tooth roots.[9]

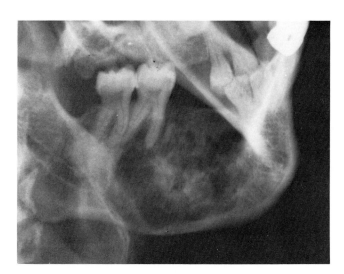

Fig SK16-4. Ossifying fibroma. Amorphous calcification with a large, well-marginated lucent mass.

Condition	Imaging Findings	Comments
Osteopetrosis	Mandible may be involved in the generalized bony sclerosis.	Rare hereditary bone dysplasia in which failure of the resorptive mechanism of calcified cartilage interferes with its normal replacement by mature bone.
Garré's sclerosing osteomyelitis	Exuberant sclerotic periosteal reaction and cortical thickening that usually involves the lower border of the mandible.	Response to a mandibular infection that is secondary to necrotic teeth in children and adolescents. There may be surprisingly little intraosseous bone destruction.
Infantile cortical hyperostosis (Caffey's disease) (Fig SK16-7)	Bilateral thickening of the inferior mandibular cortex. The deposition of layers of new bone may sometimes produce a laminated appearance.	Mandible is the most common bone involved in this condition, which occurs within the first 5 months of life.

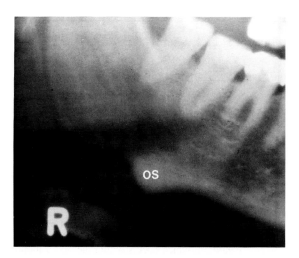

Fig SK16-5. Osteoma. The lesion (OS) is at its usual location at the inferior mandibular border just anterior to the angle. This sessile type of osteoma is seen as bulging of the cortex inferiorly.[9]

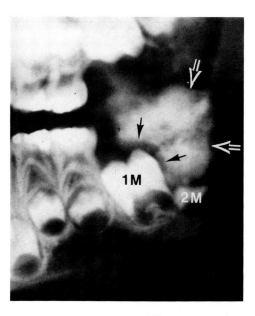

Fig SK16-6. Osteosarcoma of the mandible. The outlined arrows indicate the superior and posterior limits of the tumor, which has a fluffy radiopaque character. Superiorly, the lesion had extended past the occlusal surface of the teeth and had perforated the oral mucosa. Note that the lesion has not yet eroded through the radiolucent follicle (black arrows) of the unerupted first molar tooth (1M). (2M, second molar).[9]

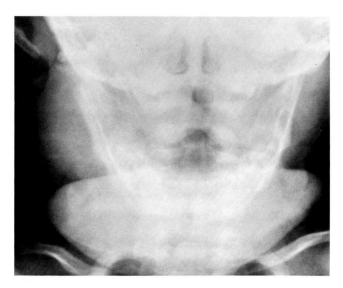

Fig SK16-7. Infantile cortical hyperostosis (Caffey's disease). Bilateral thickening of the mandibular cortex, more prominent on the right.

MASS IN A PARANASAL SINUS

Condition	Imaging Findings	Comments
Mucous or serous retention cyst	Homogeneous soft-tissue mass that usually involves the floor or lateral wall of the maxillary sinus. A dome-shaped or spherical configuration is usually diagnostic, though some cysts are broad-based and can simulate an air-fluid level.	Most common sinus complication of inflammatory sinusitis. A mucous retention cyst results from obstruction of a seromucinous gland with resulting cystic expansion (its wall is lined by epithelium of the specific gland involved). A serous cyst results from fluid accumulation and loculation in the submucosal layers of the mucoperiosteum and thus does not have an epithelial lining (the two conditions are radiographically indistinguishable).
Mucocele (Fig SK17-1)	Initially, clouding of the involved sinus with effacement of the normal mucoperiosteal line and reactive bone sclerosis. The net effect of bone destruction (with resulting decreased density) and the increased soft-tissue density of the mucocele itself makes most frontal sinus mucoceles appear radiolucent when compared to the adjacent frontal bone.	Complication of inflammatory disease that probably reflects obstruction of the ostium of the sinus and the accumulation of mucous secretions. The most clinically important cystic complication of inflammatory disease because it can expand and destroy adjacent structures. Primarily involves the frontal sinuses (65%). About 25% affect the ethmoid sinuses and 10% the maxillary sinuses. Infection of the lesion is termed a pyocele.
Sinusitis (Figs SK17-2 and SK17-3)	Soft-tissue density (mucosal thickening) lining the walls of the involved sinuses. An air-fluid level in the sinus indicates acute inflammatory disease. Most commonly affects the maxillary sinuses.	Viral infection or allergic reaction involving the upper respiratory tract may lead to the obstruction of drainage from one or more of the paranasal sinuses and the development of localized pain, tenderness, and fever. Destruction of the bony sinus wall is an ominous sign indicating secondary osteomyelitis.
Granulomatous disease (Fig SK17-4)	Various patterns of soft-tissue swelling, polypoid lesions, bone destruction, and sclerosis involving the sinuses.	Infectious causes include tuberculosis, syphilis, leprosy, glanders (*Pseudomonas mallei*), yaws, and fungal disorders (mucormycosis, actinomycosis). Granulomatous involvement of the sinuses also occurs in sarcoidosis and erythema nodosum.
Wegener's granulomatosis (Fig SK17-5)	Thickening of the mucous membranes of the paranasal sinuses that may progress to destruction of the nasal bones, orbits, mastoids, and base of the skull.	Necrotizing vasculitis and granulomatous inflammation that primarily affects the upper and lower respiratory tracts and the kidneys. The paranasal sinuses are involved in more than 90% of patients.
Midline granuloma (Fig SK17-6)	Granulomatous masses in the nose and sinuses cause clouding or complete obliteration of the air space. May progress to extensive destruction of the nasal bone and the medial walls of the maxillary antra.	Uncommon disease characterized by local inflammation, destruction, and often mutilation of the tissues of the upper respiratory tract and face. The sinus involvement is similar to Wegener's granulomatosis (but there are no pulmonary or renal lesions).
Fracture with hemorrhage	Localized submucosal hematoma may simulate a polyp (eg, blowout fracture of the orbit producing a polypoid mass on the roof of the maxillary sinus).	Partial or complete sinus opacification may be a manifestation of an acute fracture or the sequela of an old fracture.

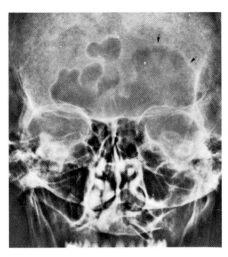

FIG SK17-1. **Mucocele** of left frontal sinus. The right frontal sinus has a normal scalloped margin with a sharp mucoperiosteal line. On the left, the frontal sinus is slightly clouded when compared to the normal right side; however, the overall appearance on the left is that of a "lucent" defect. The contour is smooth and the mucoperiosteal line is hazy or absent (arrows).[9]

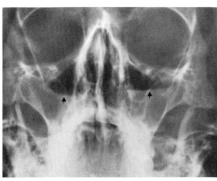

FIG SK17-2. **Acute sinusitis.** There is mucosal thickening involving most of the paranasal sinuses, and air-fluid levels (arrows) appear in both maxillary antra.

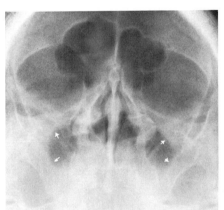

FIG SK17-3. **Chronic sinusitis.** Mucosal thickening appears as a soft-tissue density (arrows) lining the walls of the maxillary antra.

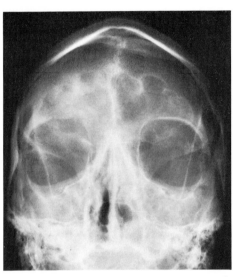

FIG SK17-4. **Mucormycosis** causing pansinusitis with osteomyelitis. There is destruction of the roof of the right orbit with a loss of the mucoperiosteal line of the right frontal sinus.

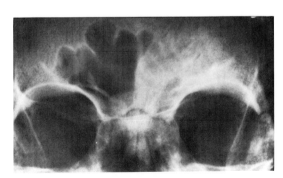

FIG SK17-5. **Wegener's granulomatosis.** Obliteration of the left frontal sinus, which has become densely opaque.[10]

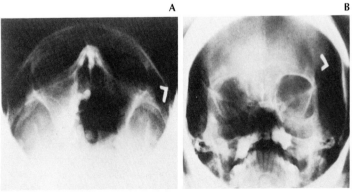

FIG SK17-6. **Midline granuloma.** (A) Extensive destruction of the palate and the left maxillary sinus with involvement of the floor of the left orbit. (B) In another patient, there is destruction of the nasal septum and the right maxillary sinus.[11]

Condition	Imaging Findings	Comments
Barotrauma	Mucosal thickening (often nodular) that may progress to complete opacification of the involved sinus.	Complication of sudden markedly negative intrasinus pressure (in airplane pilots and deep-sea divers) that causes rupture of mucosal vessels and results in subepithelial hematomas as well as free intrasinus bleeding. The radiographic changes primarily involve the maxillary sinuses (though the frontal sinuses are clinically affected more often) and may take 3 to 10 weeks to completely return to normal.
Encapsulated fluid/polyp	Localized soft-tissue mass along the wall of a sinus.	Encapsulated exudate, pus, or blood or localized inflammatory hypertrophic swelling of the mucosa.
Carcinoma (Fig SK17-7)	Soft-tissue mass with diffuse bone destruction but no sclerotic reaction.	Some 90% are squamous cell carcinomas, which are usually found in patients over age 40. About 80% arise in the maxillary sinuses.
Other malignant neoplasms (Fig SK17-8)	Appearance identical to that of carcinoma (there may be new bone formation in osteosarcoma).	Rare manifestation of sarcoma, lymphoma, extramedullary plasmacytoma, mixed salivary tumor, or melanoma.
Benign neoplasm (Figs SK17-9 and SK17-10)	Various patterns ranging from a soft-tissue mass to a dense bony lesion.	Chondroma; hemangioma; dermoid; lipoma; osteoma. Juvenile nasopharyngeal angiofibroma produces characteristic anterior bowing of the posterior wall of a maxillary sinus.
Odontogenic lesion	Mass at the base of a maxillary sinus.	Various types of cysts and tumors (see pages 828 and 832).
Extrinsic neoplasm invading sinus	Soft-tissue mass with destruction of sinus walls.	Pituitary, orbital, oral, or nasopharyngeal tumor; chordoma; Burkitt's lymphoma.
Fibrous dysplasia	Expansion and nonhomogeneous opacification of the involved sinuses with marked sclerosis and thickening of the facial bones.	Similar appearance may occur in ossifying fibroma (considered a localized form of fibrous dysplasia in the facial bones).
Surgical ciliated cyst	Various patterns (fibrosis simulating mucosal disease, a soft-tissue mass, or complete opacification of the sinus).	Follows the Caldwell-Luc procedure, in which an anterior opening is made into the maxillary sinuses between the roots of the upper canine and first molar teeth.

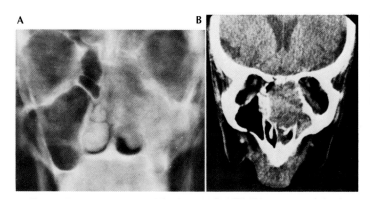

FIG SK17-7. **Malignant tumors of the paranasal sinuses.** (A) Coronal tomogram reveals a tumor mass in the left nasal cavity and ethmoid and maxillary sinuses. The lamina papyracea, orbital floor, and most of the remaining antral margins are intact (mixed tumor of minor salivary gland origin). (B) Coronal CT scan shows an expansile nonenhanced tumor of the left nasal cavity and ethmoid and maxillary sinuses (cylindroma).[9]

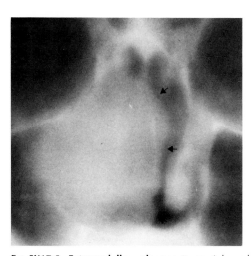

FIG SK17-8. **Extramedullary plasmacytoma.** A large lesion of the right nasal cavity (arrows) causes destruction of the medial wall of the right maxillary antrum.[12]

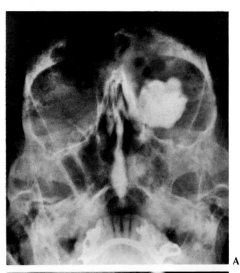

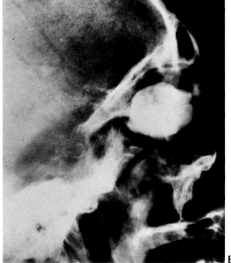

FIG SK17-9. **Osteoma** of the ethmoid sinus. (A) Frontal and (B) lateral views of the skull demonstrate a large, extremely dense osteoma filling and expanding the left ethmoid sinus.

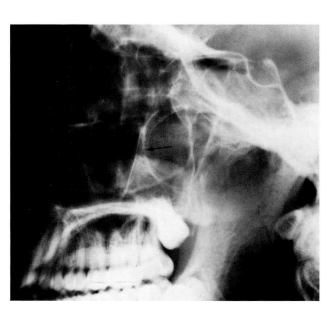

FIG SK17-10. **Juvenile nasopharyngeal angiofibroma.** Pronounced anterior bowing (arrow) of the posterior wall of the maxillary sinus.[13]

HYPODENSE SUPRATENTORIAL MASS
ON COMPUTED TOMOGRAPHY

Condition	Imaging Findings	Comments
Astrocytoma (Fig SK18-1)	Hypodense lesion with little contrast enhancement or peritumoral edema. Calcification frequently occurs.	Slowly growing tumor that has an infiltrative character and can form large cavities or pseudocysts.
Glioblastoma multiforme (Fig SK18-2)	Large inhomogeneous mass with irregular, poorly defined margins and central hypodense zones. Contrast enhancement is usually intense and inhomogeneous, and a ring with thickened irregular walls or nodules of enhancement is common.	Highly malignant lesion that is predominantly cerebral in location. Typically has low-attenuation tissue consisting of edema and malignant glial cells surrounding the enhancing portion of the tumor.
Oligodendroglioma (Fig SK18-3)	Large, irregular, inhomogeneous mass containing calcification and hypodense zones. Variable peritumoral edema and contrast enhancement.	Slow-growing tumor that originates from oligodendrocytes in the central white matter (especially the anterior half of the cerebrum). Calcification (peripheral or central, nodular or shell-like) occurs in about 90% of tumors.
Metastasis (Fig SK18-4)	Hypodense mass surrounded by edema (which usually exceeds tumor volume). Variable contrast enhancement depending on the size and type of tumor.	The density of a metastasis depends on its cellularity and neovascularity and the presence of central necrosis or hemorrhage. Epithelial tumors are typically hypodense; melanoma, choriocarcinoma, and osteosarcoma are usually hyperdense.
Ganglioglioma/ ganglioneuroma	Small, well-defined hypodense or ill-defined isodense mass. Calcified and cystic areas are frequent and most tumors show homogeneous contrast enhancement.	Rare, relatively benign, slow-growing tumors containing mature ganglion cells and stromal elements derived from glial tissue. Typically occur in adolescents and young adults in the temporal and frontal lobes, basal ganglia, and anterior third ventricle.
Epidermoid (primary cholesteatoma) (Fig SK18-5)	Round, sharply marginated, nearly homogeneous hypodense mass. May have extremely low attenuation due to a high fat content. No contrast enhancement.	The result of inclusion of ectodermal germ layer elements in the neural tube during its closure between the third and fifth weeks of gestation. Ectodermal inclusion early in this period produces a midline tumor, while later inclusion produces an eccentrically located lesion. More common in the cerebellopontine angle and suprasellar region.
Dermoid	Inhomogeneous midline mass that often contains focal areas of fat, mural or central calcification, or bone. No contrast enhancement.	Congenital inclusion of both ectodermal and mesodermal germ layer elements at the time of neural tube closure. Contains hair follicles and sebaceous and apocrine glands (derived from mesoderm) that produce a thick, buttery mixture of sweat and sebum.

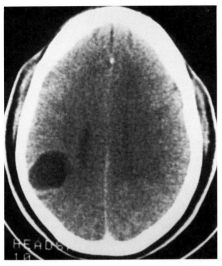

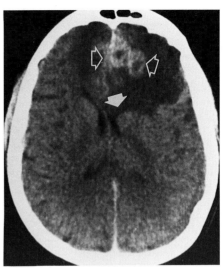

FIG SK18-1. Cystic astrocytoma. Hypodense mass with a thin rim of contrast enhancement.

◄

FIG SK18-2. Glioblastoma multiforme. Irregular enhancing lesion (open arrows). The substantial mass effect of the tumor distorts the frontal horns (closed arrow).

►

A

B

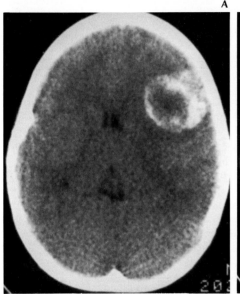

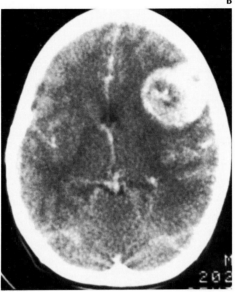

FIG SK18-3. Oligodendroglioma. (A) Nonenhanced scan showing a hypodense mass containing amorphous areas of calcification. (B) After the intravenous injection of contrast material, there is marked contrast enhancement.

A

B

FIG SK18-4. Metastasis. (A) Nonenhanced scan shows a small hypodense mass with an isodense rim (arrow) surrounded by extensive edema. (B) After the intravenous injection of contrast material, there is prominent ring enhancement (arrow) about the metastasis.

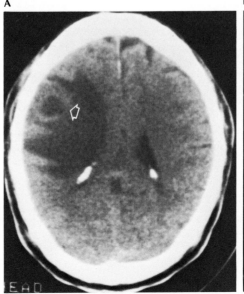

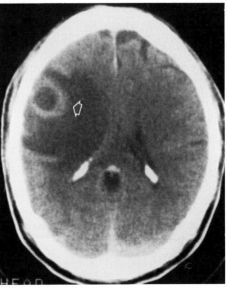

Condition	Imaging Findings	Comments
Lipoma (Fig SK18-6)	Well-defined, homogeneously hypodense fatty mass that occurs in the midline. No contrast enhancement.	Uncommon congenital tumor resulting from inclusion of mesodermal adipose tissue at the time of neural tube closure. Most commonly involves the corpus callosum (often with dense, curvilinear mural calcification).
Radiation necrosis (see Fig SK20-11)	Deep, focal, hypodense mass that is usually in or near the irradiated tumor bed. May show an irregular ring of contrast enhancement.	Develops 9 to 24 months after radiation therapy and may be impossible to differentiate from recurrent or residual tumor.
Cerebral infarction (Figs SK18-7 to SK18-10)	Triangular or wedge-shaped area of hypodensity involving the cortex and the underlying white matter down to the ventricular surface.	Unlike a hypodense glioma, an infarct has a distinctive shape that corresponds to the distribution of a specific vessel or vessels and has a characteristic pattern of peripheral, rarely central, enhancement. The clinical diagnosis is usually obvious because of the abrupt onset of symptoms.
Pyogenic abscess (Fig SK18-11)	Central hypodense zone (pus, necrotic tissue) surrounded by a thin, isodense ring (fibrous capsule) and peripheral low-density tissue (reactive edema).	Unlike intermediate-grade and highly aggressive gliomas, where enhancement is often ringlike but irregular in thickness, a cerebral abscess is characterized by a thin uniform ring of enhancement. There also is usually a strongly suggestive clinical picture of fever, leukocytosis, obtundation, extracranial infection, or a previous operation.
Hytadid (echinococcal) cyst (Fig SK18-12)	Round, sharply marginated, smooth-walled hypodense mass.	Rare manifestation of this parasitic infection. The parenchymal cysts tend to be large and multiple, with no reactive edema or contrast enhancement.
Herpes simplex encephalitis (Fig SK18-13)	Poorly defined, frequently bilateral areas of decreased attenuation, especially involving the temporal and parietal lobes.	Most common cause of nonepidemic fatal encephalitis in the United States. The putamen, which is spared by this infection, often forms the sharply defined, slightly concave or straight medial border of the low-density zone. Various patterns of contrast enhancement develop in about half the patients.
Cerebritis	Irregular, poorly marginated hypodense area (representing edema) in the white matter or basal ganglia that may behave as a mass and result in effacement of the adjacent sulci or ventricle. Unlike most cerebral abscesses, there is no discrete ringlike capsule on unenhanced scans in patients with cerebritis.	Focal inflammatory process in the brain, usually resulting from bacteria or fungi, which may progress to abscess formation (requires about 10 to 14 days). After administration of contrast material, may show a well-defined ring that tends to increase in thickness on serial scans.
Resolving intracerebral hematoma (3 to 6 weeks old) (see Fig SK20-9)	Hypodense region with a thin uniform ring of enhancement that mimics a neoplasm.	Usually a history of previous intracerebral hematoma.

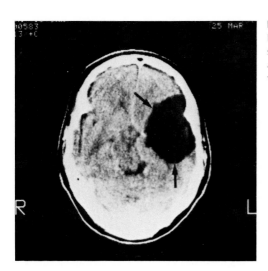

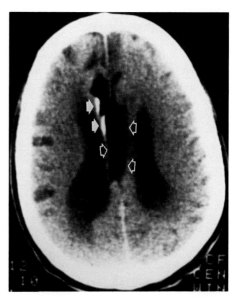

FIG SK18-5. Epidermoid. Enhanced scan shows a large, sharply marginated, low-attenuation, extra-axial sylvian mass.[8]

FIG SK18-6. Lipoma of the corpus callosum. Extremely low-density mass (open arrows) involving much of the corpus callosum. Note the peripheral calcifications (closed arrows).

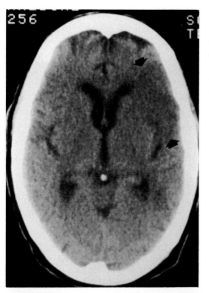

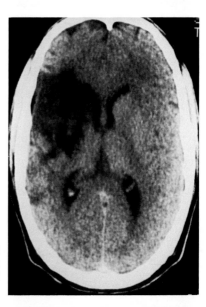

FIG SK18-7. Acute left middle cerebral artery infarct. Scan obtained 20 hours after the onset of acute hemiparesis and aphasia shows obliteration of the normal sulci (arrows) in the involved hemisphere. There is low density of the gray and white matter in the distribution of the left middle cerebral artery.

FIG SK18-8. Chronic right middle cerebral artery infarct. Low-attenuation region with sharply defined borders and some dilatation of the adjacent ventricle.

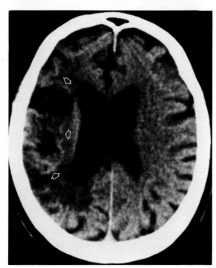

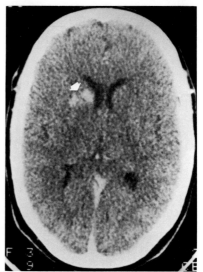

FIG SK18-9. Old infarct in the distribution of the right middle cerebral artery. There is a thin peripheral rim of contrast enhancement (arrows) about the hypodense region. Note the enlargement of the right lateral ventricle.

FIG SK18-10. Basal ganglia infarction. (A) Hypodense region (arrow) involving the right head of the caudate and putamen and passing through the anterior limb of the internal capsule. This distribution reflects a lesion of the artery of Heubner. (B) After the intravenous injection of contrast material, there is contrast enhancement of the area of infarction (arrow).

Condition	Imaging Findings	Comments
Resolving subdural hematoma (Figs SK18-14 and SK18-15)	Well-defined, hypodense, crescentic mass adjacent to the inner table of the skull.	After the injection of contrast material there is characteristic enhancement of the richly vascular membrane that forms around a subdural hematoma 1 to 4 weeks after injury. Occasionally, contrast material seeps into the hematoma and produces a fluid-fluid level.
Subdural empyema (Fig SK18-16)	Crescentic or lentiform, extra-axial hypodense collection (representing pus) adjacent to the inner border of the skull. After administration of contrast material, a narrow zone of enhancement of relatively uniform thickness separates the hypodense extracerebral collection from the brain surface.	Suppurative process in the cranial subdural space that is most commonly the result of the spread of infection from the frontal or ethmoid sinuses. Less frequent causes include mastoiditis, middle ear infection, purulent meningitis, penetrating wounds to the skull, craniectomy, or osteomyelitis of the skull. Often bilateral and associated with a high mortality rate, even if properly treated.
Epidural abscess (see Fig SK20-8)	Poorly defined area of low density adjacent to the inner table of the skull. There may be an adjacent area of bone destruction or evidence of paranasal sinus or mastoid infection. After the intravenous injection of contrast material, the inflamed dural membrane appears as a thickened zone of enhancement on the convex inner side of the lesion.	Almost invariably associated with cranial bone osteomyelitis originating from an infection in the ear or paranasal sinuses. The infectious process is localized outside the dural membrane and beneath the inner table of the skull. The frontal region is most frequently affected because of its close relation to the frontal sinuses and the ease with which the dura can be stripped from the bone.
Multiple sclerosis (Fig SK18-17)	Multifocal, nonconfluent, low-attenuation regions with distinct margins near the atria of the lateral ventricles.	Contrast enhancement in the plaques is unusual except in rapidly evolving ones with surrounding inflammatory changes.
Necrosis of the globus pallidus	Bilaterally symmetric areas of low attenuation in the basal ganglia.	Causes include carbon monoxide poisoning, barbiturate intoxication, cyanide or hydrogen sulfide poisoning, hypoglycemia, hypoxia, hypotension, and Wilson's disease.

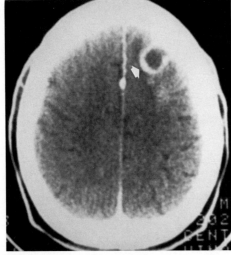

FIG SK18-11. **Pyogenic abscess.** Hypodense lesion surrounded by a uniform ring of contrast enhancement (arrow).

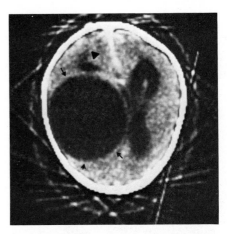

FIG SK18-12. **Echinococcal cyst.** Huge right supratentorial hypodense mass (arrows). The right ventricle is partially visible posterior and medial to the cyst (arrowhead), and the left ventricle is enlarged.[14]

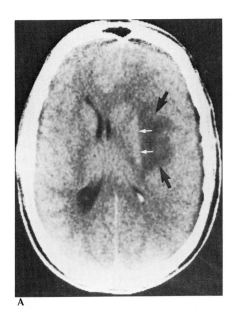

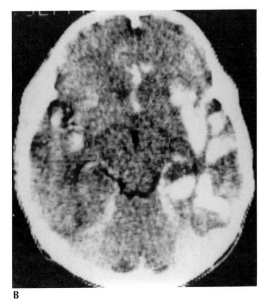

FIG SK18-13. **Herpes simplex encephalitis.** (A) Nonenhanced scan demonstrates a hypodense area deep in the left frontotemporal region (large black arrows) and a shift of midline structures. The putamen, with its well-defined lateral border (small white arrows), is unaffected by infection. (B) In another patient, there is dramatic gyral contrast enhancement that is most prominent on the left.[8]

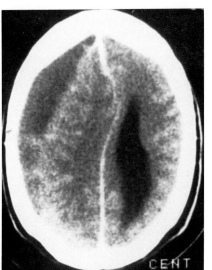

FIG SK18-14. **Right subdural hematoma.** Crescent-shaped, low-density region in the right frontoparietal area. Note the marginal contrast enhancement, dilated left ventricle, and evidence of subfalcine and transtentorial herniation.

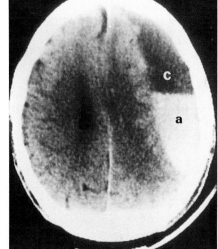

FIG SK18-15. **Mixed acute and chronic left subdural hematoma.** The high-density acute hemorrhage (a) is layered in the dependent portion of the hematoma, with the lower density chronic collection (c) situated anteriorly.

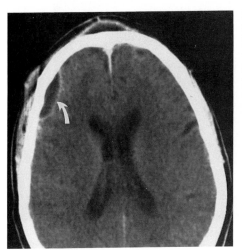

FIG SK18-16. **Subdural empyema.** Lens-shaped extra-axial hypodense collection (arrow) that complicated a severe sinus infection. Note the thin rim of peripheral contrast enhancement.

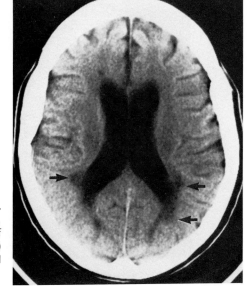

FIG SK18-17. **Multiple sclerosis.** Multiple discrete, homogeneous, and slightly irregular regions of diminished attenuation (arrows) adjacent to the slightly enlarged ventricles.[8]

HIGH-ATTENUATION MASS IN A CEREBRAL HEMISPHERE
ON COMPUTED TOMOGRAPHY

Condition	Imaging Findings	Comments
Meningioma **(Figs SK19-1 and SK19-2)**	Rounded, sharply delineated hyperdense mass in a juxtadural location. Often contains calcification and usually shows intense homogeneous contrast enhancement.	Benign tumor that arises from arachnoid lining cells and is attached to the dura. The hyperdense matrix of a meningioma is the result of diminished water content, tumor hypervascularity, and microscopic psammomatous calcification. The detection of hyperostosis is virtually pathognomonic.
Metastasis **(Fig SK19-3)**	Some dense metastases mimic meningiomas because of their superficial location and well-defined margins, though they are entirely intraparenchymal.	Metastatic colon carcinoma, which has a very dense cellular structure, and metastatic osteosarcoma, which contains osteoid and calcification, tend to be extremely dense. Melanoma and choriocarcinoma also tend to be hyperdense.
Primary lymphoma **(Fig SK19-4)**	Slightly hyperdense mass that enhances homogeneously and often intensely.	Rare malignant neoplasm derived from microglial cells (histologically similar to lymphocytes) that is often multifocal and has a markedly increased incidence in organ transplant recipients.
Acute intracerebral hemorrhage **(Fig SK19-5)**	Homogeneously dense, well-defined lesion with a round to oval configuration.	Causes include head trauma, surgery, hypertensive vascular disease, or rupture of a vascular malformation, mycotic aneurysm, or berry aneurysm.
Acute epidural hematoma **(Figs SK19-6 and SK19-7)**	Biconvex (lens-shaped), peripheral high-density lesion.	Caused by acute arterial bleeding; most commonly develops over the parietotemporal convexity.
Acute subdural hematoma **(Fig SK19-8)**	Peripheral zone of increased density that follows the surface of the brain and has a crescentic shape adjacent to the inner table of the skull.	Caused by venous bleeding, most commonly from ruptured veins between the dura and leptomeninges. Serial scans demonstrate a gradual decrease in the attenuation of a subdural lesion over several weeks.

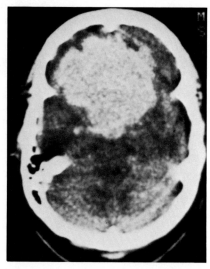

FIG SK19-1. **Meningioma.** Huge hyperdense mass in the frontal lobe.

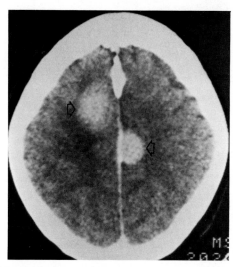

FIG SK19-2. **Meningioma.** Bilateral hyperdense masses (arrows) in juxtadural locations.

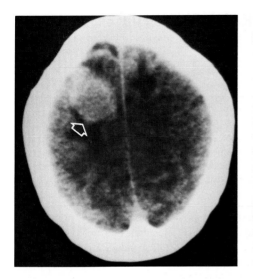

FIG SK19-3. Metastasis. Nonenhanced scan shows a hyperdense mass in the right frontal region representing a metastasis from carcinoma of the lung.

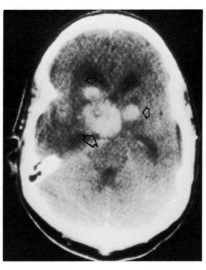

FIG SK19-4. Primary lymphoma. Multifocal hyperdense masses (arrows).

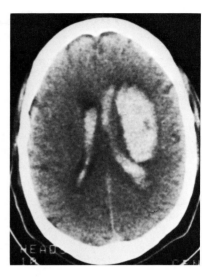

FIG SK19-5. Intracerebral hematoma. Large homogeneous high-density area with extensive acute bleeding into the lateral ventricles.

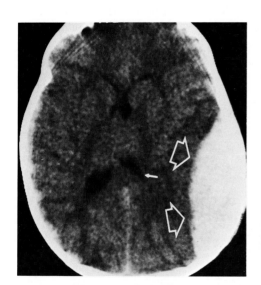

FIG SK19-6. Acute epidural hematoma. CT scan of a 4-year-old involved in a motor vehicle accident shows a characteristic lens-shaped epidural hematoma (open arrows). The substantial mass effect associated with the hematoma distorts the lateral ventricle (closed arrow).

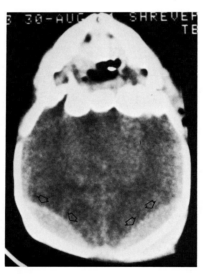

FIG SK19-7. Epidural hematoma. Bilaterally symmetric posterior high-density areas (arrows) with lens-shaped configurations.

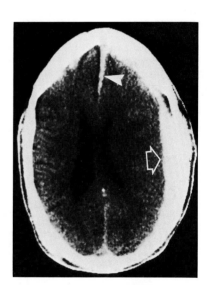

FIG SK19-8. Acute subdural hematoma. High-density, crescent-shaped lesion (open arrow) adjacent to the inner table of the skull. The hematoma extends into the interhemispheric fissure (closed arrowhead).

RING-ENHANCING LESION ON COMPUTED TOMOGRAPHY

Condition	Comments
Glioblastoma multiforme (Figs SK20-1 and SK20-2)	Thick, irregular ring enhancement in a solitary lesion that tends to be situated in a deep hemispheric location and associated with surrounding low-attenuation edema and glial cell infiltration. May occasionally have a relatively uniform rim of enhancement that mimics the capsule of an abscess.
Metastases (Fig SK20-3)	Irregular rim enhancement with a relatively lucent center due to tumor necrosis. Typically located at the gray matter–white matter junction and usually associated with surrounding low-density edema that tends to be relatively concentric and uniform in the adjacent white matter (unlike glial cell infiltration with glioblastoma multiforme, which is usually eccentric and irregular in both gray and white matter).
Lymphoma (Fig SK20-4)	Single or multiple ring-enhancing lesions that primarily affect transplant recipients (high incidence of central nervous system lymphoma in these patients).
Abscess (Figs SK20-5 to SK20-8)	Usually a relatively thin, uniform ring of enhancement associated with considerable reactive edema and a strongly suggestive clinical picture of fever, leukocytosis, obtundation, extracranial infection, or a previous operation. Some pyogenic or fungal abscesses may develop a relatively thick capsule, which resembles the periphery of a high-grade glioma or metastasis. The relatively poor inflammatory response of deep hemispheric white matter may cause the capsule of an abscess to be less developed along the medial wall than along the lateral margin, a feature that may aid in distinguishing an abscess from a neoplasm.
Resolving intracerebral hematoma (3 to 6 weeks old) (Fig SK20-9)	Thin, uniform ring of contrast enhancement that initially represents perivascular inflammation and defects in the tight capillary junctions and eventually reflects the collagenous capsule. Causes of intracerebral hematoma include trauma, surgery, hypertensive vascular disease, vascular malformation, mycotic aneurysm, and berry aneurysm.
Nonacute subdural hematoma	Occasionally produces a pattern of thick rim enhancement with loculation, reflecting its richly vascular surrounding membrane.

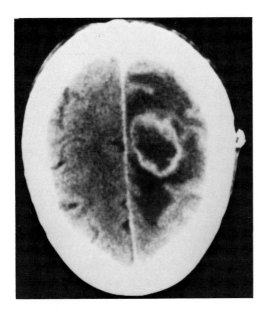

FIG SK20-1. Glioblastoma multiforme. Thick irregular ring-enhancing lesion associated with a large amount of surrounding low-attenuation edema.

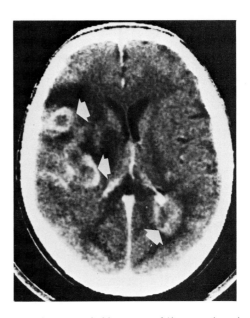

FIG SK20-2. Multicentric glioblastoma multiforme. Bilateral irregular enhancing masses (arrows) with surrounding low-density edema.

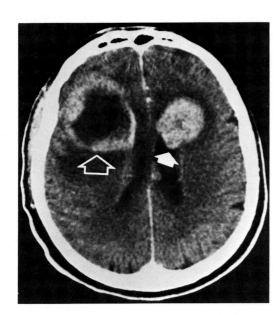

FIG SK20-3. Metastases. Enhancing metastases from squamous cell carcinoma of the lung that are both ring-enhancing (open arrow) and solid (solid arrow).

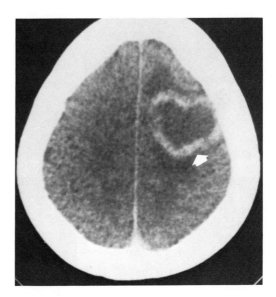

FIG SK20-4. Lymphoma developing after renal transplantation. Heart-shaped, peripherally enhancing, central lucent lesion (arrow) situated in the frontoparietal region. There is moderate surrounding edema.[15]

Condition	Comments
Atypical meningioma **(Fig SK20-10)**	A few meningiomas contain low-attenuation, non-enhancing areas (necrosis, old hemorrhage, cyst formation, or fat in the meningioma tissue) that produce a thick, often irregular, rim. This pattern, especially if associated with prominent edema, may mimic a malignant glioma or metastasis. Coronal scans demonstrating that the mass arises from a dural base suggest the diagnosis of meningioma, though superficial gliomas may invade the dura and dural-based metastases may occur.
Radiation necrosis **(Fig SK20-11)**	Occasional manifestation. Develops in the tumor bed 9 to 24 months after radiation therapy and may be impossible to differentiate from recurrent or residual tumor.

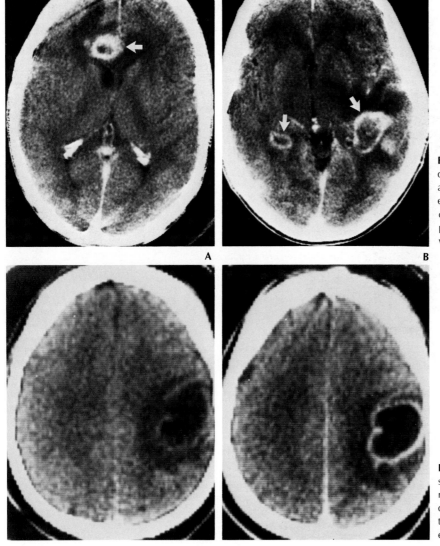

FIG SK20-5. Brain abscess in acquired immune deficiency syndrome. (A) Candidal abscess appears as a cystic lesion with a thick zone of enhancement (arrow) near the genu of the corpus callosum. (B) In another patient, multiple toxoplasmic brain abscesses appear as lucent lesions with rings of enhancement.[16]

FIG SK20-6. Cysticercosis. (A) Precontrast CT scan shows a primarily low-density area in the right frontoparietal region. The ring of increased density around the lesion is vaguely evident initially, but becomes readily apparent after contrast enhancement (B).[17]

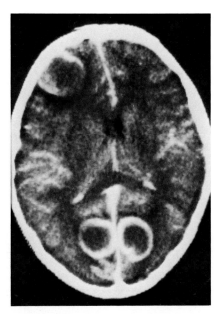

FIG SK20-7. **Pyogenic brain abscesses.** One frontal and two occipital lesions with relatively thin, uniform rings of enhancement.

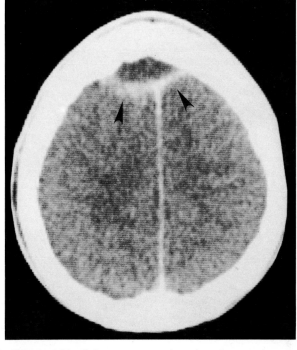

FIG SK20-8. **Epidural abscess.** Biconvex hypodense lesion with contrast-enhanced dural margin (arrowheads) that crosses the falx and displaces the falx away from the inner table of the skull.[18]

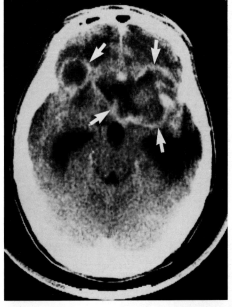

FIG SK20-9. **Resolving intracerebral hematoma.** Five weeks after the initial episode of bleeding, there has been a decrease in attenuation of the hematoma with peripheral contrast enhancement.[8]

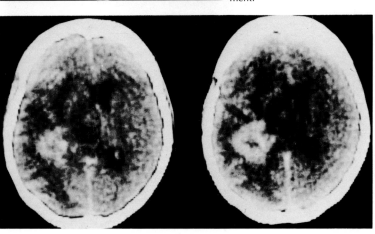

FIG SK20-10. **Atypical meningioma.** The contrast enhancement is predominantly peripheral, with the area of central necrosis remaining relatively nonenhanced. The correct diagnosis is indicated by the origin of the tumor from the thickened tentorium.

FIG SK20-11. **Radiation necrosis.** Lesion with ring enhancement and surrounding edema that could represent a primary or metastatic tumor. At autopsy the mass was found to represent postradiation necrosis with sarcomatous changes in a patient who had undergone surgery for a solitary metastasis.[18]

CEREBELLAR LESIONS ON COMPUTED TOMOGRAPHY

Condition	Imaging Findings	Comments
Astrocytoma **(Fig SK21-1)**	Cystic or hypodense solid mass. Variable contrast enhancement (cystic astrocytomas may display an enhancing rim of tissue surrounding the circumference of the cyst or an enhancing localized mural nodule along nonenhancing cyst margins).	Occurs more commonly in children (first or second most frequent tumor of the posterior fossa) than in adults. Affects the cerebellar hemispheres more commonly than the vermis, tonsils, or brainstem. About 20% of the tumors calcify. Malignant astrocytomas show edema and necrosis in addition to enhancement after the administration of contrast material.
Medulloblastoma **(Fig SK21-2)**	Sharply marginated, spherical midline mass that is hyperdense and shows uniform and intense contrast enhancement.	Embryonal tumor consisting of primitive and poorly differentiated cells that originate immediately above the fourth ventricle and migrate during gestation toward the surface of the cerebellum. One of the two most common posterior fossa tumors in children. May occur in the cerebellar hemispheres in older patients. Metastasizes along the cerebrospinal fluid pathways in about 10% of cases (abnormal contrast enhancement or irregular thickening of the lining of the subarachnoid spaces).
Ependymoma	Isodense or slightly hyperdense midline mass. Unlike medulloblastomas, ependymomas are often inhomogeneous with cystic or hemorrhagic areas and frequently calcify. The tumor margins are often irregular and poorly defined and the enhancement pattern is usually less homogeneous and intense than in medulloblastoma.	Fourth ventricular tumor that is more common in children than in adults. A characteristic finding is a thin, well-defined, low-attenuation halo that represents the distended and usually effaced fourth ventricle surrounding the tumor. The lesion frequently extends through the foramina of Luschka into the cerebellopontine angle or through the foramen of Magendie into the cisterna magna and typically causes hydrocephalus.
Hemangioblastoma **(Fig SK21-3)**	Most commonly a cystic hemispheric mass, typically with one or more small intensely enhancing mural nodules. May appear as a solid mass. Calcification is extremely rare.	Relatively uncommon tumor of the posterior fossa and spinal cord that is usually seen in adults. Hemangioblastomas tend to be smaller than hemispheric astrocytomas and almost never calcify. Characteristic intense tumor stain on angiography (more sensitive and specific than CT for this type of tumor).
Cerebellar sarcoma (lateral medulloblastoma) **(Fig SK21-4)**	Large, solid, lobulated mass that is hyperdense or heterogeneous.	Probably represents a variety of desmoplastic peripheral medulloblastoma that is never calcified or predominantly cystic (as may be a central medulloblastoma).
Metastases **(Fig SK21-5)**	Various appearances (densely enhancing nodules surrounded by edema; large, inhomogeneous, poorly enhancing mass; ring enhancement in tumors with central necrosis).	Most common cerebellar tumors of older patients. There is usually a history of an extracerebral tumor and evidence of other cerebral metastases.

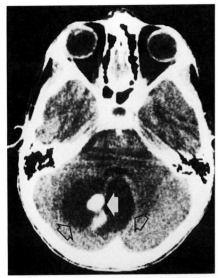

Fɪɢ SK21-1. Cystic astrocytoma. The cystic posterior fossa lesion (open arrows) contains a central nodular area of enhancement (closed arrow).

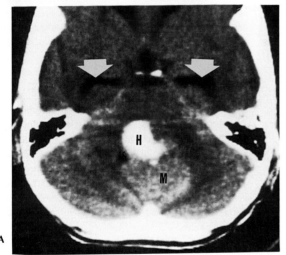

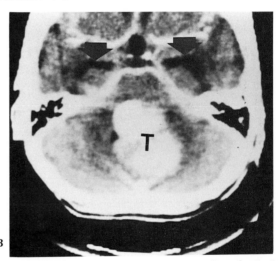

Fɪɢ SK21-2. Medulloblastoma. (A) Noncontrast scan in an 8-year-old girl shows the tumor as a mixed high-density (H) and medium-density (M) mass in the posterior fossa. (B) After the intravenous injection of contrast material there was marked enhancement of the tumor (T). The arrows point to the dilated temporal horns representing hydrocephalus.

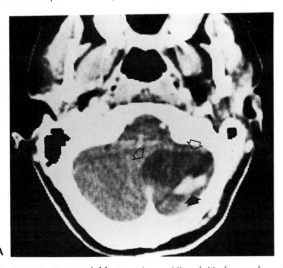

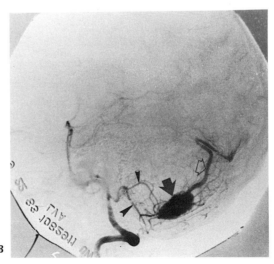

Fɪɢ SK21-3. Hemangioblastoma in von Hippel–Lindau syndrome. (A) CT scan shows a cystic lesion (open arrows) with an enhancing nodule (closed arrow) in the left cerebellar hemisphere. (B) Vertebral arteriogram shows the vascular nodule (solid arrow) of the tumor with multiple feeding arteries (black arrowheads) and a large draining vein (open arrow).

Condition	Imaging Findings	Comments
Lymphoma	Solid, hyperdense, densely enhancing mass that is located near the fourth ventricle or cerebellar surface and is usually associated with little or no edema.	Often multicentric with infiltration into adjoining tissue and across the midline (no respect for normal anatomic boundaries). Tumor margins are invariably poorly defined and irregular, probably because of the characteristic perivascular and vascular infiltration pattern of the tumor cells.
Epidermoid	Sharply marginated, nearly homogeneous, hypodense mass that may have an extremely low attenuation due to a high fat content.	Result of inclusion of ectodermal germ layer elements in the neural tube during its closure between the third and fifth weeks of gestation. Most commonly occurs in the cerebellopontine angle and suprasellar region, though it may develop in the fourth ventricle. Rupture into the ventricular system may produce a characteristic fat–cerebrospinal fluid level.
Choroid plexus papilloma	Homogeneous isodense or hyperdense intraventricular mass with smooth, well-defined, frequently lobulated margins. Intense homogeneous contrast enhancement.	Most commonly occurs in the first decade of life, usually in infancy. Typically develops in the lateral ventricles, though the fourth ventricle may be involved. In choroid plexus carcinoma, there are low-attenuation zones in the adjacent brain (representing edema or tumor invasion) and massive hydrocephalus.
Infarct (Fig SK21-6)	Well-defined, low-attenuation region in a cerebellar hemisphere.	Contrast enhancement in a subacute infarction may simulate a cerebellar tumor.
Hemorrhage (Fig SK21-7)	High-attenuation process that may appear round or irregular in shape and compress the fourth ventricle to cause hydrocephalus.	Hemorrhage into the cisterns usually produces a thin layer of higher-density tissue adjacent to the tentorium or in the pontine cistern.
Arteriovenous malformation (Fig SK21-8)	Large, tortuous, high-attenuation structures (representing serpiginous dilated vessels) that are seen after contrast enhancement.	An unruptured arteriovenous malformation may appear normal or only subtly abnormal on unenhanced CT studies, since the abnormal vessels are usually only slightly hyperdense with respect to the brain and are therefore difficult to identify. In some cases, calcification in the malformation or a low-density cyst or damaged cerebral tissue from previous hemorrhage suggests the presence of a malformation.
Abscess	Various patterns.	Pyogenic; tuberculous; fungal; parasitic; sarcoid.

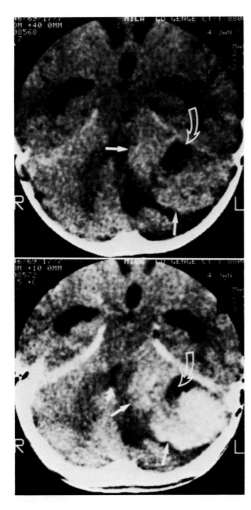

Fig SK21-4. Cerebellar sarcoma. (A) Noncontrast scan shows dense tumor (arrows) in the left cerebellar hemisphere. Note the cystic region (open curved arrow) within it. (B) After intravenous contrast infusion, the tumor is notably enhanced (arrows). The fourth ventricle is displaced severely from left to right (closed curved arrow), causing noncommunicating hydrocephalus.[8]

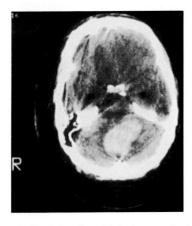

Fig SK21-7. Cerebellar infarction. Well-circumscribed, high-attenuation mass.

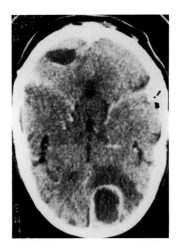

Fig SK21-5. Metastasis. Ring-enhancing lesion with surrounding edema.

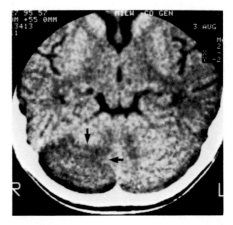

Fig SK21-6. Right cerebellar infarction. The low-attenuation process (arrows) has well-defined margins consistent with chronic infarction.[8]

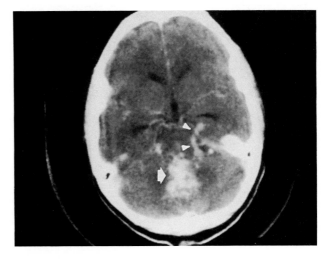

Fig SK21-8. Arteriovenous malformation. Irregular mass of increased attenuation in the vermis (arrow). Note the dilated vein (arrowheads) draining the lesion.

MULTIPLE ENHANCING CEREBRAL AND CEREBELLAR NODULES ON COMPUTED TOMOGRAPHY

Condition	Comments
Metastases **(Fig SK22-1)**	Round, well-marginated, homogeneously enhancing nodules that are typically located at the gray matter–white matter junction and are often associated with some peritumoral edema. The major malignant tumors causing intracranial metastases are, in decreasing order of frequency, lung, breast, skin (melanoma), colon, rectum, and kidney.
Primary lymphoma **(Fig SK22-2)**	Homogeneously and often intensely enhancing masses that most commonly occur in the basal ganglia, corpus callosum, or periventricular region. Peritumoral edema is usually slight. Primary lymphoma of the brain is rare in otherwise healthy individuals and is much more common in patients who are immunosuppressed (especially organ transplant recipients).
Multiple sclerosis **(Fig SK22-3)**	Contrast enhancement in plaques of demyelination is unusual except in rapidly evolving ones with surrounding inflammatory changes. The plaques in multiple sclerosis usually have a more central or periventricular location, unlike the more peripheral position of metastases near the gray matter–white matter junction.

Disseminated infection
  Cysticercosis
  (Fig SK22-4)
	Multiple small, homogeneously enhancing nodules may develop after infection by the larvae of the pork tapeworm (*Taenia solium*). Usually associated with much more extensive edema than are metastases. May demonstrate multiple enhancing rings, some of which contain focal calcification representing the scolices of degenerated larvae.

Tuberculosis	Homogeneously enhancing nodules or small rings with central punctate lucencies representing foci of cavitation surrounded by a rim of inflammatory cells.
Histoplasmosis	Pattern identical to that of multiple tuberculous abscesses.
Toxoplasmosis	Multiple densely enhancing nodules (or ring-enhancing lesions) that occur at both the gray matter–white matter junction and in a periventricular location.

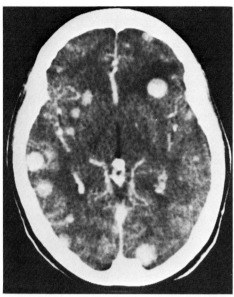

Fig SK22-1. Metastatic carcinoma. Multiple enhancing masses of various shapes and sizes representing hematogenous metastases from carcinoma of the breast.

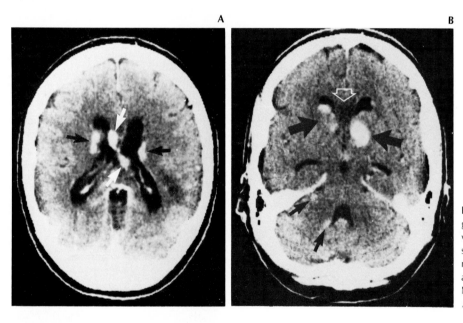

Fig SK22-2. Primary lymphoma. (A) Homogeneous enhancement of multiple periventricular nodules (arrows). (B) Another section shows additional enhancing lymphomatous nodules in the basal ganglia (large arrows) and posterior fossa (small arrows). Note the cystic cavum septi pellucidi (open arrow).[8]

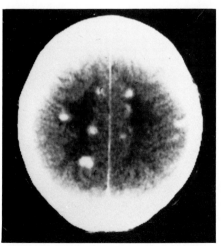

Fig SK22-3. Multiple sclerosis simulating metastases. Nodular enhancement in periventricular and subcortical white matter resulting from demyelination.[8]

Condition	Comments

Subacute, multifocal infarction
   Arterial
   (Fig SK22-5)
	Small focal enhancing lesions distributed along vascular watersheds. Underlying causes include hypoperfusion, multiple emboli, cerebral vasculitis (eg, systemic lupus erythematosus), and meningitis.

Venous	Parasagittal hemorrhages due to cortical venous infarction are a highly specific secondary finding in superior sagittal sinus thrombosis.
Sarcoidosis **(Fig SK22-6)**	Homogeneous enhancement of the noncaseating granulomas (more often affects the meninges than the brain).

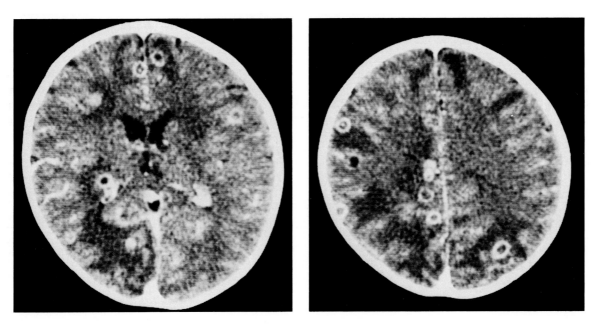

Fig SK22-4. Cysticercosis. Multiple enhancing nodules or rings, some of which contain focal calcification representing the scolices of erupted larvae. Note the zones of surrounding edema.[8]

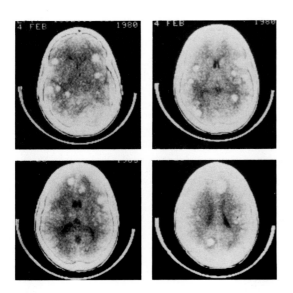

Fig SK22-5. Subacute, multifocal infarction. Multiple enhancing nodules producing a pattern mimicking metastases.

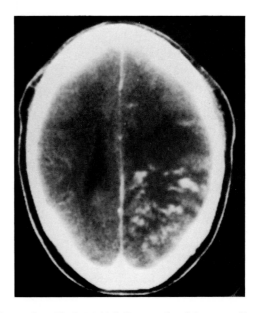

Fig SK22-6. Sarcoidosis. Multiple linear and nodular areas of increased density in the posterior half of the left cerebrum extending from the meninges to the deep white matter. This appearance represents infiltration of the Virchow-Robin space by granulomatous disease, in this case sarcoidosis. Note the associated encephalomalacia.[19]

SELLAR AND JUXTASELLAR MASSES ON COMPUTED TOMOGRAPHY

Condition	Imaging Findings	Comments
Pituitary adenoma (Figs SK23-1 and SK23-2)	Typically a well-circumscribed tumor of slightly greater than brain density that shows homogeneous contrast enhancement. Regions of necrosis or cyst formation in the tumor produce internal areas of low density. Microadenomas (< 10 mm) are usually less dense than the normal pituitary gland.	Computed tomography can demonstrate adjacent bone erosion, extension of the tumor beyond the confines of the sella, and impression of nearby structures such as the third ventricle, optic nerves, or optic chiasm.
Craniopharyngioma (Fig SK23-3)	Typically a mixed-density lesion containing cystic and solid areas and dense globular or, less commonly, rim calcification. Variable contrast enhancement of the solid portion of the tumor.	Benign congenital, or ''rest-cell,'' tumor with cystic and solid components that usually originates above the sella turcica, depressing the optic chiasm and extending up into the third ventricle. Less commonly, a craniopharyngioma lies in the sella, where it compresses the pituitary gland and may erode adjacent bony walls.
Meningioma (Fig SK23-4)	Hyperdense mass that enhances intensely and homogeneously after intravenous administration of contrast material. May have associated hyperostosis of adjacent bone.	Suprasellar meningiomas arise from the tuberculum sellae, clinoid processes, optic nerve sheath, cerebellopontine angle cistern, cavernous sinus, or medial sphenoidal ridge.
Glioma		
Optic chiasm (Fig SK23-5)	Suprasellar mass that is isodense on nonenhanced scans and shows moderate and variable enhancement after administration of contrast material.	Benign globular mass occupying the anterior aspect of the suprasellar cistern that most often occurs in adolescent girls, gradually produces bilateral visual abnormalities and optic atrophy, and is often associated with neurofibromatosis.
Hypothalamus	Usually a large, well-defined, irregularly contoured mass that is inhomogeneous with low-density and markedly enhancing regions.	Slow-growing astrocytoma that usually occurs in children and young adults. In infants, it typically produces a syndrome of failure to thrive despite adequate caloric intake, unusual alertness, and hyperactivity.
Chordoma (Fig SK23-6)	Well-defined mass with variable enhancement and homogeneity. Usually associated with destruction of the clivus and retrosellar calcification.	Locally invasive tumor that arises from remnants of the fetal notochord and most commonly occurs in patients 50 to 70 years of age.
Metastases (Fig SK23-7)	Smooth or irregular masses that usually enhance homogeneously and are associated with bone destruction.	Most metastases to the sellar and juxtasellar region originate from tumors of the lung, breast, kidney, or gastrointestinal tract or are due to direct spread from carcinomas of the nasopharynx or sphenoid sinus.
Germ cell tumor (germinoma/teratoma) (Fig SK23-8)	Various patterns of density and enhancement.	Occasionally involve the suprasellar region and frequently calcify (especially teratomas). May spread via cerebrospinal fluid pathways.

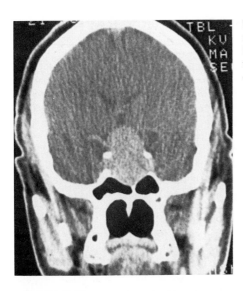

Fig SK23-1. **Pituitary adenoma.** Coronal scan shows an enhancing mass filling and extending out from the pituitary fossa. Note the remodeling of the base of the sella.

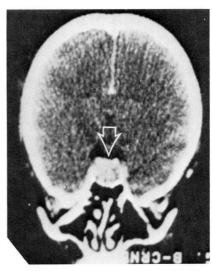

Fig SK23-2. **Nelson's syndrome.** Hyperdense tumor filling the enlarged sella (arrow) in a patient whose pituitary adenoma developed after adrenal surgery.

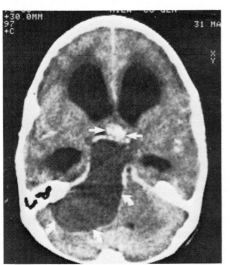

Fig SK23-3. **Craniopharyngioma.** The rim-enhancing tumor contains dense calcification (straight arrows) and a large cystic component (curved arrows) that extends into the posterior fossa. Note the associated hydrocephalus.[8]

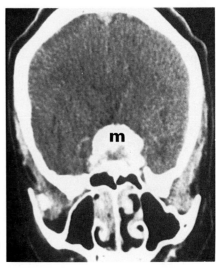

Fig SK23-4. **Meningioma.** Coronal reconstruction shows the large calcified mass (M) and associated bone destruction.

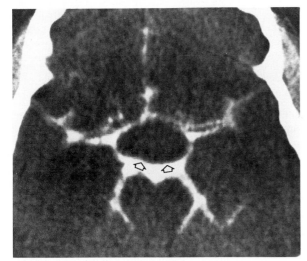

Fig SK23-5. **Optic chiasm glioma.** Axial suprasellar metrizamide cisternogram demonstrates a tumor filling the suprasellar cistern (arrows). Only faint enhancement was present on the standard contrast-enhanced CT scan.[20]

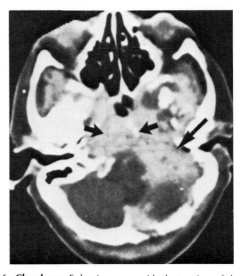

Fig SK23-6. **Chordoma.** Enlarging mass with destruction of the entire clivus (short arrows) and only small bone fractures remaining. The left petrous pyramid is also destroyed (long arrow).[18]

Condition	Imaging Findings	Comments
Epidermoid/dermoid (Fig SK23-9)	Smooth or lobulated suprasellar masses of low attenuation (usually of less than cerebrospinal fluid density). Usually nonenhancing (may have a thin peripheral rim of contrast enhancement).	Epidermoids are lined with squamous epithelium, while dermoids typically contain hair, dermal elements, calcification, and fat. Intrathecal contrast material may be required to find the margins of these lesions.
Neuroma	Inhomogeneously enhancing mass. A trigeminal tumor typically erodes the base of the skull (especially the foramen ovale and apex of the petrous pyramid).	Arises from cranial nerves III to VI. Gasserian ganglion neuroma appears as a large filling defect in the enhanced cavernous sinus.
Hamartoma of the tuber cinereum (Fig SK23-10)	Small, smooth, isodense and nonenhancing mass attached to the posterior aspect of the hypothalamus between the tuber cinereum and the pons.	Rare lesion of early childhood that usually presents with precocious puberty, seizures, and mental changes (behavioral disorders and intellectual deterioration).
Aneurysm **Intracavernous**	Well-defined, oval or teardrop-shaped, eccentric mass that is slightly denser than cerebral tissue on unenhanced scans and markedly and homogeneously enhanced after intravenous administration of contrast material.	Intracavernous internal carotid aneurysms are saccular, occasionally have an intrasellar component, and are bilateral in about 25% of cases. They may have rim calcification and contain a low-density area representing a thrombus. An aneurysm can erode bone and compress the cavernous sinus (causing cranial nerve palsy) or rupture and produce a carotid-cavernous fistula.
Suprasellar (Fig SK23-11)	Slightly hyperdense mass that enhances intensely and homogeneously. May have rim calcification and contain a low-density thrombus.	Usually most common in the fourth to sixth decades, congenital (berry aneurysm), and the result of maldevelopment of the media (especially at points of arterial bifurcation). The sudden onset of headache or neck stiffness suggests aneurysmal leakage or rupture.
Carotid-cavernous fistula	Focal or diffuse enlargement of one or both enhancing cavernous sinuses (most prominent on the side of the fistula) and enlargement of the superior ophthalmic vein (especially on the side of the fistula) and edematous extraocular muscles.	Arises from traumatic rupture of the internal carotid artery or spontaneous rupture of a carotid aneurysm. May occasionally produce a normal CT scan for a few days after head trauma because the fistula develops slowly or after a delay.
Arachnoid cyst (Fig SK23-12)	Well-defined, nonenhancing mass of cerebrospinal fluid density. Sharp, noncalcified margin.	A suprasellar cyst often causes hydrocephalus (most common in infancy), visual impairment, and endocrine dysfunction.
Inflammatory lesion	Various patterns.	Infrequent manifestation of sarcoidosis, tuberculosis, sphenoid mucocele, pituitary abscess, or lymphoid hypophysitis (an autoimmune disorder in which lymphocytes infiltrate the pituitary gland).
Histiocytosis X	Irregularly marginated, relatively well-defined enhancing suprasellar mass.	Involvement of the hypothalamus and sella turcica, which is most common in children, is usually associated with multiple destructive skeletal lesions.

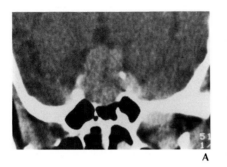
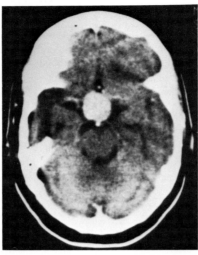
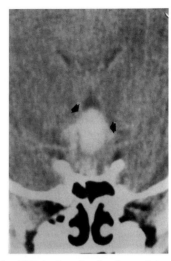

FIG SK23-7. Metastasis from oat cell carcinoma of the lung. (A) Noncontrast coronal scan shows a somewhat hyperdense mass filling the pituitary fossa and extending into the suprasellar region. (B) After intravenous injection of contrast material, there is dense enhancement of the metastasis.

FIG SK23-8. Ectopic pinealoma. Enhancing suprasellar mass (arrows).

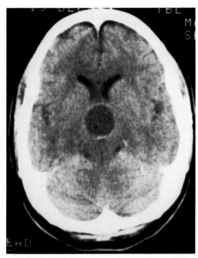
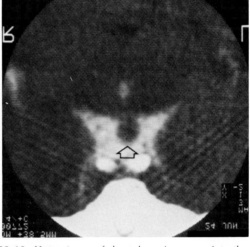

FIG SK23-9. Epidermoid. Smooth, low-attenuation suprasellar mass with a thin rim of contrast enhancement.

FIG SK23-10. Hamartoma of the tuber cinereum. Intrathecally enhanced coronal scan shows a small mass (arrow) that was isodense and nonenhancing in initial CT scans.

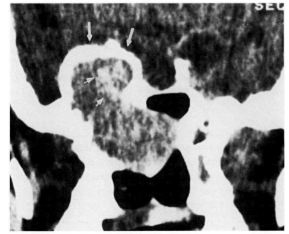
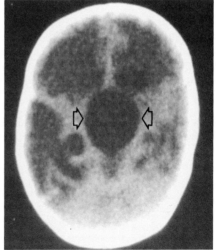

FIG SK23-11. Giant parasellar aneurysm. There is a rim of calcification (long arrows) along the superior margin of the aneurysm. Areas of enhancement in the aneurysm (short arrows) represent the patent lumen; the remainder of the aneurysm is filled with nonenhancing thrombus.

FIG SK23-12. Arachnoid cyst. Large, well-defined suprasellar mass of cerebrospinal fluid density (arrows). Note the prominent associated hydrocephalus.

MASSES IN THE PINEAL REGION
ON COMPUTED TOMOGRAPHY

Condition	Imaging Findings	Comments
Pineal tumors **Germinoma ("atypical teratoma")** **(Fig SK24-1)**	Isodense or hyperdense mass in the posterior third ventricle adjacent to or surrounding the pineal gland. Usually shows intense, homogeneous contrast enhancement.	Malignant primitive germ cell neoplasm that occurs almost exclusively in males, is usually radiosensitive, and is the most common tumor of the pineal region. May occur in association with a suprasellar germinoma. Because of their proximity to the aqueduct, these tumors frequently cause hydrocephalus. May produce ependymal or cisternal seeding.
Teratoma **(Fig SK24-2)**	Inhomogeneous mass containing regions of low and high attenuation representing fat and calcification, respectively.	Rare benign tumor that has a marked predominance in males and contains elements of all three germ layers. Usually shows minimal contrast enhancement (intense enhancement suggests malignant degeneration).
Teratocarcinoma	Irregularly marginated mass that varies in density and typically shows intense homogeneous contrast enhancement.	Malignant tumors (embryonal cell carcinoma; choriocarcinoma) that arise from primitive germ cells and are characterized by intratumoral hemorrhage, invasion of adjacent structures, and seeding via cerebrospinal fluid pathways.
Pineocytoma	Slightly hyperdense mass that often contains dense, focal calcification. Variable contrast enhancement.	Slow-growing tumor composed of mature pineal parenchymal cells and usually confined to the posterior third ventricle. Indistinct tumor margins suggest infiltration of adjacent structures. May spread via cerebrospinal fluid pathways.
Pineoblastoma **(Fig SK24-3)**	Poorly marginated, isodense or slightly hyperdense mass typically containing dense calcification. Homogeneous and intense contrast enhancement.	Highly malignant tumor of primitive pineal parenchymal cells that frequently spreads via cerebrospinal fluid pathways.
Metastasis **(Fig SK24-4)**	Indistinct hypodense or isodense mass that shows homogeneous enhancement. Occasionally hyperdense.	Infrequent manifestation that must be considered in older adults with known malignant disease.
Glioma of nonpineal origin	Low-density mass with poorly defined margins, minimal or moderate enhancement, and no calcification. May displace the normal calcified pineal gland.	Tumors arising from the thalamus, posterior hypothalamus, tectal plate of the mesencephalon, or splenium that extend into the quadrigeminal cistern. Usually occur in older patients.
Meningioma **(Fig SK24-5)**	Round, sharply delineated, isodense or hyperdense mass that is often calcified and shows intense homogeneous contrast enhancement.	Midline tumors arising from the edge of the tentorium may be difficult to distinguish from pineal tumors. However, they are usually eccentrically located and often have a flat border along the tentorium close to the dural margin.
Vein of Galen aneurysm **(Fig SK24-6)**	Mass of uniform density and intense contrast enhancement that mimics a pineal tumor.	Arteriovenous malformation that often presents in childhood, produces high blood flow, and is an important cause of neonatal heart failure.

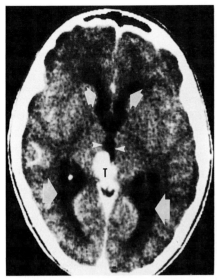

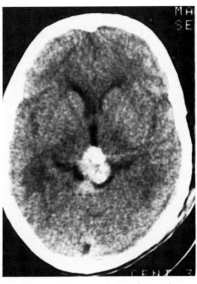

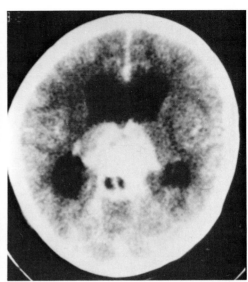

FIG SK24-1. **Germinoma.** Enhancing tumor (T) in the pineal region of a young girl with paralysis of upward gaze, headaches, and nausea (Perinaud's syndrome). The minimal dilatation of the third ventricle (arrowheads) and lateral ventricles (arrows) indicates mild hydrocephalus, which developed because of obstruction of the posterior portion of the third ventricle by the tumor.

FIG SK24-2. **Teratoma.** Nonenhanced scan shows an inhomogeneous mass containing a large amount of calcification.

FIG SK24-3. **Pineoblastoma.** Huge densely calcified mass in the pineal region causing obstructive hydrocephalus.

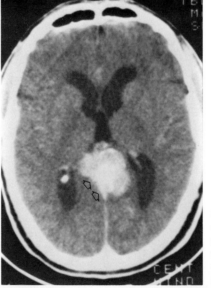

FIG SK24-5. **Meningioma.** Densely enhancing mass in the pineal region that arises from the incisura of the tentorium. Note the characteristic flat border (arrows) along the tentorium.

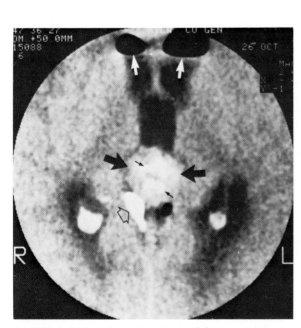

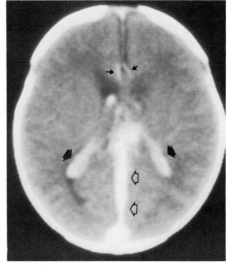

FIG SK24-4. **Metastasis.** In this patient with lung carcinoma, an unenhanced scan shows a well-circumscribed, hyperdense pineal mass (large arrows) containing dense punctate calcification (small arrows). Air in the frontal horns (white arrows) resulted from a recent ventricular shunting procedure. Note the tentorial calcification (open arrow) adjacent to the metastasis.[8]

FIG SK24-6. **Vein of Galen aneurysm.** Contrast-enhanced scan shows dilatation of the vein of Galen and straight sinus (open arrows). Note the prominent feeding vessels of the choroid plexus (closed arrows) and the anterior cerebral arteries (thin arrows).

CEREBELLOPONTINE ANGLE MASSES
ON COMPUTED TOMOGRAPHY

Condition	Imaging Findings	Comments
Acoustic neuroma (Figs SK25-1 to SK25-3)	Well-defined, uniformly enhancing tumor with smooth, rounded margins. Typically there is enlargement and erosion of the internal auditory canal. May contain low-attenuation cystic areas and simulate an epidermoid. Bilateral acoustic neuromas suggest neurofibromatosis.	Represents about 10% of primary intracranial tumors and accounts for most masses in the cerebellopontine angle. Small intracanalicular tumors confined to the internal auditory canal may cause bony changes or clinical findings suggesting an acoustic neuroma in the absence of CT evidence of a discrete mass. In such cases (if MRI not available), repeat CT examination is required after the intrathecal administration of contrast material (metrizamide or air).
Meningioma (Fig SK25-4)	Hyperdense mass on noncontrast scans that shows dense enhancement after the intravenous injection of contrast material. Unlike acoustic neuromas, meningiomas commonly show calcification and cystic changes. Typically they are larger and more broadly based along the petrous bone than neuromas.	Second most common cerebellopontine angle mass. Usually centered above or below the internal auditory meatus and infrequently associated with widening of the internal auditory canal (or hearing loss).
Epidermoid (Fig SK25-5)	Low-density mass on both pre- and postcontrast scans (though occasional high-density and enhancing lesions have been recorded). Infrequently has a calcified margin.	Most common location for these fat-containing tumors. Because the tumor tends not to stretch or distort the brainstem or cranial nerves but to surround them, an extensive neoplasm may be present before symptoms occur.
Metastasis (Fig SK25-6)	Enhancing mass with bone erosion (often without distinct margins) and sometimes edema in the adjacent cerebellum.	Usually a history of a primary neoplasm elsewhere.
Arachnoid cyst (Fig SK25-7)	Cystic structure with a density equal to that of cerebrospinal fluid. With positive contrast cisternography, there is enhancement of the adjacent cisterns without enhancement of the cyst (some intrathecal contrast eventually penetrates the cyst).	Typically displaces adjacent brainstem and cerebellar structures to a much greater degree than a cystic epidermoid tumor. Arachnoid cysts do not calcify, unlike epidermoids.
Aneurysm of basilar or vertebral artery (Fig SK25-8)	Usually has greater than brain density on precontrast scans.	The amount of contrast enhancement depends on the degree of luminal thrombosis. A characteristic appearance is concentric or eccentric circles representing the enhanced lumen, the less dense thrombus, and the dense wall of the aneurysm.
Arterial ectasia	Curvilinear, homogeneously enhancing structure that may simulate a cerebellopontine angle tumor.	Elongation and ectasia of the vertebral, basilar, or inferior cerebellar artery. Digital or conventional arteriography or dynamic CT can show the true nature of the process.

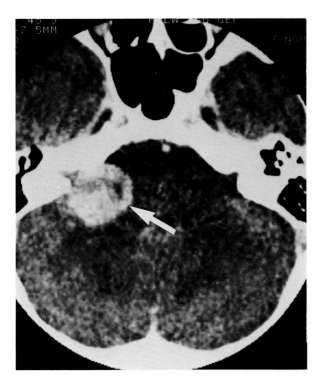

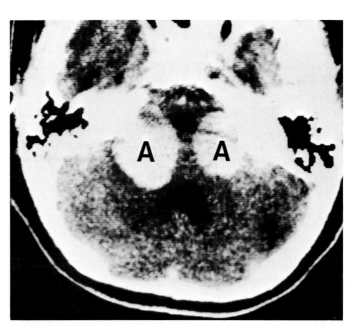

FIG SK25-2. **Neurofibromatosis.** Bilateral acoustic neuromas (A) in a young girl with progressive bilateral sensorineural hearing loss.

FIG SK25-1. **Acoustic neuroma.** Contrast-enhancing mass (arrow) in the right internal auditory canal and cerebellopontine angle cistern.[8]

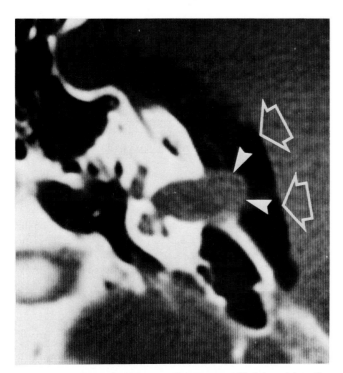

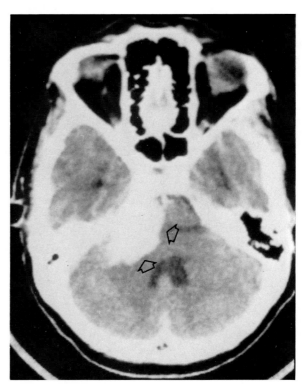

FIG SK25-3. **Intracanalicular acoustic neuroma.** Air injected into the subarachnoid space shows the cerebellopontine angle cistern (open arrows) and outlines the small tumor (closed arrows).

FIG SK25-4. **Meningioma.** Dense enhancing lesion that is more broadly based along the petrous bone than a typical acoustic neuroma.

Condition	Imaging Findings	Comments
Glomus jugulare tumor (Fig SK25-9)	Lobulated, uniformly dense, and densely enhancing mass. Although the highly vascular mass may simulate other enhancing extra-axial lesions at this site, associated erosion of the jugular foramen usually permits the diagnosis.	The tumor arises in the middle ear and produces a blue or red polypoid mass, which can be visualized otoscopically, or a mass in the jugular foramen. Although most are histologically benign, the tumor may be locally invasive and cause irregular and poorly defined bone erosion suggesting malignancy.
Extension of adjacent tumor	Various patterns.	May be secondary to brainstem or cerebellar glioma, chordoma, pituitary adenoma, craniopharyngioma, fourth ventricular tumor, choroid plexus papilloma, or neuroma of one of the lowest four cranial nerves.

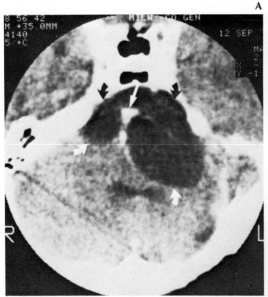
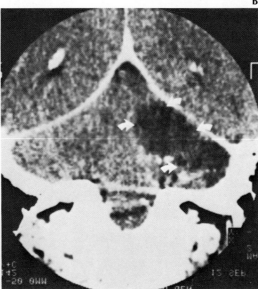

FIG SK25-5. Epidermoid. Irregularly shaped, low-density mass (curved arrows) in front of the basilar artery (arrow) and brainstem on (A) axial and (B) coronal images.[8]

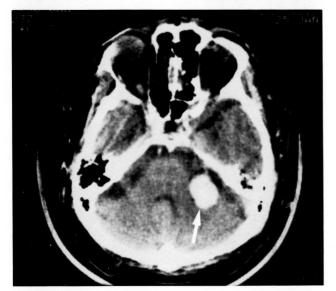

FIG SK25-6. Metastasis to left flocculus. Contrast-enhancing nodule (arrow) displaces the brainstem. It is distinguished from an acoustic neuroma by its location posterior and medial to the porus acusticus.[8]

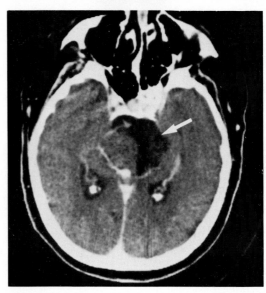

FIG SK25-7. Arachnoid cyst. Slightly irregular cystic mass (arrow) of cerebrospinal fluid density that displaces the brainstem and basilar artery to the right.[8]

Condition	Imaging Findings	Comments
Normal flocculus	Nodule along the lateral surface of the cerebellum near the internal auditory canal.	The flocculus is located posterior to the internal auditory canal, does not enhance as prominently as the usual acoustic neuroma, and is not associated with widening of the internal auditory canal.

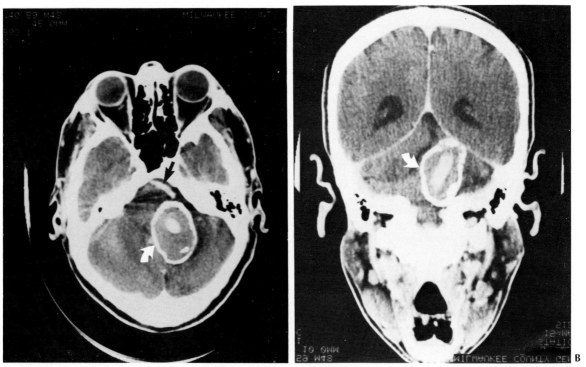

FIG SK25-8. **Giant aneurysm** with thrombus simulating meningioma. (A) Axial and (B) coronal images show the mass (curved arrow) with calcific rim and high density within it displacing the pons and cerebellum. The aneurysm fails to enhance as densely as the basilar artery (arrow).[8]

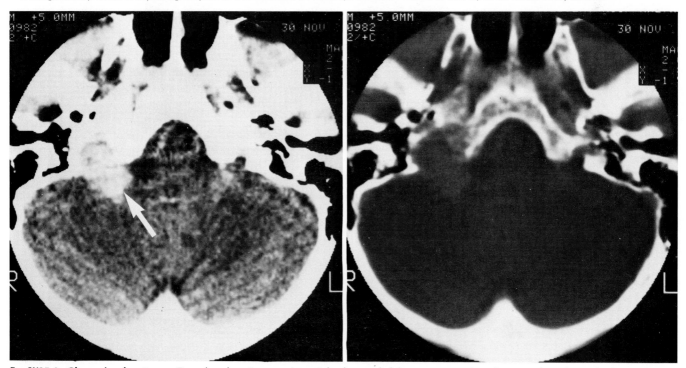

FIG SK25-9. **Glomus jugulare tumor.** Densely enhancing mass (arrow) that has eroded the osseous margins adjacent to the right jugular foramen.[8]

LOW-DENSITY MASS IN THE BRAINSTEM
ON COMPUTED TOMOGRAPHY

Condition	Imaging Findings	Comments
Glioma (Fig SK26-1)	Typically a low-attenuation area with indistinct margins in an asymmetrically expanded brainstem. The tumor may be relatively isodense (and be difficult to detect) or occasionally show increased attenuation or even gross calcification.	The mass effect depends on tumor size and may be generalized or focal. Contrast enhancement may be obvious, minimal, or absent. Cysts may occur, allowing palliative decompression.
Metastasis (Fig SK26-2)	Mass of inhomogeneous density with expansion of the brainstem and variable contrast enhancement (typically better defined than with gliomas).	More likely than primary glioma in a patient over 50 years of age with progressive brainstem signs. Usually there is evidence of other intracranial lesions (isolated metastasis to the brainstem is unusual).
Other tumors	Various patterns.	Hamartoma; teratoma; epidermoid; lymphoma.
Infarction (Fig SK26-3)	Combination of low attenuation, mass effect, and vague contrast enhancement may resemble a tumor.	Clinical information or follow-up scans can usually establish the diagnosis.
Multiple sclerosis	Combination of low attenuation, mass effect, and vague contrast enhancement may resemble a tumor.	Clinical information or follow-up scans can usually establish the diagnosis.
Central pontine myelinosis (Fig SK26-4)	Central region of diminished attenuation in the pons and medulla without marked contrast enhancement.	Characteristic clinical picture of a patient in coma with an electrolyte imbalance caused by prolonged intravenous fluid administration or alcoholism.
Syringobulbia (Fig SK26-5)	Central mass of cerebrospinal fluid density within and usually enlarging the medulla. Sharply defined margins. Does not show contrast enhancement (unlike cystic neoplasm).	Cystic process in the medulla that is most frequently found in conjunction with syringomyelia (an Arnold-Chiari malformation) and less often with a tumor or degeneration in the brain.
Granuloma/abscess	Appearance mimicking that of a neoplasm.	Rare manifestation of tuberculosis, sarcoidosis, or infection. Diagnosis may require biopsy.

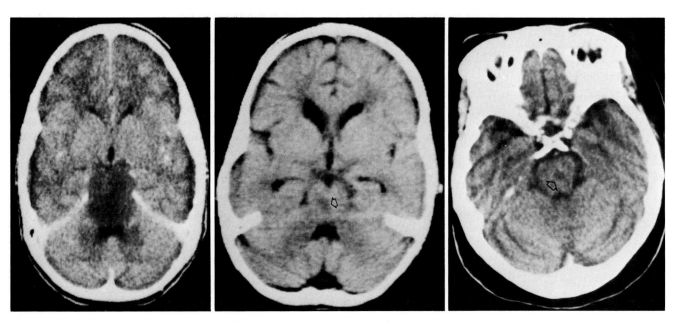

FIG SK26-1. Glioma. Poorly defined low-attenuation mass causing irregular expansion of the brainstem and compression of the fourth ventricle.

FIG SK26-2. Metastasis. Subtle, ill-defined area of low density (arrow).

FIG SK26-3. Infarction. Central low-attenuation region (arrow).

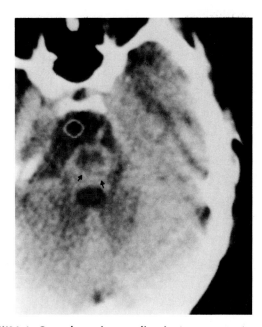

FIG SK26-4. Central pontine myelinosis. Low-attenuation region (arrows) in the center of the pons in a comatose alcoholic patient. Note the widening of the prepontine subarachnoid space, indicating loss of brainstem volume due to atrophy.

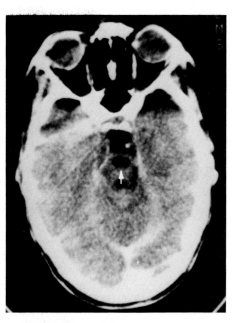

FIG SK26-5. Syringobulbia. Well-demarcated mass of cerebrospinal fluid density (arrow) in the center of the brainstem.

ENHANCING VENTRICULAR MARGINS
ON COMPUTED TOMOGRAPHY

Condition	Comments
Meningeal carcinomatosis (Fig SK27-1)	Most commonly secondary to oat cell carcinoma of the lung, melanoma, or breast carcinoma. Unlike meningitis, leukemia, or lymphoma, meningeal metastases usually occur in patients with a disseminated malignancy and are seldom associated with fever, leukocytosis, or meningismus.
Leukemia	Meningeal infiltration occurs in up to 10% of patients with acute leukemia. Although systemic chemotherapy, which penetrates the blood-brain barrier ineffectively, fails to prevent cerebral leukemia, the combination of intrathecal methotrexate and whole-brain irradiation effectively eradicates leukemic cells in the central nervous system (except for subarachnoid deposits isolated by adhesions).
Lymphoma (Fig SK27-2)	Most common form of intracranial lymphoma, which typically occurs in patients with diffuse histiocytic or undifferentiated lymphoma and poorly differentiated Hodgkin's disease.
Subependymal spread of primary brain tumor (Fig SK27-3)	Periventricular ''cast'' of tumor may reflect the ependymal seeding or subependymal spread of gliomas or other intracranial neoplasms (eg, medulloblastoma, germinoma).
Inflammatory ventriculitis (Figs SK27-4 and SK27-5)	May be secondary to bacterial, fungal, or parasitic infections or to noninfectious inflammatory disease (eg, sarcoidosis).

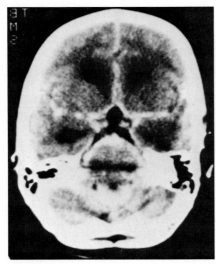

FIG SK27-1. Meningeal carcinomatosis. Generalized enhancement of the meninges with obstructive hydrocephalus.

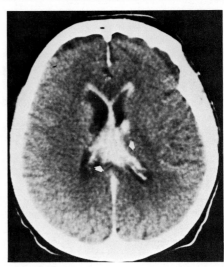

FIG SK27-2. Histiocytic lymphoma. Homogeneously enhancing lesions (arrows) deep in the brain associated with enhancement of ventricular margins.

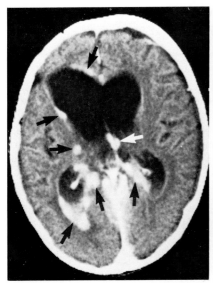
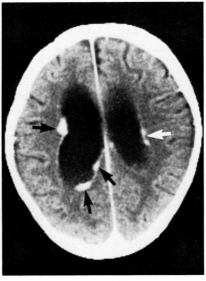

FIG SK27-3. **Subependymal metastases.** Multiple enhancing ependymal nodules (arrows) in a patient with posterior fossa ependymoblastoma and hydrocephalus.[8]

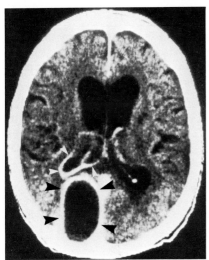

FIG SK27-4. **Brain abscess** with ventriculitis. CT scan following the intravenous injection of contrast material in a drug addict with lethargy and confusion demonstrates enhancement of the ventricular system (white arrowheads) due to extensive spread of infection. Note the ring-enhancing abscess (black arrowheads) in the right occipital lobe.

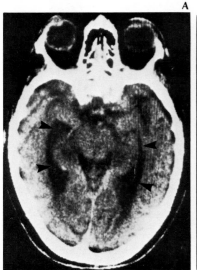
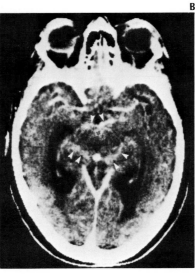

FIG SK27-5. **Pneumococcal meningitis.** (A) Noncontrast scan shows dilatation of the temporal horns of the lateral ventricles (arrowheads). (B) After the intravenous injection of contrast material, there is enhancement of the meninges in the basal cisterns (arrowheads), reflecting the underlying inflammation due to meningitis. The hydrocephalus in meningitis is due to blockage of the normal flow of cerebrospinal fluid by inflammatory exudate at the level of the aqueduct and the basal cisterns.

COMPUTED TOMOGRAPHY OF
PERIVENTRICULAR CALCIFICATION IN A CHILD

Condition	Comments
Tuberous sclerosis **(Fig SK28-1)**	Small, round, calcified nodules along the lateral wall of the frontal horn and anterior third ventricle are a hallmark of this inherited neurocutaneous syndrome, which is manifested by the clinical triad of convulsive seizures, mental deficiency, and adenoma sebaceum.
Intrauterine infection **(Fig SK28-2)**	Diffuse calcifications and ventricular enlargement associated with substantial cerebral atrophy and microcephaly typically develop in patients with congenital infections due to cytomegalovirus or toxoplasmosis.

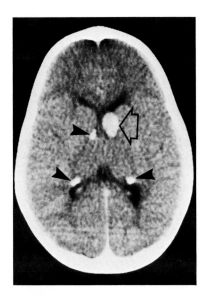

Fig SK28-1. Tuberous sclerosis. Multiple calcified hamartomas (solid black arrowheads) lying along the ependymal surface of the ventricles. The open arrow points to a giant cell astrocytoma at the foramen of Monro.

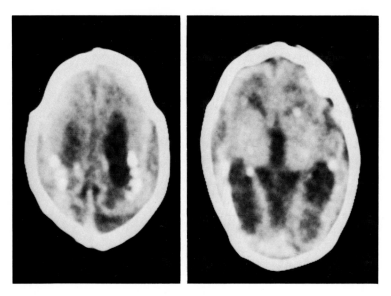

Fig SK28-2. Cytomegalovirus infection. Two scans of an infant show multiple periventricular calcifications and dilatation of the ventricular system.

THICKENING OF THE OPTIC NERVE
ON COMPUTED TOMOGRAPHY

Condition	Comments
Optic nerve glioma (**Fig SK29-1**)	Most common cause of optic nerve enlargement. Typically causes uniform thickening of the nerve with mild undulation or lobulation. In children (especially preadolescent girls), optic nerve gliomas are usually hamartomas that spontaneously stop enlarging and require no treatment. In older patients, however, these gliomas may have a progressive malignant course despite surgical or radiation therapy. Optic nerve gliomas are a common manifestation of neurofibromatosis (typically low-grade lesions that act more like hyperplasia than neoplasms).
Optic nerve sheath meningioma (**Fig SK29-2**)	Most commonly occur in middle-aged women and typically have a greater density, greater enhancement, and less homogeneous appearance than optic nerve gliomas. Other CT features include sphenoid bone hyperostosis and calcification, either eccentric when the tumor is polypoid or on both sides of the optic nerve with a tramline appearance when the tumor circumferentially surrounds the nerve.
Cyst of optic nerve sheath (**Fig SK29-3**)	Cystic dilatation of the optic nerve sheath produces a mass that is less dense than a meningioma. May develop after irradiation of an optic nerve glioma.
Optic neuritis	General term referring to thickening of the optic nerve developing from such nonneoplastic processes as multiple sclerosis, infection, ischemia (occlusion of vessels at the anterior portion of the optic nerve associated with temporal arteritis), and degenerative changes resulting from toxic, metabolic, or nutritional factors. After steroid therapy, enlargement of the optic nerve usually resolves.

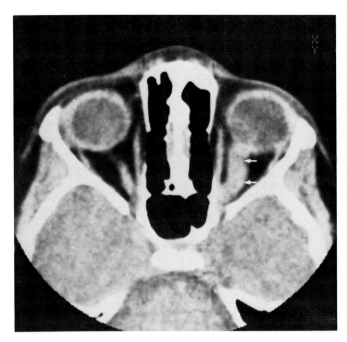

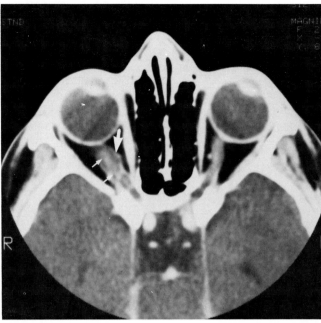

FIG SK29-1. Optic nerve glioma. Diffuse enlargement of the left optic nerve (arrows) in an 8-year-old girl.[8]

FIG SK29-3. Optic nerve sheath cyst. Large, smoothly marginated retrobulbar mass (arrows) that produced proptosis in this 43-year-old man.[8]

FIG SK29-2. Optic nerve sheath meningioma. (A) Axial scan shows the enhancing tumor (white arrows) along the entire length of the intraorbital optic nerve (black arrows). Note the intracranial portion of the tumor. (B) Coronal scan demonstrates the meningioma (white arrows) surrounding the optic nerve.[8]

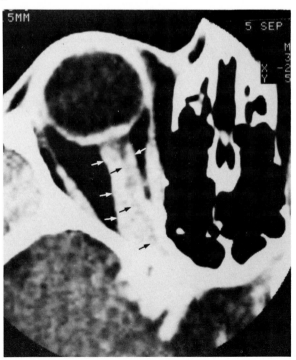

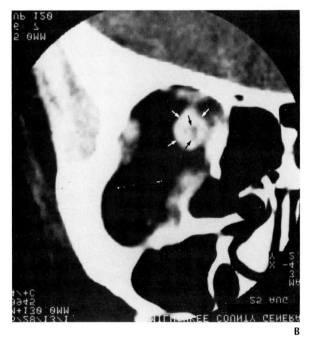

THICKENING OF THE RECTUS MUSCLES
ON COMPUTED TOMOGRAPHY

Condition	Comments
Thyroid ophthalmopathy (Graves' disease) (Fig SK30-1)	Hypersecretion by fibroblasts of mucopolysaccharides, collagen, and glycoproteins causes binding of water and increased intraorbital pressure, leading to ischemia, edema, and sometimes fibrosis of extraocular muscles. The medial and inferior rectus muscles are usually affected before and to a greater degree than the lateral rectus or superior muscle group. The two eyes may be involved symmetrically or asymmetrically.
Rhabdomyosarcoma (Fig SK30-2)	Uncommon, highly malignant orbital tumor arising from extraocular muscle that typically presents with rapidly progressive exophthalmus in boys under 10 years of age. Appears as a large, noncalcified, enhancing retrobulbar mass, often with adjacent bone destruction. The identification of a displaced, but otherwise normal, optic nerve helps to exclude an optic nerve tumor.
Metastases	Unusual manifestation of infiltration by such neoplasms as lymphoma, leukemia, and neuroblastoma. An orbital neurofibroma may rarely produce a mass thickening the contour of a rectus muscle.
Orbital myositis	Inflammatory process that usually affects multiple muscles in children and a single muscle in adults and presents with rapid onset of proptosis, erythema of the lids, and injection of the conjunctiva. In most cases, steroid therapy causes the enlarged muscles to return to a normal appearance.
Orbital pseudotumor	Inflammatory process that can affect virtually all the intraorbital soft-tissue structures. The variable CT appearances of this condition include enlargement of one or more extraocular muscles, a discrete or poorly defined intraconal or extraconal mass that may obliterate the muscle-fat planes, enlargement of the lacrimal gland, and scleral thickening. There is generally improvement after steroid therapy.
Infiltrative processes	Orbital cellulitis, Wegener's granulomatosis, lethal midline granuloma, sarcoidosis, foreign body reaction.

Condition	Imaging Findings	Comments
Carotid-cavernous fistula		Dilatation of the cavernous sinus may cause enlargement of the extraocular muscles due to venous congestion. Typical CT findings consist of unilateral proptosis and enlargement of the superior ophthalmic vein.

FIG SK30-1. Thyroid ophthalmopathy. (A) Axial view shows bilateral thickening of the inferior rectus muscles (arrows). (B) At a higher level, there is thickening of the medial rectus muscles bilaterally (arrows). (C) Coronal view shows thickening of virtually all the rectus muscles on both sides.

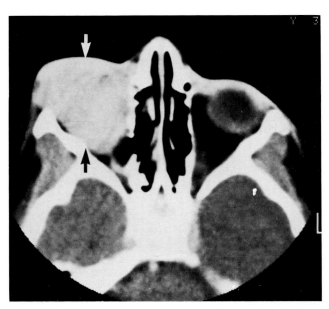

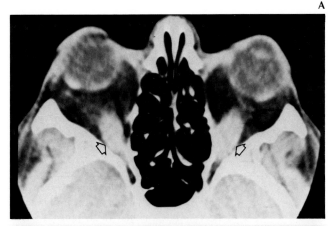

A

FIG SK30-2. Rhabdomyosarcoma. Enhancing tumor (arrows) fills virtually the entire right orbit in a 6-year-old child with rapidly progressing proptosis.[8]

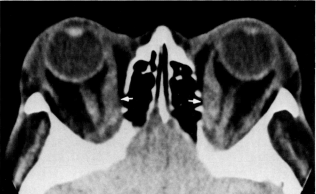

B

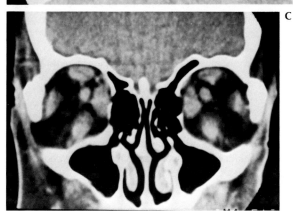

C

SOURCES

1. Reprinted with permission from ''Hypophosphatasia'' by W James and B Moule, *Clinical Radiology* (1966;17:368–376), Copyright © 1966, Royal College of Radiologists.

2. Reprinted from *Caffey's Pediatric X-Ray Diagnosis,* ed 8, by FN Silverman with permission of Year Book Medical Publishers Inc, © 1985.

3. Reprinted with permission from ''Button Sequestrum Revisited'' by SD Sholkoff and F Mainzer, *Radiology* (1971;100:649–652), Copyright © 1971, Radiological Society of North America Inc.

4. Reprinted with permission from ''The Calvarial 'Doughnut Lesion': A Previously Undescribed Entity'' by T Keats and JF Holt, *American Journal of Roentgenology* (1969;105:314–318), Copyright © 1969, Williams & Wilkins Company.

5. Reprinted with permission from ''The Small Orbit Sign in Supraorbital Fibrous Dysplasia'' by SK Tchang, *Journal of Canadian Association of Radiologists* (1973;24:65–69), Copyright © 1973, Canadian Association of Radiologists.

6. Reprinted from *Introduction to Neuroradiology* by HO Peterson and SA Kieffer with permission of JB Lippincott Company, © 1972.

7. Reprinted with permission from ''Roentgen Findings in Cerebral Paragonomiasis'' by SJ Oh, *Radiology* (1968;90:292–299), Copyright © 1968, Radiological Society of North America Inc.

8. Reprinted from *Cranial Computed Tomography* by AL Williams and VM Haughton with permission of The CV Mosby Company, St Louis, © 1985.

9. Reprinted from *Head and Neck Imaging* by RT Bergeron, AG Osborn, and PM Som (Eds) with permission of The CV Mosby Company, St Louis, © 1984.

10. Reprinted with permission from ''Paranasal Sinus Obliteration in Wegener's Granulomatosis'' by MR Paling, RL Roberts, and AS Fauci, *Radiology* (1982;144:539–543), Copyright © 1982, Radiological Society of North America Inc.

11. Reprinted with permission from ''Radiation Therapy of Midline Granuloma'' by AS Fauci, RE Johnson, and SM Wolff, *Annals of Internal Medicine* (1976;84:140–147), Copyright © 1976, American College of Physicians.

12. Reprinted with permission from ''Extramedullary Plasmacytoma'' by SI Schabel et al, *Radiology* (1978;128:625–628), Copyright © 1978, Radiological Society of North America Inc.

13. Reprinted with permission from ''Juvenile Nasopharyngeal Fibroma: Roentgenologic Characteristics'' by CB Holman and WE Miller, *American Journal of Roentgenology* (1965;94:292–298), Copyright © 1965, Williams & Wilkins Company.

14. Reprinted with permission from ''CT in Hydatid Cyst of the Brain'' by K Abbassioun et al, *Journal of Neurosurgery* (1978;49:408–411), Copyright © 1978, American Association of Neurological Surgeons.

15. Reprinted with permission from ''Lymphoma after Organ Transplantation: Radiological Manifestations in the Central Nervous System, Thorax, and Abdomen'' by DE Tubman, MP Frick, and DW Hanto, *Radiology* (1984;149:625–631), Copyright © 1984, Radiological Society of North America Inc.

16. Reprinted with permission from ''Acquired Immunodeficiency Syndrome: Neuroradiologic Findings'' by WM Kelly and MB Brant-Zawadzki, *Radiology* (1983;149:485–491), Copyright © 1983, Radiological Society of North America Inc.

17. Reprinted with permission from ''Unusual Neuroradiological Features of Intracranial Cysticercosis'' by CS Zee et al, *Radiology* (1980;137:397–407), Copyright © 1980, Radiological Society of North America Inc.

18. Reprinted from *Cranial Computed Tomography* by SH Lee and KCVG Rao (Eds) with permission of McGraw-Hill Book Company, © 1983.

19. Reprinted with permission from ''Virchow-Robin Space: A Path of Spread in Neurosarcoidosis'' by M Mirfakhraee et al, *Radiology* (1986;158:715–720), Copyright © 1986, Radiological Society of North America Inc.

20. Reprinted with permission from ''The Radiology of Pituitary Adenoma'' by SM Wolpert, *Seminars in Roentgenology* (1984;19:53–69), Copyright © 1984, Grune & Stratton Inc.

Index

A

Abetalipoproteinemia, 303, 306
Abdominal malignancy, undifferentiated, 400, *401*
Abdominal musculature, absent, 508, *509*, 512
Abdominal surgery, 137, 272, *273*
Abdominal wall, gas/abscess, 372, *373*
Abscess,
  abdominal wall, 372, *373*
  amebic, 376, *377*, 414
  brain, 806, 810, 848, *850*, *851*
  Brodie's, 578, *579*
  cerebellar, 854
  epidural, 844, *851*
  hepatic, 408, *409*, *411*, 412, *415*
  intraperitoneal, 314
  lesser sac, 370, *371*
  lung, 40, *43*, 56-69, 78, *79*, 98
  pancreatic, 370, *371*, 427, 430, *431*
  perirenal, 370, *371*, 468, *471*
  peritonsilar, 154
  pyogenic, 48, *49*, 376, *377*, 412, *415*, 842
  renal, 370, *371*, 469, *471*, 528, 536, *537*, 542, *543*
  retropharyngeal, 752
  soft tissue, 236
  splenic, 433, *435*
  subdural, 768
  subphrenic, 136, 140, *141*, 370, *371*
  tubo-ovarian, 550, *551*
Acanthosis nigricans, 97

Achalasia, 232, *233, 235*
Achondroplasia, *745*, 746, 758, *761*
Acoustic neuroma, 818, *819*, 866, *867*
Acromegaly, 462, *463*, 628, *629*, 656, 712, *713*,
  730, *731*, 746, *747*, 794
Acro-osteolysis, 638-43
Actinomycosis, 6, *13, 141*, 320
Adamantinoma, 600, 828, *829*
Adenoids, enlarged, 154, *157*
Adenolipoma, 544
Adenoma,
  adrenal, 544, *545*
  bronchial, 40, *43*, 80, *81*, 88, *89*
  liver, 410, *411*, 414, *417*
  pituitary, 816, *817*
  tracheal, 150, *151*
Adenomatous polyp, 260, *261*, 340, *341*
Adenomyoma, 356, *357*
Adenomyomatosis, 403
Adherent fecalith, 326, *327*
Adhesive bands, 338
Adrenal calcification, 388-89
Adrenal cortical carcinoma, 388
Adrenal cyst, 388, 546
Adrenal hemorrhage, neonatal, 388, *389*
Adrenal hyperplasia, 544, *545*
Adrenal masses, on computed tomography,
  544-47
Adult polycystic kidney disease, 464, *465*, 472, 526,
  527, 532, *533*

Adult respiratory distress syndrome (ARDS), 22, *23*, 148, *149*
Adynamic ileus, 294-96, *295*, *296*, 300
Aging,
    osteoporosis, 566, *567*
    parietal thinning, 784
    vas deferens calcification, 524, 525
    ventricular dilation, 822
Air-crescent sign, 98-99
Airway obstruction, upper, in children, 154-57
Albers-Schonberg disease, 584, *587*
Alcoholism, 234
    cardiomyopathy, 176, *177*, 240
    gastritis, 264, *265*
    joint damage, 648, 696
Aldosteronoma, 544, *545*
Allergic alveolitis, 52
Allergic angiitis, 458
Alpha-chain disease, 306
Alport's syndrome, 454
Alveolar cell carcinoma, 14, *17*, 42, *46*, 48, *51*, 52, 140
Alveolar microlithiasis, 24, *25*, 54, 86
Alveolar proteinosis, 24, *25*
Alzheimer's disease, 822, *823*
Amebiasis, 10, 320, *321*, 328, *329*, 334, *335*
Amebic abscess, 376, *377*, 414
Ameboma, 342
Ameloblastoma, 828, *829*
Amniotic fluid embolism, 20, *21*
Ampullary carcinoma, 360, *361*
Amyloidosis, 32, *35*, 36, *39*, 50, 54, 68, 88, *97*, 152, 258, 303, 304, *305*, 318, *319*, 332, 338, 346, 348, 456, 460, *461*, 504, 516, 650, 738
Anastomosis, surgical, 338
Anemia, 212, *213*, 568, *569*, 682, 684, *685*, 686, 794, *795*
Aneurysm,
    aortic (*see* Aortic aneurysm)
    basilar artery, 866, *869*
    carotid artery, 802, 812, *813*, 817
    dissecting, 190
    hepatic artery, 378
    iliac artery, 502
    pulmonary, 62
    renal artery, 393, *393*
    sinus of Valsalva (*see* Sinus of Valsalva)
    splenic artery, 380, *381*
    suprasellor, 862, *863*
    vang galen, 802, 864, *865*
    ventricular, 220, *222*
    vertebral artery, 750, *751*, 866, *869*
Angiomatous lesion, 602
Angiomyolipoma, 530, *531*, 534, *535*
Angioneurotic edema, hereditary, 348
Angiosarcoma, primary splenic, 434
Anisakiasis, 322, *323*

Ankylosing spondylitis, 36, 622, *625*, 632, *633*, 748, *749*, 754, *757*
Anthrax pneumonia, 6
Anticonvulsant drug therapy, 574
Antral mucosal diaphragm, 268, 270, *271*
Antral polyp, 270
Aorta,
    coarctation of (*see* Coarctation of aorta)
    corrected transposition of, 192, *195*
    prominent ascending, 190-95
    pseudocoarctation of, 192, *193*
    small ascending, 196-97
    tortuosity of 238, *239*
Aortic aneurysm, 82, 100, *103*, 108, *109*, 114, *115*, 190, *219*, 206, 218, 238, 274, 292, 502, 744
Aortic annulus/valve, 218, *219*
Aortic arch,
    anomalies of, and pulmonary artery, 198-99
    cervical, *199*, 238
    congenital heart disease and right, 200, *201*
    double, 198, *199*, 238
    prominent ascending aorta or, 190-95
    right, 238, *239*
    small ascending aorta or, 196-97
Aortic insufficiency, 174, *175*, 190, *191*
Aortic knob, 238, *239*
Aorticoduodenal fistula, 288
Aorticopulmonary window, 184, *187*
Aortic stenosis, 174, *175*, 188, *189*
    supravalvular, 196, *197*
    valvular, 190, *191*
Aortitis, syphilitic, 190, *193*, 218, *219*
Apical pleuropulmonary fibrosis, 240
Appendiceal stump, inverted, 324, *325*
Appendicitis, 320, 324, *325*
Appendicolith, 382, *383*
Appendix,
    calcified epiploicae of, 382, *383*
    intussusception of, 324, *325*
    mucocele of, 324, *325*, 382
    neoplasm of, 324, *325*
Arachnoid cyst, 766, 772, 782, *785*, 862, *863*, 866, *868*
Arachnoiditis, 766, *769*
Areae gastricae, 260
Arnold-Chiari malformation, 826
Arteriosclerosis, 174, *175*, 190, *191*, 240, 218, *219*, 454, *455*, 638, 802
Arteriovenous fistula, 208, 210, 212
Arteriovenous malformation, 392, 470, 762, *765*, 782, 802, 814, 818, 854, *855*
Arthritis, 610, *613*, 614, *622*. *See also*Ankylosing spondylitis;; Osteoarthritis; Psoriatic arthritis; Rheumatoid arthritis
    associated with inflammatory bowel disease, 624, *633*
infectious, 628, 630
Asbestosis/talcosis, 16, 26, 27, 135, 137, 142

Ascariasis, 10, 90, *92*, 358
Ascites, 274, 314, 402, *403*
Aspergillosis,
    fungal ball, 98, *99*
    hypersensitivity bronchopulmonary, 90, *93*
    pneumonia, 8, *99*
Aspiration causing pulmonary edema,
    of foreign body, 70, *123*
    of gastric contents, 18
    of hypertonic contrast material, 20
Asplenia syndrome, 211
Asthma, 76, *77*, 90, *93*, 126, *149*
Astrocytoma, 840, *841*, 852, *853*
Atelectasis, 122
Atlantoaxial subluxation, 752-53
Atrial enlargement,
    left, 172, *173*, 240
    right, 166-67
Atrial septal defect, 184, *185*, 196
Atrium, left, 220, *221*
Azygos continuation of the interior vena cava, 116,
    117, 208
Azygos vein, dilation of, 208

B

Bacterial infections, chest patterns for, 4, *5*, 6, *7, 9*,
    56, *57*, 66, *67*, 136, *139*, 140, *141*, 146
Bacteroides pneumonia, 6, *9*
Barotrauma, 838
Barrett's esophagus, 242, *243*, 246, *247*
Basal cell nevus syndrome, 672
Basal ganglia calcification, *800*, 808, *809*
Basilar artery, aneurysm of, 866, *869*
Basilar impression, 826-27
Battered child syndrome, 614, *615*
Bauxite pneumonoconiosis, 148
Behcet's syndrome, 332
Beriberi, 212, *213*
Berylliosis, *27*
Bezoar, 262, *263*, 270, *271*, 276, *277*, 297, *299*
Bile duct,
    calcification, 386-87
    cystic dilatation of, 364-65
    filling defects of, 358-59
    narrowing or obstruction of, 360-63
Biliary atresia, 362, 686
Biliary calculi, 358, *359*, 362
Biloma, 416, *419*
Bladder, urinary,
    calcification, 396-97
    carcinoma, 500
    diverticulum, 504
    filling defects of, 514-19
    fistula, 520, *521*
    gas in the lumen or wall of, 520-21
    large, 512-13
    neurogenic (*see* Neurogenic bladder)
    polyp, 514

prolapse, 512, *513*
    small, 510-11
Bladder neck obstruction, congenital,
    522
Bladder outlet obstruction, *495*, 512, *521*
Blastomycosis,
    chest, 6, *9*
    gastrointestinal, 322
Bleb/bulla, 58, *61*, 70, *71*, 76, *77*
Bleeding diathesis, 226
Block vertebrae, 730, *731*
Blood clot,
    bladder, 514
    intracavitary chest, 98
    pelvocalyceal, 484, *485*
    ureteral, 492, *493*, 502
Bochdalek's hernia, 114, *161*
Bone,
    acquired softening of, 716
    benign tumor of, 610, *612*
    bubbly lesions of, 592-603
    dysplasia, 684-91
    fracture, 610, 714, *715*, 734, *735*
    infarction, 564, *565*, 612
        in shaft, 578, *579*
    osteolytic destructive lesions of, 603-613
    overconstriction/overtubulation, 692-95
    primary malignant tumor of, 610, *611*
    secondary malignant tumor of, 610, *611*
    underconstriction/undertubulation, 682-91
Bone cyst, 688
    aneurysmal, 594, *595*, 726, *729*
    hemorrhagic/solitary, 828, *829*
    simple, 592, *594*
Bone island, 576
Bone-within-a-bone appearance, 708-11
Bowel wall,
    gas in, 368-69, 370, *373*
    hemorrhage into, *303*
    stricture, 298
    thickening/infiltration of, 314, *315*
Brain abscess, 848, *850, 851*
    healed, 806, 810
Brodie's abscess, 578, *579*
Bronchial adenoma, 40, *43*, 80, *81*, 88, *89*
Bronchial atresia, congenital, 44, 72
Bronchial injury, 126, *127*
Bronchial metastases, 80
Bronchial stricture, inflammatory, 82
Bronchiectasis, 82
Bronchiolitis,
    acute, 28, 76
    obliterans, 54
Bronchioloalveolar (alveolar cell) carcinoma, 14, *17*,
    42, *46*, 52, *55*, 140
Bronchitis, chronic, 28, *31*
Bronchogenic carcinoma, 40, *45*, 58, *59*, 66, *67*,
    78, *79*, 80, *81*, 140

Bronchogenic cyst, 44, 88, 108, *109, 110*, 112,
    113, 122
Broncholithiasis, 74, 84, 88, *89*
Bronchopleural fistula, *149*
Bronchus,
    fractured, 82
    left main stem, 238, *239*
Brown tumor, 596, *597*
Brucellosis, 376, 380, *381*, 734, *735*
Brunner's gland hyperplasia, 280, *281*
Bubonic plague. *See Yersinia pestis*
Bulla. *See* Bleb/bulla
Bull's eye lesions of the gastrointestinal tract,
    374-75, 436-37
Burkitt's lymphoma, 326, *327*
Burns, causing bone damage, 562, *563*, 616, 638,
    666
Burr hole, 784
Bursitis, calcific, 658, *659*
Busulfan-induced lung disease, *31, 97*
Button sequestrum, 788-89
Byssinosis, *29*

C

Caffey's disease. *See* Infantile cortical hyperostosis
Caisson disease, 698
Calcification,
    abdominal, 400, *401*
    adrenal, 388-89
    alimentary tract, 382-83
    appendix epiploica 382, *383*
    basal ganglia, *800*, 808, *809*
    bile duct, 386-87
    bladder, 396-97
    bursitis, 658, *659*
    cardiovascular, 218-23
    carotid artery, 800 *801*, 812
    dentate nucleus, *800*
    dura, 798, *799, 800*
    fingertips, 674-75
    gallbladder, 386-87
    genitourinary tract, female, 398-99
    habenula, 798, *799*
    intervertebral disk, 754-57
    intra-articular tumor, 652
    intracranial, 798-807
    liver capsule, 378, *379*
    mesenteric, 382, *383*
    muscular, 664-73
    pancreatic, 384-85
    periarticular, 658-63
    periventricular, in young child, 874-75
    pineal gland, 798, *799*
    placental, 398
    pleural, 134-35
    postinjection, 644, *665*
    postsurgical scar, 666, *667*

    psammomatous, 400, *401*
    pulmonnary parenchymal, 86-9
    renal, 390-93
    sellar or parasellar, 812-15
    spleen, 380-81
    subcutaneous, 664-67
    tendinous, 658, *659*
    tumoral, 660, *661*
    ureteral, 394, *395*
    vascular, 668, 670, *671*, 802, 808
    vas deferens, 524-25
Calcinosis universalis, 660, 668, *669*, 674,
    675
Calcium metabolism, disorders of, 572, *573*, 658,
    668, *671*, 796
Calcium pyrophosphate crystal dihydrate deposition
    disease, 626, *627*, 654, *655*, 658, 740,
    754
Calculus,
    bladder, 396, *397*, 514, *515*
    pelvocalyceal, 484, *485*
    renal, 390, *391*, 530
    ureteral, 394, *395*, 492, *493*, 498, *499*
Caliectasis, localized, 488
Callus formation, 576
Calvarial "doughnut", 788, *789*
Calvarial tumor, *793*, 806
Calvarium,
    generalized increased density/thickness of, 794-97
    localized increased density or hyperostosis, 790-93
Calyceal cyst or diverticulum, renal, 474
Campylobacter fetus colitis, 330
Candidiasis,
    esophagitis, 242, *243*
    pneumonia, 8, *95, 99*
Caplan's syndrome, 26, 50, *51*
Carcinoid-islet cell tumor, 282
Carcinoma. *See also* Lymphoma; Metastases;
    Neoplasm
    gastrointestinal, 254, *255*, 256, *257*, 260, *261,
        266*, 276, *277*, 278, *279*, 288, 308, *309, 311*,
        314, *315*, 320, 336, *337*, 338, 340, *341*, 350,
        351, 356, *357*, 358, *359*, 360, *361*, 376, 382,
        383, 388, 390, *391*, 416, *418*, 426, 428, *429*,
        432
    genitourinary, *469*, 484, *485, 487*, 490, *491*, 492,
        495, 500, *501*, 502, *503*, 510, 514, *515*, 528,
        530, *531*, 534, *535*, 544, *545*, 554, *555*
    skull, 838, *839*, 872
Cardiac output, decreased, 196. *See also* High-output
    heart disease
Caroli's disease, 364, *365*, 404, *405*, 412, *413*
Carotid artery,
    aneurysm, 802, 812, *813*, 817
    calcification of internal, 800, *801*, 812
Carotid-cavernous fistula, 862, 879
Castleman's disease, 102, 108
Catamenial pneumothorax, 146

Catheter, malpositioned/injury caused by, 138, *139*, *147*, 514
Cavitary lesions of the lungs, 56-61
Cecum,
    coned, 320-23
    diverticulum of, perforated, 320, *323*
    filling defects in, 324-27
    ulcer of, 326
Cementoma, 830, 832, *833*
Central venous pressure, increased, *206*, 208
Cephalhematoma, 790, *793*
Cerebellar abscess, 854
Cerebellar hemorrhage, 854, *855*
Cerebellar infarction, 854, *855*, 858, *859*
Cerebellar lesions on computed tomography, 852-55
Cerebellar nodules, 856-59
Cerebellar sarcoma, 852, *855*
Cerebellopontine angle tumors, 818, 866-69
Cerebelloretinal hemangioblastomatosis, 810
Cerebral atrophy in childhood, 794
Cerebral hemiatrophy, 792
Cerebral hemisphere, high-attenuation mass in, 846-47
Cerebral infarction, 806, 842, *843*, 858, *859*
Cerebral nodules, 856-59
Cerebral ventricles, dilated, 820-23
Cerebritis, 842
Cerebrospinal fluid, overproduction of, *822*
Ceroidosis, 296
Cervical aortic arch, 198, *199*
Cervical carcinoma, 554, *555*
Chagas' disease, 232, 302, 508, 512
Charcot's joint, 648-51, 652, *653*
Cherubism, *831*
Chest wall,
    hematoma, 132, *133*
    infection, 132
    lesion, 128
    trauma to, 126
Chicken pox. *See* Varicella
Chilaiditi's syndrome, 372, *373*
Choanal atresia, 154
Cholangiocarcinoma, 360, *361*, 416
Cholangiohepatitis, 364, *365*
Cholangiolitic hepatitis, 360, *363*
Cholangitis, 360, *363*, 364, *365*
Cholecystitis, 288, *289*, 354, *355*, 402, *403*
    emphysematous, 372, *373*
Choledochal cyst, 274, 292, 364, *365*
Choledochocele, 280, *283*, 364, *365*
Choledocholithiasis, 364
Cholesteatoma, 486, 784
Cholesterolosis, 356, *357*
Chondroblastoma, 596, *601*
Chondrodysplasia punctata, 580, *583*
Chondromyxoid fibroma, 598, *601*
Chondrosarcoma, 594, *595*, *666*
Chordoma, 726, 804, 812, *815*, 816, *817*, 860, *861*

Choroid plexus, 798, *799*
    papilloma, 804, *805*, 854
Chronic bronchitis, 28, *31*
Chronic obstructive pulmonary disease, 80
Chylothorax, 144-45
Clavicle, erosion/destruction/defect of the outer end of, 644-48
Cleidocranial dysostosis, 644, *645*, 824, *825*, 826
Coal worker's pneumoconiosis, *29*, *135*
Coarctation of aorta, 176, 188, *189*, 192, 196, 209, *211*, 216, 238, 700, *701*
Coccidioidomycosis pneumonia, 6, *11*, 56, *57*, 66, 92, *93*
Colitis,
    caustic, 330, 336, *337*
    cystic profunda, 344, *352*
    infectious, 348
    ischemic, 328, *329*, 334, *335*, 348, *349*
    pseudomembranous, 330, *331*, 348, *349*
    ulcerataive, 328, *329*, 334, *335*, 348
Collagen vascular disease, 216, 568, *571*, 658, *659*, 698, 704
Colon,
    annular carcinoma of, 336, *337*
    carcinoma of, 350, *351*
    cathartic, 336, *337*
    double tracking in, 350-51
    filling defects in the, 340-47
    ileus of, 294, *295*
    lesions, 326
    narrowing of, 334-39
    scirrhous carcinoma of, 336, *337*
    sphincters of, 336
    thumbprinting of, 348-49
    ulceration of, 328-33, 336
Common bile duct stone, 386,
    impacted, 284
Common ventricle, 210
Compensatory hypertrophy, 450, *451*
Computed tomography,
    adrenal masses on, 544-47
    anterior mediastinal chest lesions on, 104-7
    brainstem mass on, 870-71
    cerebellar and cerebral nodules on, 856-59
    cerebellar lesions on, 852-55
    cerebellopontine angle masses on, 866-69
    cystic renal masses on, 532-33
    focal solid renal masses on, 534-37
    high-attenuation mass in a cerebral hemisphere on, 846-47
    hypodense supratentorial mass on, 840-45
    middle mediastinal chest lesions on, 112-13
    optic nerve thickening on, 876-77
    pancreatic masses on, 428-31
    pineal region masses on, 864, *865*
    preventricular calcification in children on, 874-75
    rectus muscle thickening on, 878-79
    sellar and juxtasellar masses on, 860-63

ventricular margins on, 872-73
Conduction and rhythm abnormalities, 210
Congenital heart disease, 64
   acyanotic, with increased pulmonary blood flow,
     184-87
   acyanotic, with normal pulmonary blood flow,
     188-89
   cyanotic, with decreased pulmonary vascularity,
     182-83
   cyanotic, with incresed pulmonary vascularity,
     178-81
   and right aortic arch, 200-201
Congestive heart failure, 142, *143*, 174, 202, 224,
    402
   in neonates less than four weeks old, 209-11
Connective tissue disorders, 28, 36, *39*, 194, *195*,746
Constrictive pericarditis, 142, *143*
Convulsions, 738, *739*
Coronary artery, 220, *221*
   fistula, 184, *187*
Cor pulmonale, 168, *171*, 202, *203, 204*
Corpus callosum, 804, *805*
Corpus luteum cyst, 552
Cortical necrosis, acute, 460, *461*
Courvoisier phenomenon, 354, *355*
Cowden's disease, 342
Craniometaphyseal dysplasia, 588, *797*, 680, *681*,
    684
Craniopharyngioma, 812, *813*, 816, *817*, 860, *861*
Craniotomy, 784
Creeping eruption. *See* Cutaneous larva migrans
    pneumonia
Cretinism, 678, 758, 824
Cricopharyngeal muscle, 236, *237*
   achalasia, 232, *233*
Crohn's disease, 244, 256, *258, 268, 278, 279*, 286,
    287, 290, *291*, 304, *315*, 318, 320, *321*, 324,
    328, *329*, 334, *335*, 348, 350, *351, 437*
Cronkhite-Canada syndrome, 342
Croup, 154, *155*
Cryptococcosis pneumonia, 6, *11*
Cushing's syndrome, 352, 544, *545, 566*, 696, *697*
Cutaneous larva migrans pneumonia, 10, 90, *93*
Cyst
   adrenal, 388, 546
   arachnoid, 766, 772, 782, *785, 862, 863*, 866, *868*
   bone, 592, *594, 595*, 688, 726, *729*, 828, *829*
   bronchogenic, 44, 88, 108, *109, 110*, 112, *113*,
    122
   calyceal, 474
   choledochal, 274, 292, 364, *365*
   Dandy-Walker, 820
   dentigerous, 828, *829*
   dermoid, 398, *399*, 550, *551*, 782, 840, 862, *863*
   diaphragmatic, 160
   duplication, 250, *251*, 262, 282, 286, 310
   follicular, 828, *829*
   gastroenteric, 116, 118

hepatic, 412, *413*
jaw, 828-31
leptomeningeal, 784, *787*
neurenteric, 116, *117,* 118, 764
paraovarian, 548
parapelvic, 472, 490, *491*, 526, *527*, 532, 533
pelvic, 548-49
pericardial, 102, *103*, 112, *113*, 190
peridontal, 828, *829*
perinephric, 474
pleuropericardial, 108
primordial, 828
pyelogenetic, 474
radicular, 828, *829*
serous retentum, 836
splenic, 380, *381*, 434, *435*
thymic, 104, *105*
traumatic, 828, *829*
Cystadenoma/cystadenocarcinoma, 384, 426, *427*,
    428, 550, *551*
Cystic adenomatoid malformation, 60, 72, *75*, 122
Cystic bronchiectasis, 58, *61*
Cysticercosis (*Taenia solium*), 670, *673*, 808, *809*,
    856, *859*
Cystic fibrosis,
   chest patterns, 30, *35*, 60, *61*, 68, 76, *77*, 82
   gastrointestinal, 290, *291*, 346, 354, 384, *385*
Cystic lymphangioma of mesentery, 292, *293*
Cystitis, 500, 510, *511, 517*, 518, *519*
   emphysematous, *519*, 520, *521*
Cytomegalovirus, 8, 330, 808, *809*

D

Dactylitis, 718-21
Dandy-Walker cyst, 820
Davidoff-Dyke syndrome, 822, *823*
Degenerative disk disease, 754, *755*
Degenerative joint disease, 652, 654
Dentigerous cyst, 828, *829*
Dermatomyositis, 28, 94, 668, *669*, 674, *675*
Dermoid cyst, 398, *399*, 550, *551*, 782, 840, 862,
    863
Desquamative interstitial pneumonia (DIP), 32, *35*,
    36, 92, *93*
Diabetes,
   glomerulosclerosis, 460, *461*
   with hypokalemia, 300
   insipidus, 508, 512
   maternal, 211
   mellitus, 234, 272, *273*, 354, 524, *525*, 564, *565*,
    648, *649*
Diabetic gangrene, 638, *639*
Diaphragm,
   elevated, 158-61
   hernia of, 124, *125*, 160, *161*
   ruptured, 160, *161*
   tumor/cyst of, 160

Diaphyseal acalsis, 684, *687*

Diaphyseal dysplasia, 586, *589*, 684, *689*

Diastematomyelia, 742, *743*, 762, *765*

Diffuse esophageal spasm, 232, *235*

Dilantin therapy, 712, 796

Diptheria, 156

Dirofilariasis, 90, *93*

Disuse atrophy, bone, 562, *563*, 692

Diuretics, physiologic response to, 462

Diverticulitis, 338, *339*, 350, *351*
  ileocecal, *323*, 326

Diverticulosis, 348

Double-outlet right ventricle, 178, *179, 180*

Down's syndrome, 748, 752, 758

Dressler's syndrome, 137, 224, *225*

Drug-induced disorders,
  chest, 22, 24, 28, *31*, 68, 90, *91, 97*, 142
  gastrointestinal, 234, 244, 294
  genitourinary, 512
  skeletal, 566, *567*, 574, 650, 696, 712
  skull, 796

Ductus arteriosus, 222, *223. See also* Patent ductus
    arteriosus

Duodenal atresia, 286, *287*

Duodenal bulb,
  and gastric antrum, 278-79
  pseudodiverticulum of, 316

Duodenal diaphragm, 286, *287*

Duodenal diverticulum, 316, 362
  intraluminal, 316, *317*

Duodenal filling defects, 280-83

Duodenal folds, thickening of, 290-91

Duodenal narrowing/obstruction, 286-89

Duodenal stenosis, 286, *287*

Duodenal sweep, widening of, 292-93

Duodenal ulcer, 284, *285*, 316, *317*

Duodenal varices, 282, *283*, 290, *291*

Duplication cyst, 250, *251*, 262, 282, 286,
    310

Dust inhalation,
  inorganic, 26, *27, 29*
  organic, 26, *29*

Dwarfism, 694

Dysautonomia, familial, 32, *35*

E

Ebstein's anomaly, 166, 182, *183*, 210

Echinococcal (hydatid) cyst, 40, *43*, 56, *59*, 98, *99*,
    358, *359*, 380, *381*, 406, *407*, 408, *411*, 412,
    413, 424, 434, *435*, 476, 600, 672, 726, 738,
    784, 806, 810, 842, *844*

Echinococcus granulosus, 376, *377*

Echinococcus multilocularis, 376, *377*

Ehlers-Danlos syndrome, 670

Eisenmenger syndrome, 180, *181*, 202, *204*

Electric shock, causing bone damage, 562, *563*, 666

Electrolyte/acid-base imbalance, 272, 294

Emotional distress, and gastric dilatation, 272

Emphysema,
  bullous, 122
  chronic obstructive, 76, *77*
  congenital lobar, 70, *74*, 122
  localized obstructive, 70
  mediastinal, 146, 206
  unilateral or lobar, 70, *73*

Emphysematous cystitis, *519*, 520, *521*

Empty sella syndrome, 817

Empyema, 354
  old tuberculosis, 135, *135*
  organized, 134, *135*
  subdural, 844, *845*

Encephalocele, 782

Encephalotrigeminal angiomatosis, 810, *811*

Enchondroma, 594, *595*

Enchondromatosis, multiple, 684, *689*

Endocardial cushion defect, 178, *181*, 184, *186*, 196

Endocardial fibroelastosis, 172, 176, *177*, 188, *189*

Endocarditis, subacute infective, 460

Endometrial carcinoma, 554, *555*

Endometrioma, 310, 548, *549*, 550, *551*

Endometriosis, 326, 338, 344, *345*, 348, 494, 504,
    516

Endotracheal tube, malpositioned, 80, *81*

Engelmann-Camurati disease, 586, *589*, 684, *689*

Enteric gram-negative bacteria pneumonia, 4, *7*

Enterolith, 382, *383*

Eosinophilia, pulmonary disease with, 90-94

Eosinophilic enteritis, 278, *279*, 303, 304, *307*, 318

Eosinophilic granuloma, 30, *34*, 262, 374, 596, *599*,
    610, 736, *737*, 788, *789*

Eosinophilic leukemia, 90

Ependymoma, 802, 852

Epicardial fat pad, 112

Epidermoid (primary cholesteatoma) lesions, 598,
    782, *785*, 840, *843*, 854, 862, *863*, 866, *868*

Epidermolysis bullosa, 640, *641*, 674, 694

Epidural abscess, 844, *851*

Epidural hematoma, 846, *847*

Epiglottitis, 4, 154, *155*

Epiphrenic diverticulum, 252, *253*

Erythema nodosum, 96

Esophageal atresia, 156, *157*

Esophageal diverticulum, 116, 252-53

Esophageal filling defects, 248-53

Esophageal motility disorders, 232-35

Esophageal narrowing, 246-47

Esophageal neoplasm, 114, *119*, 120

Esophageal ring, 246, *247*

Esophageal ulceration, 242-45

Esophageal varices, 250, *251*

Esophageal web, 236, *237*, 246, *247*

Esophagitis, 234, *235*
  corrosive, 242, *245*, 246, *247*
  eosinophilic, 244

infectious, 242, *243*, 248, *249*
  reflux, 242, *243*, 246, *247*
Esophagogastric polyp, inflammatory, 248, *249*
Esophagus, carcinoma of, 242, *245*, 246, *247*, 248,
    249, 382, *383*
  extrinsic impressions on cervical, 236-37
  extrinsic impressions on thoracic, 238-41
  rupture of, 126, *127*
Eventration of the diaphragm, 158, *159*
Ewing's sarcoma, 604, *605, 611*
Exostoses, multiple, 684, *687*

F

Fanconi's syndrome, 572
Fat embolism, causing pulmonary edema, 20
Fatty infiltration, hepatic, 420, *421*, 422
Fecal material, 342, *345*
Fetal lobulation, renal, 478
Fibrin ball, 128
Fibrogenesis imperfecta, 574
Fibroma,
  desmoplastic, 600
  nonossifying bone, 592, *593*
  ossifying, 600, 832, *833*
  tracheal, 154, *155*
Fibromuscular hyperplasia, 214, *217*
Fibrosarcoma, 608, *609*
Fibrosis, 422, *423*
Fibrous cortical defect, bone, 592, *593*
Fibrous dysplasia, bone, 580, 592, *593*, 684, *685*,
    714, 726, 730, 782, *785*, 790, *791*, 794, *795*,
    830, *831*, 832, 838
Fibrovascular polyp, 248, *249*
Filariasis, 30, *92*, 144
Fingertips, calcification about the, 674-75
Fissural developmental cyst, 830
Flexure defect, duodenal, 280
Flocculus, normal, 869
Fluid overload, causing pulmonary edema, 18, *19*
Fuorosis, bone damage caused by, 586, *587*, 616,
  672, *673*, 796
Focal nodular hyperplasia, hepatic, 410, *411*, 414, *417*
Follicular cyst, 828, *829*
Foramen of Monro, 820, *821*
Foramen ovale, premature closure of, 210, 211
Foreign body obstruction,
  chest, 70, 80, 122, *123*, 152, 154
  gastrointestinal, 250, *251*, 262, 344, 372, 382,
    383
  genitourinary, 518, 522
Frostbite, causing bone damage, 562, *563*, 638, 666
Fundoplication, 262, *263*
Fungal infections,
  chest, 6, 8, *9, 11, 13*, 30, *33*, 40, *43*, 52, *53*, 56,
    57, 59, 86, *95*, 96, 98, *99*, 130, *131*, 136, *139*,
    140, *141*, 146
  gastrointestinal, 330

genitourinary, 486, *487*, 518, 520
  hepatic, 414, *415*
  skeletal, 600, *601*, 630
  spine, 734

G

Gallbladder,
  calcification, 386-87
  carcinoma of, 356, *357*, 403
  congenital multiseptate, 354
  filling defects in an opacified, 356-57
  hypoplasia of, 354
  mucinous adenocarcinoma of, 386
  pseudopolyp, 356
Gallbladder size, alternations in, 354-55
Gallbladder wall, thickened, 402-3
Gallstone, 344, *347*, 356, *357*, 386, *387*
  ileus, 297, *298*, 308
Ganglioglioma, 840
Ganglioneuroma, 118, *119*, 120, 840
Gangrene
  diabetic, 638, *639*
  of lung, 98
Gardner's syndrome, 342, *343*
Gargoylism. *See* Hurler's syndrome
Garre's sclerosing osteomyelitis, 578, *581*, 834
Gas,
  in biliary system, 358, 373, *373*, 424
  in bladder lumen or wall, 514, 520-21
  extension of, and pneumomediastinum, 126, *127*
  extraluminal, in upper intestinal quadrants, 370-73
  in pelvocalyceal system, 484
  in portal venous system, 372, *373*, 424
  in ureter, 492
Gastric dilatation without outlet obstruction, 272-73
Gastric duplication, 268
Gastric irradiation/freezing, 256, *259*, 264
Gastric outlet obstruction, 268-71
Gastric remnant, filling defects in, 276-77
Gastric stump carcinoma, 276, *277*
Gastric ulcers, 254-55
Gastric varices, 266, *267*, 318
Gastric volvulus, 268, *271*
Gastritis, 254, *255*
  alcoholic, 264, *265*
  antral, 264, *265*
  bile (alkaline) reflux, 276, *277*
  corrosive, 256, *259*, 264
  hypertrophic, 264, *265*
  infectious, 164
  phlegmonous, 256, *259*
Gastroenteric cyst, 116, 118
Gastrojejunal muscosal prolapse, 276, *277*
Gaucher's disease, 590, 616, 682, *683*, 696, *699*,
  710, 736
Germinal cell neoplasms, 100, *102*, 106, *107*, 860,
  863, 864, *865*

Giant cell tumor, bone, 592, *593*, 726, *729*, 830, *831*
Giardiasis, 304, *305*
Glioblastoma multiforme, 840, *841*, 848, *849*
Glioma, 802, *803*, 860, 864, 870, *871*, 876, *877*
Globus pallidus, necrosis of, 844
Glomerular abnormality, in multisystem diseases, 458
Glomerulonephritis, 454, *457*, 458, *459*, 480, *481*
Glomerulosclerosis, diabetic, 460, *461*
Glomus jugulare tumor, 868, *869*
Glycogen storage disease, 176, *17*...
Gonorrheal proctitis, 328
Goodpasture's syndrome, 22, *23*...
Gout, 624, *625*, *627*, 632, 644, ... 698
Granulomatosis, allergic, 90
Granulomatous infections, 48... 836, *837*. *See also* Coc... Tuberculosis
Graves' disease, 878, *879*
Great vessels,
  aneurysm of, 206
  transposition of, 196,
Guinea worm (*Dracunc*...
Gynecological causes f...

Habenla, 798, 799
Hamartoma, 40, *43*... 863
Hamman-Rich sy...
Hand-foot syndr...
Heavy-chain dise...
Heavy metal poison...
Heel pad thickenin...
Hemangioblastoma, 85...
Hemangioendothelioma, 410, *411*, 41...
Hemangioma, 210, 308, *309*, 602, *603*, 726, *727*, 793, 780, *783*, 792, *793*
  cavernous, 376, 408, 414, *417*
Hematogenous metastases, 42, *45*, 58
Hematoma
  cerebellar, 854, *855*
  chest wall, 132, *133*
  epidural, 846, *847*
  intracerebral, 844, 848, *851*
  intracranial, 806, *807*, 810
  intrahepatic, 416, *419*
  intramural
    abdominal, 436
    bladder, 518
    duodenal, 282, *283*, 288, *289*
  mediastinal, 102, 106, 108, *110*, 112, 114, 120
  perirenal, 214, 390
  pulmonary, 12, 42, *46*, 50

renal, 528, 536, *537*, 542, *543*
soft tissue, 236
splenic, 434, *435*
subcapsular
  hepatic, 416, *419*
  renal, 470
subdural, 844, *845*, 846, *847*, 848
vertebral body, 772, *773*
Hematopoiesis, extramedullary, 114, 118, *119*, 120
Hemochromatosis, 420, 570, 628, *629*, 654, 756
Hemophilia, 564, 570, *624*
  bleeding into joints, 624, *627*, 698
  pseudotumor, 600, *602*
Hemophilus influenzae pneumonia, 4, 7, 78, *79*, 155
...ophilus pertussis (whooping cough) pneumonia,

...ds, internal, 344, *347*
...ax, organized, *134*
...chonlein purpura, 458, *459*
...bscess, 408, *409*, *411*, 412, *415*
...arterial infusion chemotheraphy, 258
...artery aneurysm, 378
...e attenuation, generalized abnormality of, ...20-21
...ic cysts, 412, *413*
...tic fibrosis, congenital, 364, *365*, 540
...tic hematoma, 404, *405*
...atitis, 402, 424
...ecurrent pyogenic, 364, *365*
...patocellular carcinoma, 408, *409*, 416, *418*
...epatomegaly, 274, 442, *444*
...ernia, 118
  Bochdalek's, 114, *161*
  diaphragmatic, 124, *125*, 160, *161*
  external/internal small bowel, 297
  hiatal, 114, *115*
  intrapericardial, 108, *111*
  Morgagni, 100, 106, *161*
  omental, 104, 118
  retroperitoneal, 314, *315*
Herniated disk, 770, *771*
Herpes simplex encephalitis, 842, *845*
Herpes zoster, 330
Herpetic esophagitis, 242, *243*
Heterotopic gastric muscosa, 280, *281*
Hiatal hernia, 114, *115*
High altitude pulmonary edema, 20
High-output heart disease, 174, 202, *203*, 211, 212-13
Hilar enlargement,
  bilateral, 64-65
  and mediastinal lymph node enlargement, 66-69
  unilateral, 62-63
Hip, avascular necrosis of, 696-99
Histiocytosis X, 30, *34*, 36, *38*, 52, 68, *95*, 96, *599*, 608, 784, *787*, 830, 862
Histoplasmoma, 40, *41*, 66, 86, *87*
Histoplasmosis,
  brain, 856

gastrointestinal disorders, 304, 312, *313*, 376, 380, *381*
pneumonia, 6, *9*
Hodgkin's disease, 58, 100, *102*
Holt-Oram syndrome, 646
Homocystinuria, 568, 688, 692
Homogentisic acid deposition, 626, *755*
Honeycombing chest patterns, 36-39
Hookworm. *See* Cutaneous larva migrans pneumonia
Horseshoe kidney, 442, *444*
Huntington's disease, 822, *823*
Hurler's syndrome, 646, 746, *747*, 758, *759*
Hyaline membrane disease, 126, *127*, 146
Hydatid cyst. *See* Echinococcal (hydatid) cyst
Hydrocarbon poisoning, 74, *75*
Hydrocele, scrotal, 556, *557*
Hydrocephalus, 818
    atrophic, *822, 823*
    communicating, 820, *821*
    infantile, 825
noncommunicating, 820
Hydrocolpos, 548, *549*
Hydrometrocolpos, 523
Hydromyelia, 762, *765*
Hydronephrosis, 462, 468, 488, *489*, 506, 528, *529*
Hydrops, 354
Hydrosalpinx, 548, *549*
Hydroureter, 506
Hydroxyapatite deposition disease, 626
Hygroma, 100
Hypercalcemia, idiopathic, 588
Hypereosinophilic syndrome, 90
Hyperlucency of the lung,
    bilateral, 76-77
    unilateral/lobar/localized, 70-75, 122
Hypernephroma, 534, *535*
Hyperostosis,
    generalized cortical, 586, *797*
    frontalis, 790, *791*
    infantile cortical, 590, 610, *613*
    interna generalisata, 794
Hyperparathyroidism, 384, 574, *575*, 632, 638, *641*, 644, *645*, 654, 658, *659*, 678, 706, 732, 778, *779*, 786, 830, *831*
Hyperphosphatasia, 590, *591*
Hyperplastic polyp, 260, *261*, 276, 340
Hypersensitivity reaction, 97. *See also* Drug-induced disorders
Hypertensive cardiovascular disease, 174, 190, *191*, 214-17
    essential (idiopathic), 214, *215*
Hypertrophic pyloric stenosis, 258, 270, *271*, 436, *437*
Hypervitaminosis D, 588, 676, 688, 710, 756
Hypervolemia, 18, *19*, 212
Hypoalbuminemia, 402, *403*
Hypodense supratentorial mass, 840-45
Hypogenetic lung syndrome, 72

Hypoglycemia, neonatal, 211
Hypoparathyroidism, 588
Hypophosphatasia, 574, *575*, 686, 778, *779*, 824
Hypopituitarism, 694
Hypoplastic left heart syndrome, 166, *167*, 170, *189*, 196, 209, *211*
Hypoplastic lung, *71*, 122
Hypoproteinemia, causing pulmonary edema, 18, *19*
Hypothalamus, 860

I

Iatrogenic injury,
    bladder, 520
    infant heart, 210
    pneumomediastinum, 126
    pneumoperitoneum, 366
    pneumothorax, 146, *147*
    skull, 788
    thoracic duct, 144
Ileum,
    diverticulum/pseudodiverticulum of, 316, *317*
    filling defects of, 308-11
Iliac artery, aneurysm of, 502
Infantile cortical hyperostosis, 590, *613*, 610, *613*, 613, 690, 834, *835*
Infantile polycystic kidney disease, 472, *473*, 540
Infectious agents. *See also* Bacterial infections; Fungal infections; *names of specific infections, e.g.* Tuberculosis
    chest, 4-12, 30, 146, *149*
    constrictive pericarditis, 227
    gastrointestinal, 246, 256, *258*, 366
    genitourinary, 490, 506, 524, 536
    skeletal, 636, *637*, 666, 680, *681*, 718, *719, 720*
    skull, 788, *789, 793*, 806, 808, 810
    spine, 740, *741*, 764
Inflammatory bowel disease, 352, *353*
    associated with arthritis, 624, *633*
    associated with sacroiliac joint abnormality, 632, *633*
Inhalation,
    of heavy metals, 86
    of inorganic dust, 26, *27, 29*
    of noxious gases, 18, *19*
Interior vena cava, azygos continuation of, 116, *117*
Internal auditory canal, erosion and widening of, 818-19
Interpedicular distance, localized widening of, 742-43
Interstitial fibrosis, 32, *35*, 54
    idiopathic, 36, *38*
    secondary to pulmonary disease, 34, *17*
Interstitial lung disease, and pneumothorax, 146, *149*
Interstitial pulmonary edema, 28, *31*
Intervertebral disk space, narrowing of, and adjacent sclerosis, 740-41
Intervertebral foramen, enlarged cervical, 750-51

Intestinal atresia, 297, *299*

Intestinal edema, *303*

Intestinal lymphangiectasia, 303, 312, *313*

Intestinal malabsorption, and osteoporosis, 566

Intestinal pseudoobstruction, chronic idiopathic, 294, *295*, 302

Intestinal stenosis, 297, *299*

Intra-articular bodies, loose, causing skeletal damage, 652-63

Intracerebral hemorrhage, 846, *847*

Intracranial calcifications,
  multiple, 808-11
  normal (physiologic), 798-801
  solitary, 802-7

Intracranial pressure, increased, 210, 794, 816

Intracranial scarring (gliosis), 806, 810

Intrahepatic gallbladder, 404

Intramural esophageal-pseudodiverticulosis, 244, *245*, 246, *247*, 252, *253*

Intraosseous ganglion, 598

Intraosseous hemangiomatosis, 608

Intraparenchymal, 384

Intraperitoneal abscess, 314

Intrathoracic neoplasm, 206, *207*

Intrathoracic process, acute, 158, *160*

Intrauterine infection, and preventricular calcification, 874, *875*

Intubation,
  malpositioned, 80, *81*, *151*, 152, *153*
  prolonged nasogastric, 246

Intussusception, 297, *299*
  abdominal, 436, *437*
  appendix, 324, *325*
  colon, 344, *345*
  jejunogastric, 276, *277*

Ischemic bone necrosis, 578, *579*

Islet cell tumor, pancreatic, 426, 428, *429*

J

Jaccoud's arthritis, 622, *625*

Jaw,
  cystlike lesions of, 828-31
  radiopaque lesions of, 832-35

Jejunal diverticulum, 316, *317*
  pseudodiverticula, 316, *317*

Jejunogastric intussusception, 276, *277*

Jejunum, filling defects of, 308-11

Juvenile osteoporosis, idiopathic, 570

Juvenile polyps, multiple, 342

Juvenile rheumatoid arthritis, 620, *623*, 680, 694, *695*

K

Kaposi's sarcoma, 374

Kidney. *See also* Pelvocalyceal system; Renal anatomy
  bilateral large, multifocal, 464-65
  bilateral large, smooth, 458-63
  bilateral small, smooth, 454-57
  compensatory hypertrophy of, 450, *451*
  cystic diseases of, 472-77
  dense nephrogram, 480-81
  depression/scar in the renal margin, 478-79
  dysplastic, 452, 474, *475*, 532, *533*
  focal renal mass, 466-71
  hypoplasia of, congenital, 446, *447*
  misplaced, displaced, or absent, 442-45
  transplanted (*see* Transplanted kidney)
  unilateral large, multilobulated kidney, 452-53
  unilateral large, smooth, 450-51
  unilateral small, scarred, 448-49
  unilateral small, smooth, 446-47

Klebsiella pneumonia, 4, *5*, 78, *79*

Kummell's spondylitis, 738

Kwashiorkor (protein deficiency), 384

L

Lactase deficiency, 300, *301*

Lacunar skull, 782, *783*

Ladd's bands, 286, *287*

Laryngeal obstruction/compression, 76

Laryngeal web, 156

Laryngectomy, total, 232

Laryngomalacia, 156

Laryngospasm, 156

Lead poisoning, 272, 676, *677*, 690

Left-to-right intracardiac shunt, 166, 168, 172, 176, *185*, *186*, 202, *205*, 209, *211*
  reversal of, 180, *181*

Legg-Calve-Perthes disease, 696, *697*

Legionnaires' disease pneumonia, 6, *7*

Leiomyoma,
  stomach, *249*, 382
  uterus, 398, *399*, 554, *555*

Leiomyosarcoma, 554

Leprosy, 650, *651*, 666, 718

Leptomeningeal cyst, 784, *787*

Lesch-Nyhan syndrome, 638, *641*

Lesser sac abscess, 370, *371*

Leukemia, 66, *69*, 100, *102*, 462, *463*, 530, *531*, 606, *609*, 676, *679*, 680, *681*, 718, 744, 780, 872

Leukoplakia, 486

Ligamentum flavum, thickening of, 770

Lipid storage diseases, 570, *571*, 682, *683*

Lipoid pneumonia, 14, *15*, 38, 42, *46*

Lipoma, 104, 118, 128, 132, 340, *341*, 598, 766, 804, *805*, 842, *843*

Lipomatosis, 104, 112, 118
  pelvic, 338, 352, 502, *511*
Liposarcoma, 118
Listeriosis, 54, *55*
Lithopedion, 398, *399*
Liver,
  abscess, 370, 412
  calcification, 376-79, 424, *425*
  focal anechoic (cystic) masses of, 404-07
  focal decreased-attenuation masses in, 412-19
  generalized attenuation abnormality, 420-21
  generalized decreased echogeniticy of, 424
  generalized increased echogenicity of, 422-23
  increased density, 378, *379*
  shadowing lesions in, 424-25
Liver flukes, 358, *359*
Loa Ioa (*Filaria bancrofti*), 670
Lobar agenesis, congenital, 132
Lobar enlargement, 78-79
Lobar/segmental collapse, 80-85
Loeffler's syndrome, 16, 90, *91*
Lung abscess, 78, *79*
  acute, 40, *43*
  amebic, 56
  bacterial, 56, *57*
  fungal, 56, *57, 59*
  with inspissated pus, 98
Lung parenchyma, tear of, 126
Lung torsion, 14
Lymphadenopathy, 62, *63,* 64, *65,* 82, *96,* 112, *113,*
  119, 120, 744
Lymphangioma, 100, 384, *385*
Lymphangiomatosis, diffuse, 608, *609*
Lymphangitic metastases, 26, *27,* 68
Lymphatic obstruction, 403
Lymphatic stasis, 614, *617*
Lymph node enlargement, 108, *109, 239,* 248, 292
Lymphocele, 542, *543*
Lymphogranuloma venereum, 330, 334, *353*
Lymphoid follicular pattern, 344, *347*
Lymphoid hyperplasia,
  benign, 102, 108, 280, *281*
  nodular, 310, *312, 313,* 344, *347*
Lymphoma. *See also* Carcinoma; Neoplasm
  chest patterns, 14, 26, *27,* 48, 62, *65,* 66, *69,* 96,
    100, *102,* 106, 132, 136, 140
  gastrointestinal patterns, 254, *255,* 256, 260, *261,*
    264, *266,* 278, *279,* 300, 304, *305,* 308, *310,*
    318, 326, 338, 340, *343,* 348, *349,* 352, *353,*
    360, *361,* 363, *416, 426, 428, 430,* 434, *435*
  genitourinary patterns, 464, 516, 530, 534, *535*
  skeletal, *577,* 596, *599,* 606
  skull, 780, 846, *847,* 848, *849,* 854, 856, *857, 872*
  spine, 744, 770

M

Macroglobulinemia. *See* Waldenstrom's
  macroglobulinemia
Macroglossia, 156
Maffucci's syndrome, *671*
Malabsorption states, 572
Malacoplakia, 452, 494, *497,* 518, *519*
Malrotation, renal, 442, *443*
Marfan's syndrome, 194, *195,* 692, *693,* 706
Mastocytosis, 304, 312, 580, *581,* 586
Measles penumonia, *66, 95,* 97
Meatal stenosis, 522
Meckel's diverticulum, 316, *317*
Meconium ileus, 297, *299*
Mediastinal fibrosis, 206
Mediastinal hemorrhage/hematoma, 102, 106, 108,
  110, 112, 114, 120
Mediastinal lesions, anterior, 100-103
  computed tomography of, 104-7
Mediastinal lesions, middle, 108-11
  computed tomography of, 112-13
Mediastinal lesions, posterior, 114-17
  computed tomography of, 118-21
Mediastinal lymph node enlargement, 66-69
Mediastinal neoplasm, 82, 240
Mediastinitis, 102, 106, 108, *110, 111,* 112, 114, 118
Mediastinum, shift of, 122-25
Mediterranean fever, familial, 138, 626, 634, *637*
Medullary cystic disease, 456, 474, *477,* 526
Medullary sponge kidney, 390, *391,* 472, *473,* 488,
  489
Medulloblastoma, 852, *853*
Megacalyces, congenital, 488
Megacystis syndrome, 512
Megaesophagus, 114, *116*
Megaloureter, congenital, 506
Meig's syndrome, 136
Melanoma, gastrointestinal, 374, *375*
Melorheostosis, 586, *587*
Membranous lipodystrophy, 608
Mendelson's syndrome, 18
Menetrier's disease, 264, *265,* 318
Meningeal carcinomatosis, *872*
Meningioma, 766, *767,* 780, 790, *791, 803,* 804,
  812, *815, 846,* 850, *851,* 860, *861,* 864, *865,*
  866, *867*
Meningitis, 806, *807*
Meningocele, 116, 118, 742, *743,* 782
Meningomyelocele, 648
Meniscus (air-crescent) sign, 98-99
Mercury poisoning, 332
Mesenchymal tumor, 42, 100, *103,* 492, 516
Mesenteric arterial collaterals, 282, *283,* 290
Mesenteric artery syndrome, superior, 288, *289*
Mesenteric calcification, 382, *383*
Mesenteric vascular disease, 368, *369*
Mesenteritis, retractile, 314, *315,* 338
Mesothelioma, 128, *129,* 140, *141*
Metabolic disorders, 294
  calcification in, 88, *89*
Metachromatic leukodystrophy, 356
Metaphyseal dysplasia, 684, *687*

Metaphyseal injury, 686
Metaphyses,
    abnormalities, 588, *677*, *679*
    increased density zones in, 676-79
    radilucent bands, 680-81
Metastases,
    chest, 62, *63*, 88, *89*, 128, *129*, 136, 140, 150
    gastrointestinal, 254, *255*, 256, *257*, 260, 288,
        308, 326, *327*, 332, *333*, 336, *337*, 340, *341*,
        343, 356, 374, 376, *379*, 406, *407*, 408, *409*,
        416, *418*, *419*, 426, 428, 434, *435*
    genitourinary, 494, 514, 534, 544, *547*
    skeletal, 596, *598*, *599*, 604, 680
    skull, 780, 790, *791*, *793*, 794, *797*, 816, 830,
        840, *841*, 846, *847*, 848, *849*, 852, *855*, 856,
        857, 860, *863*, 864, *865*, 866, *868*, 870, *871*,
        878
    spine, 728, 732, 766, *769*, 770, *773*
Metatropic dwarfism, 686
Methotrexate-induced lung disease, 31, *91*
Middle lobe syndrome, lung, 82
Miliary nodules, 52-55
Milk of calcium,
    bile, 386, *387*
    renal, 392, *393*
Mirror-image pattern, right aortic arch, 198, 200, *201*
Mitral annulus, 218, *219*
Mitral insufficiency, 172, *173*, 176, *177*, 202
Mitral stenosis, 168, *171*, 172, *173*, 196, 202
Mitral valve, 218
Monckeberg's sclerosis, *671*
Mononucleosis, 8, *64*, 66
Morgagni's hernia, 100, 106, *161*
Morquio's syndrome, 736, *737*, 752, 758, *759*
Motility disorders, esophagus, *233*, 246
Mucocele, paranasal sinus, 836, *837*
Mucoid impaction plug, 44, *47*, 50, 80, *83*
Mucopolysaccharidoses, 688, 746, *747*, 758
Mucormycosis pneumonia, 8, 56, *59*, *837*
Mucous retention cyst, 836
Multicentric reticulohistiocytosis, 626, *629*
Multilocular cyst, renal, 468, 474
Multiple sclerosis, 844, *845*, 856, *857*, 870
Muscles, calcification or ossification in,
    generalized, 668-73
    localized, 664-67
Mycetoma, 486, *487*
Mycobacteria, atypical, 12, 56, *57*
Mycoplasma, 8, *13*, 30, *33*, 66
Mycosis fungoides, 96
Myelolipoma, 544
Myeloma,
    extramedullary, 150, *151*
    localized bone, 596, *597*
    multiple, 42, *133*, 140, 460, 580, *591*, 590, *591*,
        604, *605*, 732, *733*, 780, *781*
Myelosclerosis, 584, *585*, 796
Myocardial infarction, 174, *175*, 240

Myocardial ischemia, 174, *175*
Myocardiopathy, 176, *177*, 210
Myositis ossificans, 660, *663*, *664*, 672, *673*
Myxedema, 138, 226, 712
Myxoglobulosis, 324
Myxoma of left atrium, 172

N

Narcotic abuse, causing pulmonary edema, 22
Near-drowning, causing pulmonary edema, 20, *21*
Necrotizing enterocolitis, 368, *369*
Neonates,
    adrenal hemorrhage in, 388, *389*
    bone-within-a-bone in, 708, *709*
    congestive heart failure in, 209-11
    hypoglycemia in, 211
Neoplasm. *See also* Carcinoma; Lymphoma;
        Meningioma; Metastases; Sarcoma
    chest, 22, 98, 106
    gastrointestinal, 248, 254, 260, 268, *269*, 274,
        282, 284, *285*, 290, *291*, 297, *298*, 314, 324,
        325, 374, *375*, 396, *397*, 436, *437*
    genitourinary, 442, *445*, 466, 468, *469*, *470*, *471*,
        484, 500, *501*, 514, *515*
    hepatic, 408-11
    pericardium/heart, 224
    skeletal, 562, *565*, 568, *569*, 592, *593*, 594, *595*,
        596, *597*, 600, 610, *611*, 644, 652, 666, 688
    skull, 780, 788, *789*, 792, *793*, 802, *803*, *804*,
        806, 810, 816, 818, 830, 836-71
    spine, 114, 730, 736, 742, 750, *751*, 762, *763*,
        766, *769*, 770, 772
Nephritis, 446, *447*
    acute bacterial, 480, *481*, 540, *541*
    acute interstitial, 462
Nephrocalcinosis, 390, *391*, 538
Nephrogram, dense, 480-81
Nephromegaly, 462
Nephropathy,
    acute urate, 462
    hereditary, 454, 456
Nephroptosis, 442
Nephrosclerosis, 454, *455*, *483*, 482, *483*
Nerve root, traumatic avulsion of vertebral, 750, *751*
Neural disorders, primary, 234
Neurenteric cyst, 116, *117*, 118, 764
Neuroarthropathy (Charcot's joints), 648-51, 652,
        653, 740, *741*
Neuroblastoma, 388, *389*, 546, 680, 780
Neurofibroma, 750, *751*, 766, *767*
Neurofibromatosis, 32, 36, *39*, 94, 694, 704, *705*,
        714, *715*, *745*, *781*, *745*, 746, 780, *781*, 792,
        818
Neurogenic bladder, 506, 510, *511*, 512, *513*
Neurogenic hypertension, 216
Neurogenic neoplasm, 114, *115*, 118, *119*, 352
Neurogenic pulmonary edema, 18

Neurogenic rib notching, 702, *703*
Neuromuscular abnormalities/disease, 272, *273*,
    568, *571*, 730, 760
Neurotrophic disease, 638, *639*
Niemann-Pick disease, 32, 38, 54, *571*, 682, *683*
Nitrofurantoin-induced lung disease, *91*
Nocardiosis pneumonia, 6, *13*
Non-Hodgkin's lymphoma, 42
Nonunion of a fracture, 714, *715*

O

Obesity, 212, *213*, 274, 712
Obstructive uropathy, 450, *451*
Occupational acro-osteolysis, 642
Ochronosis, 626, 654, 660, 740, 754, *755*
Odontogenic lesions, 838
Odontoma, 832, *833*
Oil granulomas, 400, *401*
Oligodendroglioma, 802, *803*, 840, *841*
Ollier's disease, 684, *689*
Omental hernia, 104, 118
Optic chiasm, 812, 860, *861*
Optic nerve, thickening of, 876-77
Optic nerve sheath,
    cyst of, 876, *877*
    meningioma, 876, *877*
Optic neuritis, 876
Orbital myositis, 878
Orbital pseudotumor, 878
Organic dust inhalation, 26, *29*
Osteitis condensans ilii, 582, 632, *633*
Osteoarthritis, 620, *621*, 632, 636, 716
    erosive, 620, *621*
Osteoarthropathy, 614, *615*, 616, *643*
Osteoblastic metastases, 576, *577*, 584, *585*
Osteoblastoma, 596, *599*, 726, *727*, 794, 797
Osteochondritis dissecans, 652, *653*, 698, 699
Osteochondroma, 576, *578*, *579*
Osteochondromatosis, synovial, 652, *653*
Osteochondrosis, intervertebral, 740, *741*
Osteogenesis imperfecta, 568, *571*, 686, 692, *695*,
    704, 714, 716, 738, *739*, 778, 824, *825*
Osteogenic sarcoma, 608, *609*
Osteolysis, posttraumatic, 646
Osteolysis of Gorham, massive, 608
Osteolytic metastases, *598*, *599*, 604
Osteoma, 576, 832, *835*
    osteoid, 576, *577*
Osteomalacia, 572-75, 732
Osteomyelitis, 578, *579*, 600, 606, *607*, 610, *612*,
    644, 690, 698
    skull, 784, *787*, 790
    vertebral, 116, *117*, 734
Osteopathia striata, 580, *583*
Osteopetrosis, 584, *587*, 678, 686, *691*, 708, *709*,
    834

Osteophyte, 770, *771*
    anterior marginal, 236, *237*
Osteopoikilosis, 580, *583*
Osteoporosis, 732, *733*, 778
    generalized, 566-71, 817
    localized, 562-65
Osteoporosis circumscripta, 564, *779*
Osteosarcoma, 832, *835*
Osteosclerosis,
    general, 584-91
    physiologic, in newborns, 590
Osteosclerotic bone lesions, 576-83
Otto pelvis, 716, *717*
Ovarian tumors, 554, *555*
Ovarian vein syndrome, 502
Ovary,
    cyst, *548*
    cystadenoma/cystadenocarcinoma, 398, *399*
    gonadoblastoma of, 398, *399*
    neoplasm, 136
    spontaneous amputation of, 398
Oxalosis, 656
Oxygen toxicity, 26, *29*

P

Pacchionian depressions, 782, *783*
Pachydermoperiostosis, 616, 640, *643*
Page kidney, 214
Paget's disease, 212, 564, 580, 584, *585*, *731*, *779*,
    795, 710, 730, *731*, 736, 748, 772, 778, *779*,
    786, 792, 794, *795*, 830, 832
Pain, congenital indifference to, 648, *651*
Pancoast tumor, 128, *131*
Pancreas,
    abscess of, 370, *371*, 427, 430, *431*
    annular, 268, 286
    calcification of, 384, 385
    carcinoma of, 136, 288, *289*, 292, *293*, 426, 428,
        429, 432
    ectopic, 260, *262*, 280, 374, *375*
    fat necrosis of, 720
    mass on computed tomography, 428-31
    mass on ultrasound, 426-27
Pancreatic duct, dilatation of, 432-33
Pancreatic pseudocyst, 118, 282, *283*, 292, *293*,
    384, *385*, 418, *427*, 430, *431*
Pancreatitis, 136, *139*, 284, *285*, 288, *289*, 290,
    291, 292, 330, *331*, 338, 360, *363*, 384, *385*,
    430, *431*, 432, *433*, 696
Pantopaque, residual, in renal cyst,
    392
Papilla,
    aberrant, 486
    sloughed, 484, *487*, 494, 504
Papilla of Vater, 280, *281*
    enlargement of, 284-85

Papillary necrosis, 390, *391,* 454, 480, *485,* 488, *489,* 504
Papillary stenosis, 362
Papillitis, 284
Papilloma,
    bladder, 514
    ureter, 492
Papillomatosis,
    intrahepatic biliary duct, 364
    lung, 48, 60, *61,* 150
Paraesophageal hernia, 240, *241*
Paragonimus westermani, 10, 48, *49,* 56, *59,* 808, *811*
Parametrial gold therapy, complications of, 398
Paranasal sinus, mass in, 836-39
Paraovarian cyst, 548
Parapelvic cyst, 472, 490, *491,* 526, *527,* 532, *533*
Parasitic disease,
    chest, 10, 54, 56, 86, 90, *92, 93*
    gastrointestinal, 290, *307,* 308, *311,* 356, 362, 376, *377*
    skeletal, 670, 672, *673*
Parathyroid tumor, 100, 106, *107,* 236
Parietal foramina, 782, *783*
Parietal thinning, 782, 784
Partial anomalous pulmonary venous return, 186, *187,* 204
Patent ductus arteriosus, 184, *185,* 192, *193*
Pectoralis muscles, absent, 74, *75*
Pedicle, congenital absence of, 750
Pellegrini-Stieda disease, 662, *663*
Pelvic mass,
    complex, 550-53
    cystic-appearing, 548-49
Pelvic tumor, and ureteral obstruction, 500, *501,* 502, *505*
Pelvocalyceal system,
    diminished concentration of contrast material in, 482-83
    effaced, 490-91
    filling defects in, 484-87
Peptic ulcer disease, 254, *255,* 256, *257,* 262, *263,* 264, *265,* 268, *269,* 278, 290
Perforated viscus, 366, *367*
Periapical rarefying osteitis, 828, *829*
Pericardial cyst, 102, *103,* 112, *113,* 190
Pericardial effusion, 224-26
Pericardial lipoma, 112
Pericardial lesions, 240
Pericarditis,
    constrictive, 227
    infectious, 224, *225*
Pericardium, 220, *223*
    partial absence of, 124
Peridontal cyst, 828, *829*
Perinephric cyst, 474
Periosteal reaction,
    generalized, 614-19
        localized, 610-13
Periostitis of newborns, 614
Peripancreatic lymph node, 428, *429*
Perirenal abscess, 370, *371,* 468, *471*
Perirenal hematoma, 214, 390
Peritoneal dialysis, 137
Peritoneal (Ladd's) bands, congenital, 286, *287*
Peritonitis, 294
    meconium, 400
    with pneumoperitoneum, 366-67
    tuberculous, 400
Peritonsilar abscess, 154
Perivaterian neoplasm, 284, *285*
Persistent truncus arteriosus, 178, *179,* 194, 200, *201,* 209, 240
Peutz-Jeghers syndrome, *308,* 342
Phalangeal tufts, erosion of multiple terminal, 638-43
Pharyngeal airway obstruction, 154
Pharyngeal venous plexus, 236, *237*
Pheochromocytoma, 388, 544, *547*
Phleboliths, 380
Phosphorus metabolism, disorders in, 572, *573,* 658, 668, *671,* 796
Phrenic nerve paralysis, 158, *159*
Pickwickian obesity, 212, *213*
Pigeon breeder's disease, *29*
Pineal gland calcification, 798, *799*
Pinealoma, 804, *805,* 812
Pineal region, masses in, 864-65
Pineoblastoma, 864, *865*
Pineocytoma, 864
Pituitary adenoma, 804, 814, 860, *861*
Pituitary "stones," 814
Pituitary tumor, 816, *817*
Placental calcification, 398
Plasmacytoma, 596, *597,* 728, *733*
Pleural-based lesions, 124, 128-31
Pleural calcification, 134-35
Pleural effusion,
    associated with radiographic evidence of chest disease, 140-43
    large unilateral, 124, *125*
    with normal-appearing chest, 136-39
Pleural fluid, 128, *131*
Pleuropericardial (mesothelial) cyst, 108
Plombage, 60, *61*
Pneumatocele, 56, *57,* 72
Pneumatosis intestinalis, 344, 348, *349,* 368, *369,* 370, *373*
Pneumococcus pneumonia, 4, *5,* 78
Pneumoconiosis, 16, 26, *27, 29,* 36, *37,* 50, *51,* 52, *55,* 134, *135,* 148
Pneumocystis carinii pneumonia, 10, *13, 25,* 30, *33, 149*
Pneumomediastinum, 126-27
Pneumonia. *See also* Bacterial infections; Fungal infections

Pneumonia,
   anthrax, 6
   ascariasis, 10
   aspergillosis, 8, *99*
   bacteriodes, 6, *9*
   blastomycosis, 6, *9*
   candidal, 9 *95, 99*
   coccidiodomycosis, 6, *11*, 56, *57*, 66, 92, *93*
   cryptococcosis, 6, *11*
   cutaneous larva migrans, 10, 90, *93*
   cytomegalovirus, 8
   enteric gram-negative bacteria, 4, *7*
   fungal, 6, 8, *9, 11, 13*
   Hemophilus ingluenzae, 4, *7*, 78, *79, 155*
   Hemophilus pertussis, 4, 7
   histoplasmosis, 6, *9*
   klebsiella, 4, *5*, 78, *79*
   Legionnaire's disease, 6, 7
   lipoid, 14, *15*, 38, 42, 46
   measles, *66, 95*, 97
   mononucleosis, 8
   mucomycosis, 8
   mycobacteria, atypical, 12, 56, *57*
   mycoplasma, 8, *13*, 30, *33*, 66
   Paragonimus westermani, 10, 48, *49*, 56, *59*
   pneumococcus, 4, *5*, 78
   Pneumcystis carinii, 10, *13, 25*, 30, *33, 149*
   schistosomiasis, 30
   spherical, 4, *5*
   sporotrichosis, 8, 56, *57*
   staphylococcus, 4, *5*
   streptococcus, 4
   strongyloidiases, 10
   toxoplasmosis, 10
   tuberculosis, 10, 12, *15*
   tularemia, 6
   varicella, 8, 86, *87, 95*, 96
Pneumonitis, postobstructive, 12, *15*
Pneumoperitoneum, 146, 366-67, 370, *371*
Pneumothorax, 146-49
   tension, 124, *125*
Polyarteritis nodosa, 50, 92, 458, *459*, 618
Polychondritis, relapsing, 152, *153*, 634
Polycystic disease,
   kidney (*see* Adult polycystic kidney disease;
     Infantile polycystic kidney disease)
   liver, 404, *405*, 412, *413*
Polycythemia, 64, 211, 212
Polymyositis, 28
Polyomyelitis, paralytic, 704, *705*
Polyostotic fibrous dysplasia, 588, *589*
Polyposis syndromes, 308, *309*
   familial, 342, *343*
   inflammatory pseudo-, 342, *345*
Polyserositis, familial recurring, 138
Polysplenia syndrome, 211
Pontine myelinosis, central, 870, *871*
Porcelain gallbladder, 386, *387*

Porphyria, 272, *296*
Portal vein thrombus, 378
Portal venous system, gas in, 373, *373*
Postbulbar ulcer, 286, *287*
Postmyocardial infarction syndrome, 137, 224, *225*
Postobstructive atrophy, kidney, 446
Postobstructive pneumonitis, 12, *15*
Postsurgical scars, calcification/ossification, 666, *667*
Pregnancy,
   cardiac patterns and, 208, 212
   ectopic, 550, *553*
Presbyesophagus, 232
Primordial cyst, 828
Progeria, 640, *643*, 646, *647*, 694, *695*
Progressive massive lung fibrosis, 16, 46, *51*
Prostatic enlargement, 516, *517*
Protein deficiency, and osteoporosis, 566
Protrusio acetabuli, 716-17
Prune belly syndrome, 508, *509*
Psammomatous calcification, 400, *401*
Pseudoarthrosis, 714-15
Pseudocalculus, 358, *359*
Pseudogout. *See* Calcium pyrophosphate crystal
    dehydrate deposition disease
Pseudokidney sign, 436-37
Pseudolymphoma, 14, 46, 254, *255*, 266
Pseudomyxoma peritonei, 398, *399*, 400
Pseudotruncus arteriosus, 170, 182, *183*, 200, 209
Pseudotumors, 280, *281*
Pseudoxanthoma elasticum, 640, 670, *673*
Psoriatic arthritis, 622, *623*, 634, *635*, 638, *639*
Pulmonary arterial hypertension, 64, *65*
Pulmonary arteriovenous fistula, 44, *47*, 48, 62, 88
Pulmonary artery,
   aberrant left, 198, *199*, 238
   aneurysm, 62
   anomalous origin of left, from right, 72
   coarctation, 62
   corrected transposition of, 192, *195*
   dilation of the main, 202-5
   narrow/occluded, 63
Pulmonary atresia, 166, *167*, 170, 182, *193*, 210
Pulmonary blood flow,
   congenital heart disease and increased/normal,
     184-89
   decreased, and rib notching, 702
Pulmonary branch stenosis, 72
Pulmonary contusion, 12, *46, 133*
Pulmonary disease,
   with eosinophilia, 90-94
   obstructive, 152, *153*, 368
Pulmonary edema patterns,
   interstitial (*see* Interstitial pulmonary edema)
   localized alveolar pattern, 14, *17*
   symmetric bilateral alveolar patterns, 18-25
Pulmonary embolism, 62, *63*, 64, 70, *73*, 82,
    141, 142
   with infarction, causing pulmonary edema, 24

from oily constrast material, 34, 54
Pulmonary hematoma, 12, 42, *46*, 50
Pulmonary hemorrhage, nontraumatic, 22, *23*, *97*, *458*
Pulmonary hemosiderosis, 32, 54, *55*, 68
Pulmonary infarction, 12, *15*, 128, *141*, 142, 148
Pulmonary lymphangiomyomatosis, 32, *35*, 144
Pulmonary/mediastinal masses, 122, 146
Pulmonary nodules,
    multiple, 48-51
    solitary, 40-47
Pulmonary ossification, 50, 88
Pulmonary osteopathia, 88
Pulmonary parenchymal calcification, 86-89
Pulmonary stenosis, 166, *167*, 168, *169*, 182
Pulmonary thrombus, 88
Pulmonary valvular stenosis, 62, 188, 202, *205*
Pulmonary varices, 50
Pulmonary vein,
    left inferior/confluence of left, 238
Pulmonary vein varix, 44
Pulmonary venous flow,
    hypertension, 18, *19*
    malformations obstructing, 170, 210
Pulmonary venous return, anomalous, 238
Pulmonary volume,
    altered, 122, 160
    increased intra-abdominal, 158
Pulseless disease, 192
Pyelitis cystica, 486, *495*
Pyelogenic cyst, 474
Pyelonephritis, 448, *449*, 450, *451*, 478, *479*, 480, *481*, 486, *487*, 488, *489*, *536*, 540, *541*. *See also* Xanthogranulomatous pyelonephritis
Pyknodysostosis, 584, *587*, 587, 642, 646, 824
Pyle's disease, 684, *687*
Pyogenic absceses, 48, *49*, 376, *377*, 412, *415*, 842, *844*
Pyogenic arthritis, 628, *631*
Pyogenic osteomyelitis, 718, 734
Pyonephrosis, 528, *529*

Q

Q fever. *See* Rickettsial infection

R

Radiation therapy damage,
    bladder, 510
    bones, 706
    constrictive pericarditis, 227
    gastrointestinal, 254, 288, 314, 330, *335*, 334, *335*
    joints, 698, *699*
    liver, 418
    lobar collapse from, 84
    nephritis, 446, *447*

pericardial effusion, 224
    pneumonitis, 16, *17*, 22, 34
    skull, 786, 788, 792, 806, 842, 850, *851*
    ureteral, 498
Radicular cyst, 828, *829*
Radiographic technique, faulty, 74, *75*, 76
Raynaud's disease, 674
Rectus muscles, thickening of, 878-79
Reflux atrophy, renal, 446
Reflux nephropathy, renal, 448, *449*
Regional migratory osteoporosis, 562
Reiter's syndrome, *613*, 622, *624*, 634, *635*
Renal abscess, 370, *371*, 469, *471*, 528, 536, *537*, 542, *543*
Renal artery,
    aneurym, 393, *393*
    compression, 502
    hypotension, 456
    stenosis, 214, *217*
    stenosis involving opposite kidney, 482, *483*
Renal calcification, 390-93
Renal calyces, clubbing or destruction of, 488-89
Renal cell carcinoma, 390, *391*, 530, *531*, 534, *535*
Renal cortical echogenicity, with preservation of medullary sonolucency, 538-39
Renal cyst, 528
    benign, 532, *533*
    on computed tomography, 532-33
    lesions mimicking, 526, *527*, 532, *533*
    multilocular, 532
    simple, 466, *467*, 469, 472, *473*, 526, *527*
Renal ectopia, 442, *443*
Renal failure, pulmonary edema from, 18, *19*. *See also* Uremia
Renal hematoma, 528, 536, *537*, 542, *543*
Renal infarction, 478, *479*, 528, 536, *537*, 540
    acute arterial, 450
    chronic, 446, *447*
    lobar, 448, *449*
Renal ischemia, 446, *447*, 480
Renal margin, depression/scar in, 478, *479*
Renal masses,
    anechoic (cystic), 526-27
    complex, 528-29
    cystic, on computed tomography, 532-33
    focal solid, on computed tomography, 534-37
    solid, 530-31
Renal oncocytoma, 534
Renal osteodystrophy, 588, *589*, 632
Renal pseudotumor, congenital, 466, *467*
Renal sinus,
    hemorrhage into, 490
    lipomatosis, 490, *491*
Renal transplantation, delayed complication of, 366
Renal tuberculosis, 448, *449*
Renal tubular acidosis, 572, *573*
Renal vein thrombosis, 450, 480, *481*

Rendu-Osler-Weber disease, 96
Reticulohistiocytosis, multicentric, 634, 640, 644
Reticulum cell sarcoma, 606, *607*
Retrocaval ureter, 502, *503*
Retrogastric space, widening of, 274-75
Retroperitoneal fibrosis, 504, *505*
Retroperitoneal gas, 370, *371*
Retroperitoneum,
    carcinoma of, 136
    mass, 274, 292, 500
Retropharyngeal abscess, 752
Retrorectal space, enlargement of, 352-53
Retrosternal thyroid, 100, *101*, 106
Rhabdomyosarcoma, 878, *879*
Rheumatoid arthritis, 568, *571*, 620, *621*, 634, *635*,
    644, 716, 740, 748, 752, *753*. *See also* Juvenile
    rheumatoid arthritis
Rheumatoid disease, chest patterns for, 28, *31*, 54,
    94, 137, 142
Rheumatoid necrobiotic nodule, 42, 50, *51*, 58, 130
Rhinoscleroma, 152
Rib,
    lesion, 128
    neoplasm, 132, *133*
    notching of, 700-703
Rib margins, resorption or notching of superior, 704-7
Rickets, 778, 825
    healing, 618, 676, *679*, 688, *691*
    Vitamin-D resistant, 572
Rickettsial infection, 10, *13*
Right-to-left cordiac shunts, and admixture lesions,
    170, 172, 176
Riley-Day syndrome, 32, *35*
Rothmund's syndrome, 642, 674
Rubella, congenital, *681*, 688

S

Sacral fracture, 352
Sacral tumor, 352
Sacroiliac joint abnormality, 632-37
Salmonellosis, 328
Sarcoidosis, 16, 24, *25*, 30, *34*, 36, *37*, 50, *51*, 52,
    60, *65*, 68, *69*, 74, 94, *95*, 142, *143*, 152, 602,
    603, 660, 718, *721*, 784, 858, *859*
Sarcoma, 248, *249*, 254, *255*, 260, *261*, 308, *311*
    bone, 580, *581*, 604, *605*, 606, *607*, 608, *609*,
    611, 626, *721*, 780
    cerebellar, 852, *855*
    Kaposi's, 374
    synovial, 662, *666*
Schatzki's ring, 246, *247*
Scheuermann's disease, *735*, 736
Schistosomiasis, 30, 328, 334, 394, 396, *397*, 494,
    498, 510, 516
Scleroderma, 28, 36, *39*, 94, 232, *233*, 300, *301*,
    626, *675*, 638, *639*, 644, 668, *669*, 674, *675*

Scrotum,
    cysts in, 556, *557*
    fluid collections in, 556-57
Scurvy, causing bone damage, 566, *567*, 680
    healing, 618, *619*, 678, 688
Sellar and juxtasellar masses, computed tomography
    of, 860-63
Sellar or parasellar calcifications, 812-15
Sellar turcica, enlargement, erosion, and destruction
    of, 816-17
Sentinel loop, 294, *295*
Septic embolism, 58, *59*
Sequestration, bronchopulmonary, 44, *47*, 60,
    120
Serous cystadenoma, 548, *549*
Serous retention cyst, 836
Shaver's disease, 148
Shigellosis, 328
Shock lung. *See* Adult respiratory distress syndrome
    (ARDS)
Shoulder-hand syndrome, 562
Sickle cell disease, 462, 584, *586*, 618, *719*, 682,
    696, *697*, 710, 718, *719*, 736, *739*
Silicosis, 26, *27*, *51*, 58, *65*, 68, 86, *87*
Sinusitis, 836, *837*
Sinus of Valsalva, 220
    aneurysm of, 100, *103*, 184, *187*, 192
Sjogren's syndrome, 28, 640
Skin disorder, combined with lung disease, 94-97
Skin malignancy, and skull defects, 780, *781*
Skull,
    diffuse demineralization/destruction of, 778-79
    fracture, 784, *786*
    lytic defects in, 780-87
    softening of bone at the base of, 826, *827*
Small bowel,
    dilation, 300-302
    diverticula and pseudodiverticula, 316-17
    obstruction, 297, *298-99*, 300
    sandlike lucencies in the, 312-13
Small bowel folds,
    generalized, irregular, distorted, 304-7
    thickening of, 303, 318-19
Soft tissue,
    abscess/hematoma, 236
    infection, 712
Solitary rectal ulcer syndrome, 332, 336
Spermatocele, 556
Sphenoid sinus carcinoma/mucocele, 816, *817*
Spherical pneumonia, 4, *5*
Spinal bifida, 648
Spinal cord,
    extradural lesions of, 770-74
    intradural, extramedullary lesions of, 766-69
    intramedullary lesion (widening of), 742, 762-65
Spinal neoplasm/inflammation, 236
Spindle cell tumor, 150, 248, *249*, 260, *261*, 308, *309*
Spleen,

calcification, 380-81
    decreased-attenuation masses in, 434-35
    increased density of, *381*, 386
Splenic abscess, 434, *435*
Splenic artery, 380, *381*
    aneurysm, 380, *381*
Splenic capsule, calcification of, 380, *381*
Splenic cysts, 380, *381*, 434, *435*
Splenic hematoma, 434, *435*
Splenic infarction, 434
Splenomegaly, 442, *444*
Spondyloepiphyseal dysplasia, 736, *737*
Sporotrichosis pneumonia, 8, 56, *57*
Sprue, 300, *301*
    nontropical, 290
Staphylococcus infection, 4, *5, 57, 72*, 328
Steroid therapy, causing bone/joint damage, *567*,
    650, 696
Stippled epiphyses, congenital, 580, *583*
Stomach,
    carcinoma of, 382, *383, 436*
    filling defects of, 260-63
    fold thickening of, 318-19
    fundus of, malignancy in, 246, *247*, 248, *249*
    leiomyoma of, *249*, 382
    narrowing of 256-59
Streptococcus pneumonia, 4, 78, *79*
Strongyloidiasis,
    chest, 10, 90, *92*
    gastrointestinal, 278, 288, 306, *307*, 330
Sturge-Weber syndrome, 810, *811*
Subcapsular hematoma,
    hepatic, 416, *419*
    renal, 470
Subclavian artery,
    aberrant left, 198, *199*
    aberrant right, 198, *199*, 238
    isolated, 198
    obstruction of, 700
Subcutaneous tissues, localized calcification or
    ossification in, 664-67
Subdural abscess, 768
Subdural empyema, 844, *845*
Subdural hematoma, 844, *845*, 846, *847*, 848
Subhepatic gas, 370
Submucosal edema pattern, 346, *347*
Subphrenic abscess, 136, 140, *141*, 370, *371*
Subpulmonic effusion, *160*
Sudeck's atrophy, 562, *563*
Superior sulcus tumor, 128, *131*
Superior vena cava, 206-7
    occlusion of, 208
    rib notching and, 702
Superiosteal hemorrhage, 610
Surgical deformity, gastrointestinal, 276
Suture granuloma, 276, *277*
Swyer-James syndrome, 70, *73*, 122
Synovioma. *See* Sarcoma, synovial

Synovitis, pigmented villonodular, 628, *629*
Syphilis causing bone damage, 648, *649, 718*
    acquired, 582, 612, *613*
    congenital, 588, *591*, 616, 678, *681*, 796
Syringobulbia, 870, *871*
Syringomyelia, 648, *649*, 762, *765*
Systemic illness, chronic, 680, *681*
Systemic lupus erythematosus, 16, 28, 94, 137, *139*,
    142, *143, 300*, 458, 626, *629*, 670, *673*, 674

T

Tabes dorsalis, 648, *649*
Tachypnea, transient newborn, causing pulmonary
    edema, 20
Takayasu's disease, 192
Taussig-Bing anomaly, 178, *179*
Tendinitis, calcific, 658, *659*
Teratocarcinoma, 854
Teratoma, 100, *102*, 106, *107*, 864, *865*
Tetanus, 738, *739*
Tetralogy of Fallot, 168, *169*, 182, *183*, 192, 200,
    204, *205*, 209
Thalassemia, 682, *685, 795*
Thermal burn. *See* Burns; Electrical shock; Frostbite
Thoracic duct,
    iatrogenic injury to, 144
    intrinsic abnormality of, 144
    trauma to, 144, *145*
    tumor obstruction of, 144, *145*
Thoracic trauma (contused lung), 20, *23*
Thorotrast deposition, 420, *421*, 708, *711*
Thromboembolic disease, 70, *73*, 136
    pulmonary, *63*, 202
Thrombosis of superior vena cava, 206
Thrombotic thrombocytopenic purpura, 458
Thymic cyst, 104, *105*
Thymic hyperplasia, 106
Thymoma, 100, *101*, 104, *105*
Thyroid acropachy, 614, *617*, 712
Thyroid enlargement, 236, *237*
Thyroid ophthalmophathy, 878, *879*
Thyroid tumor, *101*, 116
    ectopic, 150
Thyrotoxicosis, 212, *213*
Tongue, pharyngeal airway obstruction by, 154
Tonsils, enlarged, 154, *157*
Torulosis, 806, 810
Torus mandibularis, 832, *833*
Torus palatinus, 832, *833*
Total anomalous pulmonary venous return, 178, *181*,
    204
Toxoplasmosis, 10, 30, 808, *809*, 856
Trachea,
    injury, 126, *127*
    obstruction/compression, 76, 154

saber-sheath, 152, *153*
Tracheal mass/narrowing, 150-53
Tracheoesophageal fistula, 156, *157*
Tracheopathia osteoplastica, 152
Transitional cell carcinoma, 484, *485, 492, 495,* 502,
    503, 510, 514, *515,* 534, *535*
Transplacental infection, 680, *681*
Transplanted kidney, 444, *445*
    fluid collections around, 542-43
Transposition of great artieris, 178, *179,* 196, *197,*
    200, 209
Transverse growth line, 676, 708, *711*
    Trauma,
        cardiovascular patterns, 224, 227
        chest patterns and, 20, *23,* 58, 126, 127, 132, 137,
            141, 142, *145,* 146, *147,* 152, 160, *161*
        gastrointestinal, 272, *273,* 363, *363,* 416, 418
        genitourinary, 482, 500
        skeletal, 652, 662, *663,* 696, 712, 716
        skull, 784, *786, 787,* 806, 810, 826, 828
        spine, 740, 750, 752, 754, 760
Traumatic cyst, 828, *829*
Traumatic ischemic necrosis, 738
Trichinosis (*Trichinella spiralis*), 672, 808
Tricuspid atresia, 166, 182, *183,* 200
    without pulmonary stenosis, 204, 209
Tricuspid insufficiency, 168
Tricuspid valve disease, 166, *167*
Trisomy 13/trisomy 18, 648
Trophoblastic disease, 554, *555*
Tropical ulcer, 612, *613*
Tuber cinereum, 862, *863*
Tuberculoma, 40, *41,* 806, 810
Tuberculosis,
    cardiovascular patterns, *227*
    chest, 10, 12, *15,* 30, *33,* 36, 52, *53, 57, 63,* 72,
        78, *135,* 136, *139,* 144
    gastrointestinal, 242, 278, 286, 290, 304, 320,
        328, 334, 376, 380, 388, *389,* 390, 394, *395,*
        396, 400
    genitourinary, 448, *449,* 478, 488, *489,* 494, *497,*
        498, 510, 524
    skeletal, 628, *631,* 662, 718, *719*
    skull, 856
    spine, *733,* 734
Tuberculous arthritis, 628, *631*
Tuberculous meningitis, healed, 814
Tuberculous osteomyelitis, *733,* 734
Tuberculous salpingitis, 398
Tuberous sclerosis, 32, 38, 94, *95,* 582, 616, 720,
    721, 810, 874, *875*
Tubo-ovarian abscess, 550, *551*
Tubular necrosis, acute renal, 460, 480
Tularemia pneumonia, 6, *67*
Tumor. *See* Neoplasm
Tumoral calcinosis, 660, *661*
Turcot syndrome, 342
Typhoid fever, 306, 322, *323*

U

Uhl's disease, 166, 182, 210
Ulcerative bowel disease, 366
Ulcerative colitis, 320, *321*
Ulcerative pseudopolyps proximal to an obstruction,
    346
Uremia, 18, *19,* 224, *225,* 227, 290, 482, *483*
Ureter,
    calcification of, 394, *395*
    diverticulum of, 496
    filling defects in, 492-97
    herniation, 504
    obstruction of, 498-505, 506-7
    polyp of, 492
    spasm of, 496
    stricture/compression of, 494, 496, 498, 500
    valve of, 504
Ureterectasis, 506-9
Ureteritis cystica, 494, *495*
Ureterocele, 500, *501,* 516, *517*
    ectopic, *503,* 522
Urethra,
    diverticulum of, 522
    duplication of, congenital, 522
    obstruction of, 512
    posterior valve of, 522, *523*
    stricture, 522
Urinary bladder. *See* Bladder, urinary
Urinary tract obstruction, 482
    below the bladder in children, 522-23
Urinoma, 542, *543*
"Usual" interstitial pneumonia (UIP), 32, *35*
Uterine fibroid (leiomyoma), 398, *399,* 554,
    555

V

Vagotomy, 272, 300, 354
Van Buchem's syndrome, 586, *797*
Vanishing bone disease, 738
Varicella, 8, 86, *87, 95,* 96
Varicocele, scrotal, 556, *557*
Vascular malformations/angioma, 768, *769*
Vascular ring, 154
Vasculitis, 300, *302*
Vas deferens, calcification of, 524-25
Vein of Galen aneurysm, 802, 864, *865*
Venous stasis, 616, *617,* 666, *667*
Ventricle,
    common, 178, *180*
    double-outlet right, 178, *179, 180*
Ventricular aneurysm, 220, *222*
Ventricular enlargement,
    left, 174-77, 240
    right, 166, 168-71
Ventricular septal defect, 184, *185,* 196
Ventriculitis, inflammatory, 872, *873*

Vertebral artery, aneurysm/tortuosity of, 750, *751,*
    866, *869*
Vertebral body,
    anterior scalloping of, 744
    beaked, notched, or hooked, in children,
        758-61
    cystlike lesions of, 726-29
    fracture/dislocation of, 772
    hematoma, 772, *773*
    increased size of, 730-31
    loss of height in, 732-39
    posterior scalloping of, 744-47
    squaring of, 748-49
Verumontanum, hypertrophy of, 523
Vesicoureteral reflux, 506, *509*
Villous adenoma, 248, 260, *262,* 282, *283,* 340,
    341
Viral arthritis, 630
Viral encephalitis, 808, *809*
Viral infections, chest patterns for, 8, *13,* 30, *33,* 52,
    55, 64, 66, *67*
Vitamin A, bone damage due to excessive, 616,
    617
Vitamin C deficiency, and osteoporosis, 566,
    567
Vitamin D, bone damage due to excessive, 588,
    676, 688, 756
Vocal cord paralysis, congenital, 156
Volvulus, 297
    gastric, 268, *271*
    midgut, 286
Von Hippel-Lindau disease, 810

W

Waldenstrom's macroglobulinemia, 32, 142, *312*

Water lily sign, 40, 56, *59*
Wegener's granulomatosis, 42, 48, 54, 58, *61,* 90,
    94, 142, 152, 458, 836, *837*
Werner's syndrome, 662, 672
Westermark's sign, 70, *73*
Whipple's disease, 304, *305,* 312, 318
Whooping cough. *See Hemophilus pertussis*
    (whooping cough) pneumonia
Wilms' tumor, 390, *444, 466,* 530, *531,* 534, *535, 536*
Wilson's disease, 574, *575,* 656, *657*
Wolman's disease, 388, *389*
Wormian bones, multiple, 824-25

X

Xanthogranulomatous pyelonephritis, 390, *393,*
    452, *453,* 470, 536, *537*

Y

Yaws, osteomyelitis caused by, 582, *583,* 612, *613,*
    718, *719*
Yersinia pestis,
    colitis, 330, *323*
    enterocolitis, 306, 312, 322, *323*
    pneumonia, 6, *24, 67,* 78

Z

Zenker's diverticulum, 116, *252, 253*
Zollinger-Ellison syndrome, 264, *265,* 290, *291,* 318